medicine

The National Medical Series for Independent Study

medicine

Allen R. Myers, M.D.

*Dean and Professor of Medicine
Temple University
   School of Medicine
Associate Vice President
Temple University
   Health Sciences Center
Philadelphia, Pennsylvania*

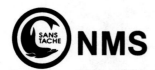

National Medical Series from Williams & Wilkins
Baltimore, Hong Kong, London, Sydney

Harwal Publishing Company, Malvern, Pennsylvania

Williams & Wilkins

Library of Congress Cataloging in Publication Data

Main entry under title:
Medicine.
(The National medical series for independent study)
(A Wiley medical publication)
Includes index.
1. Internal medicine—Outlines, syllabi, etc.
2. Internal medicine—Examinations, questions, etc.
I. Myers, Allen R. II. Series. III. Series: Wiley
medical publication. [DNLM: 1. Internal Medicine—
examination questions. 2. Internal Medicine—
outlines. WB 18 M489]
RC59.M44   1986   616'.0076   85-30554
ISBN 0-683-06232-8

Dedication

To Ellen, whose support has made it all possible.

To David, Rob, and Scott, for all of the time taken from the family over the years.

To Rosina and Ellis, for pointing me in the right direction.

To Dr. Theodore E. Woodward, for setting a standard to which to aspire.

To the medical students and residents, who have provided a constant source of stimulation and made teaching so worthwhile and pleasurable.

Contents

Contents

Contributors

E. Victor Adlin, M.D.
Associate Professor of Medicine
Endocrinology Section
Temple University School of Medicine
Attending Physician
Temple University Hospital
Philadelphia, Pennsylvania

Blase A. Carabello, M.D.
Professor of Medicine
Cardiovascular Division
Medical University of South Carolina
   College of Medicine
Attending Physician
Medical University Hospital
Veterans Administration Medical Center
Charleston, South Carolina

Douglas C. Conaway, M.D.
Assistant Professor of Medicine
Rheumatology Section
Temple University School of Medicine
Attending Physician
Temple University Hospital
Philadelphia, Pennsylvania

Marta A. Dabezies, M.D.
Assistant Professor of Medicine
Gastrointestinal Section
Temple University School of Medicine
Director, Gastrointestinal Endoscopy
Temple University Hospital
Philadelphia, Pennsylvania

Anthony J. DiMarino, Jr., M.D.
Clinical Professor of Medicine
Hospital of the University of Pennsylvania
Chief, Division of Gastroenterology
Presbyterian-University of Pennsylvania
   Medical Center
Philadelphia, Pennsylvania

Thomas Fekete, M.D.
Associate Professor of Medicine
Infectious Diseases Section
Temple University School of Medicine
Attending Physician
Temple University Hospital
Philadelphia, Pennsylvania

Stanley B. Fiel, M.D.
Professor of Medicine
Associate Chief, Pulmonary Diseases Section
Temple University School of Medicine
Director, Adult Cystic Fibrosis Program
Temple University Hospital
Attending Physician
St. Christopher's Hospital for Children
Philadelphia, Pennsylvania

Stanley Goldfarb, M.D.
Associate Professor of Medicine
Renal Electrolyte Section
University of Pennsylvania School
   of Medicine
Attending Physician
Hospital of the University of Pennsylvania
Philadelphia, Pennsylvania

Donald P. Goldsmith, M.D.
Associate Professor of Pediatrics
Robert Wood Johnson Medical School
  at Camden
University of Medicine and Dentistry
  of New Jersey
Camden, New Jersey

Carl S. Goldstein, M.D.
Assistant Professor of Clinical
  Medicine
College of Physicians and Surgeons
Columbia University
New York, New York
Director, Dialysis Services
Overlook Hospital
Summit, New Jersey

Thomas E. Klein, M.D.
Attending Allergist
Riddle Memorial Hospital
Media, Pennsylvania

Stephen J. McGeady, M.D.
Associate Professor of Pediatrics
Clinical Assistant Professor of Medicine
Jefferson Medical College
Thomas Jefferson University
Director, Allergy and Clinical Immunology
  Division
Thomas Jefferson University Hospital
Medical Director
Jefferson Park Hospital/
  Children's Rehabilitation Hospital
Philadelphia, Pennsylvania

Allen R. Myers, M.D.
Dean and Professor of Medicine
Temple University School of Medicine
Associate Vice President
Temple University Health Sciences Center
Attending Physician
Temple University Hospital
Philadelphia, Pennsylvania

Ronald N. Rubin, M.D.
Professor and Deputy Chairman
Department of Medicine
Temple University School of Medicine
Attending Physician
Temple University Hospital
Philadelphia, Pennsylvania

Preface

The easiest and surest way of acquiring facts is to learn them in groups, in systems, and systematized knowledge is science. You can very often carry two facts fastened together more easily than one by itself. . .
—Oliver Wendell Holmes, "Scholastic and Bedside Teaching" from *Medical Essays*

Internal medicine is a vast and complicated field that is based upon strong scientific and clinical foundations. While certain pedagogic learning is unavoidable, an understanding of basic sciences, particularly pathophysiology, allows some meaning to be made of seemingly unrelated facts.

Any effort to provide a comprehensive review of internal medicine is destined to fall short of its goal. Despite this limitation, the authors have provided a framework for a working knowledge of internal medicine. It is not all-inclusive but nonetheless provides the essentials of the subject in an easily read and well-organized format. By necessity, *Medicine* must be used as a companion to more extensive texts and monographs, but it can be considered a starting point. Internal medicine cannot be fully learned in a year or two, or in a lifetime, but its essence can be appreciated by students and house officers.

Medicine has been written primarily for students and residents. However, the authors believe it also can be used by family physicians, general surgeons, surgical subspecialists, obstetricians and gynecologists, physiatrists, anesthesiologists, and all others who deal with patients who have medical illnesses.

Allen R. Myers

Acknowledgments

The editor and contributing authors are grateful to Harwal Publishing Company, particularly Jim Harris for his patience and guidance and Debra Dreger for her outstanding editorial contributions.

Publisher's Note

The objective of the *National Medical Series* is to present an extraordinarily large amount of information in an easily retrievable form. The outline format was selected for this purpose of reducing to the essentials the medical information needed by today's student and practitioner.

While the concept of an outline format was well received by the authors and publisher, the difficulties inherent in working with this style were not initially apparent. That the series has been published and received enthusiastically is a tribute to the authors who worked long and diligently to produce books that are stylistically consistent and comprehensive in content.

The task of producing the *National Medical Series* required more than the efforts of the authors, however, and the missing elements have been supplied by highly competent and dedicated developmental editors and support staff. Editors, compositors, proofreaders, and layout and design staff have all polished the outline to a fine form. It is with deep appreciation that I thank all who have participated, in particular the staff at Harwal—Debra L. Dreger, Jane Edwards, Gloria Hamilton, Deborah G. Huey, Susan Kelly, Wieslawa B. Langenfeld, Keith LaSala, June Sangiorgio Mash, and Jane Velker.

The Publisher

Introduction

Medicine is one of six clinical science review books in the *National Medical Series for Independent Study*. This series has been designed to provide students and house officers, as well as physicians, with a concise but comprehensive instrument for self-evaluation and review within the clinical sciences. Although *Medicine* would be most useful to students preparing for the National Board of Medical Examiners examinations (Part II, Part III, FLEX, and FMGEMS), it should also be useful to students studying for course examinations. These books are not intended to replace the standard clinical science texts but, rather, to complement them.

The books in this series present the core content of each clinical science, using an outline format and featuring 300 study questions. The questions are distributed throughout the book, at the end of each chapter and in a pretest and post-test. In addition, each question is accompanied by the correct answer, a paragraph-length explanation of the correct answer, and specific reference to the outline points under which the information necessary to answer the question can be found.

We have chosen an outline format to allow maximal ease in retrieving information, assuming that the time available to the reader is limited. Considerable editorial time has been spent to ensure that the information required by all medical school curricula has been included and that the question format parallels that of the National Board examinations. We feel that the combination of the outline and the board-type study questions provides a unique teaching device.

We hope that you will find this series interesting, relevant, and challenging. The authors, as well as the John Wiley and Harwal staffs, welcome your comments and suggestions.

Pretest

QUESTIONS

Directions: Each question below contains five suggested answers. Choose the **one best** response to each question.

1. Which of the following findings is virtually always seen in a patient with adult respiratory distress syndrome?

(A) A small localized mass on chest x-ray
(B) Reduced lung compliance
(C) Normal oxygenation with impaired minute ventilation
(D) Increased arterial PCO_2
(E) Pulmonary embolism

2. Uncomplicated seasonal allergic rhinitis is associated with all of the following clinical findings EXCEPT

(A) nasal and palatal pruritus
(B) thin, watery nasal discharge
(C) reddened nasal mucosa and cervical adenopathy
(D) paroxysmal sneezing
(E) excess lacrimation

3. A 42-year-old woman with menorrhagia from uterine fibroid tumors presents with anemia characterized by a hemoglobin level of 8.0 g/dl. The mean corpuscular hemoglobin value is 70 μ^3, and the blood smear reveals a uniform collection of both hypochromic and microcytic cells. The most likely diagnosis is

(A) pernicious anemia
(B) sickle cell anemia
(C) iron deficiency anemia
(D) sideroblastic anemia
(E) glucose-6-phosphate dehydrogenase (G6PD) deficiency

4. A patient with lung carcinoma becomes weak and lethargic and is found to have a serum calcium level of 16.4 mg/dl. The first step in treatment should be

(A) intravenous phosphate
(B) intravenous mithramycin
(C) intravenous glucocorticoids
(D) intravenous saline and furosemide
(E) subcutaneous calcitonin

5. Which combination of findings provides a definitive diagnosis of cystic fibrosis?

(A) Family history of cystic fibrosis; abnormal pulmonary function
(B) Abnormal pulmonary function; pancreatic insufficiency
(C) Pancreatic insufficiency; high electrolyte concentration in sweat
(D) High electrolyte concentration in serum; abnormal chest x-ray
(E) Abnormal chest x-ray; family history of cystic fibrosis

6. Tumors that are somewhat responsive to therapy and should be investigated in patients with carcinoma of unknown primary origin include all of the following EXCEPT

(A) adenocarcinoma of the prostate gland
(B) adenocarcinoma of the lung
(C) adenocarcinoma of the breast
(D) germ cell carcinoma
(E) thyroid carcinoma

7. Eosinophilia is most likely to be found in which of the following settings?

(A) Pinworm infection
(B) Diarrhea caused by *Giardia lamblia*
(C) Schistosomiasis
(D) Measles
(E) Corticosteroid therapy

8. Which of the following physical signs and symptoms is indicative of left ventricular failure?

(A) Neck vein distension
(B) Ascites
(C) Anorexia
(D) Orthopnea
(E) Cardiac edema

9. The most common form of nephrotic syndrome seen in adults is

(A) primary membranous glomerulonephritis
(B) lipoid nephrosis
(C) focal glomerulosclerosis
(D) crescentic glomerulonephritis
(E) amyloidosis

10. The most potent stimulus for the development of pulmonary hypertension in chronic obstructive pulmonary disease (COPD) is

(A) obliteration of the pulmonary vascular bed
(B) alveolar membrane damage
(C) left ventricular failure
(D) hypoxia
(E) acidosis

11. Acute gastritis may be caused by all of the following agents EXCEPT

(A) alcohol
(B) aspirin
(C) acetaminophen
(D) streptococcus
(E) indomethacin

12. Which of the following statements concerning immunoglobulin E (IgE) is correct?

(A) IgE levels peak in adulthood
(B) Individuals with low IgE levels experience more infections
(C) The production of IgE is T-cell independent
(D) IgE is formed in the spleen
(E) IgE crosses the placenta

13. An 18-year-old man sustains abnormal bleeding after minor trauma. Platelet count and bleeding time are normal, prothrombin time (PT) is 12 seconds, and partial thromboplastin time (PTT) is 69 seconds. The most likely diagnosis is

(A) idiopathic thrombocytopenic purpura (ITP)
(B) factor VII deficiency
(C) factor IX deficiency
(D) factor XII deficiency
(E) aspirin ingestion

14. All of the following are important practices in the management of patients with intravenous catheters EXCEPT

(A) insertion under aseptic conditions
(B) systemic antimicrobial prophylaxis during insertion
(C) changing catheters every 48–72 hours
(D) using forearm veins in preference to femoral veins
(E) avoiding insertion through areas of diseased or infected skin

15. A 21-year-old man enters the hospital complaining that he has been passing dark reddish urine. The patient has recently recovered from a football-related knee injury, which he incurred 3 months before, and the day before entering the hospital he engaged in vigorous physical activity for the first time since his knee injury. This morning he awoke with sore, painful muscles and the aforementioned change in the character of his urine. Physical examination of the patient is essentially normal except for the painful muscles. Findings on urinalysis include: red-brown color, pH of 5.0, specific gravity of 1.02, 3^+ dipstick test for blood, and no evidence of glucose, ketones, or bilirubin. Microscopic examination of the urine reveals occasional amorphous debris and 3 or 4 granular casts but no red blood cells. The most likely explanation for this urinalysis is

(A) myoglobinuria
(B) hemolyzed blood in the urine
(C) ingestion of foodstuffs containing red dye
(D) urinary tract infection
(E) renal trauma

16. All of the following are proven mediators in the pathogenesis of asthma EXCEPT

(A) slow reacting substance of anaphylaxis (SRS-A)
(B) eosinophil chemotactic factor of anaphylaxis (ECF-A)
(C) viruses
(D) prostaglandins
(E) histamine

17. All of the following drugs show positive immediate skin tests at reasonable concentrations EXCEPT

(A) chymopapain
(B) insulin
(C) cephalosporin
(D) aspirin
(E) penicillin

18. The definitive diagnosis of pulmonary embolism is best made by

(A) arterial blood gas analysis
(B) chest x-ray
(C) electrocardiography
(D) nuclear scanning of the lung
(E) pulmonary arteriography

19. A patient with polycystic ovary syndrome is most likely to have which of the following findings?

(A) Deepening of the voice, enlargement of the clitoris, and a high testosterone level
(B) Oligomenorrhea, obesity, a high luteinizing hormone (LH) level, and a low follicle-stimulating hormone (FSH) level
(C) Amenorrhea, acne, a low LH level, and a low FSH level
(D) Facial hirsutism, acne, and increased urinary pregnanetriol and 17-ketosteroids
(E) Facial hirsutism, normal menstrual periods, and normal levels of FSH, LH, and testosterone

20. All of the following statements concerning upper respiratory infections are true EXCEPT

(A) these infections represent the most common cause of morbidity in the United States
(B) most of these infections are caused by viruses
(C) symptoms may involve the sinuses, throat, larynx, or airways
(D) treatment is primarily symptomatic
(E) prevention usually is achieved by timely immunization

21. The most helpful study in the diagnosis of allergic rhinitis is

(A) the radioallergosorbent test (RAST)
(B) immunoglobulin E (IgE) level
(C) peripheral eosinophilia
(D) the immediate hypersensitivity skin test
(E) a stained nasal smear for eosinophils

22. The hormone that is most commonly found to be elevated in patients with pituitary adenomas is

(A) growth hormone (GH)
(B) adrenocorticotropic hormone (ACTH)
(C) prolactin
(D) thyroid-stimulating hormone (TSH)
(E) follicle-stimulating hormone (FSH)

Directions: Each question below contains four suggested answers of which **one or more** is correct. Choose the answer

  A   if **1, 2, and 3** are correct
  B   if **1 and 3** are correct
  C   if **2 and 4** are correct
  D   if **4** is correct
  E   if **1, 2, 3, and 4** are correct

23. True statements concerning myocardial infarction include

(1) coronary thrombosis is important in the pathophysiology of most transmural infarctions
(2) the chest pain usually differs in quality from that occurring in angina
(3) pain persisting for longer than 30 minutes should suggest that infarction has occurred
(4) a sudden increase in myocardial oxygen demand is the most common cause of infarction

24. True statements concerning intracranial abscess include

(1) computed tomography (CT) of the brain is helpful in the diagnosis
(2) the route of infection usually is direct spread from an infected ear or sinus
(3) penicillin and chloramphenicol are effective antimicrobial agents
(4) *Toxoplasma* and *Nocardia* species are the most likely agents of infection in immunocompetent patients

25. In differentiating between type I and type II diabetes mellitus, type I diabetes is indicated if the patient

(1) is 50 pounds overweight
(2) reveals anti-islet cell antibodies in the blood
(3) requires insulin to maintain normal blood glucose levels but has never developed keto-acidosis
(4) developed diabetes at the age of 14

26. Angiodysplasia of the colon can be described as being

(1) a common cause of bleeding in older patients
(2) usually located in the descending or sigmoid colon
(3) associated with aortic stenosis in some patients
(4) a common cause of abdominal pain in patients

27. Pulmonary conditions that may be improved by the use of positive end-expiratory pressure (PEEP) ventilation include

(1) lung complications in kyphoscoliosis
(2) chronic bronchitis
(3) adult respiratory distress syndrome
(4) pulmonary emphysema

28. The causes of metabolic acidosis can be divided into those associated with a normal anion gap and those associated with an increased anion gap. Metabolic acidosis with an increased anion gap can result from

(1) renal failure
(2) diabetic ketoacidosis
(3) methanol ingestion
(4) hydrochloric acid infusion

29. The use of diuretics in the treatment of hypertension may be associated with side effects. These include

(1) hyperglycemia
(2) bronchospasm
(3) prerenal azotemia
(4) hemolytic anemia

30. Diseases that can lead to the development of infectious proctitis include

(1) syphilis
(2) lymphogranuloma venereum
(3) gonorrhea
(4) herpes zoster

31. The systolic ejection murmur in hypertrophic obstructive cardiomyopathy is diminished when the patient

(1) performs the Valsalva maneuver
(2) lies down
(3) inhales amyl nitrite
(4) assumes the squatting position

32. Conditions that can produce metabolic alkalosis in an otherwise normal individual include

(1) vomiting
(2) ingestion of sodium bicarbonate
(3) use of diuretics
(4) use of nonabsorbable antacids

33. A reduced 1-second forced expiratory volume (FEV_1) is likely to be observed in

(1) bronchial asthma
(2) pulmonary emphysema
(3) chronic bronchitis
(4) lung abscess

34. The currently used treatment for local and regional breast cancer includes

(1) Halsted radical mastectomy
(2) modified radical mastectomy
(3) radiation to the chest wall
(4) lumpectomy with regional high-dose radiation

35. A patient with chronic renal failure who is being treated with maintenance hemodialysis may develop

(1) pericarditis
(2) polycythemia
(3) urticaria
(4) pulmonary embolism

36. A 40-year-old woman has a 3-cm thyroid nodule that does not concentrate radioiodine. Associated findings that would support a decision to remove the nodule surgically include

(1) normal size and consistency of the remainder of the thyroid gland
(2) history of irradiation of the tonsils in childhood
(3) recent growth of the nodule
(4) cystic appearance of the nodule on ultrasonogram

37. The diagnosis of constrictive pericarditis is supported by which of the following findings?

(1) Neck vein distension that increases during inspiration
(2) Diminished first and second heart sounds (S_1 and S_2)
(3) Equal pressures in the four heart chambers during diastole
(4) A predominance of left-sided signs and symptoms over right-sided findings

38. Generalized lymphadenopathy rarely is found in

(1) chancroid
(2) infectious mononucleosis
(3) malaria
(4) syphilis

39. Disorders commonly treated by transsphenoidal pituitary surgery include

(1) acromegaly
(2) galactorrhea-amenorrhea syndrome
(3) Cushing's disease
(4) hyperthyroidism

40. The major constituents of an atherosclerotic plaque are

(1) smooth muscle cells
(2) red blood cells
(3) lipids
(4) fibroblasts

41. Exploratory laparotomy with splenectomy should be performed on Hodgkin's disease patients who have

(1) stage I A disease involving the neck
(2) stage II A disease involving the neck and mediastinum
(3) stage II B disease involving the neck and mediastinum
(4) stage IV A disease

42. Angioedema can be recognized clinically as

(1) colorless
(2) pruritic
(3) well demarcated
(4) pitting

Directions: The groups of questions below consist of lettered choices followed by several numbered items. For each numbered item select the **one** lettered choice with which it is **most** closely associated. Each lettered choice may be used once, more than once, or not at all.

Questions 43–46

Esophageal manometry frequently is used in the evaluation of dysphagia. For each manometric pattern described below, select the esophageal disease with which it is associated.

(A) Achalasia
(B) Scleroderma
(C) Reflux esophagitis
(D) Symptomatic diffuse esophageal spasm (SDES)
(E) Esophageal carcinoma

43. Normal peristalsis in the esophageal body; lower esophageal sphincter (LES) pressure decreased to less than one-third the lower limit of normal

44. Normal peristalsis in the upper one-third (striated muscle portion) of the esophagus but decreased amplitude of peristaltic contractions in the distal two-thirds (smooth muscle portion); decreased LES pressure

45. High amplitude repetitive contractions in the esophageal body with intermittent normal peristalsis; normal or increased LES pressure

46. Absence of normal peristalsis in the esophageal body; increased LES pressure and impaired LES relaxation

Questions 47–50

Match each of the following stages of prostatic carcinoma with its appropriate therapy.

(A) Hormone therapy
(B) Radical surgery
(C) Observation
(D) Radical radiotherapy
(E) Radical radiotherapy with boost doses to the prostate gland

47. Stage A2
48. Stage B
49. Stage C
50. Stage D

Questions 51–55

For each condition described below, select the vitamin status with which it is most closely associated.

(A) Folic acid deficiency
(B) Vitamin B_{12} deficiency
(C) Deficiency of both folic acid and vitamin B_{12}
(D) No vitamin deficiency

51. Pancytopenia with macrocytic anemia and megaloblastic marrow

52. Gastric carcinoma

53. An abnormal Schilling test

54. Neuropathy of the spinal cord

55. Alcoholism

Questions 56–60

Laboratory analysis of synovial fluid often provides valuable information for the diagnosis of arthritis. For each synovial fluid finding listed below, select the most likely diagnosis.

(A) Calcium pyrophosphate dihydrate (CPPD) deposition disease
(B) Osteoarthritis
(C) Infectious arthritis
(D) Acute gouty arthritis
(E) Rheumatoid arthritis

56. Negatively birefringent crystals

57. Chunky, rhomboid crystals

58. White cell count below 1000/mm³; good mucin clot

59. White cell count of 15,000/mm³, with 90% neutrophils

60. White cell count of 70,000/mm³, with 95% neutrophils

ANSWERS AND EXPLANATIONS

1. The answer is B. (*Chapter 2 V C, D*) Adult respiratory distress syndrome (also called wet lung) begins with a disruption of capillary integrity, which leads to extravasation of fluid, fibrin, and protein into the alveoli. As a result, the lungs become wet and stiff (i.e., noncompliant). This condition is characterized by severe hypoxia due to extreme ventilation-perfusion imbalance and shunting of blood in the fluid-filled areas of the lung. Clinical features include progressive tachypnea; patchy, diffuse, fluffy infiltrates on chest x-ray; increased minute ventilation; and decreased lung volumes. There usually is an absence of physical findings.

2. The answer is C. (*Chapter 7 III D*) Symptoms of seasonal allergic rhinitis often are severe enough to disturb normal daily activity. Intense pruritus of the nose, palate, and eyes occurs along with paroxysmal sneezing and excess lacrimation. Complications such as acute sinusitis, otitis media, and superimposed viral or bacterial infection may develop. The color of the nasal mucosa in uncomplicated allergic rhinitis most often is pale or slightly blue rather than red and is not associated with localized adenopathy.

3. The answer is C. (*Chapter 3 I A 1*) The setting and history of this case are appropriate for a diagnosis of iron deficiency anemia. The excessive menses represent a source of iron loss. The hypochromia and microcytosis revealed by the blood smear establish that there is no deficiency of vitamin B_{12}; therefore, pernicious anemia is unlikely. The blood smear also excludes sickle cell anemia. Although blood smear reveals a microcytic cell population in cases of sideroblastic anemia, it also shows a normal or slightly macrocytic population existing with the microcytic component. Glucose-6-phosphate dehydrogenase (G6PD) deficiency is unlikely because it presents as hemolysis, for which there is no evidence in this case.

4. The answer is D. (*Chapter 9 III A 7 c*) Forced diuresis with several liters of saline and intravenous furosemide is a rapid and safe way to lower serum calcium and should be tried first. Intravenous phosphate is very effective but presents the risk of metastatic calcification. Mithramycin and calcitonin may be tried if forced diuresis and phosphate therapy are inadequate. Glucocorticoids are effective in vitamin D excess and sarcoidosis but do not lower calcium levels in malignancy complicated by hypercalcemia.

5. The answer is C. (*Chapter 2 III B 5 a–c*) In virtually all cases of cystic fibrosis, sodium and chloride concentrations in sweat are increased significantly, while normal concentrations of these electrolytes exist elsewhere in the body. In order to make a diagnosis, this defect must be identified. The diagnosis of cystic fibrosis is confirmed by a positive sweat test combined with any one of the following findings: a family history of cystic fibrosis, obstructive pulmonary disease, or pancreatic insufficiency. Although chest x-ray and pulmonary function testing reveal abnormalities, the sweat test is the only objective test for cystic fibrosis.

6. The answer is B. (*Chapter 4 II D 1 a–c*) Because prostatic carcinoma has a high rate of initial response to hormone therapy, this tumor should be sought in men with disease of unknown tumor origin. Likewise, breast carcinoma should be sought in women, as this tumor responds well initially to hormone therapy, chemotherapy, or a combination of both treatments. Germ cell tumors and thyroid carcinoma also are responsive to systemic therapy in many cases. Despite unconfirmed reports of success, however, adenocarcinoma of the lung remains a fairly refractory neoplasm.

7. The answer is C. (*Chapter 8 VI B 1, 2*) Eosinophilia is a characteristic finding in infections due to multicellular, tissue-invasive parasites, such as *Schistosoma*, *Trichinella*, *Ascaris*, and *Strongyloides* species. Pinworm infestation is a purely luminal process, which does not elicit eosinophilia. Protozoal infections, such as giardiasis and amebiasis, rarely are associated with eosinophilia; the same is true of bacterial and viral infections such as measles. Corticosteroids may be administered to individuals with underlying eosinophilia due to asthma or allergy to reduce the eosinophilia.

8. The answer is D. (*Chapter 1 I D 1 b, e, f, 2 f, h*) Orthopnea is defined as dyspnea (i.e., the feeling of breathlessness) that occurs in the recumbent position. Recumbency leads to increased cardiac venous return and, thus, increased left and right ventricular volumes. The increased left ventricular volume results in increased left ventricular filling pressure, which leads to pulmonary congestion and the feeling of breathlessness. Neck vein distension, ascites, anorexia, and cardiac edema all are signs and symptoms of right ventricular failure.

9. The answer is A. (*Chapter 6 Part I: XI B 1, C 1 a, F 1 a; XIII B 4 a*) The most common form of nephrotic syndrome seen in adults is primary membranous glomerulonephritis, which accounts for 30%–50%

of cases in adults but less than 1% of cases in children. Lipoid nephrosis (also called minimal change disease) is the most common form of nephrotic syndrome seen in children, accounting for about 80% of cases in children but only about 20% of cases in adults. Focal glomerulosclerosis is seen in about 5%–12% of renal biopsies in adult patients with nephrotic syndrome. Crescentic glomerulonephritis and amyloidosis are rarely encountered forms of nephrotic syndrome.

10. The answer is D. (*Chapter 2 VI C–D*) Pulmonary hypertension in patients with chronic obstructive pulmonary disease (COPD) is due primarily to the vasoconstrictive effect of hypoxia. This response may be increased by acidosis, which also has a direct, although less dramatic, vasoconstrictive effect on the pulmonary vasculature. Pulmonary vasoconstriction puts a strain on the right ventricle, leading to its eventual failure (cor pulmonale). Left ventricular failure occurs independently of right ventricular failure and usually is caused by atherosclerotic coronary artery disease. In patients with emphysema, a loss of the pulmonary capillary bed also may contribute to pulmonary hypertension.

11. The answer is C. (*Chapter 5 II A 1 a*) Acute gastritis may be caused by accidental ingestion of caustic substances, stress, infections (e.g., the rare but fatal phlegmonous gastritis, which is caused by streptococci), and certain drugs, including alcohol. Aspirin and other nonsteroidal anti-inflammatory agents (e.g., indomethacin) probably interfere with the normal mucosal barrier to back-diffusion of acid by impairing prostaglandin synthesis. Acetaminophen, which has no anti-inflammatory properties, does not cause gastritis.

12. The answer is D. [*Chapter 7 II A 2 b (2), (3)*] B cells, in cooperation with helper T cells and suppressor T cells, produce all of the immunoglobulin isotypes, including immunoglobulin E (IgE). IgE production occurs in B cells in the spleen and lymphoid tissues of the tonsils and adenoids as well as in the bronchi, peritoneum, and the respiratory and intestinal mucosa. IgE levels peak in childhood and decline slightly in adulthood. This is in contrast to other immunoglobulin isotypes, such as IgG and IgM, which peak in the third decade and decline toward childhood levels in the sixth decade. Unlike IgG, IgE does not cross the placenta. Individuals with low IgE levels do not experience more infections.

13. The answer is C. (*Chapter 3 V D 1 a, c*) Factor IX deficiency, or hemophilia B, is an X-linked disorder of the intrinsic coagulation mechanism. This deficiency is associated with a prolonged partial thromboplastin time (PTT) but a normal platelet count and prothrombin time (PT). Factor XII deficiency causes similar coagulation profiles but is not associated with abnormal bleeding. Factor VII deficiency represents a defect in the extrinsic coagulation mechanism and is associated with a prolonged PT. Idiopathic thrombocytopenic purpura (ITP) and aspirin ingestion cause platelet disorders, which manifest as thrombocytopenia and thrombocytopathia, respectively.

14. The answer is B. (*Chapter 8 IV G 2*) The two most important factors in managing patients with intravenous catheters are insertion under sterile conditions and avoiding prolonged catheterization. The former is achieved by careful skin cleansing and avoiding sites that are diseased or infected or are prone to heavy bacterial contamination (e.g., the groin). The latter is achieved by removing catheters as quickly as feasible or by rotating sites every 48–72 hours. For practical purposes this rule is relaxed for intra-arterial and central venous catheters. Antimicrobial therapy is not indicated for prophylaxis in any "clean" procedure, including intravascular catheter insertion.

15. The answer is A. [*Chapter 6 Part I: I A 1 b, 2 a, f; II C 3 a (5)*] The finding of dark reddish urine suggests a number of possible underlying conditions. However, the absence of red blood cells on microscopic examination of the urine combined with the positive dipstick test for blood strongly suggest the possibility of myoglobinuria. Myoglobin is a pigment that is detected by the orthotoluidine reagent on the dipstick. While hemolyzed blood could be present in the urine, a few red blood cells should be noted, whereas none is seen in this patient's urine. Although foodstuffs do contain dyes that may color the urine, these do not produce positive dipstick tests for blood. This clinical picture is most consistent with myoglobinuria due to sudden, extreme physical exertion by an individual who is not well-conditioned. Such activity leads to muscle cell breakdown and the release of myoglobin into the circulation, with its ultimate filtration by the kidney and appearance in the urine.

16. The answer is C. [*Chapter 2 II C 1, 2 b (5)*] Asthma is a reversible airway obstruction characterized by hyperirritability of the airways. There are many chemical mediators of airway hyperirritability, including histamine, slow reacting substance of anaphylaxis (SRS-A), eosinophil chemotactic factor of anaphylaxis (ECF-A), and prostaglandins. These chemical mediators may be triggered by allergic as well as nonallergic stimuli (e.g., viral infections) to produce airway narrowing and edema. Therefore, viruses do not mediate but trigger the events leading to an asthmatic attack.

17. The answer is D. (*Chapter 7 V E 2 a, 4*) Of the drugs listed, all but aspirin show positive immediate skin tests at reasonable concentrations. Because anaphylaxis occurs in about 1% of herniated disk patients treated with chymopapain, skin testing is a useful screening procedure to identify those at risk for chymopapain-induced anaphylaxis. Allergy to purified bovine, porcine, and human insulin also can be identified by skin testing. Cephalosporin, at concentrations equivalent to penicillin G (benzylpenicillin) reagents, may produce wheal and flare reactions. Penicilloic acid, a major degradation product of penicillin, can react with polylysine (a synthetic polypeptide) to form penicilloyl-polylysine, which is non-immunogenic but produces a positive immediate skin test in penicillin-sensitive individuals. A definitive diagnosis of aspirin sensitivity can be made only by oral challenge with aspirin.

18. The answer is E. (*Chapter 1 VII C 4 a–e*) The most sensitive and specific test for pulmonary embolism is pulmonary arteriography. Nuclear scanning of the lung is another useful technique but is not as specific as arteriography. Although a normal scan virtually rules out pulmonary embolism, scanning results often fall into the intermediate probability range, making a definitive diagnosis impossible. In most cases of pulmonary embolism, the electrocardiogram (ECG) is normal. Acute right axis deviation noted on the ECG may lead to the erroneous diagnosis of anterior myocardial infarction. Hypoxia, hypocapnia, and respiratory alkalosis are classic findings on arterial blood gas analysis but are not specific for pulmonary embolism. The chest x-ray may be normal, especially if infarction has not occurred.

19. The answer is B. (*Chapter 9 VI C 1*) Severe virilization and marked testosterone elevation are more likely to be caused by an ovarian tumor or hyperthecosis than by the polycystic ovary syndrome. A low luteinizing hormone (LH) level and an increased urinary pregnanetriol concentration are not characteristic of the polycystic ovary syndrome. Hirsutism without other clinical or laboratory abnormalities usually is diagnosed as "idiopathic hirsutism."

20. The answer is E. (*Chapter 8 V D 1*) Upper respiratory infections (i.e., infections involving the nose, throat, larynx, airways, and adjacent structures) are the leading cause of morbidity in the United States. Viruses cause the overwhelming majority of upper respiratory infections, although bacterial complications may ensue. Prevention by immunization is not practical because of the large number of immunologically distinct agents that can cause upper respiratory disease. Infection due to influenza virus is an exception to this rule, since epidemic strains may be predicted and polyvalent killed virus vaccines administered, which can prevent such infection. Treatment usually is symptomatic, although influenza virus infections may respond to amantadine.

21. The answer is D. (*Chapter 7 III E 1*) An accurately applied immediate hypersensitivity skin test is the most valuable tool for identifying the antigen responsible for allergic rhinitis. Although the radioallergosorbent test (RAST) is accurate, studies comparing RAST to the skin test have proven the skin test to be more discriminative; it is also less expensive, with results available in 20–30 minutes. Elevated immunoglobulin E (IgE) levels are seen in only 30%–40% of patients with allergic rhinitis and may be secondary to other, unrelated disorders. Peripheral eosinophilia is an inconsistent finding, and, although eosinophils usually are identified in nasal secretions, they also may be seen in eosinophilic nonallergic rhinitis and hyperplastic sinusitis.

22. The answer is C. (*Chapter 9 I A 4*) As many as 50% of all pituitary adenomas have been found to secrete prolactin, and blood prolactin levels should be measured in any patient suspected of having a pituitary tumor. Acromegaly due to growth hormone (GH) excess and Cushing's disease due to adrenocorticotropic hormone (ACTH) excess are considerably less common, and overproduction of thyroid-stimulating hormone (TSH), luteinizing hormone (LH), and follicle-stimulating hormone (FSH) is rare. The clinical syndromes produced by prolactin excess are galactorrhea-amenorrhea in women and hypogonadism in men; however, patients with pituitary tumors may have prolactin excess with no clinical endocrine abnormality.

23. The answer is B (1, 3). [*Chapter 1 II A 5 b (1) (a)*] Coronary thrombosis currently is thought to be a major pathophysiologic mechanism of a transmural myocardial infarction. When infarction occurs, pain usually persists for a period of 30 minutes to several hours. The pain that occurs in myocardial infarction usually is similar in quality to the angina pectoris previously experienced by the patient, but it is more severe. Although myocardial infarction occasionally occurs during exercise, it is much more likely to occur at rest due to a sudden reduction in myocardial oxygen supply.

24. The answer is A (1, 2, 3). (*Chapter 8 V B 3*) Intracranial suppurative infections—whether epidural, subdural, or parenchymal—tend to arise from sinus or otic sources. The bacteriology is predominantly one of streptococci and oral anaerobes; however, cultures should be obtained in all cases to help guide therapy. Penicillin and chloramphenicol are effective against the common bacterial pathogens, and both of these drugs can penetrate intracranial abscesses. Many diagnostic procedures can be used, but computed tomography (CT) of the brain (with contrast enhancement) is the most reliable. *Toxoplasma* and *Nocardia* species and fungi rarely cause brain abscess in healthy individuals but are strongly associated with infection in immunodepressed individuals.

25. The answer is C (2, 4). (*Chapter 9 IV A 1, 2; Table 9-8*) Obesity is associated with type II (maturity-onset) but not type I (juvenile-onset) diabetes mellitus. Anti-islet cell antibodies are present at the time of diagnosis in many patients with type I diabetes, although these antibodies often disappear within a few years. The tendency to develop ketoacidosis in the absence of adequate insulin therapy indicates type I diabetes, but both type I and type II patients may require insulin treatment for optimal control of serum glucose levels. Onset at an early age is characteristic of type I diabetes.

26. The answer is B (1, 3). (*Chapter 5 V E*) Angiodysplasia refers to vascular abnormalities in the colon, which probably result from obstruction of capillaries passing through the mucosa. Angiodysplasia is a common cause of painless bleeding in elderly patients. Diagnosis can be difficult except during an active bleeding episode, when colonoscopy or angiography may show the site of bleeding. In a nonbleeding patient, colonoscopy may show the lesion in the cecum or ascending colon. Aortic stenosis is a concomitant finding in some patients.

27. The answer is B (1, 3). (*Chapter 2 V A, B, D 2; X B 3 a, 7*) Positive end-expiratory pressure (PEEP) ventilation is helpful in the treatment of pulmonary conditions that are associated with stiff, poorly compliant lungs. The mechanism of action of PEEP is to improve the functional residual capacity (FRC) in poorly compliant lungs. In adult respiratory distress syndrome (also called wet lung), the lungs stiffen and become less compliant due to increased extravascular lung water. In kyphoscoliosis, lung function is compromised as a result of reduced lung volume secondary to stiffness of the chest wall (reduced compliance and FRC). Chronic bronchitis and pulmonary emphysema are components of chronic obstructive pulmonary disease (COPD), which is associated with highly compliant lungs and increased FRC. In addition, COPD patients are at high risk for developing barotrauma.

28. The answer is A (1, 2, 3). (*Chapter 6 Part II: IV D 2 a*) An increased anion gap indicates either increased organic acid production or retention of mineral acids due to poor renal function. In renal failure, the kidney is unable to excrete phosphoric acid and sulfuric acid, which are end products of the metabolism of neutral precursors in foodstuffs. The increased anion gap represents the accumulation of the anions of these strong acids. In methanol ingestion, the increased anion gap is caused by the retention of formic acid and its anion, formate, in the plasma. In diabetic ketoacidosis, increased formation of ketone bodies (acetoacetate and β-hydroxybutyrate) is the basis for the increased anion gap. Conditions in which the chloride level of the blood is increased (e.g., as a result of hydrochloric acid administration) are not associated with an increased anion gap.

29. The answer is B (1, 3). [*Chapter 1 VIII B 2 b (2)–(4)*] Diuretic therapy generally is the first step in the treatment of hypertension. Diuretics reduce sodium and fluid excesses in the body and ultimately cause a reduction in peripheral vascular resistance. Side effects of diuretic therapy include hypokalemia, hyperglycemia, hyperuricemia, hypercalcemia, and prerenal azotemia. Also used in the treatment of hypertension is β-blockade, which may cause bronchospasm. Hemolytic anemia is a side effect of methyldopa, which is a centrally acting adrenergic antagonist that also is used to treat hypertension.

30. The answer is A (1, 2, 3). (*Chapter 5 VI B 1*) In general, any organism that can cause sexually transmitted disease also can cause infectious proctitis. These agents include *Treponema pallidum* (the organism responsible for venereal syphilis), *Chlamydia trachomatis* (the bacterium responsible for lymphogranuloma venereum), *Neisseria gonorrhoeae* (the organism responsible for gonorrhea), and Herpesvirus hominis (the virus responsible for herpes simplex). Varicella zoster virus causes varicella (chickenpox) and herpes zoster (shingles) but does not lead to the development of infectious proctitis. Homosexual men often are infected simultaneously with more than one organism linked to infectious proctitis; therefore, cultures and serologic testing for all possible organisms should be performed in these patients.

31. The answer is C (2, 4). [*Chapter 1 IV B 4 b (2)*] All maneuvers that decrease left ventricular size (e.g., the Valsalva maneuver and inhalation of amyl nitrite) bring the anterior leaflet of the mitral valve (i.e., the active obstructing body in hypertrophic obstructive cardiomyopathy) closer to the septum and increase the amount of obstruction. This, in turn, increases the intensity of the murmur. Conversely, maneuvers that increase cardiac size by increasing venous return (e.g., lying down or assuming the squatting position) tend to diminish the intensity of the murmur.

32. The answer is B (1, 3). (*Chapter 6 Part II: IV E 2*) Metabolic alkalosis is defined as an increased blood pH with an increased plasma bicarbonate concentration. Plasma bicarbonate levels may rise as a result of increased endogenous production of bicarbonate in the stomach (due to vomiting) or in the kidney (due to diuretics). In vomiting, the loss of hydrochloric acid from the stomach results in the accumulation of bicarbonate ions in plasma. The use of diuretics leads to increased renal production of bicarbonate through stimulation of hydrogen ion secretion in the distal tubule. In normal individuals, bicarbonate ingestion does not produce metabolic alkalosis, because the renal transport rate for bicarbonate maintains the serum level at 25 mEq/L. Ingestion of bicarbonate does not alter this rate, and any excess bicarbonate is excreted. Use of nonabsorbable antacids also does not produce metabolic alkalosis, because the buffering of hydrogen ions in the stomach is countered by the secretion of bicarbonate ions into the small intestine, which maintains the body fluid pH at 7.4.

33. The answer is A (1, 2, 3). (*Chapter 2 I A 1, G 1–3; II F 3; III C 4 b*) Of the disorders listed, bronchial asthma, pulmonary emphysema, and chronic bronchitis represent obstructive airway disease. The hallmark of airway obstruction is decreased airflow manifested by a decreased 1-second forced expiratory volume (FEV_1). A lung abscess usually is localized and, if large enough, may decrease the lung volumes. However, the abscess itself does not cause airway obstruction. (These patients frequently are smokers and may have independent airway obstruction not related to the abscess.)

34. The answer is C (2, 4). (*Chapter 4 VIII F 1 a*) Studies have shown that the Halsted radical mastectomy increases morbidity without providing any survival benefit over modified radical mastectomy. Furthermore, the latter procedure spares the pectoralis major and, therefore, is far less deforming than the Halsted operation. Radiotherapy alone is inadequate treatment. However, when combined with the removal of local disease by lumpectomy and axillary node sampling, high-dose regional radiation yields favorable survival rates. As a result, this therapeutic combination is gaining popularity as an alternative for breast cancer patients.

35. The answer is B (1, 3). (*Chapter 6 Part I: III E 2; IV B 4*) Pericarditis occurs in 5%–10% of patients on maintenance hemodialysis at some time during the course of treatment. Its cause remains obscure, although it may be viral in orgin. Pericarditis in this setting must be contrasted with the mild pericardial inflammation that may be seen in patients with untreated chronic renal failure, in whom the major manifestation is a pericardial rub heard on physical examination. Pericarditis in dialysis patients may progress to a hemorrhagic form with cardiac tamponade. Allergic reactions also are seen commonly in dialysis patients and may include eosinophilia, urticaria, and anaphylaxis. Pulmonary embolism is not typically seen in dialysis patients; in fact, these individuals have difficulty with coagulation, with long clotting times and severe bleeding when undergoing surgery or other trauma.

36. The answer is A (1, 2, 3). (*Chapter 9 II F 2*) A solitary nodule is more likely to be malignant than a nodule in an enlarged or multinodular thyroid gland. Head or neck irradiation in childhood and recent growth of the nodule increase the chance of malignancy. A cystic nodule is much less likely to be malignant than a solid nodule.

37. The answer is A (1, 2, 3). [*Chapter 1 V D 3 a, b (1), (3), 4 d*] In constrictive pericarditis, deep inspiration causes an increase in jugular venous distension (Kussmaul's sign). Also, the first and second heart sounds (S_1 and S_2) are reduced in intensity due to reduced sound transmission through the thickened pericardium. Equal cardiac pressures during diastole is the diagnostic sign found at cardiac catheterization. In most cases of constrictive pericarditis, the clinical findings of right-sided failure are more prominant than those of left-sided failure.

38. The answer is B (1, 3). (*Chapter 8 VI A 1 a, b, d, 2*) Although generalized enlargement of lymph nodes is a nonspecific finding, it often can lead to the diagnosis of a clinical entity. When the lymphadenopathy is coupled with fatigue and an atypical lymphocytosis, infectious mononucleosis is suggested. This syndrome most often is caused by Epstein-Barr virus, but a similar clinical picture is produced by cytomegalovirus infection. The two infections can be distinguished, however, using serologic tests (e.g., the Monospot test) or specific antibodies. Syphilis also should be considered in patients with a short duration of adenopathy and can be confirmed on the basis of serologic tests and the finding of an appropriate rash. Malaria typically is not accompanied by lymphadenopathy, although splenomegaly and fever are characteristic. Chancroid usually leads to inguinal adenopathy.

39. The answer is A (1, 2, 3). (*Chapter 9 I A 3 d, 4 b, d; II C 4; V B 4 d*) Acromegaly and galactorrhea-amenorrhea syndrome usually are caused by pituitary eosinophilic or chromophobic adenomas. Cushing's disease is caused by a pituitary basophilic or chromophobic adenoma. Transsphenoidal microsurgery is the treatment of choice for these conditions. Hyperthyroidism, on the other hand, is most commonly caused by thyroid-stimulating immunoglobulins and only rarely by pituitary overproduction of thyroid-stimulating hormone (TSH).

40. The answer is B (1, 3). (*Chapter 1 II A 1; Fig. 1-1*) Smooth muscle cells, lipids, and cholesterol are the major constituents of an atherosclerotic plaque. Smooth muscle cells proliferate probably in response to vessel wall damage. Damage also may increase the permeability of the vessel wall to cholesterol and lipids, resulting in their deposition in the plaque.

41. The answer is A (1, 2, 3). (*Chapter 4 XI D 3*) Clinical staging is not sufficient for the early stages of Hodgkin's disease. Clinically inapparent disease may exist elsewhere, which will change the therapy strategy. Therefore, patients with stage I or stage II supradiaphragmatic Hodgkin's disease require laparotomy with splenectomy to ascertain the existence of any occult disease in the abdomen.

42. The answer is B (1, 3). (*Chapter 7 IV A 2*) Angioedema presents as colorless areas of well-demarcated, nonpitting edema. The pathophysiologic changes in angioedema are confined to deep areas of the dermis and subcutaneous tissue, where there are few sensory nerve endings. For this reason, angioedema usually is not pruritic.

43–46. The answers are: 43-C, 44-B, 45-D, 46-A. [*Chapter 5 I B 1 c (6), 3 b (3), c (4) (b), d (3) (b)*] Reflux esophagitis occurs when gastric acid is allowed to enter the esophagus. Normally, the lower esophageal sphincter (LES) provides a barrier to acid reflux, but a decrease in LES pressure, an increase in abdominal pressure, or both may overcome this protective mechanism. Manometric documentation of a markedly decreased LES pressure is associated clinically with reflux esophagitis.

Scleroderma is a systemic disease that affects skin and smooth muscle. Therefore, the distal two-thirds (smooth muscle portion) of the esophagus is affected by scleroderma, whereas the upper one-third (striated muscle portion) is spared. The combination of poor esophageal clearance because of decreased peristalsis and free reflux because of decreased LES pressure leads to severe reflux esophagitis. Medical therapy aimed at decreasing gastric acid secretion and decreasing reflux into the esophagus usually is met with only limited success.

Symptomatic diffuse esophageal spasm (SDES) is a motor disorder of the esophagus characterized by high-amplitude, repetitive, simultaneous contractions (spasms) in the esophageal body. Unlike in achalasia (see below), normal peristalsis also is present in SDES. The LES pressure may be normal or increased, and there may be impaired relaxation of the LES.

In achalasia, there is no evidence of normal peristalsis, and the LES shows elevated resting pressure with incomplete relaxation. These changes probably have a neural basis. Symptoms probably are due to the impaired LES relaxation because pneumatic dilatation or surgical myotomy of the LES usually provides relief.

47–50. The answers are: 47-D, 48-B, 49-E, 50-A. (*Chapter 4 IV E 1–4*) Stage A1 prostatic tumors are low morbidity lesions that usually are found in a routine examination for benign obstructive disease. Close follow-up is adequate for stage A1 tumors. Stage A2 tumors are confined to the prostate gland and can be cured with radical radiotherapy (7000 rads).

Stage B tumors are the true, classic prostatic nodules that are found on rectal examination. These tumors are confined to the gland and, therefore, theoretically can be cured with radical prostatectomy.

Stage C tumors are cancers that are associated with metastasis to local structures (e.g., the seminal vesicles) but not to distant sites. These tumors cannot be treated surgically. However, radical radiotherapy with boost doses to the prostate gland has proved to be curative.

Stage D tumors are cancers that have distant metastases, and, therefore, local measures do not suffice as therapy. Stage D prostatic carcinoma requires systemic treatment such as hormone therapy or chemotherapy.

51–55. The answers are: 51-C, 52-B, 53-B, 54-B, 55-A. (*Chapter 3 I B 3 a–d*) Both folic acid and vitamin B_{12} deficiencies cause defective DNA synthesis and, thus, impaired cell maturation. Deficient DNA synthesis is the main characteristic of classic megaloblastic marrow (i.e., marrow cells with immature nuclei but mature cytoplasm) and macrocytic anemia. Because all marrow cell lines are affected, there is pancytopenia.

Vitamin B_{12} deficiency can result from absence of the gastric intrinsic factor needed to bind the vitamin and, thus, aid its absorption into the terminal ileum. This form of vitamin B_{12} deficiency, termed pernicious anemia, is associated with gastric atrophy, achlorhydria, and gastric carcinoma. The inability to absorb vitamin B_{12} into the ileum, which is corrected by administration of intrinsic factor, is identified by an abnormal Schilling test.

Due to the role of vitamin B_{12} in myelin metabolism, deficiency causes neuropathy in the lateral and posterior columns of the spinal cord. Folic acid deficiency causes blood findings that are similar to those caused by vitamin B_{12} deficiency; however, folic acid deficiency is not associated with neuropathy. Usually, folic acid deficiency results from dietary deficiency due to poor intake (e.g., in the case of alcoholism).

56–60. The answers are: 56-D, 57-A, 58-B, 59-E, 60-C. [*Chapter 10 I G 2 b; II A 4 b (4) (ii), B 5 a; III G 3 c*] The examination of synovial fluid often can provide a precise diagnosis of joint disease owing to the highly characteristic appearance of this fluid in each type of joint disease.

The term gout refers to a group of crystal-related joint disorders characterized by urate deposition in articular and extra-articular tissues. In acute gouty arthritis, the characteristic finding on synovial fluid analysis is the presence of needle-shaped crystals that are negatively birefringent in red-compensated, polarized light.

Calcium pyrophosphate dihydrate (CPPD) deposition disease is another crystal-related joint disease, which is characterized by deposition of CPPD crystals in cartilage and periarticular connective tissues.

The hallmark of CPPD deposition disease on synovial fluid examination is the presence of crystals that are chunky and rhomboid and that exhibit weakly positive birefringence in red-compensated, polarized light.

Osteoarthritis, also called degenerative joint disease, is a common disorder characterized by the deterioration of articular cartilage and underlying bone with age. Other factors (e.g., obesity and heredity) also contribute to the development of osteoarthritis. Osteoarthritic synovial fluid typically is slightly turbid, with a white cell count that is only mildly inflammatory (i.e., < 2000 cells/mm³), and demonstrates a good mucin clot. The mucin clot test is a gross test for the polymerization of hyaluronate in synovial fluid. When a small amount of normal, noninflammatory fluid is added to acetic acid, the hyaluronate is highly polymerized, forming a firm ("good") mucin clot.

Rheumatoid arthritis is a chronic inflammatory joint disorder characterized by polyarticular, symmetrical joint involvement as well as extra-articular involvement. The typical synovial fluid findings are those of a moderately inflammatory fluid (i.e., a white cell count of 5000–25,000/mm³, with mostly neutrophils). Urate and CPPD crystals are not present.

Infectious (pyogenic) arthritis is an acute process that occurs in a joint following infection by any of several different pathogens. Patients receiving steroid therapy and patients with existing joint disease (e.g., rheumatoid arthritis) appear to be predisposed. The diagnosis of infectious arthritis is based on synovial fluid examination for microorganisms and for evidence of severe inflammation. A white cell count of 70,000 cells/mm³ indicates a severely inflammatory fluid, which would characterize infectious arthritis. These fluids typically are neutrophil predominant.

1

Cardiovascular Diseases

Blase A. Carabello

I. CONGESTIVE HEART FAILURE

A. Definition. Congestive heart failure is the inability of the heart, working at normal or elevated filling pressure, to pump enough blood to supply the oxygen requirements of the body tissues. Congestive heart failure should never be considered a diagnosis. Rather, it is the syndrome resulting from many diseases that interfere with cardiac function.

B. Etiology

1. **Decreased contractile function.** Most cases of congestive heart failure occur when an insult to the myocardium reduces its ability to generate force, thus reducing its contractility.

    a. **Myocardial infarction.** In myocardial infarction, a portion of the myocardium undergoes necrosis and can no longer contract. These portions of the myocardium can no longer generate force, resulting in weakening of the ventricle. If the areas of infarction are extensive, congestive heart failure results.

    b. **Valvular heart disease. Stenosis** or **regurgitation** of the cardiac valves places a **pressure** or **volume overload**, respectively, on the ventricles. Initially, compensatory mechanisms accommodate these overloads and maintain normal cardiac output at acceptable filling pressure. Compensatory mechanisms include the **Frank-Starling mechanism**, development of cardiac hypertrophy, and hormonal stimulation, which increase the inotropic state. Eventually, however, these compensatory mechanisms fail and the myocardium no longer can generate adequate force to maintain cardiac output. The exact cellular malfunction producing this reduction in force-generating capacity is unknown.

    c. **Hypertension.** Seventy-five percent of patients who develop congestive heart failure have had systemic hypertension at some time in the clinical course of their illness. It is apparent that **persistent severe hypertension** is associated with a **contractile deficit** that leads to congestive heart failure.

    d. **Cardiomyopathy**

    (1) **Toxic.** Substances directly toxic to the myocardium may damage its force-generating ability. Examples of such toxins are alcohol, cobalt, and catecholamines. Prolonged exposure to these toxins may lead to the development of congestive heart failure.

    (2) **Idiopathic.** In many instances, the contractile function of the myocardium fails in the absence of a known etiology. In these circumstances a viral cause often is implied but cannot be proven.

2. **Increased afterload.** Afterload is the force that the myocardium must generate in order to shorten (i.e., the force that resists contraction of the heart). This force may become excessive and inhibit myocardial contraction, in which case the force generation of the myocardium is normal but not strong enough to overcome the excessive resistance. An example of this situation is **acute systemic hypertension**. As noted above, chronic hypertension may lead to eventual contractile failure of the myocardium. However, if blood pressure is acutely and sharply elevated, congestive heart failure ensues not because of contractile dysfunction but because the load placed on the myocardium exceeds its force-generating capacity.

3. **Abnormalities in preload.** Preload refers to the stretch of the myocardial fiber prior to myocardial contraction and is an expression of the Frank-Starling mechanism. An increased preload (i.e., a greater muscle length) increases the force-generating capabilities of the myocardium but is associated with an increased ventricular filling pressure, which leads to pulmonary congestion.

    a. **High preload states.** In the absence of contractile dysfunction or excessive afterload, preload usually is normal. An exception is the presence of severe renal failure. In such cases, the myocardium may be normal but the preload is increased because of the body's inability to rid itself of excessive intravascular volume. A patient in this condition demonstrates all of the signs and symptoms of congestive heart failure in the presence of a normally functioning myocardium.

b. **Reduced preload/reduced compliance states.** Compliance is an expression of the distensibility of the heart, which is determined as the volume change (ΔV) per unit of pressure change (ΔP), or $\Delta V/\Delta P$. If compliance is reduced, cardiac muscle that is normal or even reduced in length is associated with a very high filling pressure. An example is **constrictive pericarditis**, in which a thickened pericardium inhibits cardiac filling and a high filling pressure is required for filling to occur. Despite a high filling pressure, cardiac output is diminished because preload is diminished.

C. Terminology

1. **High-output failure** is characterized by cardiac output that may be several times higher than normal but still is not adequate to maintain tissue perfusion needs or, if adequate, is maintained with a higher than normal filling pressure. A classic example of high-output failure is **chronic severe anemia**, which causes a reduced oxygen-carrying capacity. Compensation is provided by increased forward cardiac output, which is facilitated by cardiac enlargement, decreased total peripheral resistance, and increased venous return to the heart. Thus, a volume overload to the left ventricle occurs similar to that seen in aortic insufficiency. Eventually, the demands on the heart lead to cardiac failure; cardiac output, though high, still is not adequate to meet the circulatory demands placed on the heart by the anemia.

2. **Left-sided failure** indicates that the left ventricle is the failing chamber. A disease that primarily affects the left ventricle (e.g., myocardial infarction) may reduce its contractile force, while the right ventricle continues to pump normally. Thus, left ventricular failure occurs without right ventricular failure.

3. **Right-sided failure** indicates that the right ventricle has failed together with the left ventricle or in isolation from it.
   a. The most common cause of right ventricular failure is left ventricular failure. When left ventricular failure occurs, the filling pressure in the left ventricle becomes elevated, requiring increased work of the right ventricle (i.e., the chamber responsible for filling the left ventricle). Thus overtaxed, the right ventricle eventually fails also.
   b. The right ventricle also may fail in isolation from the left ventricle. In **chronic obstructive pulmonary disease**, increased pulmonary vascular resistance occurs due to architectural changes in the lungs. The increased pulmonary vascular resistance in turn produces a pressure overload on the right ventricle, which subsequently leads to increased right ventricular work and eventual failure.

D. Clinical features

1. **Symptoms**
   a. **Dyspnea** is the most frequently encountered symptom of congestive heart failure.
      (1) The feeling of **breathlessness** is due to vascular congestion, which reduces pulmonary oxygenation. In addition, the vascular congestion diminishes lung compliance, increasing the work of breathing and thus adding to the feeling of breathlessness.
      (2) Dyspnea also results from reduced cardiac output to the periphery, which triggers the symptom through neurohumoral mechanisms. In the early stages of congestive heart failure, dyspnea occurs only with exertion. As heart failure progresses, the amount of exertion required to produce dyspnea becomes progressively less until dyspnea may occur at rest.
   b. **Orthopnea** refers to dyspnea that occurs in the recumbent position and is relieved by elevation of the head. Orthopnea results from volume pooling in the central vasculature during recumbency. Increased cardiac volume results, which in turn increases left ventricular filling pressure and leads to pulmonary congestion and the feeling of dyspnea. Orthopnea often is gauged by the number of pillows the patient sleeps on.
   c. **Paroxysmal nocturnal dyspnea** is the occurrence of sudden dyspnea that awakens the patient from sleep. Like orthopnea, it occurs during recumbency as a result of pooling in the central vasculature, which increases left ventricular filling pressure. Paroxysmal nocturnal dyspnea may occur in the orthopneic patient who inadvertently slips off the pillows used to elevate the upper body. Usually, the patient awakens from sleep and feels the need to sit upright or, not uncommonly, to go to an open window for increased ventilation. The symptom usually subsides after the patient has been in the upright position for 5–20 minutes.

    d. Nocturia occurs in congestive heart failure due to increased renal blood flow in recumbency during sleep.

        (1) During the day when the skeletal muscles are active, limited cardiac output is shifted away from the kidney toward the skeletal musculature. The kidney interprets this reduction in blood flow as **hypovolemia** and becomes sodium avid via activation of the **renin-angiotensin system**.

        (2) At night when the patient is at rest, cardiac output is shifted toward the kidney and diuresis ensues.

    e. Edema. There are many causes of peripheral edema, several of which are noncardiac. **Cardiac edema** occurs when the systemic hydrostatic venous pressure is greater than the systemic oncotic venous pressure. Thus, cardiac edema is a sign of right-sided failure since it occurs due to an increase in the systemic venous pressure as a manifestation of right ventricular failure.

    f. Anorexia may occur as a late manifestation of congestive heart failure. The exact mechanism of anorexia is unknown, but it seems to correlate with hepatic congestion and right-sided failure.

2. Physical signs

    a. Tachycardia occurs in heart failure as a compensatory mechanism for maintaining cardiac output in the presence of decreased stroke volume.

    b. Pulmonary rales. The increased left ventricular filling pressure associated with congestive heart failure is referred to the left atrium and pulmonary veins. The increased hydrostatic pressure produces transudation of fluid into the alveoli. As air circulates through the alveoli, pulmonary rales are produced. It is important to note that there are multiple causes of pulmonary rales; the mere presence of rales does not necessarily indicate congestive heart failure.

    c. Cardiac enlargement. As the failing heart relies more and more on the Frank-Starling mechanism, it dilates and may develop **eccentric hypertrophy**. Cardiac enlargement can be detected on physical examination as the point of maximal impulse of the left ventricle is shifted downward and to the left.

    d. Fourth heart sound (S_4). Patients in sinus rhythm in heart failure often have an S_4 (**atrial gallop**) produced as left atrial systole propels volume into the left ventricle just prior to ventricular systole. In congestive heart failure, the left ventricle is noncompliant and the S_4 probably is due to the reverberation of the blood ejected from the left atrium into the left ventricle. In elderly patients, however, an S_4 may indicate reduced compliance of the left ventricle due to aging rather than heart failure. The S_4 also may be heard over the right ventricle in right ventricular failure.

    e. Third heart sound (S_3). An S_3 (**ventricular gallop**), which occurs early in diastole, probably is the single most reliable sign of heart failure on physical examination. The S_3 occurs during rapid filling of the left ventricle. Noncompliance of the left ventricle together with the increased left atrial pressure that propels the blood forward at increased force are important in producing this extra sound. While an S_3 is a reliable sign of heart failure in individuals over the age of 40, it also may be heard in young, healthy athletes as a normal finding.

    f. Neck vein distension. The neck veins can be considered manometers attached to the right atrium and, as such, reflect right atrial pressure. By measuring the vertical height of the veins above the right atrium it is possible to estimate the central venous pressure. When the right ventricle fails it relies increasingly on the Frank-Starling mechanism for compensation. This results in an increase in right ventricular volume and pressure, which is referred back to the right atrium. This increased pressure can be gauged by evaluation of the neck veins.

    g. Edema. Lower extremity and presacral edema occur in right-sided failure, as increased venous pressure results in transudation of fluid into these areas. For edema to be attributable to congestive heart failure, distended neck veins indicative of elevated right-sided filling pressure also should be present.

    h. Ascites. Transudation of fluid into the **peritoneal space** also may occur due to increased systemic venous pressure. When ascites is due to congestive heart failure, the neck veins typically are elevated, and the liver is distended from passive congestion.

E. Diagnosis

    1. Etiologic considerations. Congestive heart failure is not a disease but rather a syndrome that results from a disease. In the management of congestive heart failure, the cause of the heart failure should be sought so that therapy can be directed toward the cause and not simply the relief of the heart failure symptoms. Although a careful history and physical examination of the patient are the most important tools available in arriving at a diagnosis, in many cases a diagnosis may not be reached. In these instances the following studies often are helpful.

a. The **electrocardiogram (ECG)** frequently is nonspecific. However, the presence of Q waves helps to confirm that myocardial infarction has been the cause of the patient's congestive heart failure.

b. The **chest x-ray** is useful in demonstrating cardiac chamber enlargement and in documenting congestion in the lungs. It provides objective evidence that heart failure is present.

c. The **echocardiogram** is useful in identifying chamber enlargement and in quantifying left ventricular function and valvular function. This method is particularly useful in the diagnosis of mitral valve disease.

d. **Radionuclide ventriculography.** Right and left ventricular performance can be gauged accurately by this technique. Radionuclide ventriculography is an excellent noninvasive test to quantify the degree of cardiac dysfunction present.

e. During **cardiac catheterization**, intracardiac pressures, chamber size, valvular stenosis, valvular regurgitation, and coronary anatomy can be evaluated. Usually, this is the most accurate method for determining a specific cardiac diagnosis. Unlike the noninvasive tests mentioned above, however, catheterization has a small but finite risk. Therefore, cardiac catheterization is performed in congestive heart failure patients in whom it is important to know the primary etiology in order to reverse the heart failure.

2. **Symptomatic considerations.** Even in cases in which the definitive etiology is not thought to be important in the management of congestive heart failure (e.g., a patient with terminal cancer), some objective evidence of cardiac dysfunction is advisable prior to therapy. Frequently, a patient with dyspnea on exertion and orthopnea is treated for congestive heart failure, yet the symptoms have another cause. The chest x-ray and echocardiogram are useful adjuncts to the physical examination in providing objective evidence of cardiac dysfunction prior to therapy and also for gauging the effects of therapy.

F. Therapy

1. **Etiologic therapy.** It is important, when possible, to direct therapy at the etiologic agent responsible for the congestive heart failure. For example, if aortic stenosis is the cause of congestive heart failure, aortic valve replacement is the most effective therapy.

2. **Symptomatic therapy.** If the etiologic agent cannot be found, or if the patient's condition does not permit direct intervention, or if the patient refuses to consider corrective surgery even if indicated, the physician must resort to therapy aimed at relieving the symptoms of heart failure.

a. **Increasing the contractile state**

(1) **Cardiac glycosides** (e.g., digoxin) increase the contractile state by impeding the sodium-potassium-ATPase–controlled intracellular pump. This results in the net influx of calcium into the myocardium, which increases contractile strength. Since contractile dysfunction usually is the cause of heart failure, there is a good rationale for attempting to increase the contractile state. However, the use of cardiac glycosides in the chronic treatment of congestive heart failure is controversial. Although digoxin frequently is used in the United States, it does not form the mainstay of therapy in other countries, such as Great Britain.

(2) **Beta-adrenergic agonists** (e.g., catecholamines) also increase contractile function. Chronic oral therapy with these medications currently is in the experimental stage, and the use of these drugs is limited to intravenous treatment of acute reversible heart failure (e.g., that seen following cardiac surgery).

(3) **Amrinone** is a new, potent inotropic agent that is useful in the acute treatment of congestive heart failure. Its mechanism of action is unknown but is clearly different from that of the cardiac glycosides and the β-adrenergic agonists.

b. **Reducing afterload.** Agents that cause arteriolar dilatation produce less impedance to the outflow of blood from the left ventricle. By diminishing total peripheral resistance, cardiac output rises as the left ventricle can eject more completely against a lower afterload. The net effect is increased cardiac output without a serious fall in blood pressure, leading to symptomatic improvement. Currently, several vasodilators are used in the treatment of congestive heart failure to reduce afterload, including captopril, prazosin, nitrates, and hydralazine.

c. **Reducing preload and left ventricular filling pressure.** The increased preload resulting from volume retention in the ventricles is a compensatory mechanism that helps increase forward cardiac output; however, an excessive increase in preload is associated with an increase in left ventricular and right ventricular filling pressures, which is responsible for symptoms of pulmonary and systemic congestion. Judicious reduction in filling pressures without excessive reduction in preload is indicated in the therapy of congestive heart failure.

(1) **Diuretics** reduce renal tubular absorption of sodium and water and increase the

clearance of these substances from the body. The result is a reduction in central volume and in cardiac filling pressure.

    (2) Vasodilators, which increase the capacity of the systemic venous system, transfer central volume to the periphery, thus reducing central preload and filling pressure. The nitrates, captopril, and prazosin, are effective as preload-reducing vasodilators.

  d. Physical conditioning is an important adjunct to the medical treatment of congestive heart failure. Physical conditioning permits the peripheral tissues to use cardiac output more efficiently. Thus, the patient experiences an increase in tolerance to physical activity without an increase in cardiac output.

  e. Cardiac transplantation may offer an improved quality of life to selected patients in whom control of congestive heart failure is not possible and prognosis is poor.

3. Therapy for cases involving pulmonary edema. Pulmonary edema is the most extreme example of congestive heart failure, in which profound transudation of fluid into the pulmonary alveoli occurs due to a high left ventricular filling pressure. The result is impaired oxygenation and, if untreated, death. The goal of therapy is to improve oxygenation, to reduce left ventricular filling pressure, and to increase forward cardiac output.

  a. Oxygen therapy is an important part of the treatment of acute pulmonary edema. Oxygen should be administered by face mask, since patients in pulmonary edema are so dyspneic that they breathe primarily through their mouths.

  b. Diuretics. Furosemide probably is the single most commonly used medication in the treatment of acute pulmonary edema. This rapid-acting, loop diuretic promotes an immediate diuresis in most cases. A low (20-mg) dose should be given intravenously to patients who currently are not receiving the drug since higher doses may produce excessive diuresis.

  c. Rotating tourniquets. Tourniquets are placed on three of the four limbs, with enough constriction to impede venous outflow from the limb while permitting arterial inflow. This decreases venous return to the heart and reduces preload. Tourniquets should be rotated every 20 minutes so that no limb is persistently constricted.

  d. Morphine sulfate reduces patient anxiety, which may help to relieve the arterial vasoconstriction often present in acute pulmonary edema. This, in turn, helps to increase forward cardiac output. Morphine also is a venodilator and, therefore, acts to reduce central volume and left ventricular filling pressure.

  e. Other vasodilators. Sublingual or intravenous administration of nitroglycerin or nitroprusside given intravenously often is effective in treating pulmonary edema when other therapies fail. These drugs reduce central volume by venodilatation and also increase cardiac output secondary to arteriolar vasodilatation. However, the potent vasodilating ability of these drugs requires that blood pressure be monitored constantly during their administration in order to avoid significant hypotension.

  f. Intubation and positive pressure ventilation. If the patient's level of oxygenation does not improve rapidly with the above therapies, intubation may be necessary to provide mechanical ventilation and to improve oxygenation.

  g. Cardiac glycosides are effective in increasing cardiac contractile function, which is beneficial in the treatment of heart failure. In the setting of acute pulmonary edema, however, these drugs provide only adjunctive therapy since symptomatic improvement usually occurs before the digitalis glycosides have a chance to take effect.

  h. Invasive hemodynamic monitoring. Most cases of pulmonary edema resolve quickly, making invasive hemodynamic monitoring neither necessary nor useful. However, in cases of recalcitrant pulmonary edema with severe cardiac compromise, exact knowledge of intracardiac filling pressure may be useful in guiding therapy. Hemodynamic monitoring (via Swan-Ganz catheterization) provides this information so that optimal filling pressure and cardiac output may be obtained.

II. ISCHEMIC HEART DISEASE

  A. Atherosclerotic coronary artery disease (ASCAD)

    1. Definition. ASCAD is the focal narrowing of the large and medium-sized coronary arteries due to intimal proliferation of smooth muscle cells and the deposition of lipids. The basic lesion is called a **plaque**, the chief components of which are diagrammed in Figure 1-1 and include:

      a. Intimal smooth muscle cells, which are caused to proliferate due to endothelial damage

      b. Lipids (cholesterol esters and crystals), which are deposited at the center of the plaque and also accumulate within smooth muscle cells

    2. Incidence and risk factors. Currently in the United States the incidence of death due to ASCAD is 3 in 1000 and decreasing. However, ASCAD occurs with different frequencies according to the following risk factors.

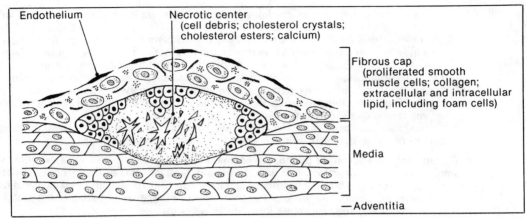

Figure 1-1. Diagrammatic representation of an atherosclerotic plaque, showing its composition. The *fibrous cap* of the plaque is linked to clinical events due to its size and tendency to fracture and ulcerate. The *necrotic core* of the plaque has clinical consequence due to its size, consistency, and thromboplastic components. (Adapted from Braunwald E: *Heart Disease*, 2nd ed. Philadelphia, WB Saunders, 1984, p 1186.)

    a. Age. The incidence of ASCAD in the United States increases progressively with age and is approximately 150 in 100,000 individuals at age 50.

    b. Sex. ASCAD is more prevalent in men than in women. This difference is most marked in premenopausal women compared to men of similar age; men in this age group are affected five times more commonly than women.

    c. Serum cholesterol. The incidence of ASCAD increases with increasing total serum cholesterol levels, as shown in Figure 1-2. Total serum cholesterol is carried in the blood by **low-density lipoprotein (LDL)**, **very low-density lipoprotein (VLDL)**, and **high-density lipoprotein (HDL)**. The higher the percentage of total cholesterol carried by LDL in relation to HDL, the higher the risk of ASCAD. Patients with LDL-to-HDL ratios of greater than 5:1 are particularly prone to ASCAD. Conversely, high levels of HDL seem to be protective. One theory is that HDL may allow for elution of cholesterol out of the coronary vessel.

    d. Smoking. Cigarette smokers are 60% more likely to develop ASCAD than nonsmokers when other risk factors are controlled. Smoking increases carbon monoxide levels in the blood, which may in turn damage the coronary endothelium. Smoking also increases platelet adhesiveness and thus the likelihood of thrombotic coronary occlusion.

    e. Hypertension. The higher either the systolic or diastolic blood pressure, the more likely the development of ASCAD. This likelihood is noted in both men and women and becomes more pronounced with advancing age.

    f. Diabetes mellitus is associated with a 50% increase in the incidence of ASCAD in men and a 100% increase in women. This correlation may be explained in part by the increased platelet adhesiveness and increased serum cholesterol levels associated with diabetes. In general, however, there is a poor correlation between the severity of the diabetes and the severity of ASCAD.

    g. Family history. A familial predisposition to coronary artery disease exists and is partially due to the fact that the above risk factors (except smoking) also are inherited.

    h. Oral contraceptives are associated with an increased incidence of myocardial infarction from 0.01% to 0.04% in nonsmoking women aged 30–40 years. In smokers who use oral contraceptives, the increase is more dramatic (0.06% to 0.25%).

    i. Other risk factors. Gout, type A personality, premature arcus senilis, obesity, hypertriglyceridemia, and a diagonal ear lobe crease also are associated with an increased risk of ASCAD.

  3. Pathogenesis. The above-mentioned risk factors do not constitute a known mechanism for ASCAD; however, three major theories of atherogenesis exist.

    a. The insudation theory was developed from the constant observation that high levels of serum cholesterol and LDL are associated with ASCAD. This suggests that increased levels of these substances lead to their increased deposition in the vessel walls.

    b. The damage thrombosis theory postulates that intermittent damage to the vessel (e.g., from hypertension or carbon monoxide) leads to platelet activation and thrombus deposition. This in turn leads to smooth muscle cell proliferation and genesis of a plaque. The damage also may increase the permeability of the vessel to cholesterol, which could increase cholesterol deposition.

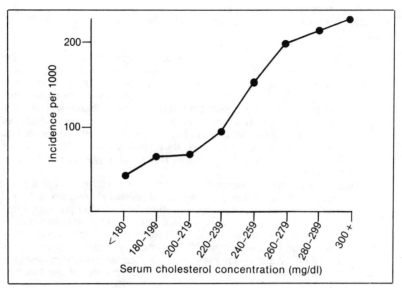

Figure 1-2. Graph showing the effect of increasing serum cholesterol concentration on the incidence of atherosclerotic coronary artery disease in men aged 30–49 years. (Adapted from Cohn PF: *Diagnosis and Therapy of Coronary Artery Disease*. Boston, Little, Brown, 1979, p 27.)

   c. The neoplasia theory. Smooth muscle cells in atherosclerotic plaques in women have the same **glucose-6-phosphate dehydrogenase** isoenzyme, suggesting a monoclonal origin of these cells. This theory postulates that a stimulus—perhaps vessel wall injury—leads to cell proliferation.

4. Pathophysiology
   a. Supply-demand relationship. The oxygen needs of the myocardium can be roughly approximated by the product of heart rate and left ventricular systolic pressure. As these variables increase (e.g., with exercise), myocardial oxygen consumption rises. This increased demand is met in normal individuals by autoregulated increases in coronary blood flow.
     (1) Increased demand. In patients with ASCAD, **stenosis** of the coronary artery prevents the increase in coronary blood flow needed to compensate for an increased demand, resulting in oxygen demand exceeding oxygen supply. Myocardial ischemia is the end product of this imbalance.
     (2) Reduced supply. The atherosclerotic stenosis was once viewed as a **fixed obstruction** to coronary blood flow. In fact, the diseased area of the coronary artery often remains dynamic, and the effective lumen of the artery undergoes constant change. Changes are produced by vasoconstriction of the coronary artery, by production and degradation of local thrombi at the site of stenosis, and by progressive enlargement of the atherosclerotic plaque. These changes may reduce the supply of coronary blood flow and, thus, produce ischemia without an increase in demand.
   b. Myocardial infarction
     (1) Although the cause of **transmural infarction** has been debated for much of the last century, recent studies demonstrate that most transmural myocardial infarctions are associated with early occlusion of a coronary artery by a **thrombus**. The thrombus usually is located adjacent to an atherosclerotic coronary stenosis. The initial events producing this thrombus are not clear. Acute lysis of the thrombus with agents such as **streptokinase** reestablishes coronary blood flow, relieves pain, reestablishes contractile function of the segment of myocardium supplied by the thrombosed artery, and may reduce myocardial damage [see section II A 5 b (5)]. These observations confirm that the thrombus is not merely a coincident event in myocardial infarction but is central to its pathogenesis. Without therapeutic or natural **recanalization**, cell death ensues. The rapidity and extent of the infarction process are determined by the extent of reduction of blood flow to the area. In some cases, **collateral flow** may supply enough blood flow to prevent infarction despite a total coronary occlusion.
     (2) The pathogenesis of **nontransmural infarction** is less clear, but total coronary occlusion is significantly less common, occurring in less than 50% of cases.

5. Clinical consequences of ASCAD
  a. Angina pectoris, in current usage, refers to chest pain or pressure produced by myocardial ischemia.
   (1) Characteristic features
     (a) Relation to exertion. The single most important feature of angina pectoris is its precipitation by exertion. Exertion increases myocardial oxygen demands beyond the supply capabilities of diseased coronary arteries, thus producing ischemia. Ischemic pain is perceived by an unknown mechanism. In some patients, angina occurs predominantly at rest, but this is unusual. When rest pain does occur, it probably is produced by a reduction in coronary blood flow as described above. However, spontaneous increases in blood pressure, heart rate, or both may increase demand at rest in some patients, thus causing angina. Ischemic pain usually is relieved by maneuvers that reduce myocardial oxygen demand, such as cessation of the precipitating activity.
     (b) Symptom quality. Although angina often is described as chest pain, many patients protest that rather than pain they feel a **pressure sensation** in their chest. Other patients complain of a **burning sensation**. In still other patients, **exertional dyspnea** may represent an anginal equivalent. Whatever the symptom quality for a given patient, it usually can be reproduced upon repeated episodes of ischemia. The symptom complex usually begins at a low intensity, increases over 2–3 minutes, and lasts a total of less than 15 minutes. Episodes longer than 30 minutes suggest that myocardial infarction may have occurred. Sudden onset of chest pain does not suggest angina.
     (c) Radiation of pain. Radiation of anginal pain to the left arm is well known. Pain also may radiate to the right arm, jaw, teeth, or throat. Occasionally, these radiation sites may be the only sites of pain, and the chest is free of discomfort. On the other hand, the chest discomfort, when present, may not radiate at all.
     (d) Unstable angina. A change in the status of a patient's angina (e.g., new-onset angina; increasing severity, duration, or frequency of angina; and angina occurring at rest for the first time) could be classified as unstable angina.
       (i) The term unstable angina implies a more serious clinical situation than chronic stable angina since unstable angina may be an immediate precursor of myocardial infarction.
       (ii) In cases of new-onset angina, it is difficult to generalize about clinical outcome. New-onset angina that progresses in frequency, severity, or duration over 1 or 2 months is worrisome. Conversely, some cases of new-onset angina may simply be the first episode in what becomes a chronic stable anginal pattern.
       (iii) Thus, it is the progressive nature of unstable angina, when present, that is ominous and should warn both the patient and his or her physician that close observation and intensive therapy are required.
     (e) Variant (Prinzmetal's) angina. The hallmark of variant angina is transient ST-segment elevation, which occurs during the attack. The ST-segment elevation represents **transmural ischemia** produced by a sudden reduction in coronary blood flow. The reduction in flow results from **transient coronary spasm**, which usually, but not always, is associated with a fixed atherosclerotic lesion. The spasm produces total but transient coronary occlusion. The cause of the spasm and its release are unknown. Variant angina usually occurs at rest instead of during exercise and often at night. Episodes frequently are complicated by complex ventricular arrhythmias.
   (2) Diagnosis. When the patient presents with the classic features of chest pain as outlined above, the diagnosis can be suspected strongly by patient history alone. The suspicion that coronary disease is present is heightened by the presence of one or more coronary risk factors. However, the following procedures are useful in confirming the diagnosis.
     (a) Physical examination during angina reveals that the patient is uncomfortable and anxious. The blood pressure and pulse usually are increased above the patient's usual vital signs. Palpation of the precordium may reveal a **dyskinetic impulse** over the apex of the left ventricle. A new S_4 may appear, and **transient mitral regurgitation** due to ischemically produced papillary muscle dysfunction may produce a **holosystolic murmur.**
     (b) Resting electrocardiography. The resting ECG in patients with angina pectoris but no history of myocardial infarction is normal in 50% of cases. However, efforts to obtain an ECG during chest pain more frequently are rewarding. The presence of new horizontal or down-sloping ST-segment depression during pain is highly suggestive of myocardial ischemia. New T-wave inversion also may occur, but this finding alone without ST-segment depression is less specific. During variant angina,

the diagnostic finding is an acute current of injury indicated by transient ST-segment elevation. The ST-segment elevation normalizes as the pain wanes and no Q waves appear.

(c) **Stress electrocardiography.** Recording the ECG during exercise substantially increases the sensitivity and specificity of this procedure.

  (i) ST-segment depression of 1 mm or more during exercise has a sensitivity of approximately 70% and a specificity of 90% for the detection of coronary disease.

  (ii) Of equal importance to the ECG, a formal exercise test permits quantification of the patient's exercise tolerance and observation of the effects of exercise on the patient's symptoms, heart rate, and blood pressure.

  (iii) The ST criteria for positivity are less accurate in women than in men. The presence of **bundle branch block** or **left ventricular hypertrophy** or the use of **digitalis** by the patient all reduce the accuracy of this test.

(d) **Stress scintigraphy.** When the radioactive isotope **thallium 201 (^{201}Tl)** is injected into the peripheral venous blood, a portion of the isotope is taken up by the myocardium. The myocardial distribution of ^{201}Tl is according to blood flow, with areas of greater blood flow taking up more ^{201}Tl than areas of lesser blood flow. Normally, blood flow and, thus, ^{201}Tl are distributed equally throughout the myocardium. With exercise, blood flow increases. In patients with coronary artery disease, exercise causes an increase in ^{201}Tl uptake in areas receiving normal blood flow. However, those parts of the myocardium supplied by diseased coronary arteries and areas of myocardial infarction take up less ^{201}Tl than normal areas, as shown in the scintigram in Figure 1-3. The combination of stress scintigraphy with the stress ECG has yielded increased sensitivity (80%) and specificity (92%) over the standard stress ECG alone. Stress scintigraphy is particularly useful when the standard stress ECG is expected to be of low yield (e.g., in women and in patients with bundle branch block) and in patients in whom a previous stress ECG has produced equivocal results.

(e) **Stress radionuclide ventriculography.** A radionuclide such as **technetium**, injected peripherally, can be bound to red blood cells by pyrophosphate. Radionuclide-tagged red blood cells in the blood pool of the left ventricle can be used to produce

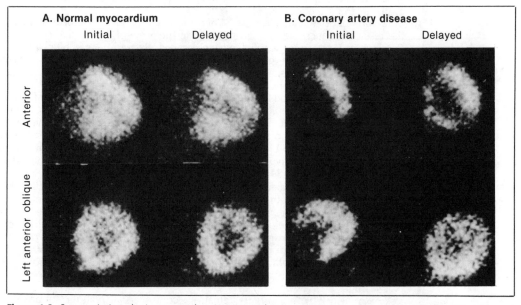

Figure 1-3. Stress scintigraphy in a normal patient (*A*) and in a patient with coronary artery disease (*B*). *A* Normal thallium study shows initial (i.e., immediately after exercise) and delayed thallium 201 (^{201}Tl) images in the anterior and left anterior oblique views. ^{201}Tl is taken up and released homogeneously throughout the myocardium, indicating equal coronary blood flow to all portions of the left ventricle. *B* A large defect (*black area from 5 o'clock to 11 o'clock*) is seen in the initial scintiscan in the anterior view. This area corresponds to the inferoapical area of the left ventricle. A defect also is seen in the left anterior oblique view (*black area from 6 o'clock to 9 o'clock*), which corresponds to the inferior portion of the left ventricular septum. Areas of decreased perfusion eventually demonstrate ^{201}Tl uptake, as seen in the delayed scintiscan. This study is consistent with exercise-induced hypoperfusion of the inferolateral and septal areas of the left ventricle and with obstructive disease of the right coronary artery. (Reprinted with permission from Johnson R, et al: *The Practice of Cardiology*. Boston, Little, Brown, 1980, p 1046.)

a scintigraphic image of the left ventricle. By gating the time that one measures the radioactivity coming from this pool for systole and diastole, a radionuclide ventriculogram can be produced.

(i) Coronary disease produces regional dysfunction by ischemia or infarction of those areas of the left ventricle not receiving an adequate blood supply. Exercise-induced ischemia produces transient regional dysfunction, which can be detected by radionuclide angiography. For example, in a patient with disease in the left anterior descending coronary artery, the anterior left ventricular wall may move normally at rest but become dyskinetic with exercise due to ischemia.

(ii) This test is sensitive (90%) for the detection of coronary artery disease but is not specific since heart disease other than coronary artery disease may produce exercise-induced regional dysfunction.

(f) **Cardiac catheterization and coronary arteriography.** Direct visualization of the coronary arteries by selective injection of radiographic contrast material is the most sensitive and specific test for coronary artery disease. Unlike the previously mentioned tests, this test is invasive and carries a small but finite risk. The overall risk of mortality during coronary arteriography is about 0.2%. Thus, cardiac catheterization is reserved for cases in which the diagnosis is uncertain after noninvasive testing or further information is needed to help determine whether medical or surgical therapy is most appropriate for the patient's coronary disease. If surgery is contemplated, the arteriograms obtained at catheterization guide the surgeon's placement of the bypass grafts.

(3) **Therapy** for angina pectoris is directed either at reducing myocardial oxygen demand to compensate for impaired flow through diseased coronary arteries or at increasing myocardial oxygen supply (i.e., blood flow).

(a) **Nitrates.** This class of drugs produces venodilatation and to a lesser extent arteriolar vasodilatation. These effects produce a decrease in blood pressure and a reduction in cardiac size, and both of these effects reduce myocardial oxygen demand. Direct coronary arterial vasodilation also may occur and may cause increased coronary blood flow, since even diseased portions of the coronary artery have been shown to dilate. Sublingual, oral, dermal, and intravenous nitrate preparations are available and are effective.

(b) **Beta-adrenergic blocking agents.** When the β-adrenergic receptor is stimulated, the result is an increase in heart rate and in the force of myocardial contraction. Both events increase myocardial oxygen demand. Beta-adrenergic blocking agents or β-blockers counteract these effects and act to limit myocardial oxygen demand. Recent evidence suggests that β-blockers also may diminish platelet activation, which could be important in stabilizing the coronary plaque and in preventing reduction in coronary blood flow. Currently, the three β-blockers approved for use in treating angina are propranolol, nadolol, and timolol. These drugs should be avoided in cases of severe left ventricular dysfunction as they may precipitate congestive heart failure, although their potential for doing so has been generally overestimated. In addition, β-blockers may precipitate bronchospasm in asthmatics and in patients with obstructive lung disease, and they may cause severe bradycardia in patients with sinoatrial (SA) node or atrioventricular (AV) node disease.

(c) **Calcium antagonists.** Calcium regulates the contraction of smooth muscle, which is present in the walls of the coronary and peripheral arteries. Calcium antagonists are particularly effective in preventing the coronary spasm that causes variant angina. They also are useful in treating cases of typical angina, in which they act as coronary and peripheral arterial vasodilators. Nifedipine, verapamil, and diltiazem are the calcium antagonists currently approved for the treatment of both typical and variant angina. Nifedipine may produce hypotension and constipation. Verapamil and, more rarely, diltiazem may precipitate congestive heart failure or severe bradycardia.

(d) **Coronary artery bypass surgery** remains a controversial treatment of angina. A discussion of the exact indications for surgery goes well beyond the scope of this text. In general, surgery offers a high incidence of symptomatic improvement (85%) at a 1%–2% operative risk and, thus, is indicated for patients whose life-styles are seriously compromised by angina despite medical therapy. Additionally, coronary bypass surgery increases longevity in most patients with severe disease of the main left coronary artery and some anatomic distributions of triple-vessel coronary disease (see section II A 6).

b. **Myocardial infarction** occurs when myocardial oxygen demand severely exceeds myocardial oxygen supply for a prolonged period of time. This usually is due to a severe reduction in coronary blood flow produced by coronary occlusion. The events leading to this sudden reduction are unclear. **Coronary thrombosis** recently has been implicated in most transmural myocardial infarctions, but the cause of this thrombosis is unknown. **Coronary spasm** with total occlusion of the vessel also may produce transmural myocardial infarction. The cause of nontransmural or **subendocardial** myocardial infarction remains unclear.

(1) Clinical features

  (a) Presenting symptoms. The patient usually presents with severe, oppressive chest pain or pressure that persists for more than 30 minutes and is unrelieved by nitroglycerin. The pain frequently is associated with nausea, vomiting, or both as well as diaphoresis and shortness of breath. Pain radiation is similar to that of angina pectoris. The pain usually occurs when the patient is at rest or involved in minimal activity. Although possible, it is unusual for myocardial infarction to be precipitated by vigorous activity such as shoveling snow. (Such activity, however, may precipitate sudden death without infarction.)

  (b) Findings on physical examination. The patient is in obvious pain, is quite apprehensive, and appears ill, frequently having an ashen coloring. If the infarction is extensive, hypotension and tachycardia may be present. There also may be signs of congestive heart failure (e.g., elevation of the neck veins, pulmonary rales, and a cardiac gallop rhythm). The new murmur of mitral regurgitation may be present.

(2) Diagnosis

  (a) Electrocardiography. The ECG is diagnostic in about 85% of cases; thus, 15% of patients may be having a myocardial infarction without clear-cut evidence on the ECG. In transmural myocardial infarction, an injury current usually is demonstrated by ST-segment elevation in those leads reflecting the area of the myocardial infarction. As the ST segments fall, Q waves appear and the T waves become inverted. In subendocardial infarction, the electrocardiographic diagnosis is less certain, and ST-segment depression may be the only finding.

  (b) Cardiac enzyme studies. As myocardial necrosis occurs, the myocardium releases **creatine kinase (CK)**, **serum glutamic oxaloacetic transaminase (SGOT)**, and **lactic acid dehydrogenase (LDH)**. Serum concentrations of these enzymes typically are elevated in patients having a myocardial infarction. CK elevation appears 6 hours after infarction, SGOT elevation appears 12 hours after infarction, and LDH elevation appears 24 hours after infarction. Although these enzymes may be elevated in other disease states, isoenzyme studies can determine with a high probability whether or not the enzymes are cardiac in origin. It is the **MB isoenzyme** (i.e., the CK isoenzyme found only in the myocardium) that is increased in myocardial infarction. The LDH_1 isoenzyme also is elevated so that it exceeds LDH_2.

  (c) Myocardial scanning. The damaged myocardium takes up a variety of agents more readily than does nondamaged myocardial tissue. The most common agent used in scanning is **technetium 99 (^{99}Tc)**. A focal area of uptake of ^{99}Tc in the myocardium confirms an infarction. Myocardial scanning may be helpful in cases in which the ECG and cardiac enzyme studies are equivocal.

(3) Complications. A myocardial infarction can occur with little clinical consequence; indeed, many are silent. The complications of myocardial infarction, however, produce clinically significant events.

  (a) Arrhythmias. A patient having an acute myocardial infarction is subject to acute, lethal ventricular arrhythmias (i.e., ventricular tachycardia or ventricular fibrillation), particularly within the first 24 hours after infarction. Lethal arrhythmias frequently occur without warning. Thus, while many patients have frequent, premature ventricular contractions as a harbinger of lethal ventricular arrhythmias, other patients have sudden arrhythmias without lesser, premonitory rhythm disturbances. Less serious atrial arrhythmias, such as atrial fibrillation and atrial flutter, also may occur. It is the detection of cardiac arrhythmias that has fostered the concept of the coronary care unit. With intensive monitoring of the patient with myocardial infarction, it is believed that severe cardiac arrhythmias can be detected and reversed before they lead to the patient's death.

  (b) Acute conduction system abnormalities. The specialized conducting system of the heart is the myocardium, which may become ischemic or infarcted during a myocardial infarction. This may lead to bradyarrhythmias, heart block, or both.

    (i) In **inferior-wall myocardial infarction**, it is the right coronary artery that usually is diseased. Since this artery supplies the SA node in 55% of patients and the AV node in 85% of patients, it is not surprising that **sinus bradycardia** and varying degrees of **AV node block** occur during inferior myocardial infarctions.

    (ii) On the other hand, **anterior myocardial infarction** usually involves the anterior descending coronary artery, which supplies the interventricular septum. Since the bundle branches course through the septum, acute **right** or **left bundle branch block** may occur during anterior myocardial infarctions. **Complete heart block** also may occur due to dysfunction of both bundle branches or the bundle of His.

(c) **Pump failure.** When 30% of the myocardium is infarcted from one or more myocardial infarctions, **congestive heart failure** is likely to ensue. If more than 40% of the myocardium becomes infarcted, **cardiogenic shock** is likely to develop. In true cardiogenic shock, there is not enough myocardium to generate enough cardiac output to sustain bodily function. One definition of cardiogenic shock is a systolic blood pressure of less than 90 mm Hg together with a urinary output of less than 20 ml/hr in the presence of adequate left ventricular filling pressure. When this complication occurs, the mortality rate is 75%.

(d) **Mitral regurgitation.** The mitral valve is tethered by the **papillary muscles**, which are myocardial projections. Dysfunction or infarction of the papillary muscles may lead to systolic prolapsing of the mitral valve into the left atrium, causing varying degrees of mitral regurgitation. If the mitral regurgitation is severe, the cardiac output is decreased profoundly since a large part of the left ventricular stroke volume is ejected backward. At the same time, there is a precipitous rise in the left ventricular filling pressure, which is transmitted to the lung, resulting in pulmonary edema.

(e) **Ventricular septal defect.** The left ventricular septum may become infarcted in either anterior or inferior myocardial infarction, leading to rupture of the septum in 2% of cases. Thus, a free communication between left and right ventricles or an acute ventricular septal defect is formed. This defect diverts a significant percentage of the ventricular stroke volume into the right ventricle, compromising forward cardiac output.

(f) **Cardiac rupture.** Myocardial infarction of the free wall may lead to eventual perforation of the heart. This complication nearly always is fatal as it results in overwhelming cardiac tamponade.

(g) **Left ventricular aneurysm.** The infarcted zone of the myocardium may evaginate and heal with fibrous connective tissue, forming a "fifth chamber" attached to the left ventricle. This chamber does not do work but rather saps a portion of the left ventricular stroke volume. Left ventricular aneurysms may produce cardiac failure and angina. They also may be the source of severe left ventricular arrhythmias and systemic emboli.

(4) **Therapy.** When a patient enters the hospital with a myocardial infarction, an intravenous cannula is placed percutaneously to provide access to medications. Intramuscular injections should be avoided because they may confuse interpretation of the cardiac enzymes. Oxygen is delivered via a nasal cannula.

(a) **Treatment of pain**

(i) **Nitroglycerin.** Since approximately 4% of all acute myocardial infarctions are thought to be due to **coronary spasm** as opposed to thrombotic occlusive disease, sublingual nitroglycerin should be administered in case the patient is suffering from coronary spasm. However, nitroglycerin should be administered only if the systolic blood pressure is greater than 100 mm Hg.

(ii) **Morphine sulfate.** If nitroglycerin is not effective, enough morphine sulfate should be given intravenously to relieve the patient's pain and anxiety.

(b) **Treatment of arrhythmias**

(i) **Prophylactic lidocaine.** Recent studies show that lidocaine given intravenously can reduce the number of episodes of serious ventricular arrhythmias during the early phases of myocardial infarction. Current electronic delivery devices allow safe administration of the drug and help prevent serious side effects. A loading dose is given, often followed by a second loading dose and then a constant intravenous infusion.

(ii) **Additional antiarrhythmic therapy.** If serious arrhythmias occur despite lidocaine infusion, additional drugs may be necessary to control the arrhythmias. Bretylium tosylate, procainamide, and phenytoin sodium all may be useful in controlling acute recalcitrant arrhythmias and can be given intravenously with caution.

(c) **Treatment of serious conduction disturbances.** As noted, high-degree AV node block may occur during acute myocardial infarction, producing significant bradycardia and hypotension. Atropine (1 mg given intravenously) may restore conduction and increase heart rate, especially in inferior infarctions. If this fails, an infusion of a positive chronotropic agent such as isoproterenol increases heart rate. These therapies are directed at maintaining heart rate until temporary transvenous pacemaking can be performed. Usually, ventricular pacing reestablishes heart rate and adequate blood pressure. In cases of severe left ventricular dysfunction, atrial systole must be preserved to maintain cardiac output, and AV sequential pacemaking is the preferred treatment. Although controversial, the occurrence of new bundle branch block—particularly the combination of right bundle branch block and left anterior hemiblock—is an indication for temporary prophylactic pacemaking since these disturbances may presage the occurrence of complete heart block.

   (d) Treatment of pump failure. Mild congestive heart failure in myocardial infarction can be treated with diuretics. The use of **digitalis** during acute myocardial infarction remains controversial. However, fears that digitalis may increase oxygen consumption and extend myocardial infarction do not appear justified if the patient is in congestive heart failure. In such cases, digitalis actually may reduce both cardiac size and myocardial oxygen consumption. In more advanced cases of congestive heart failure, vasodilators may be useful in reducing cardiac afterload, allowing increased cardiac output.

   (e) Treatment of shock. Shock in the presence of myocardial infarction usually is due to one of the following causes: inadequate left ventricular filling, severe muscle damage, or a mechanical complication of the myocardial infarction. When shock ensues, a **Swan-Ganz catheter** is placed to measure left ventricular filling pressure. If the pulmonary capillary wedge pressure is less than 18 mm Hg, volume is infused to maximize left ventricular filling and cardiac output. If a new cardiac murmur is detected, the Swan-Ganz catheter also is useful in making the diagnosis of acute mitral regurgitation or acute ventricular septal defect. Alternatively, if cardiogenic shock is due to severe muscle damage, pressor agents and **intra-aortic balloon pumping** may be used to stabilize the patient. However, the prognosis remains very poor despite therapy for such patients.

   (f) Treatment of mitral regurgitation and acute septal defect. The mainstay of medical therapy for these complications is arteriolar vasodilator therapy, which lowers systemic vascular resistance. This preferentially increases forward cardiac output and reduces nonproductive cardiac output either into the left atrium—in the case of mitral regurgitation—or through the ventricular septal defect. **Intra-aortic balloon pumping,** which accomplishes the same goal, also is useful in stabilizing patients with these complications. Subacute surgical correction of mechanical complications often is required.

(5) Reduction of myocardial infarction. In view of the limited usefulness of therapy in patients with pump failure, current efforts are being directed toward limiting the size of the myocardial infarction and preserving pump function. Under investigation are therapies that attempt either to increase myocardial oxygen supply or decrease demand. Intravenously administered **nitroglycerin** and **propranolol** are therapies that reduce myocardial oxygen demand. **Hyaluronidase** may stabilize the vascular bed and prevent reductions in blood flow due to microcirculatory abnormalities. The intracoronary and intravenous use of the thrombolytic agent **streptokinase** is under intense study. Strong evidence exists that streptokinase can acutely lyse a coronary thrombosis and reestablish coronary blood flow in the occluded artery. Early reports suggest that this therapy is useful in limiting the size of myocardial infarctions.

c. Sudden death in patients with coronary artery disease is common. Indeed, approximately one-third of patients with coronary disease have sudden death as the first manifestation, without antecedent angina or myocardial infarction. It is believed that most patients with sudden death die of acute ventricular arrhythmias precipitated by ischemia. Although sudden death may be the result of a myocardial infarction secondary to the coronary artery disease, most patients who die suddenly and are resuscitated do not have an acute myocardial infarction documented. It is believed that in these patients, ischemia produces heterogeneous depolarization of the ventricle, which leads to ventricular tachycardia and ventricular fibrillation.

(1) Acute therapy—cardiac resuscitation. Cardiopulmonary resuscitation must begin in the euthermic patient within 4 minutes after the cessation of effective ventricular contraction in order to preserve neurologic and myocardial function. Artificial respiration by mouth-to-mouth resuscitation and closed-chest compression are the cardinal facets of early resuscitation. Current evidence suggests that closed-chest cardiac massage does not produce cardiac output by external cardiac compression, as was previously thought. Rather, the valves in the systemic veins allow chest compression to produce a pressure gradient between the relatively low pressure in the extrathoracic veins and the relatively high pressure produced in the intrathoracic cavity by chest compression. This creates forward cardiac flow. Once the patient arrives at a medical care facility, electrical defibrillation and drug support of the myocardium are provided.

(2) Prevention—identifying high-risk patients. It is estimated that cardiac resuscitation of out-of-hospital cardiac arrest is fully successful in only 10%–20% of cases. The goal of therapy, then, is to prevent sudden death from occurring. Patients with the following conditions are recognized as being at high risk for an episode of sudden death.

    (a) Previous sudden death. Patients who have experienced one episode of sudden death and have been successfully resuscitated have a 30% chance of a second episode if the first episode occurred in the absence of a myocardial infarction. In such patients, intensive diagnostic work-up is indicated and should include invasive electrophysiologic testing and intensive antiarrhythmic therapy.

    (b) High-grade ventricular ectopy following myocardial infarction. Patients in whom electrocardiographic monitoring demonstrates high-grade ventricular ectopy (e.g., coupled ventricular extrasystoles, short runs of ventricular tachycardia, and R on T phenomenon) have approximately a four times greater risk for sudden death than patients without these abnormalities. This applies to patients in whom these abnormalities are found in the late period (i.e., 2 weeks or more) following the myocardial infarction but does not extend to severe ventricular arrhythmias during the acute phase. Many authorities believe that such patients should undergo intensive antiarrhythmic therapy, although conclusive evidence that this therapy prolongs life or prevents sudden death is not available.

    (c) Prolonged Q-T intervals. Patients with prolonged Q-T intervals are also at risk for sudden death. Prolonged Q-T syndromes can be congenital or acquired.

6. Prognosis. The prognosis of patients with coronary artery disease is primarily determined by two variables: the extent of coronary disease in terms of the **number of vessels affected** by the disease and the **extent of left ventricular damage** present due to previous myocardial infarctions.

    a. Patients with **main left coronary artery disease** have approximately a 20% mortality rate in the first year after its discovery.

    b. Patients with **single-vessel coronary artery disease** have approximately a 2% annual mortality rate, those with **double-vessel disease** have approximately a 3%–4% annual mortality rate, and those with **triple-vessel disease** have approximately a 5%–8% annual mortality rate.

    c. The presence of significant **left ventricular dysfunction** (as identified by an ejection fraction of less than 40%) approximately doubles the yearly mortality rate at each level of extent of coronary disease.

B. Nonatherosclerotic coronary artery disease. Although the majority of cardiac ischemic events are due to atherosclerotic coronary disease, nonatherosclerotic disease also may produce clinical ischemia.

1. Coronary embolism occurs in infective endocarditis, from mural thrombus formation following myocardial infarction, and in the presence of atrial fibrillation. When it occurs, coronary embolism frequently produces myocardial infarction.

2. Collagen vascular disease. The collagen vascular diseases that affect medium-sized arteries, including the coronary arteries, are: periarteritis nodosa, Wegener's granulomatosis, systemic lupus erythematosus and, occasionally, rheumatoid arthritis.

3. Radiation. Tumor irradiation, in which the field of radiation includes the heart, damages the coronary arteries and leads to nonatherosclerotic coronary disease.

III. VALVULAR HEART DISEASE

A. Aortic stenosis

1. Etiology

    a. Congenital aortic stenosis usually is detected in the pediatric age range, but occasionally patients present in early adulthood.

    b. Senile calcific aortic stenosis is a degenerative condition of the aortic valve, in which scarring and calcification of a tricuspid aortic valve lead to stenosis in the sixth, seventh, and eighth decades of life.

    c. Bicuspid aortic stenosis is a common congenital cardiac abnormality. The flow characteristics of the bicuspid valve are more turbulent than those of the normal valve, leading to valve degeneration, calcification, and stenosis in the fourth and fifth decades of life.

    d. Rheumatic aortic stenosis rarely occurs alone and almost always is associated with mitral valve disease.

2. Pathophysiology. Aortic valve stenosis produces a pressure overload on the left ventricle due

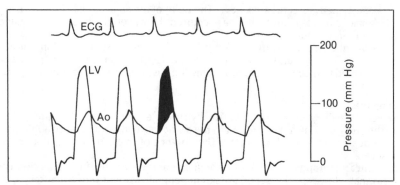

Figure 1-4. Diagram showing simultaneous recording of the electrocardiogram (*ECG*), left ventricular pressure tracing (*LV*), and aortic pressure tracing (*Ao*) in a patient with aortic stenosis. A large pressure gradient (*black area*) is evident. (Reprinted with permission from Grossman W: *Cardiac Catheterization and Angiography*, 2nd ed. Philadelphia, Lea and Febiger, 1980, p 128.)

to the greater pressure that must be generated to force blood past the stenotic valve. As shown in Figure 1-4, the systolic pressure inside the left ventricle is greater than in the aorta, producing a pressure gradient across the aortic valve. The pressure overload produced by the disease leads to the development of **concentric left ventricular hypertrophy**. Hypertrophy is a compensatory mechanism that reduces wall stress (afterload) on the left ventricle during systole. Wall stress can be expressed as:

$$\text{wall stress} = \frac{\text{pressure} \times \text{radius}}{2 \times \text{wall thickness}}.$$

Thus, increased thickness due to the development of concentric hypertrophy helps offset the increased pressure. This, in turn, reduces wall stress, which is the force each unit of myocardium must generate in order to shorten.

3. Clinical features
a. Symptoms
(1) Angina occurs frequently in patients with aortic stenosis. Fifty percent of untreated patients who develop this symptom die within 5 years after its onset. While the exact mechanism of angina is unknown, current data suggest that coronary blood flow reserve is impaired in the severely hypertrophied left ventricle. Impairment of the coronary blood flow reserve limits oxygen delivery to the myocardium and produces angina during exercise.

(2) Syncope occurs during exercise when total peripheral resistance falls due to local autoregulatory mechanisms. The mechanism for syncope is based on the following equation for blood pressure:

$$\text{blood pressure} = \text{cardiac output} \times \text{total peripheral resistance}.$$

In aortic stenosis, cardiac output across the stenotic aortic valve cannot increase during exercise. Since total peripheral resistance falls, blood pressure must also fall and syncope occurs. Other causes of syncope in aortic stenosis include atrial arrhythmias, ventricular arrhythmias, and heart block due to conduction system calcification. After syncope occurs in patients with aortic stenosis, expected survival is 2–3 years without valve replacement.

(3) Heart failure. Fifty percent of patients who develop heart failure die within 1 year after presentation if the stenosis is not corrected. Heart failure occurs because the afterload placed on the myocardium becomes excessive and because muscle dysfunction occurs when the myocardium is exposed to a prolonged, severe pressure overload.

b. Physical signs
(1) Delayed carotid upstroke. The carotid upstroke typically is delayed in its timing and reduced in volume. This finding is the most reliable physical sign in gauging the severity of the disease.

(2) Soft, single S_2. Since the aortic valve is stenotic, its motion is severely impaired. The reduction in motion of the valve causes the **aortic component (A_2)** of the S_2 to be absent. Thus, the only component of the S_2 that is heard is the **pulmonic component (P_2)**, which normally is soft.

(3) An S_4 usually is heard due to the reduction in left ventricular compliance, which occurs in left ventricular hypertrophy.

     (4) Sustained, forceful apex beat. The point of maximal cardiac impulse usually is not displaced unless heart failure has occurred. However, the impulse is sustained and forceful throughout systole.

     (5) Systolic ejection murmur. A harsh, late-peaking systolic ejection murmur is heard in the aortic area and is transmitted to the carotid arteries. The murmur also may be reflected to the mitral area, producing the false impression that mitral regurgitation also is present.

4. Diagnosis

    a. Electrocardiography. The ECG usually shows evidence of left ventricular hypertrophy.

    b. Fluoroscopy. Calcium is present in the aortic valve in most cases of aortic stenosis and can be demonstrated by fluoroscopy. The absence of calcium suggests that the stenosis is not severe.

    c. Echocardiography can rule out significant aortic stenosis if valve motion is shown to be normal. However, the echocardiogram generally cannot prove that severe aortic stenosis definitely is present.

    d. Cardiac catheterization. Precise diagnosis and evaluation of the severity of aortic stenosis currently requires cardiac catheterization, during which the pressure gradient across the valve is measured and the degree of stenosis is calculated.

5. Therapy. Medical therapy has no definitive role in the treatment of this disease. While digitalis, diuretics, and antiarrhythmic drugs may serve as palliative measures, curative therapy requires aortic valve replacement.

B. Mitral stenosis

1. Etiology. Almost all cases of mitral stenosis presenting in the adult population are secondary to rheumatic heart disease. Most cases of mitral stenosis occur in women.

2. Pathophysiology. Mitral valve stenosis impedes left ventricular filling. Increased left atrial pressure occurs as a pressure gradient develops across the mitral valve. Elevated left atrial pressure is referred to the lungs, where it produces pulmonary congestion. As the stenosis becomes more severe it may significantly reduce forward cardiac output. Since the right ventricle is responsible for filling the left ventricle, the burden of propelling blood across the stenotic mitral valve is borne by the right ventricle. The overload on the right ventricle may be increased further when secondary pulmonary vasoconstriction occurs. Thus, the right ventricle must generate enough force both to overcome the resistance offered by the stenotic valve and to propel blood through constricted pulmonary arteries. Pulmonary arterial pressure may increase to three to five times the normal level, eventually resulting in right ventricular failure.

3. Clinical features

    a. Symptoms

      (1) Left-sided failure. Dyspnea on exertion, orthopnea, and paroxysmal nocturnal dyspnea occur due to reduced left ventricular output and increased left atrial pressure. In mitral stenosis the symptoms of left ventricular failure usually are not due to left ventricular dysfunction but, rather, to the mitral stenosis itself.

      (2) Right-sided failure. When pulmonary hypertension occurs, the right ventricle may fail, producing edema, ascites, anorexia, and fatigue.

      (3) Hemoptysis. The high left atrial pressure produced in mitral stenosis may lead to rupture of anastomoses that occur between the bronchial and pulmonary systems, producing hemoptysis.

      (4) Systemic embolism. Stagnation of blood in the enlarged left atrium and left atrial appendage occurs in mitral stenosis, particularly if atrial fibrillation also is present. Under these circumstances, a thrombus may form in the left atrium and can become a source of systemic embolism.

      (5) Hoarseness may occur in mitral stenosis as the enlarged left atrium impinges upon the recurrent laryngeal nerve.

    b. Physical signs

      (1) Atrial fibrillation. An irregularly irregular cardiac rhythm indicative of atrial fibrillation frequently is present.

      (2) Carotid pulse. The carotid pulse is brisk in upstroke but diminished in volume due to reduced cardiac output.

      (3) Pulmonary rales. Bilateral pulmonary rales occur secondary to elevated left atrial and pulmonary venous pressures.

      (4) S_1 usually is increased in intensity since stenosis limits spontaneous diastolic mitral valve closure. Thus, the mitral valve remains open until ventricular systole closes it forcibly with a resultant increase in S_1 intensity. Late in the course of the disease, the valve may become so stenotic that it no longer opens or closes, reducing the intensity of S_1.

(5) The P_2 component of S_2 is increased in intensity if pulmonary hypertension has developed.

(6) An opening snap is heard following S_2 as the stenotic valve is forced open in diastole by high left atrial filling pressure. The higher the pressure, the sooner the mitral valve opens. Thus, a short S_2–opening snap interval indicates relatively high left atrial pressure and severe stenosis. An S_2–opening snap interval of greater than 0.10 second suggests relatively low left atrial pressure and mild mitral stenosis.

(7) Diastolic rumble. The murmur of mitral stenosis is a low-pitched apical rumble, which begins after the opening snap. If the patient is in sinus rhythm, atrial systole produces a presystolic accentuation of this murmur.

(8) Sternal lift. Enlargement of the right ventricle due to pulmonary hypertension produces a systolic lift of the sternum.

(9) Right ventricular failure. If right ventricular failure occurs, neck vein distension, edema, hepatic enlargement, and ascites all may be present.

4. Diagnosis

a. Electrocardiography. The ECG may show signs of left atrial enlargement and right ventricular hypertrophy.

b. Chest x-ray. Straightening of the left heart border and a double density along the right heart border, which is formed by the right and left atria, occur due to left atrial enlargement. Signs of pulmonary venous hypertension, including an increase in pulmonary vascular markings and **Kerley's line**, are likely to be present. When pulmonary hypertension leads to right ventricular enlargement, the lateral view shows a loss of the retrosternal airspace.

c. Echocardiography usually provides excellent images of the mitral valve. In mitral stenosis, the echocardiogram shows reduction in the excursion of the valve leaflets and thickening of the valve. Two-dimensional echocardiography can be used to visualize and measure the residual mitral valve orifice. Left atrial enlargement invariably is present.

d. Cardiac catheterization. Since the echocardiogram often can precisely and noninvasively quantify the severity of mitral stenosis, the need for cardiac catheterization in this disease has been challenged. In most centers, cardiac catheterization is still performed not only to confirm the severity of the mitral stenosis but also to measure the degree of pulmonary hypertension, to evaluate the aortic valve, and to perform coronary arteriography in the coronary disease–prone age-group.

5. Therapy

a. Medical therapy is reserved for patients with mild-to-moderate symptoms of left-sided failure.

(1) Diuretics are the mainstay of treatment. Diuretics are used to control pulmonary congestion and to limit dyspnea and orthopnea.

(2) Digitalis. Since left ventricular muscle function usually is normal in this disease, the use of digitalis has little rationale in patients in sinus rhythm. In patients in atrial fibrillation, however, digitalis is used to control ventricular rate.

(3) Anticoagulants. Patients with mitral stenosis and coexistent atrial fibrillation have a high incidence of systemic embolism. In such patients, anticoagulation (e.g., with warfarin) usually is indicated.

b. Surgical therapy is effective in relieving the symptoms of mitral stenosis and in prolonging life in symptomatic patients. Surgery should be performed prior to the development of pulmonary hypertension, which increases surgical risk. However, if pulmonary hypertension is present and surgery is successful, pulmonary hypertension usually regresses postoperatively.

(1) Mitral commissurotomy. In young patients without significant valvular calcification or mitral regurgitation, commissurotomy allows relief of the stenosis without valve replacement.

(2) Mitral valve replacement. If commissurotomy cannot be performed, valve replacement relieves the stenosis and the patient's symptoms.

C. Aortic regurgitation

1. Etiology

a. Hypertension. Long-standing hypertension may result in proximal aortic root dilatation with subsequent incompetence of the aortic valve.

b. Rheumatic heart disease. Aortic insufficiency usually is present to some degree in most cases of rheumatic heart disease. While mitral stenosis usually predominates, aortic insufficiency occasionally is the most severe lesion seen in this disease.

    c. Infective endocarditis. Infection of the aortic valve may lead to perforation or partial destruction of one or more aortic leaflets, producing aortic insufficiency.

    d. Marfan's syndrome may produce aortic insufficiency in two ways.

        (1) Proximal root dilatation. Extreme expansion of the proximal aortic root seen in this syndrome may produce aortic insufficiency.

        (2) Aortic root dissection. Advanced cystic medial necrosis present in Marfan's syndrome may lead to an intimal tear and dissection of the aorta. If the dissection involves the proximal aortic root, the supporting structures of the aortic valve are disrupted, and the valve is rendered incompetent.

    e. Aortic dissection. Any cause of aortic dissection may lead to aortic insufficiency.

    f. Syphilis may produce **aortitis**, which may extend to the aortic valve and produce aortic incompetence.

    g. Collagen vascular disease. Systemic lupus erythematosus and ankylosing spondylitis may produce aortic insufficiency.

2. Pathophysiology

    a. A portion of the left ventricular stroke volume ejected during systole regurgitates into the left ventricle during diastole. If no compensation occurs, left ventricular forward output decreases. However, chronic regurgitation of blood into the left ventricle is a stimulus to sarcomere replication in series, producing an increase in end-diastolic volume. Since

$$\text{stroke volume} = \text{end-diastolic volume} - \text{end-systolic volume,}$$

total stroke volume increases, helping to compensate for the volume that is regurgitated. The increase in total stroke volume leads to an increase in pulse pressure. The additional volume and pressure that the left ventricle must generate eventually lead to left ventricular dysfunction and failure.

    b. An additional pathophysiologic consequence of aortic insufficiency is a reduction in systemic diastolic blood pressure.

3. Clinical features

    a. Symptoms

        (1) Left ventricular failure. Dyspnea, orthopnea, and paroxysmal nocturnal dyspnea all may occur when left ventricular dysfunction occurs in chronic aortic insufficiency. In acute aortic insufficiency, normal muscle function may coexist with heart failure. In this circumstance, reduced forward output and elevated left ventricular filling pressure occur prior to compensatory left ventricular enlargement.

        (2) Syncope. Reduction in diastolic systemic arterial pressure produces a reduction in mean arterial pressure. If mean arterial pressure is reduced significantly, cerebral perfusion is compromised and syncope may occur.

        (3) Angina occurs less commonly in aortic insufficiency than in aortic stenosis and, in part, is due to reduced diastolic systemic pressure. Since most of coronary blood flow occurs in diastole, a reduction in diastolic pressure reduces coronary blood flow and produces angina.

    b. Physical signs

        (1) Left ventricular impulse. The point of maximal impulse is hyperdynamic and is displaced downward and to the left due to left ventricular enlargement.

        (2) Diastolic murmur. The murmur of aortic insufficiency is a high-pitched, diastolic blowing murmur heard along the left sternal border. Often the murmur is heard best when the patient is sitting up and leaning forward.

        (3) Austin Flint murmur. A low-pitched diastolic rumble similar to that heard in mitral stenosis may be present in patients with aortic insufficiency. The Austin Flint murmur usually indicates moderate-to-severe insufficiency. The murmur generally is believed to be caused by reverberation of the regurgitant flow against the mitral valve, although the exact mechanism is unclear.

        (4) Stroke volume is increased in chronic aortic insufficiency. Since

$$\text{pulse pressure} = \frac{\text{stroke volume}}{\text{aortic elasticity}},$$

pulse pressure also increases. The increased stroke volume and pulse pressure lead to many physical signs, some which are listed below. These signs may be absent in acute aortic insufficiency because compensatory increases in end-diastolic volume and stroke volume have not yet occurred.

        (a) Corrigan's pulse. The carotid pulse has a rapid rise and full upstroke with a rapid fall in diastole.

        (b) Hill's sign refers to a disproportionate (i.e., 20 mm Hg) increase of systolic blood pressure taken in the leg as compared to systolic blood pressure measured in the arm. Its presence suggests severe aortic insufficiency.

  (c) **Pistol-shot femoral pulses.** Auscultation over the femoral arteries reveals a pistol-shot pulse.

  (d) **Duroziez's sign.** A stethoscope is placed over the femoral artery with enough pressure to produce a systolic bruit. The concomitant occurrence of diastolic bruit constitutes Duroziez's sign.

  (e) **de Musset's sign** refers to a bobbing movement of the head caused by the increased stroke volume and pulse pressure.

  (f) **Quincke's pulse** is systolic blushing and diastolic blanching of the nail bed when gentle upward traction is placed on the nail.

  4. **Diagnosis**

   a. **Electrocardiography.** The ECG usually shows left ventricular hypertrophy.

   b. **Chest x-ray.** Unless the lesion is mild or acute, cardiac enlargement should be present. The absence of cardiac enlargement militates against the diagnosis of severe chronic aortic insufficiency. Also, the proximal aorta frequently is dilated.

   c. **Echocardiography.** An enlarged left ventricular cavity is the rule. Diastolic vibration of the mitral valve frequently is present and is produced by regurgitant flow striking the mitral valve.

   d. **Cardiac catheterization.** Aortography is performed during cardiac catheterization. Contrast material is injected into the aorta, and the amount that regurgitates into the left ventricle is analyzed qualitatively. The regurgitant volume also can be calculated.

  5. **Therapy.** If aortic insufficiency is severe, aortic valve replacement eventually is necessary. Timing of surgery is difficult, however, since the lesion may be tolerated for several years. Careful follow-up is required to detect early signs of decompensation. When such signs are noted, valve replacement is advisable. If surgery is not considered, therapy with digitalis, diuretics, and vasodilators may afford symptomatic relief.

D. Mitral regurgitation

  1. **Etiology**

   a. **Rheumatic heart disease.** Scarring and retraction of the mitral leaflets secondary to rheumatic involvement may lead to mitral regurgitation.

   b. **Ruptured chordae tendineae.** Spontaneous rupture of the chordae tendineae may occur in otherwise healthy individuals. Chordal rupture permits prolapse of a portion of a mitral valve leaflet into the left atrium, rendering the valve incompetent.

   c. **Coronary artery disease** may lead to ischemia or infarction of the papillary muscles to which the mitral valve is tethered, thereby producing mitral incompetence.

   d. **Infective endocarditis.** Infection of the mitral valve may lead to its destruction with subsequent regurgitation.

   e. **Mitral valve prolapse and click-murmur syndrome** are terms that describe a group of diseases in which the mitral valve or chordae are redundant, permitting systolic prolapse of the mitral valve into the left atrium with resultant mitral regurgitation. This syndrome usually is benign but in some cases may be associated with significant mitral regurgitation. Additional features include atypical chest pain and cardiac arrhythmias. A midsystolic click and a late systolic murmur typically are heard on physical examination.

  2. **Pathophysiology.** In mitral regurgitation, a portion of the left ventricular stroke volume is pumped backward into the left atrium instead of forward into the aorta, resulting in increased left atrial pressure and decreased forward cardiac output. Preload is increased by the volume overload, and afterload is decreased as the left ventricle empties a portion of its contents into the relatively (i.e., compared to the aorta) low-pressure left atrium. This augments ejection performance and helps to compensate for the regurgitation.

   a. Initially, compliance of the left atrium is low, and the regurgitant volume produces high left atrial pressure with resultant congestive symptoms. With time, the left atrial compliance and volume may increase, allowing accommodation of the regurgitant volume at more physiologic filling pressures.

   b. After a prolonged period of compensation, left ventricular muscle dysfunction eventually occurs, resulting in a fall in ejection performance from supranormal levels to normal or even subnormal levels.

  3. **Clinical features**

   a. **Symptoms** of mitral regurgitation include those of left ventricular failure (i.e., dyspnea, orthopnea, and paroxysmal nocturnal dyspnea). If mitral regurgitation is severe and chronic, pulmonary hypertension and symptoms of right-sided failure also may occur. Patients in atrial fibrillation may experience symptoms of systemic embolism.

b. **Physical signs**
   (1) **Left ventricular impulse.** The point of maximal impulse is hyperdynamic and displaced downward and to the left.
   (2) **Carotid upstroke.** The upstrokes are brisk but diminished in volume due to reduced stroke volume.
   (3) **Murmur.** The murmur of mitral regurgitation is a holosystolic apical murmur that radiates to the axilla and frequently is accompanied by a thrill.
   (4) **An S_3 usually is heard** in mitral regurgitation and may occur even in the absence of overt heart failure. The S_3 is caused by the rapid filling of the left ventricle by the large volume of blood accumulated in the left atrium during systole.

4. **Diagnosis**
   a. **Electrocardiography.** ECG shows signs of left ventricular hypertrophy and left atrial enlargement.
   b. **Chest x-ray** shows cardiac enlargement. Vascular congestion occurs when the regurgitation has led to heart failure.
   c. **Echocardiography.** In cases of a ruptured chorda or mitral valve prolapse, the mitral valve can be seen prolapsing into the left atrium during systole. In endocarditis, vegetations on the cardiac leaflets frequently are seen. Regardless of the cause of the mitral regurgitation, left atrial and left ventricular enlargement occurs if the condition is chronic.
   d. **Cardiac catheterization.** Right-heart catheterization yields a pulmonary capillary wedge tracing that usually displays a **large v wave**. This is due to systolic volume overload on the left atrium. Left ventriculography demonstrates systolic regurgitation of contrast material into the left atrium.

5. **Therapy**
   a. **Medical therapy.** The goal of medical therapy is to relieve symptoms by increasing forward cardiac output and reducing pulmonary venous hypertension.
      (1) **Digitalis** is not indicated in acute mitral regurgitation in which no inotropic deficit exists. If atrial fibrillation occurs, digitalis is useful in controlling heart rate. In chronic mitral regurgitation with muscle dysfunction, digitalis may be useful in increasing the inotropic state.
      (2) **Diuretics** are used to reduce central volume overload, which in turn reduces pulmonary venous hypertension and congestion.
      (3) **Vasodilators.** Arteriolar vasodilators are particularly useful in managing this disease. These agents reduce resistance to aortic outflow and, thereby, preferentially increase forward output and reduce the amount of regurgitation. Vasodilators also reduce left ventricular size, which helps to reestablish mitral competence.
      (4) **Anticoagulants.** Patients with mitral regurgitation and atrial fibrillation are at high risk for systemic embolism; thus, anticoagulants (e.g., warfarin) usually are indicated.
   b. **Surgery.** Mitral valve replacement or repair is indicated for chronic mitral regurgitation, even if symptoms are relatively mild. Valve replacement must be performed prior to the onset of significant muscle dysfunction. Muscle dysfunction is largely irreversible and limits the success of operative intervention.

E. **Tricuspid regurgitation**

1. **Etiology**
   a. **Infective endocarditis** is a common cause of tricuspid regurgitation in drug abusers who inject drugs under septic conditions.
   b. **Right ventricular failure.** Sustained pressure or volume overload on the right ventricle leads to right ventricular dilatation and improper alignment of the papillary muscle, which produces tricuspid regurgitation.
   c. **Rheumatic heart disease.** In rheumatic heart disease, tricuspid regurgitation may occur secondary to right ventricular pressure overload from left-sided valvular lesions. Tricuspid regurgitation also may occur due to primary rheumatic involvement of the tricuspid valve.
   d. **Right ventricular infarction.** Right coronary artery occlusion with subsequent right ventricular infarction may lead to papillary muscle dysfunction and ventricular dilatation, which in turn may produce tricuspid regurgitation.

2. **Pathophysiology.** During systole the dysfunctioning tricuspid valve allows blood to be pumped backward into the right atrium, leading to systemic venous congestion and venous hypertension.

3. **Clinical features**
   a. **Symptoms** of tricuspid regurgitation include those of right-sided failure (i.e., edema and ascites). In severe and acute cases, hepatic congestion may be extensive enough to pro-

duce right upper quadrant pain. Passive hepatic congestion also may lead to hepatocellular damage and jaundice.

  b. **Physical signs**
    (1) **Right ventricular lift.** The enlarged right ventricle may be palpated as a systolic lift of the sternum.
    (2) **Murmur.** A holosystolic murmur that increases with inspiration is heard along the left sternal border.
    (3) **Jugular venous pulsation.** A large v wave is seen in jugular veins during systole.
    (4) **Pulsatile liver.** Systolic expansion of the liver frequently is present.

4. **Diagnosis**
  a. **Electrocardiography** reveals signs of right ventricular and right atrial enlargement.
  b. **Chest x-ray.** Right ventricular enlargement is seen as an obliteration of the retrosternal airspace on the lateral view.
  c. **Echocardiography** demonstrates enlargement of the right atrium and right ventricle. An injection of saline into a systemic vein inevitably carries microbubbles of air with it. The microbubbles may be seen as **echo bright spots** that reverberate between the right ventricle and right atrium.

5. **Therapy.** Left-sided failure frequently is the cause of right-sided failure and tricuspid regurgitation. Effective treatment of left-sided failure produces a secondary reduction in the right ventricular pressure overload. This reduction may be adequate to decrease right ventricular size, thus restoring valvular competence. If tricuspid regurgitation is due to organic valvular disease, surgical repair or replacement of the tricuspid valve may be necessary.

IV. CARDIOMYOPATHIES

  A. **Congestive cardiomyopathy**

   1. **Definition.** Congestive cardiomyopathy is a diminution in the contractile function of the left, right, or both ventricles in the absence of external pressure overload, volume overload, and coronary artery disease. This loss of muscle function results in congestive heart failure.

   2. **Etiology.** The cause of most cases of congestive cardiomyopathy is unknown. Viral infection has been implicated in the pathogenesis of this disease, but proof of cause generally is lacking. In addition, the following conditions have been linked to cardiomyopathy.
     a. **Prolonged ethanol abuse** is the most common cause of cardiomyopathy.
     b. **Doxorubicin therapy.** Doxorubicin (Adriamycin) is a commonly used antitumor drug that has severe cardiac toxicity. High doses may result in an irreversible congestive cardiomyopathy.
     c. **Exposure to toxins** such as cobalt, mercury, and lead and high-dose catecholamines may lead to myocardial damage and congestive cardiomyopathy.
     d. **Endocrinopathies**, including thyrotoxicosis, hypothyroidism, and acromegaly have been reported to cause congestive cardiomyopathy. In thyrotoxicosis and in hypothyroidism, the myopathy usually is reversed when the endocrinopathy is corrected.
     e. **Metabolic disorders** such as hypophosphatemia, hypocalcemia, and thiamine deficiency may produce reversible cardiomyopathy.
     f. **Hemoglobinopathies** such as sickle cell anemia and thalassemia are associated with myocardial dysfunction.

   3. **Clinical features**
     a. **Symptoms** of cardiomyopathy are those of both left- and right-sided congestive heart failure as described in section I D 1. Generally, the symptoms of left-sided failure (i.e., orthopnea, paroxysmal nocturnal dyspnea, and dyspnea on exertion) precede those of right-sided failure. Chest pain may occur in the absence of obstructive coronary disease. The cause of the chest pain may be the excessive oxygen demands of an enlarged, thin-walled ventricle.
     b. **Physical signs** in cardiomyopathy are those of congestive heart failure. The murmur of mitral regurgitation also may be present. Mitral regurgitation occurs due to ventricular dilatation and the improper alignment of the papillary muscles.

   4. **Diagnosis**
     a. **Electrocardiography.** Left ventricular hypertrophy and nonspecific ST- and T-wave abnormalities frequently are seen. Left bundle branch block is common.
     b. **Chest x-ray.** The heart almost always is enlarged in congestive cardiomyopathy, and there is evidence of pulmonary vascular congestion.
     c. **Echocardiography** reveals dilated and poorly contracting left and right ventricles. In addition, secondary left and right atrial enlargement usually is seen.

    d. Gated blood pool scanning in congestive cardiomyopathy reveals a reduction of the ejection fraction of both ventricles. There usually is global dysfunction, but regional contractile abnormalities also may exist.

    e. Cardiac catheterization usually is not necessary to make the diagnosis of congestive cardiomyopathy. However, since surgical correction of aortic stenosis or ischemic heart disease could significantly improve left ventricular function, these diagnoses should be excluded prior to making the diagnosis of cardiomyopathy. In such cases, cardiac catheterization may be indicated to exclude or to confirm these diagnoses.

  5. Therapy

    a. Removal of an offending agent. The most hopeful situation is one in which a known toxin has caused ventricular dysfunction. In such cases, removal of the toxin (e.g., alcohol) from the patient's environment may lead to significant improvement in ventricular function.

    b. Supportive therapy. When congestive cardiomyopathy is idiopathic, the symptoms of congestive heart failure can be improved by such measures as salt restriction and administration of cardiac glycosides, diuretics, and vasodilators. However, there is no evidence that supportive therapy increases longevity.

    c. Cardiac transplantation. Immunologic rejection and the limited supply of cardiac donors have restricted cardiac transplantation as a form of therapy for congestive cardiomyopathy. In selected cases, however, cardiac transplantation may improve the quality of and prolong life.

B. Hypertrophic obstructive cardiomyopathy

  1. Definition. Hypertrophic obstructive cardiomyopathy, which also is called **idiopathic hypertrophic subaortic stenosis** and **asymmetric septal hypertrophy**, is a disorder in which the interventricular septum hypertrophies excessively. The hypertrophied septum together with the anterior leaflet of the mitral valve produce left ventricular outflow obstruction.

  2. Etiology. Most cases are inherited through an autosomal dominant mode of transmission, but sporadic cases also occur.

  3. Pathophysiology

    a. As shown in Figure 1-5, the hypertrophied septum encroaches upon the left ventricular outflow tract and comes into close approximation with the anterior leaf of the mitral valve. During systole a low-pressure zone may develop as blood flow accelerates through the narrowed area between the septum and the anterior leaflet, generating a **Bernoulli effect**. Thus, the anterior leaflet of the mitral valve is drawn into the septum (systolic anterior motion), leading to outflow obstruction. The septum itself shortens very little during systole because of its catenoid shape, and since it does not shorten it cannot thicken. Therefore, it is the anterior leaflet of the mitral valve that plays the active role in creating the obstruction.

    b. The degree of outflow obstruction varies from patient to patient and from time to time in the same patient. Physiologic conditions that enlarge the left ventricle (e.g., increases in preload and afterload) separate the septum and anterior leaflet of the mitral valve and reduce the obstruction. Physiologic conditions that make the ventricle smaller or that increase the velocity of blood flow (e.g., dehydration and positive inotropic drugs) increase the degree of obstruction. The obstruction to outflow may cause secondary cardiac hypertrophy of the nonseptal portions of the ventricle, but septal thickness generally remains greater than that of the free wall of the ventricle.

  4. Clinical features

    a. Symptoms

      (1) Angina. Patients with obstructive cardiomyopathy frequently complain of chest pain. The pain usually has atypical features; that is, the pain may occur at rest and is not always related to exercise. The pathophysiology of angina in hypertrophic obstructive cardiomyopathy is unclear, but coronary blood flow is subnormal, suggesting that ischemia could occur.

      (2) Syncope usually occurs after exercise in patients with obstructive cardiomyopathy. After exercise, afterload is reduced because of peripheral vasodilatation. Preload is reduced because of the decreased activity of the muscular pumps provided by the leg muscles, which return blood to the heart. The inotropic state remains elevated due to an increased catecholamine level after exercise. All three mechanisms reduce left ventricular size and, therefore, increase left ventricular obstruction to outflow. Increased obstruction to outflow decreases cardiac output, producing syncope. Arrhythmias, which are common in this disorder, also may precipitate syncope.

      (3) Congestive heart failure. Dyspnea on exertion, orthopnea, and paroxysmal nocturnal dyspnea occur in patients with obstructive cardiomyopathy. Systolic function usually is

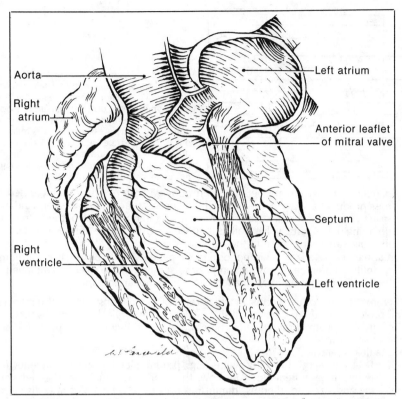

Figure 1-5. Cardiac cross section cut from the apex to the base in a patient with hypertrophic obstructive cardiomyopathy. The upper portion of the septum is thickened and comes into close proximity with the anterior leaflet of the mitral valve. (Adapted from Johnson R, et al: *The Practice of Cardiology*. Boston, Little, Brown, 1980, p 648.)

normal or supranormal with ejection fractions often in excess of 80%. The symptoms of heart failure usually are not due to systolic malfunction but rather to severe diastolic noncompliance. The thickened myocardium requires increased filling pressure for adequate diastolic distension. Increased filling pressure is reflected to the lungs and produces pulmonary congestive symptoms. In the later stages of the disease, however, systolic dysfunction also may occur, contributing to the symptoms of congestive heart failure.

  b. **Physical signs**
    (1) **Carotid upstroke.** In patients with the obstructive form of the disease, the carotid upstrokes have a **spike and dome configuration**, as seen in Figure 1-6. A spike and a dome occur due to early systolic outflow followed by a period of obstruction, during which outflow falls. The dome portion of the curve occurs during ventricular relaxation when obstruction diminishes and aortic outflow again commences at the end of systole.
    (2) **Murmur.** The murmur is a systolic ejection murmur, heard along the left sternal border. Unlike the murmur in valvular aortic stenosis, radiation into the neck is not the rule. Maneuvers that diminish left ventricular size (e.g., the Valsalva maneuver) cause an increase in both the obstruction to outflow and the intensity of the cardiac murmur. Thus, the Valsalva maneuver, which diminishes the murmur in valvular aortic stenosis due to diminished flow, increases the murmur in obstructive cardiomyopathy due to increased obstruction. Having the patient stand or inhale amyl nitrite also diminishes left ventricular size and, therefore, increases the intensity of the murmur. Squatting, which increases myocardial afterload and venous return to the heart, increases cardiac size and, therefore, diminishes the murmur.

 5. **Diagnosis**
    a. **Electrocardiography.** The ECG almost always is abnormal, usually showing evidence of left ventricular hypertrophy, nonspecific ST- and T-wave abnormalities, and left atrial enlargement.
    b. **Echocardiography** provides the diagnosis in patients who can be imaged adequately. In

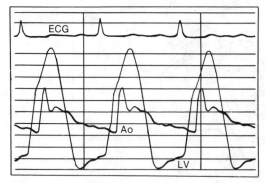

Figure 1-6. Diagram showing simultaneous recording of the electrocardiogram (*ECG*), left ventricular pressure tracing (*LV*), and aortic pressure tracing (*Ao*) in a patient with hypertrophic obstructive cardiomyopathy. A large pressure gradient exists between the left ventricle and aorta. The aortic pressure tracing (similar to the carotid pulse) demonstrates a spike and dome configuration. (Reprinted with permission from Cohn PF, Wynne J: *Diagnostic Methods in Clinical Cardiology.* Boston, Little, Brown, 1982, p 147.)

patients with asymmetric septal hypertrophy without obstruction, increased septal thickness produces a septum–to–free wall thickness ratio of 1.3 or greater. Findings in the obstructive form of the disease include systolic anterior motion of the mitral valve, systolic fluttering of the aortic valve leaflets, and early closure of the aortic valve, corresponding to the spike and dome seen in the carotid pulse.

    c. Cardiac catheterization is performed in patients with obstructive cardiomyopathy to quantify the degree of obstruction prior to surgery. It also may be employed in those patients who cannot be imaged adequately by echocardiography.

  6. Therapy. Unlike aortic stenosis, in which relief of valvular obstruction also relieves symptoms and prolongs life, there is no conclusive evidence that surgical relief of obstruction in obstructive cardiomyopathy prolongs life. Therefore, medical therapy is employed in an attempt to relieve symptoms.

    a. Medical therapy

      (1) Beta-adrenergic blocking agents (e.g., propranolol) are effective in relieving symptoms in this disease. Beta-blockade slows the heart rate, which increases left ventricular filling and size and, thereby, diminishes obstruction. Beta-blockade also diminishes the vigor of left ventricular contraction and, thus, diminishes the velocity of blood flow. This also reduces the degree of obstruction.

      (2) Calcium channel blocking agents. Although currently not approved for treatment of obstructive myopathy, calcium channel blockers have been shown to improve left ventricular compliance and to diminish the left ventricular outflow gradient. Verapamil is the calcium channel blocker most widely used in the treatment of this disease. Caution must be exercised in congestive heart failure patients as verapamil may worsen failure and precipitate acute pulmonary edema.

      (3) Digitalis is contraindicated in the hyperdynamic phase of the disease when obstruction is present and the left ventricular cavity is small, as digitalis increases the vigor of left ventricular contraction and, thus, increases the outflow obstruction. In the end stages of the disease when ventricular dilatation has occurred, standard therapy for congestive heart failure (i.e., digitalis and diuretics) may be beneficial.

    b. Surgical therapy

      (1) Myomectomy. Surgical reduction of the thickness of the left ventricular septum has been shown to be useful in relieving the outflow gradient and symptoms in those patients who have not responded to medical therapy.

      (2) Mitral valve replacement. Since it is the anterior leaflet of the mitral valve that produces the obstruction, mitral valve replacement is effective in relieving obstruction.

C. Restrictive cardiomyopathy

  1. Definition. Restrictive cardiomyopathy refers to a condition in which the composition of the myocardium has changed so that it becomes noncompliant. The noncompliance of the myocardium restricts left ventricular filling, reducing stroke output and increasing left ventricular filling pressure.

  2. Etiology. Infiltrative diseases of the myocardium, which produce restrictive cardiomyopathy, include amyloidosis, hemochromatosis, idiopathic eosinophilia, carcinoid syndrome, sarcoidosis, and endomyocardial fibroelastosis.

  3. Pathophysiology. Systolic function usually is normal in the early stages of the disease, but the altered properties of the myocardium produce severe diastolic noncompliance. Thus, left ventricular pressure is above normal at any diastolic left ventricular volume. Increased filling pressure produces pulmonary congestion. As the infiltrative process progresses, systolic function also is compromised.

4. Clinical features
- **a. Symptoms** of both left-sided and right-sided congestive heart failure usually are present, with the symptoms of right-sided failure usually more prominent.
- **b. Physical signs** include those present in left-sided and right-sided congestive heart failure.

5. Diagnosis
- **a. Electrocardiography.** The ECG frequently shows low QRS voltages and nonspecific ST- and T-wave abnormalities.
- **b. Chest x-ray.** Signs of pulmonary vascular congestion may coexist with a normal heart size because, even when left ventricular systolic function fails in the later stages of the disease, the restriction to cardiac filling reduces cardiac dilatation.
- **c. Echocardiography.** The echocardiogram demonstrates thickening of the left and right ventricles. Left and right ventricular chamber sizes usually are normal, while the left and right atria are increased in size. In amyloidosis, the myocardium may appear brighter than normal. The combination of increased left ventricular thickness with decreased left ventricular voltages on the ECG aids in making the diagnosis.
- **d. Cardiac catheterization.** Often it is difficult to distinguish restrictive cardiomyopathy from constrictive pericarditis at cardiac catheterization. A **dip and plateau** in the left and right ventricular filling pressures may be seen in both diseases. In restrictive cardiomyopathy, left and right atrial pressures and left and right ventricular filling pressures usually are not identical, as they are in constrictive pericarditis. Endomyocardial biopsy during cardiac catheterization may help to establish the diagnosis.

6. Therapy for this disease is limited.
In cases with a known specific etiology (e.g., hemochromatosis), direct therapy such as iron chelation may result in improvement. When the cause of the disease is unknown or cannot be treated, symptomatic therapy with diuretics to reduce the symptoms of congestion is indicated. Vasodilators must be used with caution since a reduction in preload causes a reduction in both left ventricular filling and cardiac output.

V. PERICARDIAL DISEASE

A. Acute pericarditis

1. Etiology
- **a. Myocardial infarction.** Pericarditis may occur in the first 24 hours following transmural myocardial infarction, as the inflamed surface of the infarcted area of myocardium produces pericardial irritation. A second type of pericarditis, called **Dressler's syndrome**, also may be seen from 1 week to several months after myocardial infarction and may occur due to an autoimmune reaction produced by the myocardial infarction.
- **b. Viral infection.** Many cases of acute pericarditis have no known etiology. However, because pericarditis frequently follows upper respiratory tract viral infections, a viral etiology has been implicated.
- **c. Collagen vascular disease.** Acute pericarditis may be a manifestation of rheumatoid arthritis, systemic lupus erythematosus, and scleroderma.
- **d. Infectious pericarditis.** Tuberculosis, streptococcal infection, staphylococcal infection, and the sequelae of infective endocarditis all may produce pericarditis.
- **e. Drugs.** Commonly used drugs that may produce acute pericarditis include procainamide, hydralazine, and isoniazid.
- **f. Malignancy.** Pericarditis may occur secondary to metastatic involvement of the pericardium. Pulmonary and breast carcinomas are the most frequently involved primary sites.
- **g. Uremia.** Pericarditis is common in severe chronic renal failure.

2. Clinical features
- **a. Symptoms.** The most common symptom in pericarditis is **inspiratory chest pain**. The pain is located in the left side and often is lessened when the patient sits up and leans forward. Occasionally, the pain may be similar to that of myocardial ischemia and may radiate to the neck and arm.
- **b. Physical signs.** The classic sign of acute pericarditis is the **pericardial friction rub**, which is a scratchy, leathery sound heard in both systole and diastole. Atrial contraction may add a third component to the rub.

3. Diagnosis
- **a. Physical examination.** The presence of a pericardial friction rub confirms the diagnosis of pericarditis.
- **b. Electrocardiography.** Epicardial inflammation occurs in pericarditis and produces a diffuse current of injury with ST-segment elevation throughout the ECG. There is no reciprocal ST-segment depression, as is seen in acute myocardial infarction.

    c. Echocardiography. The echocardiogram frequently demonstrates a pericardial effusion, which helps confirm the diagnosis.

  4. Therapy
    a. Specific therapy is directed toward the cause of the pericarditis. Thus, if procainamide use has produced the pericarditis, removal of the offending agent is appropriate.
    b. Nonsteroidal anti-inflammatory drugs such as aspirin, indomethacin, and ibuprofen usually are effective in reducing the inflammation and relieving the chest pain produced by the pericarditis.
    c. Steroid therapy. Intractable cases of pericarditis, such as may occur with Dressler's syndrome and postpericardiotomy syndrome, may require glucocorticoid therapy for relief of symptoms.

B. Pericardial effusion

  1. Pathophysiology. The inflammation caused by acute pericarditis often produces exudation of fluid into the pericardial space. When fluid accumulates slowly the pericardium expands to accommodate it. When fluid accumulates rapidly, however, it compresses the heart and, thus, inhibits cardiac filling. This latter condition is known as **cardiac tamponade** (see section V C).

  2. Clinical features
    a. Symptoms. The mere presence of a pericardial effusion does not cause symptoms. However, symptoms of acute pericarditis may coexist with a pericardial effusion.
    b. Physical signs. As the effusion accumulates it acts as a cushion around the heart. The precordium becomes quiet, palpation of the point of maximal impulse becomes difficult, and the heart tones become distant and soft. Although the accumulation of fluid between the layers of pericardium may diminish a pericardial friction rub, a friction rub still may exist in the presence of a large effusion.

  3. Diagnosis
    a. Electrocardiography. The ECG demonstrates low voltage, and electrical alternans often is present.
    b. Chest x-ray. Cardiac enlargement occurs as the effusion develops. Typically the cardiac silhouette has a "water bottle" appearance. The presence of an extremely enlarged heart without signs of vascular congestion suggests the diagnosis of pericardial effusion.
    c. Echocardiography. An echocardiogram demonstrating an echo-free space between the two layers of the pericardium is diagnostic of a pericardial effusion.
    d. Pericardiocentesis. The presence of a pericardial effusion is confirmed by the aspiration of fluid from the pericardial sac. Examination of the fluid helps to establish the cause of the effusion.
      (1) The fluid should be sent for cell count and differential, bacterial and fungal cultures, stains and cultures for *Mycobacterium tuberculosis*, protein content, and LDH content.
      (2) An additional aliquot of fluid should be centrifuged and examined for tumor cells.
      (3) If collagen vascular disease is suspected, fluid should also be sent for antinuclear antibody and LE preparation.
      (4) If the effusion is bloody, it may be difficult to determine if the effusion has been tapped or if the needle has passed too far and ventricular blood has been aspirated by mistake. It is possible to make a distinction, however, because ventricular blood clots whereas an effusion does not.
    e. Therapy for a pericardial effusion, with the exception of aspiration, is the same as that for acute pericarditis.

C. Cardiac tamponade

  1. Definition. Cardiac tamponade is a life-threatening condition in which a pericardial effusion has developed so rapidly or has become so large that it compresses the heart. The heart cannot fill adequately, and since the heart only can pump out what it takes in, impaired filling causes profound reduction in cardiac output. The external pressure produced by the fluid on the four chambers of the heart is dispersed equally. Since external pressure usually rises to a greater level than the normal cardiac filling pressures, intrapericardial pressure, left and right atrial pressures, and left and right ventricular pressures all become equal in diastole.

  2. Clinical features
    a. Symptoms. Most patients with cardiac tamponade complain of dyspnea, fatigue, and orthopnea.
    b. Physical signs
      (1) Pulsus paradoxus of more than 10 mm Hg occurs in 95% of patients with cardiac tam-

ponade. The presence of pulsus paradoxus implies that stroke volume is falling during inspiration due to the following mechanisms.

   (a) **Septal shift.** During inspiration right ventricular filling is augmented due to negative intrathoracic pressure, which increases venous return. This causes transient enlargement of the right ventricle and pushes the ventricular septum into the left ventricle, thus reducing the size and output of the left ventricle.

   (b) **Tensing of the pericardium.** Inspiration produces downward traction on the pericardium, further compressing the cardiac structures and reducing left ventricular output.

   (c) **Right ventricular enlargement.** The enhanced right ventricular filling during inspiration also distends the right ventricle, causing it to take up more room in the pericardial space. This further limits left ventricular filling.

   (d) **Negative intrathoracic pressure.** During inspiration the negative pressure inside the chest subtracts pressure from the extrathoracic vasculature, further reducing blood pressure.

   (e) **Expansion of the pulmonary vascular bed.** During inspiration the pulmonary vascular bed expands, increasing its capacity and, thus, reducing left atrial filling.

   (2) **Neck vein distension.** The intrapericardial pressure and right atrial pressure are reflected by extreme elevation of the jugular venous pressure. However, **Kussmaul's sign** (i.e., increased neck vein distension with inspiration) usually is absent in this condition.

   (3) **Pulse pressure.** Reduction in left ventricular stroke volume leads to a reduction in systolic pressure; the tachycardia that usually occurs as a compensatory mechanism diminishes diastolic runoff and maintains diastolic pressure. Thus, pulse pressure is narrowed. However, less severe cases of cardiac tamponade may coexist with a normal pulse pressure.

   (4) **Shock.** The carotid upstroke is diminished in volume, systolic blood pressure is reduced, and the periphery is cold and clammy due to the vasoconstriction present in reduced cardiac output states.

3. **Diagnosis.** Elevated neck veins and pulsus paradoxus in a patient with findings consistent with compromised cardiac output strongly suggest the diagnosis. A chest x-ray that shows an enlarged heart and an echocardiogram that confirms the presence of a pericardial effusion, together with the above clinical findings, make the presumptive diagnosis of cardiac tamponade. The diagnosis is strengthened further by catheterization that confirms that left and right atrial pressures are equal.

4. **Therapy.** The only effective therapy for cardiac tamponade is removal of fluid from the pericardial sac. Thus, emergency pericardiocentesis is indicated. The use of pressor agents and vasodilators together with volume expansion are of limited benefit until pericardiocentesis can be performed.

D. Constrictive pericarditis

1. **Definition.** Constrictive pericarditis is the diffuse thickening of the pericardium in reaction to prior inflammation, which results in reduced distensibility of the cardiac chambers. Cardiac output is limited, and filling pressures are increased to match the external constrictive force placed on the heart by the pericardium.

2. **Etiology.** Nearly all conditions that cause acute pericarditis may lead to chronic constrictive pericarditis.

3. **Clinical features**
   a. **Symptoms.** Most patients with constrictive pericarditis complain of dyspnea on exertion due to limited cardiac output. While orthopnea occurs in about 50% of cases, paroxysmal nocturnal dyspnea is rare. Symptoms related to systemic venous hypertension frequently are reported and include ascites, edema, and jaundice. Thus, the clinical picture typically is dominated by symptoms of right-sided failure rather than left-sided failure.
   b. **Physical signs**
      (1) **Jugular venous distension.** The jugular veins are distended, indicating systemic venous hypertension. Neck vein distension increases with inspiration (**Kussmaul's sign**).
      (2) **Carotid pulse.** The carotid upstroke is normal, but the volume may be decreased due to decreased stroke volume.
      (3) **Heart sounds.** The heart sounds are distant. Early in diastole a pericardial knock may be heard, which falls in the same cadence as an S_3 but is higher pitched.
      (4) **Other signs of systemic venous hypertension** frequently present include ascites, edema, hepatic tenderness, and hepatomegaly.

4. Diagnosis
a. **Electrocardiography.** The ECG shows low voltage in the limb leads. Atrial arrhythmias are common.

b. **Chest x-ray** reveals pericardial calcification in 50% of patients. This finding is seen as a radiopaque ring around the heart in the lateral view. The heart usually is normal in size, although cardiomegaly occasionally is noted.

c. **Echocardiography.** Although pericardial thickening often can be detected, reliable diagnosis of constrictive pericarditis by echocardiography is difficult.

d. **Cardiac catheterization** reveals equal pressures in the four cardiac chambers during diastole; in addition, all pressures usually are elevated. A marked **Y descent** is present in the right atrial pressure tracing. Left and right ventricular pressure tracings demonstrate a characteristic **dip and plateau** or **square root sign**.

5. Therapy.
Surgical removal of the pericardium is curative. However, immediate relief of constrictive symptoms may not occur for up to 6 weeks after pericardiectomy.

VI. CONGENITAL HEART DISEASE IN THE ADULT

A. Atrial septal defect

1. **Pathophysiology.** In atrial septal defect, left and right atrial pressures usually are equal; thus, no pressure gradient exists between the atria. However, the increased thickness of the left ventricle as compared to the right ventricle makes the left ventricle less compliant and, therefore, harder to fill. Blood flow takes the path of least resistance and, thus, is shunted from the left atrium to the right atrium. The net effect is to increase the volume work of the right ventricle. The increased volume pumped through the pulmonary vasculature may lead to architectural changes in the pulmonary vasculature and to the development of irreversible pulmonary hypertension—a serious but rare complication.

2. **Classification**
a. An **ostium secundum atrial septal defect** occurs in the midportion of the intra-atrial septum and is due to failure of the septum secundum to form properly.

b. An **ostium primum atrial septal defect** results from improper septation by the endocardial cushion portion of the septum. It invariably involves the mitral valve, which is cleft and often regurgitant.

c. A **sinus venosus–type atrial septal defect** frequently is associated with anomalous drainage of one or more of the pulmonary veins into the right atrium.

d. **Holt-Oram syndrome** is characterized by the presence of a secundum defect together with bony abnormalities of the forearms and hands. Holt-Oram syndrome is a hereditary disease that is transmitted as an autosomal dominant trait.

3. **Clinical features**
a. **Symptoms.** Patients with atrial septal defect may have a prolonged symptom-free period. Eventually, symptoms develop and may include palpitations due to atrial arrhythmias, fatigue, dyspnea on exertion, orthopnea, frequent respiratory tract infections, and symptoms of right ventricular failure.

b. **Physical signs**
(1) **S_2.** The increased cardiac flow through the right ventricle delays pulmonic valve closure, widening the normal splitting of the S_2. Inspiration produces relatively little change in right-sided flow, so there is little respiratory variation in the splitting of the S_2. Thus, the classic finding in atrial septal defect is a widely split and fixed S_2.

(2) **Murmur.** Under low pressure, blood flow from the left to the right atrium occurs through a wide aperture and produces no turbulence or murmur. However, the increased pulmonary blood flow in atrial septal defect produces a systolic ejection murmur, which is heard in the pulmonic area. The increased flow also may produce a diastolic rumble across the tricuspid valve if the left-to-right shunt ratio is greater than 3:1.

(3) **Right ventricular failure**, if it occurs, is followed by neck vein distension, ascites, and edema.

4. **Diagnosis**
a. **Electrocardiography.** In ostium secundum defects, incomplete right bundle block and right axis deviation are common findings. Ostium primum defects usually involve the anterior fascicle of the left bundle, producing left anterior hemiblock and left axis deviation.

b. **Chest x-ray.** Increased pulmonary blood flow produces increased pulmonary vascular markings in the lungs, called **shunt vascularity**. Right ventricular enlargement may encroach on the retrosternal airspace, reducing it in the lateral view. Enlargement of the pulmonary artery segment in the posteroanterior view also may be seen.

   c. Echocardiography. The echocardiogram shows enlargement of the right ventricle. The atrial septal defect itself may be seen in some cases. A saline injection, which carries with it microbubbles of air, shows a negative-contrast image at the site of the defect.

   d. Radionuclide studies. Quantification of first-pass radionuclide activity demonstrates recirculation of blood in the pulmonary circuit.

   e. Cardiac catheterization. During cardiac catheterization, the diagnosis can be confirmed by passage of the catheter across the atrial septal defect. Left and right atrial pressures usually are equal. Oxygen samples drawn from the superior vena cava and right atrium demonstrate a **step-up in oxygen concentration** in the right atrium, as highly oxygenated left atrial blood is shunted into the right atrium. Oxygen saturations can be used to quantitate the magnitude of the left-to-right shunt.

5. Therapy. Surgical correction is indicated for shunts with a pulmonary-to-systemic flow ratio of greater than 2:1 since shunts of this magnitude may lead to the development of pulmonary hypertension, usually become symptomatic, and worsen with age. Closure of the atrial septal defect, which has a low operative mortality rate, is indicated prior to the development of such complications.

B. Ventricular septal defect

1. Pathophysiology. In ventricular septal defect, blood is shunted from the left to the right ventricle, producing an increase in pulmonary blood flow. Unlike atrial septal defect, in which shunting of blood is passive, in ventricular septal defect, the left ventricle propels the blood from the left to the right ventricle. Thus, pulmonary hypertension is more severe and more frequent in ventricular septal defect than in atrial septal defect. Since most ventricular septal defects lead to symptoms and are corrected in childhood, significant congenital ventricular septal defect rarely is diagnosed for the first time in adulthood. In ventricular septal defect, both the left and right ventricles pump the increased volume and, thus, are volume overloaded. This is in contrast to atrial septal defect, in which only the right ventricle is volume overloaded.

2. Clinical features
   a. Symptoms of ventricular septal defect are those of both left- and right-sided congestive heart failure.
   b. Physical signs
      (1) Murmur. A harsh, holosystolic murmur is heard along the left sternal border. The murmur often is accompanied by a thrill and radiates to the right of the sternum.
      (2) Aortic regurgitation. Ventricular septal defects may involve the right coronary cusp of the aortic valve, producing insufficient support for this valve leaflet and, hence, aortic regurgitation. About 6% of patients with ventricular septal defect have signs of aortic insufficiency.

3. Diagnosis
   a. Electrocardiography. The ECG typically shows biventricular hypertrophy.
   b. Chest x-ray. Cardiac enlargement is the rule. If the shunt is greater than 2:1 in magnitude, **shunt vascularity** usually is present.
   c. Echocardiography. The septal defect frequently can be demonstrated during two-dimensional echocardiography. Left and right ventricular enlargement also is seen.
   d. Radionuclide studies. As with atrial septal defect, first-pass radionuclide studies can be used to detect and quantify the left-to-right shunt.
   e. Cardiac catheterization. During cardiac catheterization an oxygen step-up occurs at the level of the right ventricle, and pulmonary hypertension, if present, can be quantified. A left ventriculogram obtained in the left anterior oblique position demonstrates flow of contrast from the left ventricle across the septum into the right ventricle.

4. Therapy. Because of the propensity for patients to develop pulmonary vascular complications and bacterial endocarditis, ventricular septal defects with a magnitude of 2:1 or greater should be corrected surgically.

C. Patent ductus arteriosus

1. Pathophysiology. In patent ductus arteriosus, blood flows from the aorta into the pulmonary artery after the takeoff of the left subclavian artery. Volume overload is imposed on the left ventricle, which must pump blood into both the systemic and pulmonary circulations, and in time may lead to left ventricular failure. The increased pulmonary blood flow created by this lesion may lead to the development of pulmonary hypertension, imposing a pressure overload on the right ventricle.

2. **Physical signs**
   a. **Murmur.** Throughout the cardiac cycle, the vascular resistance and pressure in the pulmonary circuit are lower than pressures in the aorta. Therefore, blood is shunted from left to right in both systole and diastole, and a **continuous murmur** with systolic and diastolic components is heard.
   b. **Pulses.** The presence of a low-pressure, low-resistance pathway allows for increased aortic runoff in diastole, which produces bounding, full pulses similar to those found in aortic insufficiency.

3. **Diagnosis**
   a. **Chest x-ray** shows an enlarged cardiac silhouette with the presence of shunt vascularity. In adults, the patent ductus may become calcified and be visible on chest x-ray.
   b. **Cardiac catheterization.** During cardiac catheterization the catheter usually can be passed from the pulmonary artery into the descending aorta, confirming the presence of a patent ductus arteriosus. The magnitude of the left-to-right shunt can be quantified by oximetry. Aortography demonstrates the flow of contrast from the aorta through the patent ductus into the pulmonary artery.

4. **Therapy.** Surgical closure of the patent ductus is indicated in adults with a shunt ratio of greater than 2:1.

D. **Coarctation of the aorta**

1. **Pathophysiology.** Coarctation of the aorta is a stenosis of the aorta, usually at the site of the ductus arteriosus. If severe, the stenosis limits aortic blood flow distal to the constriction. Tissues distal to the coarctation are perfused by an extensive collateral arterial circulation. If the coarctation does not cause heart failure due to pressure overload in childhood, it may not be detected until it presents as hypertension in the adult. While renal blood flow and renal function usually are normal in the adult with coarctation of the aorta, the kidneys still are perfused at a subnormal blood pressure. Some investigators have found elevated renin levels and activation of the renin-angiotensin system in adults with coarctation, which helps to explain the hypertension.

2. **Clinical features**
   a. **Symptoms.** Patients with coarctation may complain of headache, claudication, and leg fatigue.
   b. **Physical signs**
      (1) **Blood pressure** determined in the arms usually is elevated, whereas pulses in the legs usually are reduced or absent, representing the gradient across the coarctation.
      (2) **Habitus.** The upper body usually is well developed, while the legs appear underdeveloped.
      (3) **Murmur.** Typically a midsystolic murmur is heard over the back. If the stenosis is severe, a continuous murmur may be heard. Continuous murmurs also may be heard diffusely over the chest cavity due to increased flow through collateral vessels.

3. **Diagnosis**
   a. **Electrocardiography.** The ECG shows left ventricular hypertrophy.
   b. **Chest x-ray.** Cardiac enlargement usually is seen. Dilatation of the aorta proximal and distal to the coarctation with indentation at the site of the coarctation may cause the aorta to assume a **figure 3 appearance**. Dilatation of chest wall arteries forming the collateral pathways produces rib notching.
   c. **Cardiac catheterization.** During cardiac catheterization the gradient across the coarctation can be measured. Aortography also allows visual demonstration of the coarctation.

4. **Therapy.** Surgical correction of the coarctation is the only effective therapy.

5. **Complications.** Hypertension, infective endocarditis, dissection of the thoracic aorta, and rupture of cerebral (berry) aneurysms frequently are seen in patients with coarctation of the aorta. Hypertension may persist even after the coarctation is repaired.

E. **Ebstein's anomaly of the tricuspid valve**

1. **Pathophysiology.** In Ebstein's anomaly, the tricuspid valve is situated abnormally low in the right ventricle. Part of the tricuspid valve is tethered directly to the right ventricle. Thus, a portion of the right ventricle actually lies above the AV groove and is "atrialized," reducing the size of the right ventricle and usually resulting in tricuspid regurgitation. A coexistent atrial septal defect occurs in about 75% of cases.

2. **Clinical features**
   a. **Symptoms.** Depending on the degree of tricuspid regurgitation and whether an atrial sep-

tal defect exists, a patient's status may range from asymptomatic to cyanotic. Dyspnea on exertion, peripheral edema, and other symptoms of right ventricular failure frequently are encountered; palpitations also are common in this anomaly, which is associated with **Wolff-Parkinson-White syndrome** in about 10% of cases.

- **b. Physical signs**
  - **(1) Tricuspid regurgitation.** A **large v wave** in the neck veins and a pulsatile liver reflect tricuspid regurgitation.
  - **(2) Cardiac sounds.** Wide splitting of the S_1 and S_2 is heard. Since an S_3 and an S_4 often exist also, a quadruple or quintuple cadence is a common auscultatory finding.
  - **(3) Murmur.** The holosystolic murmur of tricuspid regurgitation is heard along the sternal border and may be accompanied by a systolic thrill.

- **3. Diagnosis**
  - **a. Electrocardiography.** The ECG may show evidence of Wolff-Parkinson-White syndrome. Other findings include **giant P waves** and right bundle branch block.
  - **b. Echocardiography.** The echocardiogram in Ebstein's anomaly shows delayed closure of the tricuspid valve in relation to the mitral valve. The inferior and leftward displacement of the tricuspid valve usually can be demonstrated.
  - **c. Cardiac catheterization.** At cardiac catheterization, the simultaneous demonstration of a right atrial pressure tracing with a right ventricular electrogram in the "atrialized" portion of the right ventricle is pathognomonic.

- **4. Therapy.** Tricuspid valve replacement and closure of the atrial septal defect may be useful in patients who have developed early signs of right ventricular failure.

F. Eisenmenger's syndrome

- **1. Pathophysiology.** In Eisenmenger's syndrome, which can occur with any intracardiac shunt, the left-to-right shunt is reversed to produce a right-to-left shunt. This occurs due to the development of pulmonary vascular disease and increased pulmonary vascular resistance. These changes in turn lead to decreased right-sided compliance and increased right-sided pressures, which produce right-to-left shunting. Right-to-left shunting results in cyanosis.

- **2. Clinical features**
  - **a. Cyanosis** may be constant or noted only during exercise. Differential cyanosis may occur in the presence of a patent ductus arteriosus, with preductal tissues (including the upper trunk) being pink and postductal tissues becoming cyanotic.
  - **b. Angina.** Patients with Eisenmenger's syndrome may suffer from exertional chest pain, which occurs even in the presence of normal coronary arteries. Reduced myocardial oxygenation and increased right ventricular wall stress may be factors leading to angina in this condition.
  - **c. Heart failure.** Dyspnea on exertion, ascites, and peripheral edema are common.

- **3. Diagnosis**
  - **a. Electrocardiography.** Right ventricular hypertrophy invariably is present.
  - **b. Echocardiography.** Saline injection demonstrates right-to-left shunting of microcavitations in the presence of either an atrial or a ventricular septal defect.
  - **c. Hemogram.** Patients with Eisenmenger's syndrome are polycythemic. Hemoglobin levels in excess of 20 g/dl are common.
  - **d. Cardiac catheterization.** Right-sided pressures are extremely elevated. Oximetry is used to quantitate the right-to-left shunt. Administration of 100% oxygen via a rebreathing mask does not significantly correct the arterial desaturation.

- **4. Therapy.** Surgical therapy generally is not successful. Closure of the shunt site, which acts as an escape valve for the right ventricle, increases right ventricular pressures and causes worsening of right ventricular failure. Phlebotomy may be necessary to maintain the hemoglobin level at less than 20 g/dl to avoid hyperviscosity.

VII. VENOUS THROMBOSIS AND PULMONARY EMBOLISM

A. Deep venous thrombosis

- **1. Definition.** Deep venous thrombosis occurs when a blood clot forms in the lower extremities or in the pelvic veins. The exact initiating events are unknown.

- **2. Predisposing factors**
  - **a. Immobilization.** The muscles in the legs act as pumps to maintain venous return from the lower extremities. Inactivity of these muscles leads to venous stasis, with subsequent de-

velopment of thrombophlebitis. Stasis is likely to occur during surgery, prolonged bed rest, and prolonged periods in one position.

b. Venous incompetence. Venous valvular incompetence and the presence of varicose veins increases the incidence of thrombophlebitis.

c. Congestive heart failure. In congestive heart failure, cardiac output is reduced as is venous return from the legs.

d. Injury. Direct mechanical injury to the lower extremities may lead to blood clot formation and the development of thrombophlebitis.

e. Hypercoagulable states. Malignancy, estrogen use, and hyperviscosity syndrome may produce a hypercoagulable state, increasing the risk of thrombophlebitis.

3. Clinical features

a. Symptoms. The patient usually presents with unilateral leg pain and swelling.

b. Physical signs. In general, the physical examination for deep venous thrombosis is unreliable. Tenderness upon compression of the calf muscles, dorsiflexion of the foot (**Homans' sign**), and an increase in the circumference of the affected leg by at least 1 cm suggest the presence of deep venous thrombosis.

4. Diagnosis

a. Noninvasive studies. Impedance plethysmography, Doppler ultrasonography, and nuclear scanning with ^{125}I-tagged fibrinogen are useful tests for the detection of deep venous thrombosis.

b. Invasive studies. Contrast venography currently is the most effective way to demonstrate the area of blood clot. This technique is associated with complications such as an adverse reaction to the contrast agent and post-venography thrombophlebitis.

5. Therapy

a. Anticoagulants. Anticoagulation with intravenous heparin is indicated in the treatment of deep venous thrombosis. Anticoagulation prevents further clot formation and allows the body's autolytic system to be effective in lysing and healing deep venous thrombosis. After adequate treatment with heparin, oral anticoagulation with warfarin is begun. Anticoagulation therapy usually is maintained for 3 to 6 months.

b. Thrombolytic agents. Streptokinase and urokinase activate the conversion of plasminogen to the autolytic agent, **plasmin**. Whereas heparin can only prevent new clot formation, streptokinase and urokinase lyse an already formed clot. Thrombolytic agents result in more rapid resolution of the thrombus with improved late competency of venous valves. This helps to prevent future venous stasis. However, bleeding complications with thrombolytic agents tend to be more severe than with anticoagulants. Currently there is no consensus on whether anticoagulation or thrombolysis is the preferred therapy for deep venous thrombosis.

6. Prophylaxis. There is substantial medical evidence that the incidence of deep venous thrombosis can be reduced by the following methods.

a. Rapid mobilization. Prolonged bed rest should be avoided when possible. The increasingly rapid mobilization of patients following myocardial infarction has significantly reduced the incidence of thromboembolic complications following this disease.

b. Thromboembolic stockings compress the superficial veins, thereby increasing deep venous flow and reducing stasis and the incidence of thromboembolism. Foot exercises and avoidance of leg crossing are further methods of preventing deep venous thrombosis.

c. Minidose heparin. Intermittent doses of subcutaneous heparin given at 8- to 12-hour intervals inhibit factors X and XI in the clotting cascade without producing overt anticoagulation. This treatment significantly reduces the incidence of deep venous thrombosis in patients put to bed rest.

B. Superficial thrombophlebitis. Unlike deep venous thrombosis, in which a thrombus may break off and become a pulmonary embolism, superficial thrombophlebitis has little potential for embolic complications. Patients with superficial thrombophlebitis may present with a painful tender cord that can be easily palpated in the lower extremities. In the absence of concomitant deep venous thrombosis, anticoagulation is not indicated. Superficial thrombophlebitis is treated with elevation of the legs, heat, and administration of salicylate.

C. Pulmonary embolism

1. Definition. Pulmonary embolism occurs when a thrombus, usually arising from deep venous thrombosis in the lower extremities or in the pelvic veins, breaks off, travels through the right-sided circulation, and becomes lodged in a pulmonary artery.

2. Pathophysiology

a. Effect on oxygen exchange. The obstruction itself causes areas of the lung to be ventilated but not perfused, which is not deleterious. However, intrapulmonary reflexes and the release of humoral substances, including histamine, lead to heterogeneous areas of bronchial and arterial constriction, which cause ventilation-perfusion mismatches throughout the lungs. Ventilation-perfusion mismatches cause parts of the lungs to be perfused but not well ventilated, thus producing venous admixture and hypoxemia.

b. Direct obstructive effect. The obstruction of the pulmonary arteries by the embolus increases resistance to blood flow through the pulmonary circuit and increases right ventricular afterload. However, the direct obstructive effect usually is not significant unless 75% of the pulmonary vasculature has been occluded by the embolus. Thus, in experimental animals, even if the right or left main pulmonary artery is tied off, there is little change in right ventricular pressure.

c. Indirect obstructive effects. As noted above, pulmonary embolism may cause local vasoconstriction in parts of the lungs not affected by the embolus directly. This vasoconstrictive effect increases pulmonary vascular resistance and the work of the right ventricle.

d. Pulmonary infarction. By compromising pulmonary blood flow to a segment of the lung, a pulmonary embolus may cause pulmonary infarction. However, since the lungs also have a systemic arterial blood supply via the bronchial circulation, tissue viability may be preserved. In general, patients who have significant antecedent left ventricular dysfunction also have poor bronchial circulation and are more likely to suffer a pulmonary infarction during pulmonary embolism than patients with normal left ventricular function.

3. Clinical features

a. Symptoms

(1) Dyspnea. Nearly all patients with pulmonary embolism complain of dyspnea, which usually is acute in onset and occurs at rest. Dyspnea is due to the hypoxia created by the pulmonary embolus. In some cases, frequent small emboli may produce a more insidious onset of dyspnea, which presents initially on exertion. This syndrome can easily be mistaken for congestive heart failure.

(2) Chest pain. Patients with pulmonary embolism may suffer severe, oppressive chest pain similar to that of myocardial infarction. However, the pain usually does not radiate and is less frequently associated with epiphenomena such as nausea and diaphoresis. Patients with pulmonary embolism also are likely to complain of pleuritic pain, particularly if a pulmonary infarction has occurred.

(3) Hemoptysis is common when pulmonary infarction has occurred.

(4) Syncope may occur in patients with pulmonary embolism as cardiac output falls due to impedance of blood flow across the pulmonary bed.

b. Physical signs

(1) Respiratory rate is greater than 20 breaths/min in 90% of patients with pulmonary embolism.

(2) Pulse rate. Tachycardia is common in pulmonary embolism.

(3) Fever. Many patients with pulmonary embolism have a low-grade fever with temperatures usually not exceeding 37.5° C.

(4) Physical examination of the chest reveals signs of pleural effusion if pulmonary infarction has occurred. Diffuse wheezing due to bronchoconstriction is caused by the release of humoral agents. If pleuritic pain is present, splinting may occur in the affected side.

(5) Physical examination may show the cardiovascular system to be within normal limits in cases in which little obstruction to pulmonary blood flow has occurred. If moderate obstruction has occurred, evidence of pulmonary hypertension and right-sided failure may be noted, including a loud P_2 of the S_2 and elevation of the neck veins. In massive pulmonary embolism, signs of right-sided failure together with cardiovascular collapse are present.

(6) Examination of the extremities. Signs of deep venous thrombosis may suggest that pulmonary embolism has occurred. However, pulmonary emboli frequently occur without overt evidence of deep venous thrombosis on physical examination.

4. Diagnosis

a. Electrocardiography. In most cases of pulmonary embolism the ECG is normal. However, in cases of significant right-sided obstruction the ECG may indicate acute right axis deviation by the development of an S wave in lead I and a Q wave in lead III. The acute right axis deviation also may cause poor R-wave progression in the anterior chest leads, which may lead to the misdiagnosis of an anterior myocardial infarction.

b. Chest x-ray. A decrease in vascular markings in the area of the pulmonary embolism may be present due to decreased pulmonary flow. If pulmonary infarction has occurred, a wedge-shaped, pleural-based density is the classic finding. It may be associated with a loss of lung volume on the affected side and with pleural effusion.

    c. **Arterial blood gas analysis.** Hypoxia [indicated by a fall in oxygen tension (PO_2)], hyperventilation [indicated by a fall in carbon dioxide tension (PCO_2)], and respiratory alkalosis are the classic changes in the arterial blood gases following pulmonary embolism. However, these findings are not specific for pulmonary embolism, and pulmonary embolism may occur without these changes.

    d. **Nuclear scanning**

        (1) The principle of **perfusion scanning** in pulmonary embolism is that areas not well perfused do not receive tracer-labeled blood and show up as relatively inactive areas on the scan. Perfusion scanning is highly sensitive to diminished pulmonary blood flow and, thus, to pulmonary emboli; however, it is not specific. Pneumonia and chronic obstructive lung disease, which also may affect local perfusion, produce perfusion defects. A lobar area of hypoperfusion is highly suggestive of pulmonary embolism as are multiple segmental areas of hypoperfusion.

        (2) **Ventilation scanning** added to perfusion scanning increases the specificity of the test. Areas of the lung that are well ventilated but not well perfused are suggestive of pulmonary embolism. Scans showing a lobar perfusion defect, multiple segmental perfusion defects, or segmental perfusion defects that are well ventilated (i.e., ventilation-perfusion mismatches) are highly suggestive of pulmonary embolism. In such cases, if the clinical presentation is concordant with the diagnosis, further diagnostic tests are unnecessary.

        (3) Normal scans virtually rule out pulmonary embolism, making further diagnostic procedures unnecessary. However, scanning results often fall into an intermediate probability range, and the diagnosis can be neither confirmed nor ruled out. In such cases **pulmonary arteriography** usually is indicated.

    e. **Pulmonary arteriography.** A catheter inserted into a vein, which is maneuvered through the right atrium and ventricle and into the pulmonary artery, is used to measure pulmonary arterial pressures and to infuse contrast media. The angiograms obtained by this method provide the most sensitive and specific test for pulmonary embolism. However, since this is an invasive test, it carries a finite risk.

    f. **Digital subtraction angiography.** In this test, computer techniques are used to enhance the image produced by a small amount of radiographic contrast injected intravenously. This technique produces a pulmonary angiogram with less contrast than is needed for a standard pulmonary angiogram and without the need for a pulmonary artery catheter.

5. Therapy

    a. **Anticoagulants.** If there is no serious contraindication to anticoagulation, heparin therapy currently is the drug of choice. Heparin does not dissolve the embolus but prevents further clot formation while the body's fibrinolytic system produces clot lysis. Clot resolution by this method takes from one to several weeks. After intravenous heparin therapy is begun, therapy is changed to oral anticoagulation with warfarin.

    b. **Thrombolytic agents.** Active thrombolysis with streptokinase or urokinase is indicated in submassive pulmonary embolism, when rapid clot resolution is important. Since these drugs also increase the incidence of significant hemorrhage, they are reserved for pulmonary emboli that have led to enough pulmonary vascular occlusion to produce right-sided heart failure and hemodynamic instability.

    c. **Caval interruption.** In patients in whom anticoagulation or thrombolysis is contraindicated due to the presence of a bleeding diathesis or in whom anticoagulation has failed to protect against recurrent embolism, inferior vena caval interruption is indicated to prevent further episodes of pulmonary embolism.

    d. **Embolectomy.** In massive pulmonary embolism with intractable shock, it may be possible to remove the embolus surgically from the pulmonary artery.

VIII. SYSTEMIC HYPERTENSION

A. General considerations

1. Definition. Hypertension is present when the blood pressure exceeds 140/90 mm Hg. This is an arbitrary definition as a diastolic pressure of even 85 mm Hg may be associated with increased cardiovascular morbidity and mortality.

2. Consequences of hypertension. In general, the mortality rate over 20 years among patients with a systolic blood pressure of greater than 160 mm Hg or a diastolic blood pressure of greater than 100 mm Hg is increased 100% in those who are untreated. The increased mortality rate is due to stroke, coronary artery disease, and congestive heart failure.

    a. **Stroke.** Patients with a systolic blood pressure of greater than 160 mm Hg have a fourfold increased risk of stroke if untreated.

    b. **Coronary artery disease.** Patients with a diastolic pressure of greater than 95 mm Hg have a more than twofold increased risk of coronary artery disease as compared to normotensive patients.

   c. **Congestive heart failure.** Patients with a blood pressure of greater than 160/95 mm Hg have a fourfold increased incidence of congestive heart failure. In 75% of patients with congestive heart failure, hypertension occurs at some time during the course of their illness. Figure 1-7 shows the interaction of hypertension with other risk factors in the development of cardiovascular disease.

B. Primary (essential) hypertension. Hypertension that has no known cause is labeled as **primary** or **essential hypertension**.

   1. **Possible mechanisms of primary hypertension**
      a. **Cardiac output and peripheral resistance.** Blood pressure is the product of cardiac output and total peripheral resistance. Thus, in order for hypertension to occur there must be an elevation in cardiac output, total peripheral resistance, or both. Some studies have indicated that patients with hypertension initially have elevated cardiac output and normal peripheral resistance, which progress to reduced cardiac output and high total peripheral resistance. However, this pattern is not invariable; many patients with hypertension may have either persistently elevated cardiac output or elevated total peripheral resistance early in the course of the disease. Since an elevation in cardiac output physiologically should cause a fall in peripheral resistance, patients with elevated cardiac output and "normal" peripheral resistance actually have abnormally high peripheral resistance for their physiologic state. An abnormality in peripheral resistance is a major problem in most cases of hypertension.
      b. **Impaired pressure natriuresis.** In normal individuals, an elevation in blood pressure leads to increased renal peritubular hydrostatic pressure. This leads to a decrease in sodium reabsorption, which in turn causes a diuresis and a fall in blood pressure. In essential hypertension, the kidney fails to control blood pressure. There is evidence that hypertensive patients have an abnormally high plasma volume for their blood pressure level, suggesting

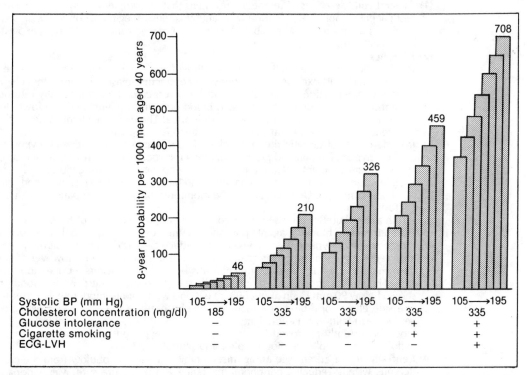

Figure 1-7. Graph showing the interaction of systolic blood pressure with other cardiac risk factors in the development of coronary artery disease in 40-year-old men. Specifically, these data (taken from the Framingham study) indicate the probability of these men developing cardiovascular disease over a period of 8 years. As systolic blood pressure increases, the probability of coronary disease also increases for any combination of cardiac risk factors. *BP* = blood pressure; − = the absence of the given risk factor; + = the presence of the given risk factor; and *ECG-LVH* = electrocardiographic criteria for left ventricular hypertrophy. (Reprinted with permission from *Hypertension: Pathophysiology and Treatment.* Edited by Genest J. New York, McGraw-Hill, 1977.)

impaired natriuresis. The cause of the failure of normal pressure natriuresis is unknown, but heredity may play a role.

c. **Natriuretic hormone.** The increased plasma volume found in hypertensive patients triggers the release of a yet uncharacterized hormone known as **natriuretic hormone**. Natriuretic hormone inhibits the sodium-potassium-ATPase mechanism in the kidney and leads to sodium and water excretion. Release of this hormone does not, however, return the plasma volume to normal. Unfortunately, the hormone also inhibits sodium-potassium-ATPase activity elsewhere in the body and may result in retention of sodium and water in the erythrocytes, arteries, and arterioles. Vascular retention of sodium and water may in turn lead to increased vascular resistance. Thus, natriuretic hormone together with high sodium intake may result in increased vascular tone and reactivity, leading to increased total peripheral resistance and further reinforcing the hypertension.

d. **Baroreceptor resetting.** Baroreceptors in the carotid arteries and the aorta are important in the regulation of blood pressure. In hypertensive patients, the baroreceptors are "reset" so that higher pressures are required to exert an influence toward lowering blood pressure.

e. **The role of renin.** Most patients with essential hypertension have renin levels within the normal range. It is likely that the normal renin levels in these patients contribute to the reabsorption of sodium and water and help to reinforce the hypertension.

2. **Therapy** in hypertension is aimed at reducing the diastolic blood pressure to less than 90 mm Hg. Whether all patients with a blood pressure of 140/90 mm Hg or greater should be treated is controversial. Some physicians withhold therapy as long as there is no end-organ involvement and observe the patient for 1 to 2 years, since many patients return to a normotensive state spontaneously. It is currently believed that most patients with a blood pressure of greater than 140/90 mm Hg should be treated.

a. **Nonmedical therapy.** Sodium restriction alone may be sufficient to lower blood pressure in many hypertensive patients, particularly those with a high sodium intake. Limitation of sodium intake to no more than 2 g/day has been shown to reduce blood pressure significantly. Weight reduction in obese patients also significantly reduces blood pressure.

b. **Medical therapy**

(1) **General considerations.** Therapeutic regimens that are simple to follow often have the best patient compliance. In choosing an antihypertensive regimen, consideration should be given not only to side effects but to the number of medications and doses per day that the patient must take.

(2) **Diuretics**

(a) Diuretics, which generally are the first line of antihypertensive therapy, reduce sodium and fluid excesses in the body by contracting plasma volume. Initially, this causes a reduction in cardiac output; however, cardiac output usually returns to normal during diuretic therapy, and blood pressure is maintained at a lower level primarily due to decreased vascular resistance. The exact mechanism whereby diuretics reduce peripheral vascular resistance is unknown.

(b) Side effects of diuretic therapy include hypokalemia, hyperglycemia, hyperuricemia, hypercalcemia, and prerenal azotemia. Hypokalemia may be avoided by oral potassium supplementation and by the use of potassium-sparing diuretics. Periodic laboratory determination of potassium and blood urea nitrogen is indicated during diuretic therapy. Uric acid should be monitored periodically in patients with a history of gout.

(c) Thiazide diuretics are used most commonly in the treatment of hypertension.

(3) **Beta-adrenergic blocking agents** probably are the next most commonly used drugs in the treatment of hypertension. These agents reduce cardiac output and blunt the renin-angiotensin mechanism for the reabsorption of sodium and water. However, it is not clear that these are the primary mechanisms by which β-blockers reduce blood pressure. The combination of a β-blocker and a diuretic reduces the diastolic blood pressure to below 90 mm Hg in about 80% of patients with mild-to-moderate hypertension. The side effects of β-blockade include bronchospasm, a worsening of existing congestive heart failure, occasional impotence, fatigue, depression, and nightmares. Beta-blockers currently approved for the treatment of hypertension include propranolol, nadolol, metoprolol, atenolol, timolol, and pindolol.

(4) **Centrally acting adrenergic antagonists** inhibit sympathetic outflow from the central nervous system, reducing peripheral resistance and blood pressure. Methyldopa and clonidine are the most commonly used centrally acting drugs. The side effects of methyldopa include somnolence, orthostatic hypotension, Coombs'-positive hemolytic anemia, impotence, and hepatic injury. With clonidine, the major but rare side effect is a rebound phenomenon that produces severe hypertension after withdrawal of the drug.

(5) **Peripherally acting sympathetic nerve antagonists** cause blood pressure to fall by reducing catecholamine release from peripheral sympathetic nerves. The most commonly used drugs in this category are reserpine and guanethidine. Reserpine depletes nerve storage vesicles of norepinephrine and, thus, limits norepinephrine secretion. The major side effect with reserpine is depression; it also may increase the incidence of gastric ulceration. Guanethidine directly inhibits the release of norepinephrine from adrenergic neurons. Orthostatic hypotension is the most common side effect with guanethidine therapy.

(6) **Alpha-adrenergic blocking agents** pharmacologically antagonize stimulation of alpha-adrenergic receptors by norepinephrine, reducing blood pressure by reducing total peripheral resistance. Prazosin and phenoxybenzamine are the most commonly used α-blockers.

(7) **Vasodilators** directly dilate arteries and arterioles, reducing blood pressure by reducing total peripheral resistance. Hydralazine and minoxidil are the most commonly used vasodilators. They are particularly effective when used with a β-blocker that inhibits the reflex tachycardia caused by direct vasodilation. The major side effects of hydralazine are headache and a lupus-like syndrome, the latter of which is reversed when the drug is discontinued. The major side effects of minoxidil are orthostatic hypotension and facial hirsutism.

(8) **Angiotensin-converting–enzyme inhibitors** inhibit the conversion of angiotensin I to angiotensin II (a vasoconstrictor) and, thus, reduce total peripheral resistance. In addition, aldosterone production is decreased, reducing the retention of sodium and water. Both mechanisms act to lower blood pressure. Captopril is the currently available agent in this category. The major side effects with captopril are rashes, leukopenia, and proteinuria, which disappear with discontinuation of the drug.

(9) **Therapeutic approach.** Generally, patients are begun on diuretics, which can be taken once or twice daily. If diuretics fail to control blood pressure, the addition of a β-blocker usually is the next step in antihypertensive therapy. If the combination of a β-blocker and a diuretic is ineffective in controlling blood pressure, a vasodilator is added. If these agents fail to control blood pressure, the addition of captopril or an α-blocker then is indicated.

C. Secondary hypertension. In 5%–10% of patients with hypertension the hypertension is secondary to a definitely diagnosable disease.

   1. Diagnosable causes of secondary hypertension

   a. Renovascular hypertension involves obstruction of renal blood flow at the level of the renal artery. The affected kidney interprets this obstruction as volume depletion and inadequate cardiac output. This stimulates the renin-angiotensin system, causing an increase in circulating angiotensin, the retention of sodium and water, and, thus, hypertension.

   (1) Renovascular hypertension occurs due to atherosclerotic involvement of the renal arteries in elderly patients or due to fibromuscular disease of the renal artery in young women. Renovascular hypertension may be suspected when the hypertension is persistent and difficult to control. The presence of an abdominal bruit or the presence of hypertension in a young woman should suggest the presence of renovascular hypertension.

   (2) Currently, screening tests for renovascular hypertension include intravenous pyelography, peripheral blood renin assays, testing for a response to a converting enzyme inhibitor, renal vein renin sampling, and renal arteriography. As digital subtraction angiography improves technically, it may be possible to visualize the renal artery quite adequately with only a small dose of intravenously injected contrast and at a low risk to the patient.

   (3) Since most cases of renovascular hypertension are suspected and investigated because the hypertension is difficult to control medically, surgical reconstruction of the affected artery or percutaneous transluminal angioplasty is indicated in most uncomplicated cases.

   b. Renal parenchymal diseases. Diseases that reduce kidney function often produce hypertension. Hypertension probably occurs because of the kidney's inability to excrete sodium and water properly. Concomitant activation of the renin-angiotensin mechanism also may be responsible. Since most renal diseases are not directly reversible, therapy for hypertension in these conditions is the same as for primary hypertension.

   c. Endocrinologic causes

   (1) **Oral contraceptives** cause hypertension in about 5% of patients who use them. Hypertension occurs due to stimulation of the renin-angiotensin mechanism by the

estrogens in the pill. The hypertension is reversed by discontinuing use of the oral contraceptives.

(2) **Primary aldosteronism.** Mineralocorticoid excess produced by an adrenal adenoma or by stimulation of the adrenal glands by an unknown mechanism leads to hypertension due to the retention of sodium and water promoted by excess aldosterone. This syndrome also is complicated by hypokalemia. Patients with a solitary adenoma should undergo resection of the tumor, while patients with bilateral adrenal hyperplasia are treated with spironolactone.

(3) **Cushing's syndrome.** Glucocorticoid excess due to exogenous glucocorticoid therapy, a pituitary tumor, or an adrenal adenoma produces hypertension in about 80% of patients who have the syndrome. Hypertension occurs because cortisol has mineralocorticoid effects and, therefore, leads to the retention of sodium and water. Additionally, adrenocorticotropic hormone (ACTH or corticotropin) may stimulate the renin-angiotensin system. Cushing's syndrome usually can be suspected in patients with a history of taking exogenous glucocorticoids and in those with a cushingoid appearance. In patients not taking exogenous glucocorticoids, the syndrome can be confirmed by the measurement of either plasma cortisol or urinary 17-hydroxycorticoids.

(4) **Pheochromocytoma.** This tumor of the adrenal medulla produces an increased secretion of catecholamines, leading to hypertension. Approximately 50% of patients have episodic hypertension; the remaining 50% have constant hypertension. Episodes of flushing, diaphoresis, weight loss, and diarrhea may suggest the diagnosis. Measurement of urinary catecholamines and catecholamine metabolites, including metanephrine and vanillylmandelic acid, also is useful in making the diagnosis. The tumor may be located in the adrenal medulla by the use of computed tomography. Therapy includes stabilizing the patient with α- and β-blockade followed by surgical removal of the tumor.

(5) **Miscellaneous causes.** Acromegaly, hyperparathyroidism, and hyperthyroidism also may produce hypertension.

d. **Coarctation of the aorta**, as noted in section VI D, is a correctable cause of hypertension.

2. **Approach to the diagnosis of secondary hypertension.** Since most hypertensive patients have primary rather than secondary hypertension, extensive screening for secondary hypertension in all hypertensive patients is impractical and unwarranted. A careful history and physical examination can readily detect most endocrinologic causes of hypertension. A simple determination of serum potassium should be useful in screening out most cases of primary aldosteronism. A history and physical examination indicating episodic flushing, diaphoresis, and other signs of pheochromocytoma suggest the need for further workup for this disease. Physical examination should be adequate to determine whether further workup for Cushing's syndrome or acromegaly is indicated. In young patients and patients whose hypertension has been difficult to control medically, a pursuit of the diagnosis of renovascular hypertension is warranted. Coarctation of the aorta usually can be ruled out by physical examination of the pulses and the distal extremities.

D. **Hypertensive crises**

1. **Definition.** Severe hypertension with a diastolic blood pressure of greater than 140 mm Hg is a life-threatening situation. Blood pressure elevation to this degree can cause vascular damage, encephalopathy, retinal hemorrhages, renal damage, and death.

2. **Diagnosis.** A diastolic blood pressure of greater than 140 mm Hg, funduscopic findings of papilledema, changes in neurologic and mental status, and an abnormal renal sediment are the hallmarks of hypertensive crises.

3. **Therapy.** Immediate lowering of the blood pressure is indicated. Infusion of sodium nitroprusside under constant blood pressure monitoring is an effective treatment for hypertensive crises. The dose can be adjusted to maintain the blood pressure within the desired range. An excessive reduction in blood pressure can be reversed rapidly by reducing the dose of the infusion. **Labetalol**, a new antihypertensive agent with both α- and β-blocking properties, also is effective in treating this condition.

E. **Pseudohypertensive crises.** Measurement of blood pressure by an improperly fitting cuff may cause the recorded blood pressure to be significantly higher than it actually is. Another cause of very high blood pressure is pain. Large elevations of blood pressure due to trauma and other pain-producing situations (e.g., the passage of a renal calculus) are best treated with analgesia as opposed to direct antihypertensive therapies.

STUDY QUESTIONS

Directions: Each question below contains five suggested answers. Choose the **one best** response to each question.

1. All of the following mechanisms may lead to the development of congestive heart failure EXCEPT

(A) decreased contractile function
(B) decreased ventricular filling pressure
(C) decreased ventricular compliance
(D) increased afterload
(E) high cardiac output states

2. The single most reliable physical sign of congestive heart failure in patients over the age of 40 years is

(A) a third heart sound (S_3)
(B) a fourth heart sound (S_4)
(C) pulmonary rales
(D) ascites
(E) edema

3. All of the following factors contribute to an increased risk for the development of coronary artery disease EXCEPT

(A) diabetes mellitus
(B) high levels of high-density lipoprotein (HDL)
(C) hypertension
(D) family history
(E) cigarette smoking

4. The etiology of acute pericarditis includes all of the following agents EXCEPT

(A) myocardial infarction
(B) malignancy
(C) collagen vascular disease
(D) exposure to toxins (e.g., ethanol)
(E) uremia

5. A 65-year-old man is admitted to the hospital complaining of dyspnea on exertion (i.e., after walking a distance of 50 feet), orthopnea, and peripheral edema. The clinical evaluation reveals the following findings: blood pressure of 90/60; regular pulse at a rate of 100 beats/min; neck vein distension with central venous pressure estimated at 12 cm H_2O; a systolic ejection murmur that radiates to the neck; a markedly delayed carotid upstroke; and 2+ peripheral edema. All of the following statements concerning this case are true EXCEPT

(A) diuretic therapy may ameliorate the patient's orthopnea and edema
(B) afterload reduction therapy with captopril should be employed
(C) a diagnostic workup for the cause of the patient's heart failure is indicated
(D) increased afterload is a likely mechanism for the patient's left ventricular heart failure
(E) the patient has evidence of biventricular failure

6. Which of the following statements best characterizes tricuspid regurgitation?

(A) Infective endocarditis is a common cause
(B) The murmur heard in tricuspid regurgitation decreases with inspiration
(C) Large a waves in the jugular venous pulse are characteristic
(D) Correction of coexistent left ventricular failure rarely improves the condition
(E) Cardiac catheterization is required for the diagnosis

Directions: Each question below contains four suggested answers of which **one or more** is correct. Choose the answer

A   if **1, 2, and 3** are correct
B   if **1 and 3** are correct
C   if **2 and 4** are correct
D   if **4** is correct
E   if **1, 2, 3, and 4** are correct

7. True statements concerning the pathophysiology and clinical presentation of restrictive cardiomyopathy include

(1) systolic cardiac function is normal in the early stages of the disease
(2) signs of pulmonary vascular congestion may coexist with a normal heart size
(3) cardiac filling pressures are elevated but cardiac volumes are normal
(4) signs of left-sided failure often are more prominent than those of right-sided failure

8. Hemodynamic abnormalities in the pathophysiology of mitral valve stenosis include

(1) increased left ventricular filling
(2) increased left atrial pressure
(3) increased forward cardiac output
(4) increased right ventricular pressure

9. Congestive cardiomyopathy is reversible when it is due to

(1) endocrinopathies (e.g., thyrotoxicosis)
(2) metabolic disorders (e.g., hypophosphatemia)
(3) prolonged ethanol abuse
(4) high-dose doxorubicin therapy

10. Signs of cardiac tamponade include

(1) pulsus paradoxus
(2) narrow pulse pressure
(3) hypotension
(4) elevated neck veins

11. Renovascular hypertension can be described as being

(1) associated with an increased renin release
(2) expected to respond to treatment with captopril
(3) relatively common in young women
(4) easy to control

12. Clinical characteristics of variant (Prinzmetal's) angina include

(1) ST-segment depression
(2) occurrence at rest
(3) occurrence in patients with normal coronary arteries
(4) coronary artery spasm

Questions 13 and 14

A 27-year-old woman enters the emergency ward complaining of dyspnea and pleuritic chest pain. She also complains that over the past 4 days her right calf and thigh have become swollen and tender. Deep venous thrombosis, which may have led to pulmonary embolism, is suspected on the basis of the clinical presentation.

13. Information in the patient history that would support the diagnosis of deep venous thrombosis includes

(1) use of oral contraceptives
(2) history of prolonged lower limb immobilization
(3) history of lower extremity injury
(4) history of hypertension

14. Techniques that would be useful for establishing the diagnosis of deep venous thrombosis include

(1) Doppler ultrasonography
(2) contrast venography
(3) impedance plethysmography
(4) nuclear scanning with ^{125}I-tagged fibrinogen

Directions: The groups of questions below consist of lettered choices followed by several numbered items. For each numbered item select the **one** lettered choice with which it is **most** closely associated. Each lettered choice may be used once, more than once, or not at all.

Questions 15–19

Match each physical sign of congenital heart disease with the lesion it best characterizes.

(A) Atrial septal defect
(B) Ventricular septal defect
(C) Patent ductus arteriosus
(D) Coarctation of the aorta
(E) Ebstein's anomaly

15. Absent femoral pulses

16. Fixed, widely split second heart sound (S_2)

17. Quintuple cardiac cadence on auscultation

18. Continuous murmur

19. Holosystolic murmur

Questions 20–24

Match each physical sign of valvular heart disease with the lesion it best characterizes.

(A) Mitral stenosis
(B) Mitral regurgitation
(C) Tricuspid regurgitation
(D) Aortic stenosis
(E) Aortic regurgitation

20. Pulsatile liver

21. Loud first heart sound (S_1)

22. Soft, single second heart sound (S_2)

23. Third heart sound (S_3, or ventricular gallop)

24. Systolic blood pressure that is 20 mm Hg higher in the leg than in the arm (Hill's sign)

ANSWERS AND EXPLANATIONS

1. The answer is B. (*I B 1–3, C 1*) Congestive heart failure is defined as the inability of the heart, working at normal or elevated filling pressure, to pump enough blood to supply the oxygen requirements of the body tissues. While decreased ventricular filling pressure might reduce cardiac output, this simply represents inadequate preload and, thus, does not fulfill the definition of congestive heart failure. Decreased contractile function, increased afterload, reduced compliance, and high cardiac output states, on the other hand, all can lead to inadequate cardiac output at normal or increased filling pressure.

2. The answer is A. (*I D 2 b, d, e, g, h*) Although it is a normal finding in some young, healthy athletes, a third heart sound (S_3) is the most reliable physical sign of congestive heart failure in individuals who are older than 40 years. A fourth heart sound (S_4) can be a normal finding in older patients. Pulmonary rales, while often the result of heart failure, may have many noncardiac causes. Ascites and edema can result from hepatic, neoplastic, or local factors not associated with cardiac pathology.

3. The answer is B. (*II A 2 c–f, i*) There are several risk factors noted for the development of atherosclerotic coronary artery disease (ASCAD). Cigarette smoking, hypertension, diabetes mellitus, and family history are only a few of these risk factors. High serum cholesterol levels also have been associated with an increased incidence of ASCAD. The higher the amount of cholesterol carried by low-density lipoproteins (LDL) in relation to that carried by high-density lipoproteins (HDL), the higher the risk of ASCAD. High levels of HDL, on the other hand, seem to protect against ASCAD.

4. The answer is D. (*IV A 2 c; V A 1 a, c, f, g*) Acute pericarditis may occur in the first 24 hours following a myocardial infarction or may occur 7–10 days after an infarction. This later occurrence, called Dressler's syndrome, is thought to be an autoimmune phenomenon. Pericarditis may occur secondary to metastatic involvement of the pericardium and may be a manifestation of collagen vascular disease. It also is common in severe chronic renal failure. The development of congestive cardiomyopathy, not acute pericarditis, has been linked to exposure to toxins such as ethanol and cobalt.

5. The answer is B. [*I F 2 a (1), b, c (1); III A 3 b (1), (5)*] The systolic ejection murmur and delayed carotid upstroke suggest that this patient has aortic stenosis. Vasodilator therapy (e.g., with captopril) in such a patient would decrease total peripheral resistance without necessarily increasing cardiac output, resulting in a serious fall in blood pressure. Thus, vasodilator therapy would not be indicated until an adequate workup ruled out aortic stenosis as a possible cause of the patient's congestive heart failure. On the other hand, diuretic therapy and digitalization (e.g., with digoxin) should be useful in reducing the patient's congestive symptoms.

6. The answer is A. [*III E 1 a 3 b (2), (3), 4, 5*] Infective endocarditis is a common cause of tricuspid regurgitation. The murmur of tricuspid regurgitation typically increases with inspiration. Large v waves are seen in the jugular venous pulse. Since a common cause of right ventricular failure and secondary tricuspid regurgitation is left ventricular failure, correction of left ventricular failure, when present, often is useful in the treatment of tricuspid regurgitation. Diagnosis of tricuspid regurgitation usually is made on the basis of clinical or echocardiographic evidence. Cardiac catheterization rarely is used to make the diagnosis.

7. The answer is A (1, 2, 3). (*IV C 3, 4 a, 5 b*) In the early phases of restrictive cardiomyopathy, systolic function usually is normal. The major disorder is that of reduced compliance, which causes increased filling pressures at normal cardiac volumes. The signs of pulmonary vascular congestion noted on chest x-ray may coexist with a normal heart size. Although symptoms of both left- and right-sided congestive heart failure exist, those of right-sided failure often are more prominent.

8. The answer is C (2, 4). (*III B 2*) Left ventricular filling is decreased in mitral valve stenosis, and a pressure gradient develops across the stenotic valve, increasing left atrial pressure. With increasing severity, the stenotic mitral valve may seriously decrease forward cardiac output. Because the right ventricle must fill the left ventricle, a stenotic mitral valve imposes a pressure overload on the right ventricle, which must generate enough force to push blood through the constricted valve.

9. The answer is A (1, 2, 3). (*IV A 2 a, b, d, e*) In most cases of congestive cardiomyopathy, no cause can be identified; however, several conditions have been linked with the development of cardiomyopathy. The most common cause of cardiomyopathy is alcohol abuse, the cessation of which can lead to significant improvement in ventricular function. Thyrotoxicosis and hypothyroidism are endocrine disorders that have been linked to congestive cardiomyopathy, which is reversible with correction of the underlying endocrinopathy. Metabolic disorders such as hypophosphatemia and hypocalcemia also produce reversible cardiomyopathy. Doxorubicin—an antitumor medication—causes irreversible congestive cardiomyopathy when administered in large doses.

10. The answer is E (all). [*V C 2 b (1)–(4)*] Recognition of any or all of the signs listed should lead to the diagnosis of cardiac tamponade. Pulsus paradoxus occurs in 95% of patients with cardiac tamponade. Impairment of cardiac filling causes a decrease in stroke volume, which produces a narrow pulse pressure and hypotension. Neck veins are elevated due to the increase in pressure that is required to fill the heart.

11. The answer is A (1, 2, 3). (*VIII C 1 a*) In renovascular hypertension, diminished renal blood flow stimulates the kidney to release increasing amounts of renin, which activate the renin-angiotensin-aldosterone axis, leading to hypertension. Since captopril prevents the conversion of angiotensin I to angiotensin II, this drug would be expected to be particularly effective in this disease. Young women develop fibromuscular obstruction of the renal arteries as a cause for renovascular hypertension. Renovascular hypertension is notoriously difficult to control; this difficulty often raises the suspicion that it is present.

12. The answer is C (2, 4). [*II A 5 a 1 (e)*] Prinzmetal's angina typically occurs at rest and is due to coronary artery spasm. Although patients with Prinzmetal's angina occasionally have ST-segment depression as well as elevation, it is the ST-segment elevation on which the diagnosis is based. Prinzmetal's angina occasionally occurs in patients with "normal" coronary arteries, but the majority of patients have atherosclerotic disease.

13. The answer is A (1, 2, 3). [*VII A 2 a, d, e, 3 a, C 1, 3 a (1), (2)*] Factors that contribute to the development of deep venous thrombosis include the use of estrogen-containing compounds (e.g., oral contraceptives); lower limb immobilization (e.g., during surgery or prolonged bed rest), which leads to venous stasis; and lower limb injury, which may lead to blood clot formation. Hypertension has no association with deep venous thrombosis. The dyspnea and pleuritic pain in this patient suggest that the suspected deep venous thrombosis has led to pulmonary embolism—the most common cause of which is the migration of a thrombus from the veins in the lower extremities or pelvis to the pulmonary artery.

14. The answer is E (all). (*VII 4 a–b*) Doppler ultrasonography, impedance plethysmography, and nuclear scanning with ^{125}I-tagged fibrinogen all are useful techniques for the diagnosis of deep venous thrombosis. These tests have the added advantage of being noninvasive. Contrast venography provides a definitive diagnosis in almost every case. However, this invasive test actually can cause thrombophlebitis in a minority of cases.

15–19. The answers are: 15-D, 16-A, 17-E, 18-C, 19-B. [*VI A 3 b (1), B 2 b (1), C 2 a, D 2 b (1), E 2 b (2)*] Coarctation of the aorta is a stenosis of the aorta, distal to which there is limited aortic blood flow. This diminishes transmission of the pulse from the aorta to the distal extremities, usually resulting in absent femoral pulses.

In atrial septal defect, both ventricles fill from a common cardiac reservoir—the combined left and right atria. With inspiration, there is little differential in total pulmonary blood flow; thus, closure of the pulmonic valve does not change in its timing with reference to closure of the aortic valve. The classic finding in atrial septal defect, therefore, is a fixed and widely split second heart sound (S_2).

In Epstein's anomaly of the tricuspid valve, the first heart sound (S_1) is split and the usual presence of an atrial septal defect causes wide splitting of the S_2. These sounds together with the frequent occurrence of a third heart sound (S_3 or ventricular gallop) or a fourth heart sound (S_4 or atrial gallop) produce a quintuple cadence on auscultation.

In patent ductus arteriosus, the pressure in the aorta is higher than the pressure in the pulmonary artery throughout both systole and diastole. This produces continuous flow from the aorta to the pulmonary artery and, thus, a continuous murmur.

In ventricular septal defect, left ventricular pressure is higher than right ventricular pressure throughout systole. Thus, the murmur heard is holosystolic.

20–24. The answers are: 20-C, 21-A, 22-D, 23-B, 24-E. [*III A 3 b (2), B 3 b (4), C 3 b (4) (b), D 3 b (4), E 3 b (4)*] A pulsatile liver often is felt in patients with tricuspid regurgitation as the mechanical effects of right ventricular systole are transmitted back to the hepatic veins.

In mitral stenosis, the mitral valve remains open during most of diastole, due to the pressure gradient across the stenotic mitral valve. Ventricular systole then closes the valve forcibly, with a resultant increase in the intensity of the first heart sound (S_1).

A soft, single second heart sound (S_2) often is noted in aortic stenosis due to the severely impaired motion of the stenotic aortic valve. The reduced motion causes the aortic component (A_2) of the S_2 to be absent. Thus, only the pulmonic component (P_2) is heard, which is soft.

Although a third heart sound (S_3) could be heard in any cardiac condition, it is most prominently heard in mitral regurgitation, even in patients without congestive heart failure.

In aortic regurgitation, a disproportionate (i.e., 20 mm Hg) increase in systolic blood pressure is noted in the leg as compared with the arm. This finding, called Hill's sign, usually indicates that the aortic regurgitation is severe.

2
Pulmonary Diseases
Stanley B. Fiel

I. CHRONIC OBSTRUCTIVE PULMONARY DISEASE

A. Introduction

1. **Definition.** Chronic obstructive pulmonary disease (COPD) is a common disorder usually characterized by progressive obstruction to airflow and a history of inhalation of such irritants as tobacco smoke. COPD also is referred to as **chronic obstructive lung disease (COLD)**, **chronic airways obstruction (CAO)**, and, either individually or together, chronic bronchitis and emphysema.

   a. **Chronic bronchitis** can be defined in terms of clinical symptoms (i.e., excessive mucus secretion in the bronchial tree leading to productive cough for at least 3 months during each of 2 successive years).

   b. **Emphysema** can be described in terms of morbid anatomy showing destruction of alveolar walls and abnormal enlargement of airspaces distal to the terminal nonrespiratory bronchiole.

   c. It has become apparent that many patients develop, to varying degrees, a combination of these two entities. The more general terminology of COPD, therefore, may be indicated and is used in this chapter.

2. The **social and economic consequences of COPD** are staggering. Screening studies of the general population suggest that 11%–13% of individuals have significant airflow obstruction.

3. The **death rate due to COPD** has doubled every 5 years in the past 2 decades. COPD now is the sixth leading cause of death in the United States.

B. Etiology. On a precise scientific level, the etiology of COPD is unknown. However, on an environmental basis, the single most important etiologic agent is chronic inhalation of tobacco smoke.

1. **Tobacco smoke.** Smoking in **pack years** (i.e., the number of years a patient has smoked × the number of packs smoked per day) is quantitatively related to varied ventilatory dysfunction and pathologic changes in the lung. Smoking also depresses alveolar macrophages, reduces the functional integrity of pulmonary surfactant, retards mucus transport, enhances the release of lysosomal enzymes, and produces numerous other effects believed to be involved in the pathogenesis of COPD.

2. **Other environmental factors**

   a. The extent that **urban and industrial air pollution** contributes to the pathogenesis of COPD is not entirely known. Studies comparing patients who live in areas of clean air to those who reside in highly polluted areas indicate a higher incidence of COPD in the latter group.

   b. The role of **viral infections** in the development and progression of COPD is unproven. However, evidence suggests that upper respiratory viral infections in childhood may predispose to COPD in adulthood, and viral infections are frequent precipitating factors in symptomatic exacerbations of COPD.

   c. **Bacterial infections** are even less implicated.

3. **Alpha₁-antitrypsin deficiency** is a well-recognized genetic factor predisposing to human emphysema.

   a. Presumably, this deficiency causes the patient to be susceptible to autodigestion of pulmonary tissue by naturally occurring proteases.

   b. Individuals with homozygous deficiency may develop emphysema early in life. Cigarette smoking accelerates the process. In its pure form, α_1-antitrypsin deficiency presents as hepatic cirrhosis, absence of the α_1-globulin peak on serum protein electrophoresis, negligible amounts of serum α_1-antitrypsin, and advanced panlobular emphysema predominantly in the base of the lungs.

C. **Pathogenesis.** Recent evidence suggests that COPD begins in the small airways (i.e., those less than 2 mm in diameter), which normally contribute only a small amount of the total resistance to airflow in the tracheobronchial tree. In COPD, however, the small airways are the sites of extensive disease and airflow limitation.

1. Histopathologic abnormalities of the small airways are common findings at autopsy in young smokers. This small airway disease is presumed to progress over about 30 years to the characteristic clinical picture of disabling COPD.

2. In young smokers, the abnormalities noted in tests of small airway function tend to resolve with cessation of smoking. It is unclear at what point during the course of the disease the changes become irreversible and inevitably progress to COPD.

D. **Pathology and pathophysiology.** The pathology of COPD reflects those changes seen in both the **airways** and the **pulmonary parenchyma**.

1. **The bronchitic component**
   a. Early in the disease, the small airways demonstrate mucous plugging, inflammation, peribronchiolar fibrosis, narrowing, and obliteration.
   b. In established disease, the bronchitic component includes varying degrees of mucous gland hyperplasia, mucosal inflammation and edema, bronchospasm, and impacted secretions. These elements contribute to airway narrowing and increased airway resistance.

2. **The emphysematous component** includes the destruction of alveolar walls and the supporting structure of the airways, which produces widely dilated airspaces.
   a. The loss of tissue support for the airways is believed to contribute to airway narrowing by a tendency for the unsupported airways to collapse dynamically during expiration to low volumes. In addition, the loss of the alveolar capillary membrane causes a reduction in carbon monoxide diffusing capacity.
   b. Anatomically, emphysema is classified as either **centrolobular** or **panlobular**.
      (1) **Centrolobular emphysema** is believed to represent a destructive lesion of the respiratory bronchiole; it originates at the center of the lobule and is distinct from the periphery of the acinus with its septae and vessels.
         (a) Centrolobular emphysema is variable and patchy and has a predilection for upper lung zones. The greatly dilated respiratory bronchioles in centrolobular emphysema and may produce **bullous cysts**.
         (b) Centrolobular emphysema often is associated with **chronic bronchitis** and **bronchial inflammation**. It is the most common type of emphysema encountered in clinical practice, and it is rare in nonsmokers.
      (2) **Panlobular emphysema**, in contrast to the centrolobular type, is thought to evolve from dilated alveolar ducts at the periphery of the lobules to markedly enlarged airspaces. It has little association with chronic bronchitis and is seen commonly in patients with α_1-**antitrypsin deficiency**.

E. **Clinical features**

1. **Typical course.** COPD is an insidious, long-term process that typically occurs as follows.
   a. A teenager who smokes develops mild but asymptomatic changes in the small airways.
   b. As an adult, this smoker experiences chronic cough and symptoms that suggest an upper respiratory infection.
   c. By middle age, the smoker has significant bronchial disease characterized by progressive airway obstruction that produces dyspnea on exertion. (This occurs in 25%–50% of smokers and frequently goes unrecognized as the patients develop a more sedentary lifestyle.)
   d. When the smoker's respiratory system is placed under stress from an unrelated health problem, the presence of COPD becomes evident. Pneumonia, surgery, and trauma are common precipitating events.

2. **Clinical syndromes**
   a. Two classic types of COPD exist and are given various names. Patients with "emphysematous," "dyspneic," or "type A" COPD are referred to as **pink puffers**; those with "bronchitic," "tussive," or "type B" COPD are referred to as **blue bloaters**.
      (1) **Pink puffers** have predominant emphysema and show symptoms at a relatively old age

(often greater than 60 years). There is progressive exertional dyspnea, weight loss, and little or no cough and expectoration.

    (a) Pulmonary function testing reveals mild hypoxia, hypocapnia, hyperinflation, decreased diffusing capacity, only a mild increase in airway resistance, and little improvement in airflow after treatment with bronchodilators.

    (b) These patients usually undergo a slowly progressive downhill course.

  (2) Blue bloaters have predominant chronic bronchitis and, at a relatively young age, experience chronic cough and expectoration, episodic dyspnea, and weight gain. Wheezing and rhonchi frequently are heard in the chest, and cor pulmonale often is seen accompanied by edema and cyanosis.

    (a) Pulmonary function testing reveals severe hypoxia, hypercapnia, polycythemia, elevated airway resistance, improved airflow after treatment with bronchodilators, and relatively preserved lung volumes and diffusing capacity.

    (b) Pathologically, there is minimal emphysema but significant bronchiolitis, bronchitis, mucous gland hyperplasia, and right ventricular hypertrophy. This is in contrast to the pathologic findings in pink puffers, in whom the major finding is emphysema with little or no airway inflammation.

  b. Patients with emphysema have proportional and matched losses of ventilation and perfusion and, hence, are spared severe hypoxia; in contrast, patients with chronic bronchitis have marked ventilation-perfusion mismatch, resulting in severe hypoxia. The hypoxia in chronic bronchitis is worsened by the hypercapnia, which may be the result of an acquired or congenital reduction in central respiratory drive or respiratory muscle fatigue.

  c. Although the definitions for the two types of COPD are useful concepts, such pure entities largely represent extremes of the spectrum of COPD and rarely are encountered in clinical practice. Most COPD patients actually present with a mixture of emphysema and chronic bronchitis in various proportions.

F. Diagnosis. The diagnosis of COPD may be suspected on the basis of patient history, symptoms, and physical signs, or it may become obvious through chest x-ray and clinical circumstances.

  1. COPD in middle-aged smokers can be diagnosed by **spirometric screening**.

  2. On **physical examination**, the findings might include hyperinflation, poor diaphragmatic movement, the use of accessory muscles of respiration, and decreased breathing sounds and wheezing on auscultation.

  3. The **chest x-ray** may show hyperinflation, a loss of vascularity, a flattened diaphragm, and a small heart. In addition, patients with chronic bronchitis often show thickened bronchial walls and "dirty" lung fields. Diagnosis should not rest solely on the basis of x-ray findings.

  4. Objective documentation of expiratory flow obstruction by **pulmonary function testing** remains a necessary criterion for the diagnosis of COPD.

G. Clinical course and prognosis. COPD tends to be a progressive disorder unless there is some form of intervention (i.e., cessation of smoking, removal of other irritants, or medical therapy).

  1. The loss of **1-second forced expiratory volume (FEV_1)** is about 50–75 ml/yr in a typical patient with COPD, as compared with a normal decline in pulmonary function of approximately half that rate.

  2. It is unclear whether any specific medical therapy can slow the progression of disease once the process is well advanced. However, cessation of smoking may alter the decline in pulmonary function in all but far-advanced disease.

  3. Survival is statistically dependent on the degree of ventilatory function that exists when the patient is first evaluated. For example, patients with an initial FEV_1 of less than 0.75 L have a 5-year survival rate of 25%, whereas those with an initial FEV_1 of 1 L have a 5-year survival rate of approximately 50%.

H. Therapy

  1. Bronchodilation

    a. COPD often is viewed erroneously as an irreversible process. It is now known that even patients with nonreversible airflow obstruction on postbronchodilator pulmonary function studies may have airflow reactivity. It appears that 15%–20% of COPD patients in this category have reversible airflow obstruction. Overall, most patients with COPD show improvement in pulmonary function after sufficient bronchodilator therapy.

    b. The two major classes of bronchodilators currently available are **xanthines** (theophylline-type agents) and β-**adrenergic agonists**. These agents may be used separately or in combination. The newer, selective β_2-adrenergic agonists offer advantages over the older β-blockers in terms of longer duration of action and reduced cardiac side effects.

2. **Corticosteroid therapy.** The use of corticosteroids to treat the bronchospasm associated with COPD is controversial. However, some of these patients clearly have an asthma-like component to their disease and would likely respond to steroid therapy to some extent.

3. **Sputum mobilization.** Little objective evidence is available to suggest that traditional expectorants and mucolytic agents have beneficial effects in COPD patients. Bland hydrating aerosols and physical therapy may improve bronchial drainage transiently, but the long-term benefit is not known. Postural drainage usually is reserved for patients with bronchiectasis.

4. **Management of infection.** There has been a long-standing empiricism in the use of broad-spectrum antibiotics during exacerbations in patients with COPD. In addition, COPD patients should receive annual vaccination against influenza; a vaccine for pneumococcal infection also should be given.

5. **Pulmonary rehabilitation** programs are prescribed for the purpose of decreasing morbidity and improving the quality of life. Patients are instructed in exercise programs aimed at increasing exercise tolerance and respiratory muscle stamina. Counseling and nutritional guidance also are given to patients.

6. **Surgery.** The only currently accepted surgical procedure for the management of COPD is the resection of large localized bullae, which is performed only in carefully selected patients. In the future, lung transplantation may offer the ultimate cure.

I. **Prevention.** Avoidance of smoking is by far the best means of disease prevention. In addition, patients should avoid chronic exposure to bronchial irritants. Simple spirometric screening of high-risk patients can help to detect early disease and to prevent further deterioration.

J. **Complications** of COPD include cor pulmonale, polycythemia, infection, respiratory failure, bronchogenic carcinoma, nocturnal hypoxia, general disability, and a proclivity for peptic ulcer disease.

1. **Pneumonia** occurring in a COPD patient is of special concern because of its relative severity and its potential for precipitating respiratory failure.

2. **Respiratory failure** may be precipitated by many conditions, including heart failure, sedation, infection, acute bronchospasm, and trauma.

3. Although **bronchogenic carcinoma** is not strictly a complication of COPD, it occurs in COPD patients with high frequency, presumably because of the common denominator of tobacco smoking.

4. The predisposition for **peptic ulcer disease** in COPD patients is not well understood.

5. Concomitant **left ventricular dysfunction** appears to be due to independent primary myocardial disease, not pulmonary disease.

II. ASTHMA

A. **Definition.** Asthma is a **reversible airway obstruction** that is characterized by hyperirritability of the airways. Substances that have no effect when inhaled by normal individuals cause bronchoconstriction in patients with asthma. Asthma does not cause emphysema or other chronic diseases but alone may be a significant cause of disability. A principal feature of asthma is its extreme variability, both from patient to patient and from time to time in the same patient.

B. **Incidence and etiology.** Asthma occurs in 3%–8% of the population. Etiologic or pathologic classification of the disease is difficult; however, asthma traditionally is divided into two forms.

1. An **allergic form** is responsible for most of childhood asthma and is due to an immunologically mediated hypersensitivity to inhaled antigens.

2. An **intrinsic form** occurs in adults and shows no evidence of immediate hypersensitivity to specific antigens.

3. In patients in whom the evidence of immediate hypersensitivity to antigen is equivocal, most attacks do not appear to be provoked by inhalation of antigens, and there is a poor correlation between the severity of symptoms and the levels of specific antigens circulating as airborne particles. These observations indicate that asthmatic bronchospasm may not necessarily require an immunologically mediated hypersensitivity reaction.

C. Pathogenesis

1. Chemical mediators of immediate hypersensitivity include histamine, slow-reacting substance of anaphylaxis (SRS-A), and eosinophil chemotactic factor of anaphylaxis (ECF-A). Other mediators, such as prostaglandins, platelet activating factor (PAF), and neutrophil chemotactic factor (NCF), also are released from sensitized lung tissue on exposure to antigens that are not as well understood.

    a. Histamine, the best characterized of the mediators, is released when immunoglobulin E (IgE)-mediated reactions are triggered. Histamine causes rapid contraction of smooth muscle and an increase in capillary permeability and, therefore, is thought to mediate the bronchoconstriction and mucosal edema associated with asthmatic bronchospasms.

        (1) Smooth muscle contraction is caused by stimulation of **histamine$_1$ (H$_1$) receptors** and can be blocked by standard antihistamines.

        (2) Histamine also stimulates **histamine$_2$ (H$_2$) receptors**, which trigger relaxation of smooth muscle and exert anti-inflammatory effects. Specific antagonists for H$_2$ receptors have been developed and include cimetidine.

    b. SRS-A, another mediator released from sensitized mast cells, provokes gradual but sustained traction of airway smooth muscle in guinea pigs. Its role in human asthma is unknown.

    c. ECF-A and **NCF**, released by the antigen-antibody interaction, attract different cell types at the site of the immune response and presumably account for the cellular infiltration of the airway walls seen in patients with asthma. Neutrophils probably release lysozymes, which cause further inflammation; eosinophils may inhibit inflammation by releasing chemicals that inhibit or inactivate other mediators.

    d. Other chemicals released or synthesized, including serotonin, prostaglandins, thromboxanes, and endoperoxides, may cause further tissue inflammation. Some of these mediators may be particularly important in the pathogenesis of some nonallergic forms of asthma.

2. Theories regarding the mechanism of airway hyperirritability

    a. One theory regarding the pathogenesis of asthma is that the observed physiologic changes result in the direct effects of the chemical mediators that diffuse locally to mucous glands, vessels, and smooth muscle. It is clear, however, that the simple release of mediators is not sufficient to cause an asthmatic attack.

    b. A possible explanation is abnormally exaggerated reactivity of the tracheobronchial tree of asthmatic individuals. This increased reactivity sometimes is called **nonspecific bronchial hyperreactivity** to distinguish it from the bronchospasm provoked by immunologically specific antigens. The ubiquity of bronchial hyperreactivity has caused pathogenetic theories to shift in focus from the **nature of the mediators** released from mast cells to the **responsiveness of the end organ**.

        (1) Muscle reactivity. The mechanism underlying bronchial hyperreactivity is unknown but may result from a change in the contractile mechanisms of airway smooth muscle.

        (2) Parasympathetic stimulation. Another explanation for bronchial hyperreactivity is that the abnormality exists in the nerves that regulate the tone of the muscle, not in the muscle itself. The airways are supplied by both the parasympathetic and sympathetic systems. The parasympathetic system appears to mediate the reflex bronchial constriction caused by inhalation of nonspecific irritants such as dust and sulfur dioxide.

        (3) Sympathetic deficiency. There is evidence that a deficiency in the sympathetic nervous system may be responsible for bronchial hyperreactivity.

        (4) Nonadrenergic inhibitory system. A third system of autonomic innervation may exist in the bronchial muscles, as it does in the gut muscles. This system sometimes is called the **inhibitory nervous system** and, in the gut, seems to regulate or inhibit spontaneous constriction of intestinal smooth muscle. The congenital absence of this system leads to **Hirschsprung's disease**, in which the distal portion of the bowel is intensely constricted. A similar deficiency in the innervation of the airway conceivably could cause recurrent episodes of abnormal constriction of bronchial smooth muscle.

        (5) Environmental factors. Recently it has been shown that bronchial reactivity varies in degree and is temporarily increased by upper respiratory viral infections and exposure to pollutants such as ozone, nitrogen dioxide, and industrial fumes. By amplifying the response to the materials released from the mast cells, this increased reactivity could be responsible for the exacerbations of asthma seen with viral infections, occupational exposures, and severe pollution.

D. Pathophysiology

1. Pathophysiologically, asthma is characterized by constriction of airway smooth muscle, hypersecretion of mucus, edema and inflammatory cell infiltration of the airway mucus, and thickening of the basement membrane underlying the airway epithelium.

2. These pathophysiologic changes are not uniformly distributed. Some airways may display a predominance of bronchospasm, others may be occluded by mucous plugging, and still others may appear unaffected.

E. Clinical features

1. Asthma classically presents as episodic bouts of coughing, dyspnea, chest tightness, and expiratory wheezing. Physical examination typically reveals tachycardia, tachypnea with prolonged expiration, overinflation of the chest with poor movement of the diaphragm, and diffuse, high-pitched expiratory wheezing. Attacks may be provoked by upper respiratory viral infection, exposure to allergens, emotional stress, and many nonspecific precipitating events.

2. The symptoms of asthma exhibit a wide spectrum of severity, reflecting the variability of the underlying airway obstruction. Some patients display only occasional attacks of exertional dyspnea and wheezing, which respond to inhaled bronchodilators alone; other patients have chronic symptoms requiring continuous use of orally inhaled medications. Although this latter group of patients may have irreversible thickening of the airway walls, their illness still is episodic in occurrence. Asthma that is characterized by a prolonged, very severe attack is termed **status asthmaticus**.

  a. The term status asthmaticus usually is reserved for patients who do not respond to initial treatment and who have bronchospasm so severe that the patients are at risk for ventilatory failure.

  b. The clinical manifestations of severe asthma include fatigue, a pulse rate of more than 100 beats/min, and cyanosis. The use of accessory muscles frequently is noted. An inspiratory decrease of more than 20 mm Hg in systolic blood pressure (i.e., **pulsus paradoxus**) indicates gross overinflation of the lung and wide swings in pleural pressure.

F. Diagnosis

1. Sputum analysis. Sputum may appear purulent due to an increased eosinophil content or to an inflammatory response to a viral tracheal bronchitis. Sputum smears may reveal **Curschmann's spirals** (i.e., mucus that forms a cast of the small airways) and **Charcot-Leyden crystals** (i.e., breakdown products of the eosinophils).

2. Hematologic studies reveal a modest leukocytosis and eosinophilia in both the allergic and intrinsic forms of the disease.

3. Pulmonary function testing. Spirometry reveals a reduction in **forced vital capacity (FVC)**. The **FEV_1/FVC ratio** is reduced but may improve after inhalation of a bronchodilator. **Residual volume (RV)**, **total lung capacity (TLC)**, and **lung compliance** usually are increased, and the diffusing capacity frequently is increased. After symptomatic recovery, TLC and lung compliance return to normal, but maximal expiratory flow rate may remain reduced at low lung volumes and an abnormal distribution of ventilation may persist, reflecting resistant obstruction of small airways.

4. Chest x-ray usually shows nothing more than overinflation. Occasional findings include localized density due to a large mucous plug and the ominous sign of pneumothorax or pneumomediastinum, reflecting the rupture of alveolar tissue caused by high intra-alveolar pressure.

5. Arterial blood gas studies usually reveal a low **carbon dioxide tension (PCO_2)**, that is, a PCO_2 of less than 36 mm Hg. An increased PCO_2 or a normal PCO_2 of 40 mm Hg indicates severe obstruction. Arterial hypoxia is common despite the increased ventilation and is due to underventilation of lung segments supplied by narrowed airways (i.e., ventilation-perfusion mismatch).

G. Therapy.
Several therapeutic approaches are implied by the conceptual model for the pathogenesis of asthma. Therapy may be directed at preventing the union of antigen with IgE antibody, at blocking the release of chemical mediators, and at reducing the responsiveness of the tracheobronchial tree.

1. Preventing antigen-antibody union

  a. With this form of therapy, the simplest approach is **avoidance of exposure** to allergens.

  b. Hyposensitization is another means of attempting to prevent the union of antigens with specific IgE antibodies. This therapeutic approach is based on the belief that repeated injections of small amounts of an antigen cause the antigen to produce circulating antibodies before it reaches the IgE of mast cells. The efficacy of hyposensitization in adults has not been established for treatment of asthma.

2. Blocking mediator release. Pretreatment of an asthmatic individual with **cromolyn sodium** prevents the bronchospasm that ordinarily would be induced by inhalation of the antigen.

Cromolyn sodium inhibits the release of mediators from synthesized cells in vitro, and its effectiveness as a prophylactic medication is believed to depend on the same mechanism in the airways.

  a. Because cromolyn sodium is not readily absorbed into the gastrointestinal tract, it is inhaled as a fine powder from capsules. The usual dose is 1 or 2 capsules, four times daily.

  b. Cromolyn sodium is most effective in young patients with allergic asthma but may be effective in older patients with the intrinsic form of the disease. It also may be useful in patients with exercise-induced asthma.

  c. It should be remembered that cromolyn sodium is a prophylactic agent. It does not reverse bronchospasm once it develops, and it is usually started only after adequate control has been achieved with other medications.

3. Reducing responsiveness of the tracheobronchial tree

  a. Aminophylline should be given intravenously at a loading dose of 5–6 mg/kg of body weight over a 30-minute period. Provided there is no toxicity, the loading dose should be followed by continuous infusion of aminophylline at a rate of 0.5–0.9 mg/kg/hr.

  b. Sympathomimetics

    (1) Subcutaneous sympathomimetics such as **epinephrine** have been used in the treatment of severe attacks of bronchospasm. A dose of 0.3–0.5 ml of 1:1000 epinephrine is given initially and may be repeated two or three times at 20- to 30-minute intervals.

    (2) Nebulized sympathomimetics such as **metaproterenol** are given as supplements or substitutes for subcutaneous sympathomimetics. In addition, chronic outpatients can use hand-held nebulized sympathomimetics.

  c. Corticosteroids should be used when symptoms persist after treatment with the above agents.

  d. Newly available agents that are being used include anticholinergic agents and more selective β_2-sympathomimetics.

III. BRONCHIECTASIS, CYSTIC FIBROSIS, AND LUNG ABSCESS

A. Bronchiectasis

  1. Definition. Bronchiectasis is a pathologic dilatation of the bronchi caused by destruction of the bronchial wall. Destruction of the bronchial wall and permanent dilatation are produced when suppurative infection occurs in an obstructed bronchus.

  2. Etiology and pathogenesis

    a. Bronchi are most susceptible to bronchial infection and obstruction during childhood. A child's small bronchi are more easily obstructed by impacted secretions, foreign bodies, and compressing lymph nodes. Seventy-five percent of patients can recall symptoms of bronchiectasis as early as the age of 5 years.

    b. The most common cause of bronchiectasis is bacterial pneumonia, which may be primary or may be a complication of measles, aspiration of gastric contents or particulate matter, or tumor.

    c. Congenital disorders that may predispose to bronchiectasis include congenital cystic disease of the lung, congenital bronchial stenosis, and compression of bronchi by anomalous arteries to the lung.

    d. Hypogammaglobulinemia and IgA deficiency result in inadequate antibody protection, leading to pneumonia and, subsequently, bronchiectasis.

    e. Cystic fibrosis also can lead to bronchiectasis.

  3. Clinical features. The symptoms of bronchiectasis include chronic cough productive of purulent sputum, recurrent chest colds or pneumonias, occasional hemoptysis, and pleuritic pain. These symptoms cannot be differentiated from those of chronic suppurative bronchitis. Progressive dyspnea, cyanosis, digital clubbing, and cor pulmonale are seen in advanced cases.

  4. Diagnosis

    a. Physical examination reveals rales over the area of involvement on repeated examinations.

    b. Chest x-ray usually shows peribronchial fibrosis in the involved segment. Segmental lung collapse in areas of bronchiectasis is common.

    c. Bronchography can provide a definitive diagnosis if the patient is stable and not actively infected or coughing up blood. Secretions and clots block the entry of contrast medium, and pneumonia causes temporary dilatation of the bronchi.

    d. Pulmonary function testing produces normal results in mild cases but in moderate or severe cases may reveal either restrictive or a mixture of restrictive and obstructive ventilatory patterns.

5. Therapy. The proper therapy can markedly improve a patient's symptoms.
  a. Medical treatment is the mainstay and consists of antibiotics on a regular basis, postural drainage, and immunization against influenza and pneumococcal pneumonia. The antibiotics of choice for outpatients are ampicillin, tetracycline, and erythromycin.
  b. Lung surgery. Attempts at resection generally have not proven to be effective for eliminating chronic cough and sputum unless the operation is performed in early childhood for single local airway disease.

B. Cystic fibrosis

  1. Definition. Cystic fibrosis is an autosomal recessive disease characterized by dysfunction of the exocrine glands leading to obstruction in such organs as the lungs, pancreas, and gastrointestinal tract. Once thought to be unique to children, cystic fibrosis now is recognized as the most common cause of obstructive airway disease among individuals up to age 30 years. The median age of patients with cystic fibrosis has risen from the teens in the 1960s to almost 21 years in 1980. In 99% of cases, death from cystic fibrosis is due to respiratory failure, with portal hypertension secondary to biliary cirrhosis accounting for the remainder of cases.

  2. Incidence. An estimated 20,000 cystic fibrosis patients live in the United States. The disease is most common in whites, occurring in 1 of 1500 births. Five percent of the white population are carriers. Because of the recessive nature of the inheritance of this disease and the fact that heterozygotes have no disease, a negative family history does not rule out the disease.

  3. Pathophysiology
  a. No single biochemical or structural defect has been identified to explain the clinical manifestations of cystic fibrosis. The disease is best characterized in pathophysiologic terms as an exocrine gland dysfunction whereby glandular ducts become obstructed by abnormal secretory products.
  b. In addition, much evidence favors an associated abnormality of mucociliary transport.
  c. No well-defined immunologic abnormalities have been described.

  4. Clinical features
  a. Pulmonary manifestations. The manifestations of cystic fibrosis are quite varied, with pulmonary abnormalities being the overriding clinical concern.
    (1) The earliest pulmonary manifestation is peripheral airway obstruction resulting from plugged bronchi. Repeated bouts of infection lead to a vicious circle of obstruction, tissue damage, and infection, which ultimately progresses to a loss of pulmonary function.
    (2) The predominant organism to colonize the lung is the highly resistant mucoid strain of *Pseudomonas aeruginosa*. Initial infections may be due to *Staphylococcus aureus*. Complete eradication of the organisms is virtually impossible.
  b. Nonpulmonary manifestations also are common and include meconium ileus, malabsorption, fatty infiltration of the liver, focal biliary cirrhosis, glucose intolerance, sterility in the male, and a predilection for heat prostration due to severe salt depletion.

  5. Diagnosis
  a. Sweat test. An abnormal sweat test is observed in virtually all cases of cystic fibrosis and, in combination with certain clinical hallmarks, confirms the diagnosis.
    (1) It is known that in cystic fibrosis the sodium and chloride concentrations in sweat are elevated drastically, while normal concentrations of these ions exist elsewhere. The sweat test, which conventionally is performed via the **quantitative pylocarpine iontophoresis method**, defines the upper limit of normal as a sweat chloride concentration of 60 mEq/L.
    (2) A positive sweat test is diagnostic in the presence of at least one of the following three criteria:
      (a) A reliable family history of cystic fibrosis
      (b) Obstructive pulmonary disease
      (c) Pancreatic insufficiency
  b. Pulmonary function testing shows limitation of maximal expiratory flow rate, elevated RV, and, later, a decreased diffusing capacity.
  c. Chest x-ray reveals striking manifestations, which are more pronounced at the apices, particularly on the right. Findings include hyperinflation, cyst formation, atelectasis, bronchiectasis, and segmental infiltration.

  6. Therapy
  a. In the early stages of the disease, therapy must be individualized according to specific clinical manifestations.
    (1) Salt depletion is a potential problem in warmer climates.
    (2) Nutritional supplementation and pancreatic enzyme replacement often are indicated.

(3) Pulmonary infections may require hospitalization and vigorous treatment with parenteral antibiotics, hydration, humidification, and supplemental oxygen.

(4) Older children and adolescents have problems referable to the cardiopulmonary system, and most patients die from respiratory complications.

b. In the late stages of the disease, therapy is aimed at suppressing the infection with specific
antibiotics, inducing sputum through physical manipulation, and administering supplemental oxygen as required.

7. Complications

a. Cor pulmonale that is only partially responsive to oxygen therapy develops late in the disease, with all of the manifestations of right-sided heart failure (e.g., hepatomegaly and peripheral edema).

b. Pulmonary complications of cystic fibrosis often include hemoptysis and pneumothorax.

c. Many cystic fibrosis patients develop sinusitis and nasal polyps, and virtually all have clubbing of the digits.

C. Lung abscess

1. Definition. A lung abscess is a localized area of infection within the lung parenchyma, which
develops from an initial pneumonic stage. The center of the infected area first becomes gan-
grenous, necrotic, and purulent and then becomes well demarcated from the surrounding
lung tissue. The wall of the abscess becomes intensely inflamed and lined with fibrous and
granulation tissue and abundant blood vessels.

2. Etiology

a. A solitary lung abscess most commonly results from aspiration of secretions in the upper
respiratory tract.

b. Other major but less common causes include bronchial obstruction, bacterial pneumonia,
pulmonary embolism with infection, spread from transdiaphragmatic infections, chest
trauma, and bacteremic infection.

3. Clinical features

a. Initially, patients present with symptoms that are similar to those of acute pneumonia.

b. Chronically, however, lung abscess is associated with constitutional symptoms that include:

(1) Weight loss

(2) Low-grade fever

(3) Fatigue

(4) Malaise

4. Diagnosis

a. Physical examination may reveal relatively normal findings, although clubbing of the nail-
beds occasionally is noted. Amphoric breath sounds may be heard over the abscess cavity.

b. Pulmonary function testing usually is not affected by a lung abscess.

5. Therapy

a. The treatment of choice is antibiotics, either penicillin or clindamycin. The total duration
of therapy may be 4–8 weeks.

b. Bronchoscopy is indicated for patients whose abscesses do not resolve completely with
antibiotic therapy, for those who are suspected of having a foreign body, and for those
who are at high risk for developing cancer.

IV. ACUTE RESPIRATORY FAILURE

A. Definition. Acute respiratory failure is defined as **hypoxia** [i.e., arterial oxygen tension (PaO_2)
below 50 mm Hg)] with or without associated **hypercapnia** [i.e., arterial PCO_2 ($PaCO_2$) above 45
mm Hg].

B. Classification. Acute respiratory failure can be divided into two types.

1. Type I: respiratory failure without carbon dioxide retention (i.e., low PaO_2 with low or normal $PaCO_2$). This type of respiratory failure is characterized by marked ventilation-perfusion
abnormalities and intrapulmonary shunting. Type I respiratory failure occurs in such clinical
settings as:

a. Adult respiratory distress syndrome (see section V)

b. Diffuse pneumonia (viral and bacterial)

c. Aspiration pneumonitis

d. Fat embolism

e. Pulmonary edema

   2. Type II: respiratory failure with carbon dioxide retention (i.e., low PaO_2 with elevated $PaCO_2$). This type of respiratory failure has two basic physiologic abnormalities: ventilation-perfusion imbalance and inadequate alveolar ventilation. Patients with type II respiratory failure are divided into two categories.

     a. One category includes **patients with intrinsically normal lungs but inadequate ventilation** due to:

      (1) Disorders of respiratory control [e.g., drug overdose, central nervous system (CNS) disease, trauma, and cerebrovascular accident (CVA or stroke)]

      (2) Neuromuscular abnormalities (e.g., poliomyelitis, myasthenia gravis, and Guillain-Barré syndrome)

      (3) Chest wall trauma

     b. The other category includes **patients with intrinsic lung disease characterized by both ventilation-perfusion imbalance and inadequate alveolar ventilation**. Respiratory failure is precipitated by additional clinical insult, usually infection, which worsens the physiologic abnormalities. Examples of such lung diseases include:

      (1) COPD, chronic bronchitis, emphysema, and cystic fibrosis

      (2) Acute obstructive lung disease, asthma, and severe acute bronchitis

C. Pathophysiologic mechanisms of hypoxia

   1. Decreased inspired oxygen concentration. The most common cause of a lowered inspired oxygen concentration is high altitude.

   2. Ventilation-perfusion imbalance is the most common pathophysiologic cause of hypoxia. Hypoxia results when decreased alveolar ventilation occurs with respect to perfusion in the lung.

   3. Intrapulmonary shunt. Hypoxia resulting from a moderate decrease in the ventilation-perfusion relationship can be reversed with relatively small increases in the inspired oxygen concentration (i.e., 24%–40% inspired oxygen). However, ventilation approaches or is zero in the presence of an intrapulmonary shunt. Hypoxia due to a shunt frequently cannot be corrected even with 100% inspired oxygen.

   4. Abnormal diffusion. An abnormality in the diffusion of oxygen across the alveolar capillary membrane may contribute to hypoxia during exercise or in conditions of lowered inspired oxygen content. However, its contribution to respiratory failure, if any, is insignificant.

   5. Hypoventilation, with resulting hypercapnia, may contribute to hypoxia. This represents type II respiratory, or ventilatory, failure.

D. Therapy. In both forms of respiratory failure, therapy is directed toward the underlying diseases as well as the ventilatory and hypoxic components. In addition to these components, there is an acute and a chronic component to respiratory failure. Patients with chronic respiratory failure frequently can maintain lower PO_2 and higher PCO_2 than patients with acute respiratory failure.

   1. Treatment of type I respiratory failure is administration of high concentrations of inspired oxygen, which may be delivered by mask or nasal cannula. These high concentrations are safe to administer to patients with type I respiratory failure because there is no risk of carbon dioxide retention in these individuals.

   2. Treatment of type II respiratory failure depends upon recognition of its cause.

     a. In the common variety arising from exacerbations of COPD, the basis of therapy is controlled administration of oxygen (i.e., low-flow oxygen treatment).

     b. Type II respiratory failure that arises from causes other than COPD usually is an indication for mechanical ventilation.

V. ADULT RESPIRATORY DISTRESS SYNDROME

A. Definition. An important form of hypoxic respiratory failure is commonly called adult respiratory distress syndrome. The synonym, **wet lung**, emphasizes the increased extravascular lung water, which is the basic pathophysiologic mechanism of this condition.

B. Etiology. Adult respiratory distress syndrome can be initiated by many different events and conditions, including:

   1. Disseminated intravascular coagulation (DIC)

   2. Bacterial septicemia

   3. Trauma

4. Blood transfusion

5. Pancreatitis

6. Smoke inhalation

7. Heroin overdose

C. Pathogenesis and pathophysiology

    1. Adult respiratory distress syndrome is initiated by an insult to the capillary epithelium or alveolar endothelium, which results in capillary congestion and interstitial edema.

    2. This is followed by disruption of capillary integrity, with extravasation of fluid, fibrin, red cells, and white cells into the lung interstitium, lymphatics, and ultimately the alveoli.

    3. The severe hypoxia in this condition is caused by extreme ventilation-perfusion imbalance and shunting of blood in the fluid-filled areas of the lung.

    4. The lungs stiffen and become less compliant. This results in difficulty with mechanical ventilation and subsequent high peak airway pressures.

D. Clinical features. Symptoms may develop immediately after the insult but usually are delayed 24–48 hours.

    1. Progressive tachypnea usually is the earliest sign, followed by dyspnea.

    2. Physical findings often are absent or limited to bronchial breath sounds and rales.

    3. Chest x-ray shows patchy, diffuse, bilateral, fluffy infiltrates.

    4. Minute ventilation is increased and lung volumes are decreased when measured.

    5. Cardiac output usually is increased somewhat, although terminally it may decrease and be accompanied by metabolic acidosis and tissue hypoxia.

E. Therapy

    1. Oxygenation
        a. The ultimate goal of therapy is to provide adequate tissue oxygenation. Hypoxia can be corrected by maintaining the PaO_2 at about 60–80 mm Hg, which results in about a 90% oxygen saturation. In a patient with a normal cardiac output and hemoglobin level, the maintenance of a 90% saturation assures that tissue oxygen needs are met.
        b. Overall tissue oxygenation can be estimated by the **mixed venous oxygen content ($C\bar{v}O_2$)**. (The $C\bar{v}O_2$ actually is an average of overall tissue oxygen delivery.) In addition, concomitant measurement of cardiac output by thermodilution can aid in the correction of abnormal oxygen transport.

    2. Mechanical ventilation is required by most patients with acute respiratory failure. In patients with adult respiratory distress syndrome, **positive end-expiratory pressure (PEEP)** commonly is used to increase lung volume [i.e., **functional residual capacity (FRC)**] and to improve ventilation-perfusion relationships. PEEP usually is effective in reducing intrapulmonary shunt but may cause barotrauma or a reduction of cardiac output. In cases in which cardiac output is compromised, the PaO_2 increases but oxygen delivery may decrease. Therefore, it is important to measure **mixed venous PO_2 ($P\bar{v}O_2$)** and cardiac output when using PEEP. PEEP usually is not helpful in treating the respiratory failure of COPD.

    3. Other measures
        a. In addition to monitoring oxygenation and tissue oxygen delivery, the underlying disease process must be carefully and specifically treated.
        b. Alimentation, preferably through the gastrointestinal tract, should be begun in patients who require more than 24–48 hours of mechanical ventilation.

VI. COR PULMONALE

A. Definition. Cor pulmonale refers to a structural or functional alteration of the right ventricle as a result of pulmonary disease.

B. Etiology. Pulmonary disease does not affect the heart directly but leads to **pulmonary hypertension**, which may cause right ventricular dilatation, hypertrophy, and, eventually, failure. Pulmonary hypertension is the central controlling factor in the development of cor pulmonale.

C. Pathophysiologic mechanisms of pulmonary hypertension

1. **Hypoxia and acidosis.** The most potent stimulus for the development of pulmonary hypertension is the vasoconstrictive effect of hypoxia. Although the mechanism of this response is not clear, it may be augmented by acidosis, which also has a direct but less dramatic effect on the pulmonary vasculature.

    a. The vasoconstrictive effects of hypoxia and acidosis are believed to be of primary importance in the development of cor pulmonale in COPD patients.

    b. The most important aspect of hypoxic vasoconstriction is its potential to be reversed with increased concentrations of inspired oxygen.

2. A less common mechanism of pulmonary hypertension is **obliteration and obstruction of the pulmonary vascular bed**, such as is seen in recurrent pulmonary embolism and primary pulmonary vascular diseases (e.g., primary pulmonary hypertension and pulmonary fibrosis).

D. **Clinical course of cor pulmonale**

1. Although acute hypoxia elicits approximately the same pressor response, each bout of pulmonary hypertension predisposes to progressively higher levels of residual hypertension after recovery.

2. This leads to sustained pulmonary hypertension, which causes hypertrophy of the muscular pulmonary arteries and extension of the smooth muscle to the peripheral pulmonary vessels, resulting in a pulmonary vascular bed that is more rigid and less reactive to change in cardiac output than in a normal circulation.

3. This, in turn, affects the performance of the right ventricle, causing right ventricular hypertrophy and right-heart failure (cor pulmonale).

4. Early in the course, patients may demonstrate pulmonary hypertension only in association with exercise.

5. No firm evidence supports the claim that cor pulmonale causes left ventricular failure.

E. **Clinical features and diagnosis**

1. The **physical findings** of peripheral edema, liver enlargement, and neck vein engorgement usually are associated with cor pulmonale but are nonspecific and invalid except in advanced disease.

2. **Roentgenographic findings**, such as widening of the pulmonary arteries, are insensitive and unreliable indicators of pulmonary arterial pressure.

3. An **oxygen saturation** of less than 85% usually causes pulmonary arterial pressure to rise above 25 mm Hg. Acidosis and exercise cause further elevations.

4. **Electrocardiography.** The electrocardiogram (ECG) shows the appearance of flat or inverted T waves in the right ventricular precordial leads, right axis deviation of greater than 30° in the mean electrical axis of the QRS, transient ST depression of leads II, III, and aVF, and transient right bundle branch block.

5. **Cardiac catheterization** provides definitive diagnosis but rarely is necessary.

F. **Therapy.** Treatment and prevention of cor pulmonale are focused on correction of hypoxia and acidosis, control of hypervolemia, and improvement of right ventricular failure when it is present.

1. **Supplemental oxygen.** The obvious first step in treatment of cor pulmonale is administration of supplemental oxygen and improvement of ventilatory status by treatment of the underlying lung disease. Because many patients are oxygen-sensitive, it is imperative not to give high-flow oxygen but to give just enough to keep the saturation at approximately 90%.

2. **Diuretics.** Fluid retention is common and can compromise pulmonary gas exchange and heighten pulmonary vascular resistance. Improved oxygenation and salt restriction may be all that is needed, but diuretics frequently are necessary.

3. **Phlebotomy** provides a short-term effect and may be useful when hematocrit levels are greater than 55%–60%.

4. **Digitalis.** It is generally agreed that, unless left ventricular failure is associated with cor pulmonale, digitalis has no benefit.

5. **Vasodilators.** A variety of vasodilator agents have been used to treat cor pulmonale, especially when it is associated with obliterative vascular disease or fibrotic lung disease. Although a

few studies using calcium channel blockers have been promising, the practical value of these agents is unknown.

VII. PULMONARY EMBOLISM

A. Definition. In pulmonary embolism, a thrombus arises elsewhere in the body and migrates to the pulmonary vascular tree, where it causes obstruction. Rarely (e.g., in sickle cell disease), pulmonary arterial thrombosis occurs as a primary event without discernible clots elsewhere.

B. Incidence. Acute pulmonary embolism is a major cause of morbidity and mortality in the United States. Each year as many as 500,000 individuals sustain pulmonary emboli, an estimated 50,000 of whom die as a result. (This mortality figure has not changed during the past 20 years.)

C. Etiology

  1. Site of thrombus formation
   a. Stasis in the **iliofemoral venous system** with subsequent **deep venous thrombosis** is the most common precursor of pulmonary embolism.
     (1) In most cases, untreated venous thrombosis resolves spontaneously without causing clinical sequelae or disease.
     (2) Occasionally, however, repeated bouts of deep venous thrombosis may damage venous valves and lead to insufficiency, stasis, leg edema, and ulceration of the involved extremity, thus predisposing the patient to further episodes of thrombophlebitis and thrombosis.
     (3) Fifty percent of cases of deep venous thrombosis are complicated by pulmonary embolism.
   b. Other common sites of thrombus formation include the **prostatic and pelvic veins**.
   c. Except in drug abusers, pulmonary emboli generally do not originate in the **upper extremities**.

  2. Predisposing conditions
   a. Prolonged bed rest due to severe illness, trauma, or surgery is the most frequent clinical setting.
   b. Other predisposing conditions include:
     (1) Disturbances of flow causing venous stasis (e.g., cardiac failure, obesity, and pregnancy)
     (2) Disturbances of coagulation and thrombolysis (e.g., tumor, estrogen excess, and hemoglobinopathy)
     (3) Crises and vascular injuries (e.g., burns, soft tissue trauma, and vasculitis)
   c. Advancing age, diabetes mellitus, and peripheral arterial disease also contribute to an increased risk for pulmonary embolism.

  3. Precipitating factors. The factors that control the tethering of a thrombus to the wall of a vein and the dislodging of a thrombus into the circulation are not well understood. It is well known, however, that exercise and straining at defecation, with consequent changes in venous flow and pressure, are precipitating events.

D. Pathology

  1. Most pulmonary emboli are sterile, bland clots consisting primarily of platelets and fibrin. Those occurring with septic abortion or right-sided infective endocarditis may become infected. Autopsy studies indicate that pulmonary emboli undergo thrombolysis and organization in the same manner as other blood clots that occur in the circulation.

  2. When a thrombus is released from its site of origin, it is carried through the inferior vena cava and right ventricle to the pulmonary arteries, where it lodges. Large thrombi may be fragmented while passing through the heart or after lodging in a major pulmonary vessel.

  3. Pulmonary emboli may occur singly or multiply and vary in size from microscopic particles to large **saddle emboli** that completely block the major branches of the pulmonary artery.

  4. It is surmised that recurrent pulmonary emboli progressively occlude the pulmonary vascular bed and lead to chronic progressive pulmonary hypertension and, ultimately, cor pulmonale.

E. Pathophysiology. Regardless of the source of the embolus, once it lodges in the pulmonary vascular bed, a uniform pathophysiologic disturbance occurs. The mechanical, reflexive, and humoral components of this disturbance are categorized as either **hemodynamic** or **pulmonary** consequences of pulmonary embolism.

1. Hemodynamic consequences
   a. The magnitude of hemodynamic consequences is determined by the state of the underlying cardiopulmonary circulation and the severity of the embolism.
   (1) In **massive pulmonary embolism** (i.e., when more than 50%–60% of the pulmonary perfusion is impeded), severe pulmonary hypertension, right ventricular strain, and cardiac failure ensue and are manifest as cyanosis, peripheral venous engorgement, and hepatic congestion.
   (2) In **submassive pulmonary embolism**, less profound hemodynamic changes are produced. These changes may be transient, so that hypotension, tachycardia, and hypoxia may not be noted at the time of initial examination.
   (3) Less than 10% of cases of pulmonary embolism progress to pulmonary infarction (i.e., lung tissue death) because the lung parenchyma has three sources of oxygen (i.e., the airways, the bronchial circulation, and the pulmonary circulation).
   b. It is strongly suspected that neurocirculatory reflexes and humoral substances (e.g., histamine, serotonin, and prostaglandins) are involved in episodes of pulmonary embolism.

2. Pulmonary (mechanical) consequences
   a. The pulmonary consequences of embolism primarily result in ventilation-perfusion mismatch.
   (1) "**Dead space**" or "**wasted**" **ventilation** occurs in those lung segments in which vascular supply is obstructed by emboli.
   (2) Conversely, **overperfusion and diminished vascular resistance** in the remaining lung segments cause profound physiologic right-to-left intrapulmonary shunting, with inadequate oxygenation of a large portion of perfused blood.
   b. Other pulmonary responses include congestive atelectasis of the ischemic segment of the lung, reflex bronchiolar constriction and vascular constriction, and the loss or malfunction of alveolar surfactant.

F. Diagnosis

1. Physical examination
   a. Auscultation reveals percussion dullness and decreased breath sounds over the involved base but usually normal findings over the remaining lung segments. Occasionally, a pleural friction rub is heard; wheezes are heard less commonly.
   b. Evidence of deep venous thrombosis is noted in 50% of patients. Evidence of cor pulmonale is seen only in massive pulmonary embolism.

2. Chest x-ray results are normal in most patients with pulmonary embolism. When they are abnormal, the results usually include plate-like atelectasis, a unilaterally high diaphragm, and a small pleural effusion of hemorrhagic fluid that ranges from a clear yellow transudate to an exudate. Other, occasional findings include a bulging pulmonary artery, a wedge-shaped pleural-based density, and a large oligemic lung segment.

3. Electrocardiography. The ECG usually is not specific but may help to support the diagnosis of embolism and to exclude myocardial infarction.
   a. The most common finding is sinus tachycardia with or without premature atrial and ventricular contractions. The mean P axis commonly shifts to the right.
   b. Other electrocardiographic findings usually are due to right ventricular strain and include intermittent right bundle branch block, P pulmonale, an abnormal S wave in lead I, an abnormal Q wave in lead III, and marked clockwise rotation of the ECG.

4. Blood gas analysis
   a. Most patients with pulmonary embolism have some degree of hypoxia; however, a normal PO_2 does not rule out pulmonary embolism. A more sensitive indicator of abnormal gas exchange is the **alveolar-arterial PO_2 gradient**; a normal gradient essentially rules out pulmonary embolism.
   b. Often the PCO_2 is low and the pH is slightly elevated, causing a mild acute respiratory alkalosis.

5. Pulmonary scanning
   a. The results of **perfusion lung scanning** must be correlated with the patient's clinical picture and with the chest x-ray results. Scanning abnormalities are not always diagnostic of pulmonary embolism; however, normal results virtually exclude the diagnosis.
   b. **Xenon ventilation scanning** often is performed in conjunction with perfusion scanning to decrease the instances of nondiagnostic results and to correlate areas that have matching defects of both perfusion and ventilation (the finding in parenchymal lung disease but not in pulmonary embolism).

    c. Diagnostic accuracy may be increased by obtaining ventilation and perfusion scans in four positions and then comparing scanning results with concurrent chest x-ray results.

    d. Scanning results frequently are divided into low, moderate, and high **probability** of pulmonary embolism. The probability of the scan must be evaluated in light of the clinical situation.

  6. Pulmonary angiography is considered the standard test for the diagnosis of pulmonary embolism and is unequivocally diagnostic if emboli are visualized. It is the author's belief that pulmonary angiography should be performed in all cases in which the ventilation and perfusion scans are equivocal or the risk of long-term anticoagulation is greater than usual.

  7. Further diagnostic methods. When the diagnosis of pulmonary embolism remains in question despite many diagnostic studies, corroborative evidence of venous disease in the lower extremities is sought.

    a. The **noninvasive methods** of impedance plethysmography, radioiodine fibrinogen leg and thigh scanning, and Doppler ultrasonography have been developed to demonstrate stasis and thrombosis in leg veins. In addition to producing a significant proportion of false-positive results, these techniques cannot be used to evaluate pelvic veins.

    b. The **invasive technique** of contrast venography evaluates the veins of the pelvis, thigh, and leg and is helpful in the diagnosis of venous occlusion. This diagnostic method is not without morbidity, however, and has been associated with phlebitis, hypersensitivity reactions, and local pain.

G. Therapy

  1. Anticoagulants

    a. Unless contraindicated, the specific acute treatment for documented or suspected pulmonary embolism is **heparin**. Although the preferred regimen is continuous intravenous administration, intermittent bolus injections or subacute heparin may be effective. Heparin should be given to maintain the **partial thromboplastin time (PTT)** at 2 to 2½ times the normal value.

    b. After anticoagulation with heparin has been achieved for a few days, the patient can be switched to oral **warfarin** to maintain the **prothrombin time (PT)** at 2 to 2½ times the normal value. Heparin then can be discontinued and the oral anticoagulants continued for 6–8 weeks. **Oxygen** is given routinely to correct hypoxia, and **bed rest** ordinarily is prescribed until the dyspnea and pain resolve, after which patients can ambulate while remaining on anticoagulant therapy.

  2. Thrombolytic agents. Streptokinase is superior to heparin, in that it causes substantial and rapid lysis of clots in most patients. The present data suggest that long-term physiologic improvement occurs in the pulmonary vascular bed of patients treated with thrombolytic agents. The long- and short-term mortality rates are unchanged, however.

  3. Surgery

    a. Inferior vena caval ligation, clipping, and plication and, more recently, percutaneous "umbrella" insertion are surgical remedies for pulmonary embolism, which preclude embolic recurrence for finite periods of time. All of these procedures produce only short-term results, with modest morbidity. Patients with chronic vena caval obstruction may develop venous channels or collaterals in the pelvis or lower abdomen, which may find routes around the obstruction to the pulmonary artery, eventually negating the effectiveness of the procedure.

    b. Vena caval occlusion should be reserved for the following groups of patients:

      (1) Patients in whom embolism occurs despite anticoagulation with heparin

      (2) Patients who have the syndrome of recurrent pulmonary embolism despite chronic anticoagulation

      (3) Patients in whom heparin is contraindicated (e.g., patients with active bleeding)

    c. Embolectomy remains an alternative treatment for patients in whom effective cardiac output cannot be maintained. Embolectomy, which on occasion is lifesaving, has a survival rate of about 10%.

  4. Prevention of pulmonary embolism in high-risk patients has received much recent attention. The efficacy and safety of prophylactic **minidose heparin** have been thoroughly documented. The regimen customarily is subcutaneous heparin given 2 hours prior to surgery and continued—at a dosage of 5000 units every 12 hours—until the patient is ambulatory.

    a. Prophylactic minidose heparin therapy is particularly applicable for older patients who undergo lower abdominal or pelvic surgery and who are at bed rest postoperatively. It also is recommended for obese patients and for patients at prolonged bed rest from stroke, myocardial infarction, cardiac failure, and cancer. There is little risk of hemorrhage in these circumstances.

b. Minidose heparin has not been shown to be effective for major orthopedic, prostatic, ocular, and neurosurgical procedures.

VIII. DISEASES OF THE PLEURA

A. Introduction

1. In health, the pleural cavity contains a small volume of thin serous fluid that acts as a lubricant during inflation and deflation of the lung. This fluid is formed mostly by transudation from the parietal pleural surface, and water and small molecules are absorbed primarily by the capillary bed of the visceral pleura. Protein, particulate matter, and debris are removed by the lymphatics of the parietal pleura and are returned to the circulation via the thoracic duct.

2. The balance between the formation and removal of this fluid may be compromised by any disorder that causes partial or complete obstruction of the lymphatic circulation, by a rise in the pulmonary or systemic venous pressure, or by a decrease in the plasma oncotic pressure.

B. Pleural effusion

1. **Definition.** A pleural effusion is an abnormal accumulation of fluid in the pleural space.

2. **Etiology**
   a. **Noninflammatory pleural effusions** may occur in any condition that causes ascites, obstruction of the venous or lymphatic outflow from the thorax, or isolated left- or right-sided congestive heart failure. In addition, a severe reduction in the plasma protein concentration may contribute to the accumulation of noninflammatory pleural fluid.
   b. **Inflammatory pleural effusions** result from inflammation of structures adjacent to the pleural surface. The site of inflammation usually is just beneath the visceral pleura within the lung but occasionally is within the mediastinum, diaphragm, or chest wall. Removal of this fluid by the normal clearing mechanisms may be considerably retarded by the presence of inflammatory obstruction of the lymphatics that drain the thorax. Secondary inflammation of larger areas of the pleural surface may result in rapid outpouring of exudate.

3. **Clinical features**
   a. **Symptoms** of pleural effusions are associated with inflammation of the parietal pleura and compression of the lung.
      (1) **Pleuritic pain** is encountered most commonly in conditions that produce an inflammatory effusion, and often it is accompanied by a friction rub.
         (a) The pain commonly is characterized as a sharp, stabbing sensation that is absent or minimal during quiet respiration but appears or is intensified abruptly during full inflation of the lungs.
         (b) Pleuritic pain should be differentiated from the pain of rib fracture, costochondritis, compression of intercostal nerve roots, herpes zoster, acute bronchitis, and various cardiovascular and esophageal conditions.
      (2) **Dyspnea.** The accumulation of pleural fluid, with the resulting compression of the lung and interference with the movement of the diaphragm, may result in dyspnea.
   b. **Physical signs.** Accumulation of fluid usually occurs first at the base of the lung, where the earliest physical signs are noted.
      (1) Auscultation usually reveals a dull-to-flat percussion over the area of the effusion as well as reduced-to-absent breath sounds in this region. An area of **bronchial breathing** sometimes is heard over the adjacent compressed lung and may be accompanied by an altered voice quality or frank **egophony**.
      (2) The mediastinum usually shifts away from the side of a large effusion unless either the mediastinum has become fixed in position by a tumor or a portion of the lung on the infected side has become completely atelectatic.
   c. **Radiographic appearance.** The earliest signs of effusion that can be appreciated on plain chest x-ray are blunting of the costophrenic angle and indistinct demarcation of the posterior portion of the diaphragm in the lateral view.
      (1) Posterior-anterior roentgenography may show no abnormality in the presence of less than 300 ml of pleural fluid. The lateral decubitus film may help to differentiate free fluid from previous inflammatory adhesions.
      (2) The use of diagnostic ultrasonography may help to localize the effusion more accurately when complete removal by thoracentesis is difficult.

4. **Diagnosis.** Unless an etiology has been established, the presence of fluid in the pleural cavity is an indication for thoracentesis. The fluid should be removed, the gross appearance should be noted, and specimens should be sent to the laboratory for examination.
   a. Routine laboratory procedures include measurement of the **total protein** and **lactate dehy-**

drogenase **(LDH)** content and examination of the spun specimen for cells. Further information can be gained by appropriate bacteriologic and cytologic examination. Under certain circumstances, it is necessary to analyze the fluid for glucose, amylase, and pH. In cases in which an inflammatory effusion is known or suspected to be present, **needle biopsy** may be performed at the time of initial thoracentesis.
   b. When ordinary measures fail to establish a definitive diagnosis and needle biopsy of the pleura is negative, **thoracotomy** with exploration of the lung and biopsy of the involved areas of the pleural surface may be essential for accurate diagnosis.

5. **Differential diagnosis.** In determining the etiology of a pleural effusion, it is useful to establish whether the fluid is a **transudate** or an **exudate**.
   a. Pathology
      (1) Transudates are caused by elevated systemic or pulmonary venous pressure or by decreased plasma oncotic pressure; the primary pathologic process does not directly involve the pulmonary surface. Common causes of transudates include congestive heart failure and nephrotic syndrome.
      (2) Exudates are caused by inflammation or disease of the pleural surface or by lymphatic obstruction. Common causes of exudates include tuberculosis, bronchogenic carcinoma, pneumonia, pulmonary infarction, lymphoma, metastatic tumor, trauma, and abdominal surgery. Less common causes include pancreatitis, collagen vascular diseases, asbestos-related pleural effusions, and hypothyroidism.
   b. Composition
      (1) Most transudates have a **protein content** of less than 3 g/dl, whereas exudates usually have a protein content of more than 3 g/dl.
      (2) A more reliable comparison can be made on the basis of **LDH content**, the pleural fluid-to-serum protein ratio, and the pleural fluid-to-serum LDH ratio. The following laboratory data indicate the presence of an exudate:
         (a) A high LDH content
         (b) A pleural fluid-to-serum LDH ratio of greater than 0.6
         (c) A pleural fluid-to-serum protein ratio of greater than 0.5
      (3) The presence of **gross blood** in the pleural fluid is most common when the effusion is due to tumor, trauma, or pulmonary infarction.
      (4) Pleural fluid **glucose** rarely is significantly lower than serum glucose when the effusion is caused by tuberculosis or tumor but usually is very low in effusions that are due to rheumatoid arthritis.
      (5) Moderate elevation of pleural fluid **amylase** occasionally is seen in malignant effusions; amylase levels are elevated more frequently when the effusion is due to pancreatic disease or rupture of the esophagus.
   c. pH. The pH of pleural fluid usually is 7.3 or greater; lower values occasionally are seen in tuberculosis and malignant effusions. A pH of less than 7.2 in a parapneumonic effusion often is associated with an **empyema**.

6. **Therapy.** Effective management requires that the etiology of the effusion be established so that specific treatment can be applied.
   a. In **transudative pleural effusions**, the underlying disease process must be treated, with thoracentesis occasionally used to treat symptoms.
   b. In **exudative pleural effusions**, the underlying etiology must be sought to determine the proper therapy, that is, chest tube placement, antituberculous therapy, or repeated thoracentesis and subsequent pleurodesis with chemotherapeutic agents.

C. Empyema

1. **Definition and description.** An empyema is an accumulation of pus in the pleural space; it is an occasional complication of both bacterial pneumonia and lung abscess. The fluid usually is thick and has the appearance of frank pus. As previously stated, pleural fluid with a pH below 7.2 strongly suggests an empyema.

2. **Therapy.** An empyema almost always requires chest tube drainage as well as effective antibiotic therapy. After several days without adequate drainage, most empyemas become loculated, so that tube drainage is not effective and rib resection is necessary to allow open drainage.

D. Pneumothorax

1. **Definition and description.** Pneumothorax is an accumulation of air or gas in the pleural space.
   a. Pneumothorax is a common medical problem. The most common type, **spontaneous**

pneumothorax, occurs with the rupture of bullae in the upper lobes. It occurs more frequently in men than in women and is most common in individuals who are 20–40 years of age.

b. Pneumothorax also may occur secondary to lung involvement in many diseases, such as tuberculosis, trauma, malignancy, emphysema, histiocytosis X, interstitial pneumonitis and fibrosis, and pulmonary infarction.

2. **Clinical features.** The major symptoms of pneumothorax are **pain** and **dyspnea**. The pain may be either sharp and severe or mild and dull.

3. **Diagnosis**
   a. **Physical examination** reveals hyperresonance and decreased breath sounds over the involved side.
   b. **A film taken during expiration** may help to demonstrate small pneumothoraces as this technique increases the contrast between the lung and the pleural space.

4. **Therapy**
   a. Treatment of an episode of spontaneous pneumothorax involves reexpansion of the lung via placement of an intercostal chest tube and application of appropriate negative pressure. The treatment is continued for 24–48 hours after the lung is reexpanded with the hope that the pleural space will seal and that pleural adhesions will prevent recurrence.
   b. Spontaneous pneumothorax has a tendency to recur. There are no firm guidelines for treatment of recurrences; however, surgical treatment should be considered at the time of a third pneumothorax on a given side. Therapy involves an open thoracotomy and abrasion of the pleural surfaces, which produces symphysis of the parietal and visceral pleurae.

5. **Complications.** Although pneumothorax is regarded as a relatively benign condition, serious complications can result.
   a. **Bilateral simultaneous pneumothorax** is rare but can cause prompt death.
   b. Pneumothorax may be accompanied by hemorrhage into the pleural space, which results in **hemopneumothorax**.
   c. **Tension pneumothorax** is another complication, which rapidly produces severe respiratory embarrassment.
      (1) Tension pneumothorax presumably occurs due to a valvular mechanism at the site of the air leak, which allows air to move progressively from the lung into the pleural space.
      (2) This leads to progressive collapse of the lung, shift of the mediastinal structures away from the involved side, and impairment of the contralateral lung function as well as cardiovascular function. Prompt decompression of the involved pleural space is indicated.

E. **Chylothorax.** When the thoracic duct is lacerated or interrupted by trauma or obstructed by tumor, lymph may accumulate in the pleural space. This condition, termed chylothorax, is identified by a murky appearance of the fluid, demonstration of fat droplets on staining with Sudan III, and a total neutral fat content of more than 0.5 g/dl.

F. **Primary pleural neoplasia**

1. **Localized fibrous mesothelioma.** This uncommon tumor arises from the pleural surface and most commonly is attached to the visceral pleura.
   a. **Symptoms**
      (1) The lesion may cause chest discomfort and dyspnea if it becomes very large; however, most tumors are discovered before these symptoms develop.
      (2) The syndrome of **hypertrophic pulmonary osteoarthropathy**, which is associated with **arthralgia** involving the hands, ankles, wrists, and knees and with **clubbing of the fingers**, may occur secondary to pleural-based tumors.
   b. **Diagnosis.** The chest x-ray reveals a mass lesion; a pleural effusion occasionally is present.
   c. **Therapy** is surgical resection, which also relieves the symptoms of the hypertrophic pulmonary osteoarthropathy.
   d. **Prognosis.** Most of these tumors are benign on pathologic examination, and patients have an excellent prognosis. A few of these tumors are malignant, but with favorable courses.

2. **Diffuse malignant mesothelioma**
   a. **Incidence.** This malignant tumor occurs over a wide age range, with the average patient age at onset being 55 years. The incidence of this tumor is increased in workers who have been exposed to asbestos; generally, the malignancy develops 20 or more years after exposure.
   b. **Symptoms.** Chest pain and dyspnea are the predominant symptoms.

    c. Diagnosis. The diagnosis is difficult to establish by cytologic examination; open pleural biopsy frequently is necessary. The chest x-ray may reveal pleural thickening, pleural effusion, or both.

    d. Therapy involves radiotherapy or chemotherapy, the results of which are uniformly dismal.

IX. PULMONARY NEOPLASMS

A. Introduction

1. Pulmonary neoplasms may be benign or malignant. Benign lung tumors are scarce in comparison with malignant tumors and include such neoplasms as hamartomas, lipomas, and papillomas. Malignant lung tumors may be **primary**—arising from cells in the bronchi, lung parenchyma, or pleura—or **metastatic**—reaching the lung via the bloodstream or lymphatics or by direct invasion.

2. Of the various primary pulmonary neoplasms, the most common by far is **bronchogenic carcinoma.** The term "bronchogenic carcinoma" commonly is used to designate nearly all types of malignant lung tumors and in this chapter is used interchangeably with "lung cancer."

B. Incidence.
In the United States, bronchogenic carcinoma is the number-one cause of cancer-related deaths in men and soon may overtake breast and colon cancers as the leading cause of cancer deaths in women. It is the only common cancer that is associated with steadily increasing mortality rates. (The annual mortality rate for men, which was approximately 5 per 100,000 in 1935, rose to 54 per 100,000 by 1975.)* Presently in the United States, the lung cancer mortality rate approaches 100,000 individuals per year and has a male-to-female ratio of about 3.5 to 1. Lung cancer usually appears between the sixth and seventh decades of life and rarely occurs before the age of 35 years.

C. Etiology

1. **Cigarette smoking**
   a. In virtually all populations studied, death from lung cancer has been shown to be strongly associated with cigarette smoking. Indeed, it is the major etiologic factor in 80%–85% of all bronchogenic cancers.
      (1) Although all histologic types of bronchogenic carcinoma are associated with cigarette smoking, squamous cell carcinomas and small cell differentiated (oat cell) carcinomas are most strongly associated. Adenocarcinomas, which once were weakly associated with this habit, recently have been shown to have a definite link with cigarette smoking.
      (2) The incidence of lung cancer is linearly related to the quantity of tobacco smoked.
   b. In addition to nicotine, carbon monoxide, noxious gases, and particulate matter, cigarette smoke yields tars that contain **carcinogens** (e.g., benzpyrene) as well as other compounds recognized as **cocarcinogens.**

2. **Occupational exposure**
   a. Occupational exposure to asbestos fibers and to radioactive gases—especially radon 222 in the mining of uranium-containing ores—has been linked to an increased incidence of lung cancer.
   b. Similarly, coke-oven workers and individuals exposed to arsenic, beryllium, chromates, nickel, zinc, and chloromethyl ether have an increased risk for developing lung cancer.

3. **Air pollution** may play a small part in the risk for developing lung cancer as the mortality rates for lung cancer are higher among urban dwellers than among rural inhabitants.

4. **Other factors**
   a. **Preexisting lung damage.** Several studies have indicated that scars within the lungs and diffuse pulmonary fibrosis are associated with a slightly increased incidence of lung cancer.
   b. **Genetic influences** also may play a part in host susceptibility to the development of lung cancer.

D. Pathology.
Most pulmonary neoplasms are carcinomas. Four major cell types of bronchogenic carcinoma are recognized; mixed cell types also are noted. The four major histologic varieties

---

*Data taken from Sartwell PE and Last JM: Epidemiology. In *Public Health and Preventive Medicine*, 11th ed. Edited by Maxcy KF and Rosenau MJ. New York, Appleton-Century-Crofts, 1980, p 23.

are discussed below in terms of their comparative incidence, site of origin, and growth and metastatic characteristics.

1. **Squamous cell carcinomas** account for about 35%–40% of lung cancers. Squamous carcinomas arise proximally, most often in the upper lobes and usually in the main stem lobar segmental bronchi. These tumors grow rather slowly; it takes approximately 5 years for a squamous cell cancer to reach 2 cm in diameter. Squamous carcinomas tend to metastasize late in their course.

2. **Adenocarcinomas** (including **bronchiolo-alveolar carcinomas**) account for 30% of lung cancers. Adenocarcinomas tend to arise more peripherally than squamous cell carcinomas and grow even more slowly; it takes 9 years for an adenocarcinoma to reach 2 cm in diameter. These tumors metastasize relatively early in their course. Bronchiolo-alveolar carcinomas sometimes have a multicentric origin.

3. **Small cell undifferentiated (oat cell) carcinomas** account for 25% of lung cancers. These tumors also arise more peripherally than squamous cell cancers, and they grow much more rapidly. By the time the diagnosis is made, it is felt that micrometastasis is well established.

4. **Large cell undifferentiated carcinomas** account for 5% of lung cancers. These tumors occur more centrally and tend to metastasize early in their course.

E. **Clinical features**

1. **Early presentations**
   a. **Symptoms.** Most patients have pulmonary symptoms, constitutional (systemic) symptoms, symptoms of metastatic spread, or a combination of these. The most common symptom is an **increase or change in the nature of a chronic cough**. Mild **hemoptysis** occurs less frequently. **Pneumonia** and **pleurisy** also may occur.
   b. **Signs.** Physical examination of the chest may be normal or—depending on the behavior of the underlying tumor—may show signs of **pleural effusion**, **atelectasis**, or **consolidation**.

2. **Late presentations.** Once a primary pulmonary neoplasm has spread beyond the lung, a patient may present with a host of diverse symptoms.
   a. **Symptoms of tumor spread within the chest**
      (1) Pleuritic pain with dyspnea suggests that the tumor has invaded the pleura and caused a pleural effusion.
      (2) Persistent local chest pain over one or two ribs suggests invasion of the ribs.
      (3) Hoarseness may indicate involvement of the left recurrent laryngeal nerve.
      (4) A bloated feeling in the head and neck accompanied by swelling of the arms, neck, and face is consistent with the diagnosis of superior vena caval obstruction due to tumor extension into the mediastinum.
      (5) Dysphagia suggests malignant invasion or compression of the esophagus.
      (6) **Pancoast's syndrome** occurs with tumors in the apex of the lung and is characterized by pain in the ipsilateral shoulder. As the pain worsens it may spread down the inner part of the arm and be accompanied by numbness and weakness. **Horner's syndrome** [i.e., ptosis, pupil constriction, (occasionally) anhidrosis, and (more rarely) enophthalmus] also may develop.
   b. **Symptoms of tumor spread outside the chest**
      (1) An enlarged lymph node in the neck may be the first sign of a bronchial carcinoma.
      (2) Bone pain in the back, pelvis, or ribs—due to bony metastasis—also may be the first manifestation.
      (3) Convulsions and other neurologic signs may occur due to cerebral metastasis.
   c. **Nonmetastatic, systemic symptoms**
      (1) **Neurologic syndromes** that have been described in association with bronchogenic carcinoma include cerebellar degeneration, peripheral neuropathies, and the myasthenia-like **Eaton-Lambert syndrome**.
      (2) **Endocrinopathies** also are recognized in association with bronchogenic carcinoma, especially small cell varieties. These tumors produce hormones and hormone-like substances, giving rise to the syndrome of inappropriate secretion of antidiuretic hormone (SIADH), Cushing's syndrome, carcinoid syndrome, gynecomastia, and secretion of parathyroid hormone–like substances.
      (3) **Other presentations**
         (a) **Myositis** sometimes is associated with bronchogenic carcinoma, and a rare skin disorder, **acanthosis nigricans**, may coexist.
         (b) **Digital clubbing** is noted in about one-third of lung cancer patients.
         (c) **Pulmonary hypertrophic osteoarthropathy** almost always is associated with carcinoma of the bronchus and is characterized by digital clubbing as well as pain, ten-

derness, and swelling (commonly) around the wrists and (uncommonly) around the knees and ankles.

F. Diagnosis

1. Chest x-ray

  a. Radiographically, neoplasms may present as a solitary pulmonary nodule or, more commonly, as multiple nodules ranging in size from micronodules to well-defined masses.

  b. Lymphatic spread to the lungs usually is seen at the bases and appears as a coarse reticulo-nodular pattern on the x-ray.

  c. Cavitation is noted in some neoplastic lesions.

2. Sputum cytology is an effective method of establishing the diagnosis, particularly if the lesion is proximal or endobronchial.

3. Percutaneous needle aspiration of peripheral tumors usually is done under the guidance of fluoroscopy or CT. Although it is a reliable cytologic method, tissue core cannot be obtained by percutaneous needle aspiration. Pneumothorax, a complication that occurs in up to 25% of patients, requires a chest tube in only half of these cases.

4. Biopsy. Diagnosis is made most definitely by tissue biopsy, which can be either an open-lung or transbronchial procedure. If patients have palpable lymph nodes, these also can be biopsied.

G. Therapy. There are several approaches to the treatment of bronchogenic carcinoma.

1. Surgery remains the most effective therapy for bronchogenic carcinoma.

  a. One exception is patients with small cell anaplastic carcinoma, for whom treatment consists of chemo- and radiotherapy. Curative surgery can be attempted in only about 15% of such cases, but the 5-year survival rate for these patients is 40%.

  b. In addition, surgery should not be considered in any patient with evidence of metastatic disease, such as pleural effusion, vocal cord paralysis, Horner's syndrome, superior vena caval syndrome, or tumor spread to the brain, bone, liver, or skin.

  c. Pulmonary dysfunction (i.e., inadequate FEV_1) also precludes surgery.

2. Radiotherapy usually is used as a palliative measure. Traditionally, radiotherapy has been used to treat hemoptysis, cough, obstructive pneumonia, and pain. Squamous cell carcinoma is more radiosensitive than the other non–oat cell lung cancers.

3. Chemotherapy has been extremely disappointing except in some cases of oat cell carcinoma. Most squamous cell carcinomas show little or no response, and adenocarcinomas are almost uniformly unresponsive.

4. Immunotherapy. Many studies suggest that cellular immunity is impaired in patients with lung cancer. Because of this, attempts have been made to bolster the immune defense of patients using bacille Calmette-Guérin (BCG) vaccine and other nonspecific antigens. There has been no definitive improvement noted with this treatment; however, experimental clinical studies continue.

5. Other measures

  a. Analgesics and appropriate radiotherapy can be used palliatively in patients with advanced disease.

  b. Antibiotics sometimes are useful for obstructive pneumonia, and the new technique of neodymium: YAG laser therapy recently has been used for special cases of tracheobronchial obstruction.

  c. Recurrent pleural effusion may be improved by injection of sclerosing agents into the pleural space.

H. Prognosis depends on the extent of spread at the time of diagnosis and the nature of the tumor. The overall 5-year survival rate for all patients with bronchogenic carcinoma is approximately 10%. Patients with early stage I disease may have survival rates of up to 40%–50%. All cell types of bronchogenic carcinoma are associated with similar mortality rates, with the exception of small cell carcinoma, which is associated with higher death rates.

X. CHEST WALL DISORDERS

A. Introduction. Chest wall disorders are both **mechanical** and **neuromuscular** in origin. They may cause respiratory dysfunction and, in severe cases, respiratory failure.

1. **Mechanical disorders** affecting the chest wall include scoliosis, obesity-associated hypoventilation, fibrothorax, thoracoplasty, ankylosing spondylitis, and chest wall trauma.

2. **Neuromuscular diseases** affecting the chest wall are polyneuropathies, motor system diseases, muscular dystrophies, spinal cord injuries, multiple sclerosis, and myasthenia gravis.

B. **Kyphoscoliosis**, the most common and best understood chest wall disease, is used here as a prototype for discussing the natural history, pathophysiology, and management of all of these disorders.

1. **Definition.** Kyphoscoliosis is a disorder characterized by posterior curvature (**kyphosis**) and lateral curvature (**scoliosis**) of the spine. These processes alone and in combination decrease the volume and mobility of the lung and chest wall.

2. **Incidence**
   a. Kyphoscoliosis is a common skeletal abnormality that affects 1% of the United States population and occurs predominantly in females. The prevalence of clinically significant deformity (i.e., an angle of greater than 10°) is 23 in 1000 individuals.
   b. The etiology of kyphoscoliosis is not clear in 80% of cases. A major known cause is childhood **poliomyelitis**. Congenital abnormalities with or without bone defects are uncommon.

3. **Pathophysiology**
   a. Derangement of lung function in kyphoscoliosis predominantly results from reduced lung volume, which is caused by stiffness of the chest wall (reduced compliance) and reduction of FRC. The pressure-volume curve of the lung is nearly normal, but the chest wall is displaced downward and to the right, thus decreasing total respiratory compliance. Forced expiratory flow is preserved relative to lung volume.
   b. Gas exchange usually is preserved until alveolar hypoventilation occurs. Mild widening of the alveolar-arterial PO_2 gradient is seen and is the result of ventilation-perfusion inequality due to the compressive effect of atelectasis and inadequate periodic hyperinflation.
   c. Pulmonary hypertension eventually is present at rest as well as during exercise with moderate chest wall deformity and in the absence of clinical signs of cardiac dysfunction.

4. **Clinical features and diagnosis**
   a. **Symptoms**
      (1) **Exertional dyspnea** is the outstanding respiratory symptom of kyphoscoliosis. The onset and severity of dyspnea correlate with the degree of the spinal angulation.
         (a) Patients with a deformity of less than 70° have no respiratory symptoms.
         (b) Patients whose deformity exceeds 70° have a risk of becoming symptomatic.
         (c) Dyspnea is the rule in patients with a deformity of more than 100°, and hypoventilation supervenes in those whose deformity exceeds 120°.
      (2) **Bronchitic symptoms** are unusual in the absence of chronic bronchitis or atelectasis.
      (3) Sequelae of prolonged arterial hypoxia may develop, including pulmonary hypertension, right ventricular dysfunction, and cor pulmonale. These are late manifestations.
   b. **Radiographic appearance.** The degree of kyphoscoliosis is determined by measuring the angle formed by converging line segments drawn on the upper and lower limbs of the primary curves. Ribs on the convex portion of the spine are widely spaced and rotated posteriorly, causing a characteristic hump. Ribs on the concave aspect are crowded and displaced anteriorly and encroach on the apex of the secondary curve.

5. **Therapy.** Early identification of kyphoscoliosis in adolescence is the key to prevention of symptomatic disease. Therapeutic intervention is considered in cases in which the angulation is greater than 40°. There are two forms of intervention.
   a. A mechanical device (e.g., the **Milwaukee brace**) can be applied externally during the early stages of the disease.
   b. An operative procedure (e.g., the **Harrington procedure**) can be performed using metallic rods and focal spinal fusion, after which the patient wears a plaster-of-Paris jacket cast for several months. Surgery does not improve the maximal breathing capacity but may improve arterial oxygen and oxygen desaturation. At best, surgery appears to preserve whatever pulmonary function is present at the time of intervention.

6. **Complications. Respiratory failure** and **cor pulmonale** are the major complications of kyphoscoliosis. These conditions result from respiratory infection and ventilatory suppression by uncontrolled oxygen therapy and sedatives. **Periodic hyperinflation** with positive or negative pressure devices appears to increase lung compliance and PO_2 in outpatients.

C. **Chest trauma**

1. **Blunt trauma**

a. Blunt chest trauma causes injury either by direct application of sudden force to the chest wall and indirect transmission of these forces to the intrathoracic structures or by secondary visceral destruction by chest wall structures.

b. Injury of extrapulmonary organs often accompanies blunt chest trauma. Disruption of the chest wall may cause rib fractures, hemothorax, pneumothorax, and flail chest. Inertial injury may cause rupture of the bronchial, diaphragmatic, or great blood vessels.

c. Flail chest most commonly results from motor vehicle injury or overzealous cardiac resuscitation. The chest wall, or at least one hemithorax, is rendered unstable by multiple fractures of the ribs, sternum, or costochondral joints. The injured portion moves paradoxically, that is, inward on inspiration as the intrapleural pressure becomes subatmospheric and outward on expiration as the intrapleural pressure increases toward atmospheric. Respiratory failure is treated with volume-cycled mechanical ventilation, pain control, and oxygen supplementation.

2. Penetrating trauma is characterized by puncture or laceration of the chest wall and intrathoracic fistulae. Knife and missile wounds are the usual causes. Exploratory thoracotomies are indicated for persistent hemothorax and sucking chest wounds and to determine the likelihood of mediastinal, diaphragmatic, or cardiac disruption.

XI. MEDIASTINAL DISEASES

A. Mediastinal masses. The mediastinum is divided into three parts: the **superior mediastinum**, the **anterior and middle mediastinum**, and the **posterior mediastinum**. Mediastinal masses can occur at any age and are characteristically associated with the mediastinal compartment in which they occur. The lateral chest x-ray often is the most important initial diagnostic measure.

1. Masses in the superior compartment most often are thymus-derived tumors (i.e., **thymomas**).

a. Thymomas frequently present as cough, chest pain, and superior vena caval obstruction. Myasthenia gravis occurs in approximately one-third of patients with a thymoma. Red blood cell aplasia and hypogammaglobulinemia are other recognized but rare associations. Surgical excision is recommended.

b. Hodgkin's disease and **non-Hodgkin's lymphomas** rarely present as mediastinal masses.

c. Intrathoracic goiters may occur, particularly in middle-aged women, and usually are asymptomatic. However, stridor, hoarseness, and dysphagia all are recognized presentations.

2. Masses in the anterior and middle mediastinum

a. Dermoid cysts appear as dense, homogeneous lobular shadows in the anterior mediastinum, often with calcifications in the walls. Teeth may be recognized within the tumor. Dermoid cysts usually are symptomless unless infection or malignant change develops.

b. Pleuropericardial cysts occur in the middle mediastinum at the right cardiophrenic angle. These tumors characteristically appear as smooth, sharply demarcated masses of uniform density.

c. Bronchogenic cysts and reduplication of the esophagus are other rare causes of middle mediastinal masses.

3. Masses in the posterior mediastinum. Neurogenic tumors are the most common mediastinal tumors and characteristically occur in the posterior mediastinum along the paravertebral border. These tumors often are asymptomatic in the adult but may cause chest pain with stridor, breathlessness, cough, and tracheal compression. **Horner's syndrome** and spinal cord compression also may occur.

a. Generalized neurofibromatosis occurs in about 25% of patients with a primary posterior mediastinal **neurofibroma**.

b. Catecholamine secretion may be associated with the rare **pheochromocytoma** in the posterior mediastinum and with other neurogenic tumors.

B. Mediastinitis

1. Acute mediastinitis is a severe, life-threatening illness that occurs most often following rupture of the esophagus. It may follow vomiting, dental work, endoscopy, and trauma and is characterized by fever, chest pain, and variable mediastinal enlargement. The disease progresses very rapidly and requires emergency medical and surgical treatment.

2. Chronic mediastinitis and mediastinal fibrosis. Histoplasmosis can produce a chronic granulomatous process in the mediastinum, which often is characterized by extensive scar tissue contracting to cause narrowing of the trachea, bronchi, vena cava, pulmonary arteries, and pulmonary veins. In rare cases there is recovery of other organisms, including fungi and atypical bacteria. Mediastinitis that occurs without any known cause is referred to as **idiopathic mediastinal fibrosis**.

C. Pneumomediastinum refers to the presence of air in the mediastinum. Air is presumed to leak from alveoli and to dissect along bronchi to the hilum, from which it may enter the mediastinum. If pressure builds in the mediastinum, air may expand into the neck, producing subcutaneous emphysema. However, if the mediastinal air is confined, the increasing pressure may interfere with circulation. When this occurs, tracheostomy usually is adequate therapy. Intervention is unnecessary in the absence of circulatory problems.

XII. DIFFUSE INTERSTITIAL LUNG DISEASE

A. Definition. Diffuse interstitial lung disease is a broad term designating a group of related disorders that represent the lung's response to diffuse infiltration. The disease begins acutely and progresses to a chronic condition; that is, potentially reversible interstitial pneumonitis progresses to diffuse pulmonary fibrosis. The terminology for this disease is controversial. In North America the term **idiopathic pulmonary fibrosis** is favored, whereas in Great Britain **cryptogenic fibrosing alveolitis** is preferred.

B. Etiology. Approximately 50% of cases of interstitial lung disease occur spontaneously and are classified as idiopathic. The remaining cases are associated with known or suspected causes, some of which are described below. Regardless of their various etiologies, these entities share certain clinical, roentgenographic, pathologic, and physiologic characteristics.

1. **Environmental or occupational exposure** to certain organic and inorganic substances is known to cause interstitial pulmonary fibrosis. These substances include the gaseous phases of such heavy metals as cadmium and mercury. In addition, silica and asbestos are important sources of mineral dust exposure in the industrial setting (see section XIII B 1–2).

2. Certain **viral infections** and **recurrent bacterial pneumonias** also have been implicated.

3. Of increasing importance are a multitude of **drug-induced diseases**. The interstitial pneumonitis and fibrosis that result may be secondary to a direct cytotoxic effect of the drug or to a hypersensitivity reaction.

4. Many cases of interstitial lung disease are associated with connective tissue disease, sarcoidosis, and chronic hypersensitivity pneumonitis.

C. Pathogenesis. The pathologic changes in this disease have a highly variable time course, depending on the degree of exposure to either endogenous or exogenous inciting antigens or to the type of injurious agent. The clinical course may run from a few weeks to many years.

1. **Acute stage**
   a. The earliest stage of diffuse interstitial lung disease is characterized by acute cellular damage, with disruption of the normal alveolar epithelial cells, interstitial and intra-alveolar edema secondary to damaged capillary and alveolar epithelia, and subsequent formation of hyaline membranes. This stage may either resolve completely or progress to the stage of **acute interstitial pneumonia**.
   b. Acute interstitial pneumonia is characterized by proliferation of the alveolar epithelial cells with some desquamation of these cells into the alveolar space, inflammation with round cells accompanied by alveolar interstitial edema and intra-alveolitis, and proliferation of fibrin with increased production of reticular fibers. Large numbers of macrophages also are present in the intra-alveolar space.

2. **Chronic stage.** In many patients the disease progresses to a chronic stage, in which extensive deposition or alteration of collagen results in widespread fibrosis. In addition, this stage is marked by smooth muscle hypertrophy and profound disruption of the alveolar spaces, which are lined with atypical cuboidal cells.

3. **End stage.** The disease eventually progresses to "honeycombed" or **end-stage lung**. In this stage, the entire alveolar and capillary network is replaced with fibrous tissue and dilated spaces, the capillary bed is decreased, and the lung has no remaining gas exchange function.

D. Pathology

1. Several names have been given to this disease in an attempt to describe the various pulmonary changes noted.
   a. The histologic classification most commonly used consists of the following five categories:
      (1) Usual interstitial pneumonitis (UIP)

    (2) Desquamative interstitial pneumonitis (DIP)

    (3) Lymphocytic interstitial pneumonitis (LIP)

    (4) Giant cell interstitial pneumonitis (GIP)

    (5) Bronchiolitis obliterans with interstitial pneumonia (BIP)

   b. Many authorities feel that these classifications are somewhat artificial and may represent various stages or different pathways in the progression from acute to end-stage pulmonary fibrosis.

  2. The histologic pattern observed at biopsy depends largely on the stage of the disease at which the specimen is obtained. In addition, because this is a heterogeneous pathologic process, different areas within a given specimen may show varied stages of anatomic alteration.

E. Pathophysiology

  1. The early stage of disease is characterized by **hypoxia** and an increase in the alveolar-arterial PO_2 gradient with exercise. Only as the disease progresses does resting hypoxia occur. These abnormalities of gas exchange are almost certainly the result of ventilation-perfusion abnormalities. Although diffusing capacity usually is decreased as the disease progresses, this becomes significant in causing hypoxia only during exercise, not at rest.

  2. The **restrictive ventilatory pattern** characteristically seen in patients as a late manifestation of the disease is characterized by a decrease in all subdivisions of lung volume.

   a. The pressure-volume compliance curve is shifted downward and to the right, and the lung compliance is decreased.

   b. Expiratory flow rates (i.e., FEV_1/FVC ratio) usually are well preserved.

   c. Recent studies have demonstrated that several tests for airway function are abnormal in a significant number of patients with pulmonary fibrosis, indicating that the peripheral airways are significantly involved in this pathologic process.

F. Clinical features

  1. Symptoms. Dyspnea on exertion and nonproductive cough are the most common symptoms of infiltrative lung disease. In addition, increased fatigability, fever, and weight loss frequently are seen.

  2. Physical findings include tachypnea, digital clubbing, and late inspiratory dry rales. If the disease is severe, cyanosis and evidence of right ventricular failure also may be present.

  3. Laboratory findings, including the results of pulmonary function testing, are nonspecific. Tests for antinuclear antibodies, rheumatoid factor, and immunoglobulins are positive with relative frequency.

  4. Chest x-ray usually reveals a diffuse reticulonodular pattern throughout both lung fields, which frequently is more pronounced at the lung bases. In some cases, however, clinical evidence of disease may exist without roentgenographic confirmation.

G. Diagnosis. The diagnosis of diffuse infiltrative lung disease is made on the basis of appropriate clinical, roentgenographic, and physiologic findings. Definitive diagnosis requires tissue confirmation, which is obtained most satisfactorily at **open lung biopsy**. Because of the heterogeneous nature of the histologic changes, **transbronchial lung biopsy** is of limited usefulness unless there is clear-cut evidence of sarcoid granuloma, infection, or carcinoma.

  1. Open-lung biopsy is perhaps the most useful technique for determining the stage of the disease, the appropriate therapy, and the probable prognosis. Whether or not the disease responds to therapeutic intervention appears to correlate well with pathologic evidence of fibrosis. Specimens showing active cellular infiltrates and minimal fibrosis are associated with a much better prognosis than those showing extensive fibrosis.

  2. Bronchoalveolar lavage is an experimental diagnostic procedure that has gained recent interest. Analysis of the cellular elements of the fluid lavaged from the lung indicates that infiltrative lung disease is associated with an increased number of polymorphonuclear leukocytes and hypersensitivity pneumonitis is associated with an increased number of lymphocytes.

  3. Gallium 67 imaging is another experimental, but nonspecific, technique that measures the degree of the patient's inflammatory response.

H. Therapy

  1. Corticosteroids have been the mainstay of therapy and are clearly indicated when open-lung biopsy reveals an active cellular process without extensive fibrosis. Large doses (i.e., 1 mg/kg of body weight/day) are employed initially, and physiologic and x-ray parameters should be monitored carefully. If there is improvement after 6 weeks, the dosage should be tapered gradually with frequent monitoring to detect physiologic relapse.

2. If no improvement occurs with steroids alone, consideration should be given to administration of additional drugs, either alone or in combination with steroids. **Azathioprine** is the most widely used alternative drug. **Cyclophosphamide** and **chlorambucil** also have been used.

I. Prognosis

1. Interstitial lung disease has a variable course, with some cases resolving or arresting spontaneously. Sometimes these changes occur in relation to removal of a known causative agent (e.g., a drug or environmental factor). Immunologic or genetic factors of the host also may be important in these changes.

2. Progressive interstitial lung disease can be an insidious, devastating disease with considerable morbidity and mortality. The average survival after diagnosis in untreated cases is 4–5 years.

XIII. OCCUPATIONAL LUNG DISEASE

A. Introduction. Unlike other organ systems, the respiratory system has continuous, active, and mandatory contact with the environment. Many respiratory illnesses are caused by inhalation of impure air. To produce lung disease, an injurious inhalant must:

1. Exist in a form that is capable of reaching the lower respiratory tract

2. Be deposited on or absorbed into bronchial or alveolar surfaces

3. Remain in the respiratory tract for a sufficient time to produce injury

B. Pulmonary response to mineral dusts

1. Asbestos-related disease
   a. Physical and pathogenic properties of asbestos
   (1) Asbestos is the term applied to naturally occurring fibrous silicates, of which there are several forms. **Chrysotile**, the most plentiful and most widely used form, occurs as long, curled, flexible fibers. The **amphiboles**, in comparison, are straight brittle fibers.
   (2) Inhaled fibers assume longitudinal orientation, which explains how fibers that are 50 μ or more in length can penetrate the peripheral airways.
   (3) The mechanism whereby asbestos enters the lung and causes disease is uncertain. However, several distinct types of lesions may be produced, and a given patient may show only one of these many forms of injury.
   b. Asbestosis is a diffuse, interstitial cellular and fibrotic reaction of the lung to inhaled asbestos fibers. Affected patients complain of breathlessness, and physical signs include digital clubbing and basilar rales. The chest x-ray shows small lungs containing hazy infiltrates composed of small irregular or linear opacities; lower lung zones are more heavily affected. A restrictive ventilatory impairment and a reduced diffusing capacity are the expected abnormalities.
   c. Cancer. Exposure to asbestos at sufficient concentrations also may cause cancer.
   (1) Bronchogenic carcinoma is a recognized complication of asbestosis and asbestos exposure. The risk for developing this cancer is much greater in individuals who smoke than in nonsmokers.
   (2) Pleural and peritoneal mesotheliomas are rare tumors. They are not associated with smoking.
   d. Other effects. Asbestos also may cause nonneoplastic pleural disorders, including pleurisy with effusion, pleural plaques, and diffuse pleural thickening.

2. Silica-related disease. Free silica and silicates are abundant components of the earth's crust. Quartz is composed largely of **free crystalline silica**, and beach sand is mostly quartz. To be injurious to the lungs, these particles must exist as aerosols at a respirable size of 3–5 μ.
   a. Silicosis is a diffuse fibrotic reaction of the lungs to inhalation of free crystalline silica. When silica particles reach the periphery of the lungs, they are ingested by alveolar macrophages. These macrophages rupture soon after, die, and release the engulfed silica particles for reingestion by other macrophages. This cycle continues and eventually stimulates collagen formation by fibroblasts in the area of macrophage death. The final result is the formation of the relatively acellular **fibrous silicotic nodule** that characterizes this disease.
   (1) Simple silicosis. In this stage, the chest x-ray appearance is that of numerous, small, rounded opacities (isolated nodules) scattered throughout the lungs. Simple silicosis usually is not associated with ventilatory impairment.

       (2) Complicated silicosis. If the fibrosis continues, isolated nodules may coalesce to form larger masses of fibrotic tissue, which distorts the lungs and causes a progression from simple to complicated silicosis. This may occur due to increased silica exposure or to mycobacterial or mycotic infections. Complicated silicosis often produces a mixture of restrictive and obstructive ventilatory impairment.

   b. Nonfibrotic effects. Silicates such as talc, kaolin, fuller's earth, and bentonite can produce simple or complicated pneumoconiosis, without diffuse pulmonary fibrosis.

3. Coal worker's pneumoconiosis (CWP) shares with silicosis the x-ray appearance of small, rounded opacities in the simple stage and large, conglomerate masses in the complicated stage. **Simple CWP** has no characteristic functional abnormality; a chronic bronchitis probably accounts for most of the respiratory disability in these patients. Only rarely does simple CWP develop into **complicated CWP**.

4. Beryllium-related disease. Beryllium compounds can produce both acute and chronic lung disease. The metal, which once was used to coat fluorescent tubes, now is used in alloys, certain plastics and ceramics, rocket fuels, and x-ray tubes.

   a. Acute beryllium lung disease occurs following heavy exposure. This diffuse, airspace-filling pneumonitis is similar to an acute phosgene inhalation that develops into an acute, noncardiogenic pulmonary edema.

   b. Chronic beryllium lung disease, by definition, is a disease of at least 1-year duration. This multisystem disorder is strikingly similar to sarcoidosis in that noncaseating granulomas are present throughout the body (see section XIV A 1). A major difference is the lack of eye involvement in chronic beryllium lung disease.

5. Pulmonary response to other mineral dusts. Some dusts are deposited and retained in the lung and are cleared into aggregations in the pulmonary lobules, causing little or no host reaction. Minerals that elicit this type of reaction include tin oxide, iron oxide, and barium sulfate. These dust collections do not physically interfere with ventilatory function or perfusion.

C. Pulmonary response to organic dusts. The pulmonary parenchymal reaction to inhalation of organic dusts (e.g., fungal spores, thermophilic actinomycetes, and fragments of animal and vegetable matter) is known as **hypersensitivity pneumonitis** or **extrinsic allergic alveolitis**. Patients often have antibodies against the offending substances, and the reactions suggest a type III hypersensitivity. This represents a deposition of antigen-antibody complex, which leads to tissue damage.

1. Farmer's lung is a typical example of hypersensitivity pneumonitis.

   a. Thermophilic actinomycetes grow in moldy hay and are inhaled when the hay is disturbed. Several hours after exposure, patients suffer malaise, fever, and chills. Chest tightness and persistent dry cough also develop. Symptoms abate one to several days after exposure and recur with subsequent exposures.

   b. X-rays taken during acute attacks show pulmonary infiltrates. Repeated exposures may lead to a fixed restrictive lung disease. Pathologically, mononuclear interstitial infiltrates and fibrosis predominate.

   c. Therapy includes avoidance of exposure and corticosteroid treatment for acute attacks.

2. Other forms of hypersensitivity pneumonitis include:

   a. Bagassosis, due to colonization of the fibrous residue of sugarcane by thermophilic actinomycetes

   b. Bird-breeder's lung, due to hypersensitivity to bird sera, feathers, and droppings

   c. Mushroom worker's lung, due to colonization of compost by thermophilic actinomycetes

   d. Malt worker's lung, due to contamination of the grain by aspergilli

   e. Humidifier lung and **parakeet fancier's lung,** which are more domestic than occupational

D. Obstructive airways disease due to inhalants

1. Occupational asthma

   a. Definition. Occupational asthma refers to asthma that is induced by occupational inhalants. Affected individuals usually are not atopic, and the reaction usually is not immediate. The diagnosis is strongly suggested by a history of coughing fits that occur at two or three o'clock in the morning on workdays but not on weekends nor during vacation from work.

   b. Etiologic agents. Heavy exposure to several different organic and inorganic substances can cause occupational asthma, often without a demonstrable immunologic mechanism. Agents of occupational asthma include:

   (1) Simple inorganic chemicals (e.g., platinum salts)

      (2) Simple organic chemicals (e.g., diisocyanates, formaldehyde, and phthalic anhydrides)
      (3) Detergent enzymes derived from the bacterium, *Bacillus subtilis*
      (4) Wood dust, especially western red cedar
      (5) Fungal antigens and grain weevil antigens
      (6) Animal dander and excretions
      (7) Grain and grain contaminants
  c. Diagnosis and therapy. Direct confirmation by challenge testing is the most convincing demonstration of the relationship with symptoms of the inhalant. Avoidance of exposure is the most effective treatment. Acute attacks may respond to standard asthma medication.

  2. Byssinosis is occupational asthma induced by respirable cotton dust that is generated in the early steps of textile production.
    a. The disease has an early phase, in which the affected worker experiences chest tightness and shortness of breath at the beginning of the workweek but feels well later in the workweek. With years of exposure, the symptoms may last later into the week, until symptoms and signs of chronic fixed airway obstruction finally prevail.
    b. The amount of cotton dust responsible for this disease has not been determined, and it is uncertain whether the pathogenetic mechanism is immunologic or pharmacologic.

  3. Industrial bronchitis refers to chronic obstructive bronchitis caused by occupational inhalants.
    a. Recognition of the disorder is hindered by the lack of a conspicuous marker. Symptoms of bronchitis (e.g., chronic cough) are prevalent in the general population, and identification of an occupational inhalant requires careful and extensive epidemiologic studies. Cigarette smoking, which also is associated with chronic cough, is the major confounding variable.
    b. Studies linking chronic bronchitis to exposure to inert dust (e.g., coal dust) as well as foundry and gold mine dust have yielded equivocal results.

E. Pulmonary response to irritant gases

  1. Irritant gases inflame the respiratory tract and, in high concentrations, can cause pulmonary edema.
    a. Such agents include:
      (1) Ammonia (NH_3)
      (2) Hydrochloric acid (HCl)
      (3) Sulfur dioxide (SO_2)
      (4) Nitrogen dioxide (NO_2)
      (5) Phosgene (Cl_2CO)
    b. These agents can cause upper and lower airway disease.

  2. Often there is a latent period of up to 12–24 hours before the onset of chest symptoms.

  3. The pulmonary edema due to any irritant gas is treated with supportive measures and corticosteroids. In some cases, follow-up reveals bronchiolitis obliterans.

XIV. PULMONARY DISEASES OF UNKNOWN ETIOLOGY. Except for sarcoidosis, pulmonary diseases of unknown etiology are encountered infrequently by clinicians.

A. Sarcoidosis (see also Chapter 6, Part I: section XIII B 4 b)

  1. Definition. Sarcoidosis is a systemic disease characterized by the presence of noncaseating granulomas in the lung and other organs. This multisystem granulomatous disorder usually presents as mediastinal or hilar lymphadenopathy with pulmonary infiltration and cutaneous or ocular lesions. Less common but important manifestations include peripheral adenopathy, erythema nodosum, arthritis, splenomegaly, hepatomegaly, hypercalcemia, diffuse or localized CNS involvement, and cardiomyopathy. A consistent immunologic feature is depression of delayed-type hypersensitivity.

  2. Incidence
    a. Sarcoidosis can occur at any age but appears most commonly in the third to fifth decades of life. There is no sex predilection.
    b. The disease occurs worldwide, but substantial differences in incidence exist among countries and in any one country among ethnic groups.
      (1) In the United States, the incidence of sarcoidosis is estimated to be from 11 to 71 individuals per 100,000 population, with the large range reflecting racial differences.
      (2) American blacks have a 10- to 18-fold higher incidence of clinically recognized sarcoidosis as compared with whites.

3. Possible etiologic factors

a. Clinical and pathologic similarities have suggested a connection with *Mycobacterium tuberculosis* infection and other mycobacterial disease. However, failure to identify any infectious agents consistently and lack of an epidemiologic association have made this and other infectious etiologies unlikely.

b. Patients with sarcoidosis show impaired cellular immunity characterized by a complete skin anergy to tuberculin and other common skin antigens. Circulating T lymphocytes are decreased, possibly due to sequestration in the lung, and bronchoalveolar lavage typically reveals marked increases in these cells. These findings are not associated with increased susceptibility to infection as humoral immunity is normal.

(1) The significance of these immunologic abnormalities is unknown. One hypothesis is that sarcoidosis represents an atypical response to a variety of pathogens by a host whose immunologic responsiveness is fundamentally abnormal.

(2) It is also possible, however, that the immunologic changes are secondary phenomena and that the primary pathologic process remains to be discovered.

4. Pathology. The fundamental lesion of sarcoidosis is a **noncaseating granuloma.**

a. This cluster of **epithelioid cells** suggests a tissue response to some focal insult. **Giant cells** frequently are present and contain several types of inclusions. **Lymphocytes** and rare **plasma cells** may be present at the periphery of the granuloma; neutrophils and eosinophils are not contained in the lesion.

b. Granulomas may remain unchanged in tissue for many years, they may regress, or they may organize. Organization results in tissue fibrosis. Chronic inflammation and fibrosis in the lung cause serious structural distortion and loss of function.

c. The noncaseating granuloma of sarcoidosis is indistinguishable from that occurring in other diseases such as fungal disease, mycobacterial disease, and Hodgkin's disease.

5. Clinical features. The clinical findings in sarcoidosis vary considerably, depending on the site and extent of involvement.

a. Pulmonary involvement. The lungs are involved in more than 90% of reported cases.

(1) Symptoms of fatigue and exertional dyspnea are common. Cough, if present, usually is nonproductive. Hemoptysis is rare. Chest pain occurs infrequently, and pleurisy is uncommon.

(2) Pulmonary function testing may produce normal results but usually shows some impairment of gas exchange and a tendency toward lung restriction with reduced vital capacity and diffusing capacity. In many cases, small airway function also is abnormal.

(3) Chest x-ray. Enlarged intrathoracic lymph nodes are the rule, particularly early in the course of the disease. Parenchymal manifestations vary from a faint interstitial infiltrate, to well-developed diffuse nodular infiltrates, to varying degrees of lung fibrosis, including honeycombing. The radiographic staging of pulmonary involvement in sarcoidosis is as follows:

(a) Stage 1: Bilateral hilar adenopathy and normal lung parenchyma

(b) Stage 2: Bilateral hilar adenopathy and interstitial infiltrate

(c) Stage 3: Interstitial infiltrate only

(d) Stage 4: Fibrosis

b. Systemic involvement

(1) Uveitis is a common presentation; this condition may progress to blindness.

(2) Skin involvement occurs in one-third of patients and may manifest as a variety of infiltrative lesions. Skin lesions often portend chronic progressive sarcoidosis. An exception is **erythema nodosum**, which may occur early in the disease and is associated with a good prognosis.

(3) Bone and joint involvement. Transient **polyarthritis** is associated with erythema nodosum, but a chronic form of arthritis also occurs. Bones may be involved, producing cystic destruction and disability.

(4) CNS involvement may present as **Bell's palsy** and other cranial neuropathies, peripheral neuropathies, and (rarely) granulomatous meningitis.

(5) Cardiac involvement manifests as arrhythmias and conduction disturbances and carries a high risk for sudden death.

(6) Liver function abnormalities may occur.

(7) Disturbances in calcium metabolism (e.g., hypercalciuria, renal stones, and hypercalcemia) occur in up to 25% of patients with sarcoidosis. These metabolic abnormalities result from increased intestinal absorption of calcium due to a hypersensitivity to vitamin D.

6. Diagnosis. Sarcoidosis should be suspected in any patient with mediastinal or hilar adenopathy and interstitial lung disease (e.g., pulmonary fibrosis). Erythema nodosum, uveitis, skin lesions, hypercalcemia, multisystem disease, and granulomas of any organ should suggest sarcoidosis.

    a. Diagnostic confirmation requires **tissue biopsy** demonstrating typical granulomas in a patient with consistent clinical presentations. Since sarcoidosis is a diagnosis of exclusion, all tissue samples should be cultured to rule out infectious etiologies and specially stained for identification of fungal disease.

    b. Transbronchial biopsy offers a high diagnostic yield.

    c. Serum angiotensin-converting enzyme (ACE) assay, gallium 67 lung scanning, and bronchoalveolar lavage all are nonspecific procedures that should not be used in diagnosing sarcoidosis but are appropriate indicators of disease activity for use in follow-up (see section XIV A 7 b).

7. Therapy

    a. Corticosteroid administration is the principal treatment for sarcoidosis. However, not all patients require steroid treatment; therefore, a decision must be made as to whether a patient's symptoms warrant therapy that has proven hazards.

        (1) Sarcoidosis that carries a threat of disability should be treated. Indications include symptomatic pulmonary disease, uveitis, hypercalcemia, cardiac sarcoidosis, and neurologic sarcoidosis.

        (2) There are few well-controlled series of corticosteroids in sarcoidosis. However, the above indications generally are felt to warrant their use.

    b. The therapeutic regimen must be assessed periodically to determine whether continuation of treatment is warranted. Clinical observation, pulmonary function testing, and chest x-ray analysis frequently are used to follow patients. However, these procedures often are not good indicators of disease activity. More recently used parameters of disease activity (e.g., bronchoalveolar lavage, serum ACE assay, and gallium scanning) are better indicators.

8. Prognosis. The course of sarcoidosis is variable.

    a. In most patients, the disease regresses within 2 years and does not recur. Any tissue destruction that occurs is permanent but usually causes no major disability.

    b. In approximately 25% of patients, the disease is more progressive and does cause serious disability. In this more severely affected group, multisystem involvement is common, with skin sarcoidosis and hypercalcemia particularly prominent. Approximately 5% of patients die with respiratory failure.

B. Goodpasture's syndrome (see also Chapter 6, Part I: section XI G)

1. Definition. Goodpasture's syndrome is a progressive disease of the lungs and kidneys, which produces intra-alveolar hemorrhage and glomerulonephritis. The disease is rare, occurs at all ages, and is predominant in males.

2. Etiology and pathology

    a. Goodpasture's syndrome is caused by an anti-glomerular basement membrane (anti-GBM) antibody, usually IgG, which reacts with glomerular and alveolar basement membranes.

    b. Linear deposition of the antibody, characteristic of a type II hypersensitivity reaction, occurs along the basement membrane of glomeruli, alveoli, and capillaries.

        (1) The pathologic result in the lung is diffuse capillary leakage and intra-alveolar hemorrhage but little or no inflammation.

        (2) The renal lesion is a proliferative glomerulonephritis that progresses to renal failure.

3. Clinical features

    a. The initial presentations usually are hemoptysis and dyspnea; however, renal failure without pulmonary complaints can be an initial finding.

    b. A history of respiratory illness often precedes the onset of pulmonary hemorrhage. Iron deficiency anemia may occur following prolonged pulmonary hemorrhage; azotemia also may be present.

    c. Bilateral alveolar infiltrates on chest x-ray and hypoxia and restriction on pulmonary function testing are characteristic.

4. Diagnosis

    a. Goodpasture's syndrome should be suspected in patients with hemoptysis and diffuse pulmonary infiltrates, particularly in the presence of anemia and nephritis.

    b. The diagnosis is based on demonstration of anti-GBM antibody in either the serum or a biopsy specimen from the kidney or lung.

    c. Differential diagnosis includes Wegener's granulomatosis (see below), systemic lupus erythematosus, and idiopathic pulmonary hemosiderosis.

        (1) Systemic lupus erythematosus is distinguished from Goodpasture's syndrome by the absence of anti-GBM antibody and the findings of free DNA, various antinuclear antibodies, and depressed serum levels of complement.

    (2) Idiopathic pulmonary hemosiderosis is characterized by repeated pulmonary hemorrhage but no nephritis. Death from massive hemorrhage may occur at any time, but prolonged survival with or without symptoms of pulmonary insufficiency is common. In contrast to Goodpasture's syndrome, idiopathic pulmonary hemosiderosis has no known immune mechanisms for pathogenesis, and no successful therapy has evolved.

  5. Therapy. Untreated Goodpasture's syndrome is rapidly fatal as a result of renal failure or asphyxia from pulmonary hemorrhage.

    a. High-dose steroid therapy often controls episodes of lung hemorrhage but not the progressive renal disease. This treatment does not prevent the ultimately fatal outcome.

    b. Bilateral nephrectomy with hemodialysis has been used to control life-threatening lung hemorrhage.

    c. Currently, the combination of **plasmapheresis and immunosuppressant therapy** with steroids and alkylating agents appears to give the best results.

C. Wegener's granulomatosis (see also Chapter 6, Part I: section XI N 3)

  1. Definition. This disease is the prototype of a group of rare disorders characterized by granulomatous inflammation and necrosis of the lung and other organs. All ages are affected; men are affected more commonly than women.

    a. The syndrome was originally described by Wegener as being a destructive granulomatosis of the upper respiratory tract combined with granulomatous infiltration of the lung parenchyma and glomerulonephritis.

    b. Today, the disease is recognized as a systemic vasculitis with a predilection for the respiratory tract. Other commonly involved sites are the skin, joints, and peripheral nerves. Involvement of the eyes, heart, and CNS occurs frequently by extension of the primary sites.

  2. Etiology and pathology

    a. The etiologic mechanism is thought to involve an immunologic injury of vessels with secondary inflammatory changes.

    b. The pathologic lesion is an angiitis of small vessels with infiltration of surrounding tissues by lymphocytes, plasma cells, and histiocytes. Tissue necrosis is characteristic, and mononuclear inflammatory cells surround the necrotic areas, forming noncaseating granulomas.

    (1) In the lung, this process results in the formation of infiltrates, nodules, or tumors, which commonly excavate and destroy the lung parenchyma causing hemoptysis and pulmonary insufficiency.

    (2) The renal lesion is a focal glomerulonephritis that can progress to renal failure.

  3. Diagnosis

    a. Wegener's granulomatosis is identified by a classic triad of findings, that is, upper and lower respiratory involvement and glomerulonephritis. The disease should be suspected in individuals with either single or multiple noninfectious focal lesions of the lung, particularly in association with hemoptysis or cavitation.

    b. Unlike Goodpasture's syndrome, Wegener's granulomatosis usually does not produce diffuse parenchymal infiltrates.

    c. The diagnosis is made by biopsy of the involved tissue. Correct interpretation of the pathologic findings sometimes is difficult, and clinical correlation may be necessary to distinguish Wegener's granulomatosis from other vasculitides.

  4. Therapy and prognosis

    a. Correct diagnosis is critical because of the remarkable efficacy of cytotoxic therapy. **Cyclophosphamide** alone or with steroids produces rapid reversal of the disease.

    b. The untreated disease is fatal in most patients within a month to several years. Some forms of the disease are associated with longer survival rates, particularly those involving active nephritis.

D. Histiocytosis X

  1. Definition. Histiocytosis X is a generic term for a group of systemic disorders characterized by varied degrees of fibrosis with focal histiocyte accumulations and infiltrations of tissue by nonmalignant histiocytes and eosinophils. The disease is rare, affects males more commonly than females, and occurs at any age, although children and young adults are affected more commonly than other age-groups.

  2. Etiology and pathology

    a. An abnormality of the immune system is suspected. Ultrastructural studies of the proliferating histiocytes have shown cytoplasmic inclusions, the so-called **X bodies**, which suggest a relationship to epithelial Langhans' cells.

b. The disease can be localized to one area (e.g., bone or lung) or can be widely disseminated. **Eosinophilic granuloma** and **Letterer-Siwe disease** refer to the localized and disseminated syndromes, respectively.

c. Pulmonary histiocytosis X produces bilateral, reticulonodular infiltrates, with a predilection for the upper lobes and typical progression to cyst formation, fibrosis, and honeycombing.

3. Clinical features. Patients commonly have bone pain, pneumothorax, and dyspnea. Pulmonary function testing indicates restriction and impaired gas exchange. In advanced cases, severe obstruction may dominate.

4. Diagnosis
   a. The diagnosis is suggested by a characteristic combination of findings, including lytic bone disease, diabetes insipidus, exophthalmos, chronic otitis, gingivitis or chronic dermatitis, hepatosplenomegaly, anemia, fever, spontaneous pneumothorax, and a honeycomb appearance on chest x-ray.
   b. Definitive diagnosis requires biopsy of involved tissue. Electron-microscopic demonstration of X bodies in bronchoalveolar lavage fluid may be useful.

5. Therapy and prognosis
   a. Therapy includes surgery or radiotherapy for localized bone disease. Steroids are useful for disseminated disease, but their efficacy is uncertain.
   b. The prognosis of the disease is variable and difficult to predict.

E. Alveolar proteinosis

1. Definition
   a. This disease is characterized by massive accumulations of a phospholipid-rich material in alveoli. The substance is closely related in its chemical and physiologic properties to pulmonary surfactant and probably accumulates as a result of impaired clearance. Macrophages engorged with the substance also are present, but other inflammatory cells are lacking. The interstitium usually is not involved.
   b. Alveolar proteinosis is more common in males than in females and has been described in all ages.
   c. There is no consistent association with underlying disease or other organ involvement.

2. Clinical features
   a. Dyspnea and nonproductive cough are the major symptoms, and pulmonary rales and cyanosis are the most common findings.
   b. Chest x-ray demonstrates an alveolar infiltrate, which usually is bilateral and in the perihilar butterfly distribution similar to pulmonary edema.
   c. Pulmonary function testing shows a restrictive ventilatory pattern and hypoxia.
   d. Patients are predisposed to lung infection, possibly because of a functional impairment of alveolar macrophages. **Nocardiosis** and fungal infections occur with increased frequency.
   e. The disease may progress to respiratory insufficiency and death, but spontaneous resolution is just as common. Pulmonary fibrosis has been described as a late complication.

3. Diagnosis
   a. Alveolar proteinosis should be suspected in patients with persistent alveolar infiltrates, particularly if the infiltrates are bilateral and congestive heart failure is not present.
   b. Lung biopsy is necessary to demonstrate the periodic acid-Schiff (PAS) positive material in the alveoli.

4. Therapy
   a. Bronchoalveolar lavage is the only effective treatment for the dyspneic patient. Lavage of the material produces remarkable reversal of the physiologic abnormality.
   b. Steroids may increase the risk of infection and are contraindicated since they do not alter the underlying dysfunction.

F. Pulmonary alveolar microlithiasis

1. Definition. This rare and mysterious disorder results from the formation of calcific bodies within the alveoli of otherwise normal lungs. The disease is not associated with systemic hypercalcinosis. The disorder often occurs among multiple siblings, suggesting a congenital metabolic disturbance.

2. Clinical features and diagnosis
   a. Pulmonary alveolar microlithiasis usually is discovered by chest x-ray in asymptomatic in-

dividuals in the third decade of life. The x-ray shows extensive infiltration of both lungs. The x-ray is pathognomonic.

    b. The disease progresses slowly to pulmonary insufficiency, cor pulmonale, and death 10–20 years later.

3. Therapy. No effective therapy has been found. Chelating agents and steroids are ineffective.

STUDY QUESTIONS

Directions: Each question below contains five suggested answers. Choose the **one best** response to each question.

1. Shortly after symptomatic resolution of an asthmatic attack, pulmonary function testing is most likely to show

(A) normal values for peak expiratory flow
(B) decreased lung compliance
(C) increased residual volume
(D) no change in peak expiratory flow after inhalation of a bronchodilator
(E) decreased diffusing capacity

2. What percentage of patients with cystic fibrosis live to be 18 years of age or older?

(A) < 10
(B) 10–20
(C) 20–30
(D) 30–40
(E) > 40

3. All of the following are components of airway obstruction in asthma EXCEPT

(A) mucous plugging
(B) laryngospasm
(C) inflammation of airways
(D) bronchospasm
(E) edema of airways

4. All of the following findings are clinical evidence of pulmonary embolism EXCEPT

(A) hypoxia
(B) pleural friction rub
(C) hypercapnia
(D) right ventricular failure
(E) deep venous thrombosis

5. All of the following are complications of chronic obstructive pulmonary disease (COPD) EXCEPT

(A) cor pulmonale
(B) polycythemia
(C) respiratory failure
(D) left ventricular failure
(E) bronchogenic carcinoma

6. All of the following statements regarding cystic fibrosis are true EXCEPT

(A) cystic fibrosis is most common in whites
(B) a negative family history of cystic fibrosis rules out this diagnosis
(C) intestinal malabsorption is seen commonly in affected individuals
(D) the most frequent cause of death in cystic fibrosis is respiratory failure
(E) cystic fibrosis is inherited as an autosomal recessive trait

7. Which of the following diagnostic techniques is most specific for pulmonary embolism?

(A) Pulmonary angiography
(B) Ventilation lung scanning
(C) Perfusion lung scanning
(D) Arterial blood gas analysis
(E) Chest x-ray

8. Chronic obstructive pulmonary disease (COPD) is classified as either emphysematous or bronchitic, depending on the pathologic changes that occur in the lung. Although these two COPD syndromes rarely exist as pure entities, by definition they can be differentiated on the basis of their clinical presentation. Which of the following clinical features is common to both the emphysematous and bronchitic types of COPD?

(A) Polycythemia
(B) Improved airflow with bronchodilators
(C) Dyspnea
(D) Chronic cough
(E) Hypercapnia

Directions: Each question below contains four suggested answers of which **one or more** is correct. Choose the answer

    A if **1, 2, and 3** are correct
    B if **1 and 3** are correct
    C if **2 and 4** are correct
    D if **4** is correct
    E if **1, 2, 3, and 4** are correct

9. A 42-year-old man who does not smoke is referred for pulmonary function testing because a routine chest x-ray revealed a reticulonodular (interstitial) infiltrate throughout both lung fields. The only symptom is mild dyspnea on exertion, and physical examination reveals only late inspiratory rales at both lung bases. Pulmonary function testing is likely to demonstrate

(1) resting hypoxia
(2) increased alveolar-arterial PO_2 gradient with exercise
(3) decreased FEV_1/FVC ratio
(4) decreased lung compliance

10. Digital clubbing may be demonstrated by patients with

(1) bronchogenic carcinoma
(2) lung abscess
(3) bronchiectasis
(4) chronic obstructive pulmonary disease (COPD)

11. A 62-year-old woman who has congestive heart failure develops pneumonia and a large pleural effusion. Thoracentesis is performed in an effort to establish the etiology of the pleural effusion (i.e., congestive heart failure or pneumonia). Pleural fluid findings that would indicate that the pleural effusion is due to congestive heart failure include

.(1) a protein content of 6 g/dl
(2) a pH of 7.13
(3) a glucose content of 20 mg/dl
(4) a lactate dehydrogenase (LDH) content of 100 mg/dl (with a serum LDH level of 420 mg/dl)

12. Clinical features of lung cancer that indicate tumor spread beyond the lung include

(1) back pain
(2) a change in a chronic cough
(3) hoarseness
(4) pleurisy with signs of pleural effusion

13. Adult respiratory distress syndrome (also referred to as wet lung) is a severe form of acute respiratory insufficiency characterized primarily by severe hypoxia. Events and conditions that may precipitate adult respiratory distress syndrome include

(1) disseminated intravascular coagulation
(2) bacterial septicemia
(3) trauma
(4) blood transfusion

14. In a patient suspected of having a pleural mesothelioma, the diagnostic workup may reveal evidence of

(1) cigarette smoking
(2) asbestos exposure
(3) silica exposure
(4) pleural effusion

15. Even when arterial PO_2 is normal, inadequate tissue oxygenation may occur if

(1) severe anemia is present
(2) cardiac output is low
(3) local vasoconstriction is present
(4) the percent saturation of oxygen in the blood is decreased

Directions: The group of questions below consists of lettered choices followed by several numbered items. For each numbered item select the **one** lettered choice with which it is **most** closely associated. Each lettered choice may be used once, more than once, or not at all.

Questions 16–20

Match each of the following statements to the pulmonary disease of unknown etiology it best describes.

(A) Sarcoidosis
(B) Goodpasture's syndrome
(C) Wegener's granulomatosis
(D) Alveolar proteinosis
(E) Alveolar microlithiasis

16. This progressive disease of the lungs and kidneys can produce intra-alveolar hemorrhage and glomerulonephritis.

17. Granulomatous inflammation and necrosis of the lung and other organs are characteristic of this disease.

18. This disease is characterized by massive accumulations of a phospholipid-rich material in alveoli.

19. This systemic disease is characterized by the presence of noncaseating granulomas in the lung and other organs.

20. Cardiac involvement in this disease may manifest as arrhythmias and conduction disturbances.

ANSWERS AND EXPLANATIONS

1. The answer is C. (*II F 3*) In patients who have had recent asthmatic attacks and are asymptomatic there is a residual airflow obstruction. This obstruction may take a couple of months to disappear, during which time patients still have a bronchodilator sensitivity but show abnormal peak expiratory flow, increased lung compliance, and continued maldistribution of ventilation. Diffusing capacity is decreased in abnormalities of capillary blood volume due to either destruction of the alveolar capillary membrane (e.g., in emphysema) or to a thickened interstitial membrane (e.g., in diffuse interstitial lung disease). Neither of these abnormalities exists in asthma.

2. The answer is E. (*III B 1*) Until the 1960s, cystic fibrosis was purely a pediatric disease. At that time, the median age of cystic fibrosis patients shifted to the teens. This was primarily due to the availability of antibiotics that are more specific to the pathogenic bacteria and due to the better understanding of the need for nutritional supplementation and exogenous pancreatic replacement. In 1980, the median age of patients with cystic fibrosis was 21 years.

3. The answer is B. (*II D*) The mediators of asthma produce mucous plugging, inflammation, and edema of the airways; these effects account for the bronchospasm that characterizes asthmatic attacks. The upper airways (i.e., the trachea and larynx) are not involved in any major way in asthma. Laryngospasm usually is an allergic phenomenon that occurs secondary to a bee sting or is a manifestation of anaphylaxis, which may have a component of bronchospasm.

4. The answer is C. (*VII F 1, 4*) Clinical evidence of pulmonary embolism includes hypoxia, a pleural friction rub, right ventricular failure, and deep venous thrombosis—but not hypercapnia. Hypoxia occurs on the basis of ventilation-perfusion mismatch due to atelectasis in the embolized areas. Auscultation occasionally reveals a pleural friction rub and wheezing. Evidence of deep venous thrombosis is noted in 50% of patients, and right ventricular failure is seen in massive pulmonary embolism, when more than 50% of the pulmonary vasculature is compromised. Hypercapnia does not occur since pulmonary embolism causes nonspecific chemical stimuli to trigger hyperventilation.

5. The answer is D. (*I J*) Chronic obstructive pulmonary disease (COPD) may be associated with several complications, including cor pulmonale, polycythemia, respiratory failure, and bronchogenic carcinoma. In addition, a predisposition for peptic ulcer disease is noted in COPD patients. Even in cases of advanced COPD, there is no concomitant left ventricular failure. When it occurs, left ventricular dysfunction is due to an independent etiology (i.e., a myocardial, not a pulmonary, disease).

6. The answer is B. (*III B 1, 2, 4 b*) Among whites, cystic fibrosis occurs in 1 in 1500–1800 live births and is carried by 4%–5% of the population. Cystic fibrosis follows a classic pattern of autosomal recessive inheritance; however, a man and a woman with no family history of cystic fibrosis can have a child with cystic fibrosis. Respiratory failure is the most common cause of death in cystic fibrosis. A less common cause is portal hypertension from a form of biliary cirrhosis.

7. The answer is A. (*VII F 2, 4–6*) Pulmonary angiography is the standard test for the diagnosis of pulmonary embolism. Algorithms have been developed for patients with appropriate clinical data and high-probability results on ventilation and perfusion lung scanning; in such cases, this combined technique has almost the diagnostic accuracy of pulmonary angiography. Abnormal results on arterial blood gas analysis and chest x-ray are too nonspecific to be helpful. When ventilation and perfusion scanning, arterial blood gas analysis, or both produce perfectly normal results and the alveolar-arterial PO_2 gradient is normal, pulmonary embolism is extremely unlikely.

8. The answer is C. (*I E 2*) The two classic types of chronic obstructive pulmonary disease (COPD)—emphysematous and bronchitic—represent extremes of the spectrum of COPD and rarely are encountered in their pure form in clinical practice. By definition, the emphysematous type of COPD presents at a relatively old age (older than 60 years) and is characterized by progressive exertional dyspnea, weight loss, little or no cough, mild hypoxia, hypocapnia, and only a mild increase in airway resistance, which shows little improvement with bronchodilation. The bronchitic type of COPD presents at a relatively young age and is characterized by episodic dyspnea, weight gain, chronic cough, severe hypoxia, hypercapnia, polycythemia, and an increase in airway resistance, which improves with bronchodilation.

9. The answer is C (2, 4). (*XII E 1–2*) This patient has idiopathic pulmonary fibrosis. In its early stage this disease is characterized by mild, not profound, hypoxia and an increase in the alveolar-arterial PO_2 gradient with exercise. The mechanism of these abnormalities is a ventilation-perfusion mismatch. Pulmonary function testing in these patients reveals reduced lung volume and normal airflow. Lung compliance also is decreased. The absolute FEV_1 may be decreased secondary to loss of lung volume, but the FEV_1/FVC ratio should be normal. The hallmark of idiopathic pulmonary fibrosis is oxygen desaturation with exercise.

10. The answer is A (1, 2, 3). [*III A 3, C 4 a; IX E 2 c (3) (b)*] The cause of clubbing of fingers and toes is not known. Digital clubbing is seen in advanced cases of bronchiectasis and in some cases of lung abscess and lung cancer. It also may be a physical finding in patients with infiltrative lung disease (interstitial fibrosis). Digital clubbing is not seen in patients with chronic obstructive pulmonary disease (COPD).

11. The answer is D (4). (*VIII B 2 a, 4–5*) In establishing the etiology of a pleural effusion, it is useful to determine whether the fluid is a transudate or an exudate. This determination often can be made on the basis of a chemical analysis of the pleural fluid. A pleural fluid protein content of more than 3 g/dl and a lactate dehydrogenase (LDH) content of more than 250 mg/dl usually indicate the presence of an exudate. In addition, an exudate usually is associated with a pleural fluid-to-serum protein ratio of less than 0.5 and a pleural fluid-to-serum LDH ratio of less than 0.6. Pleural fluid pH values below 7.2 and a pleural fluid glucose content of less than 20 mg/dl also are associated with inflammatory effusions (exudates). With the exception of the LDH findings, all of the pleural fluid findings listed indicate the presence of an exudate. Exudates are caused by inflammation or disease of the pleural surface or by lymphatic obstruction (e.g., due to tuberculosis, lung cancer, or pneumonia). Transudates are caused by elevated systemic or pulmonary venous pressure or by decreased plasma oncotic pressure (e.g., due to congestive heart failure or nephrotic syndrome).

12. The answer is B (1, 3). (*IX E 1, 2 a–b*) The early clinical features of lung cancer reflect the more local nature of the tumor and, therefore, include predominantly pulmonary symptoms. The most common symptom noted early in the disease process is an increase or a change in the nature of a chronic cough. Mild hemoptysis, pneumonia, and pleurisy also may occur, and physical examination at this time may show signs of pleural effusion. Clinical features noted later in the disease process reflect the tumor's spread beyond the lungs and, consequently, include a host of diverse, systemic symptoms. Tumor spread within the chest may be evidenced by pleuritic pain, hoarseness, and dysphagia. Symptoms of tumor spread outside the chest include bone pain in the back, pelvis, or ribs and convulsions and other neurologic signs.

13. The answer is E (all). (*V B*) Adult respiratory distress syndrome may be caused by many dissimilar factors, with the common denominator of its precipitation believed to be a complement-mediated mechanism. Although such a mechanism does not completely explain the etiology in all cases, it provides an explanation in most cases. Consequently, adult respiratory distress syndrome is associated with events that trigger the complement system. It also is associated with conditions (e.g., tissue trauma) that trigger the release of tissue thromboplastin and, thereby, factors that initiate the clotting cascade or precipitate disseminated intravascular coagulation (DIC). Sepsis and blood transfusion also may precipitate DIC.

14. The answer is C (2, 4). [*VII F 2 a, c; XIII B 1 c (2)*] Pleural and peritoneal mesotheliomas are believed to be the result of asbestos exposure. There is a long latent period from the time the patient first is exposed until the onset of the disease. The association is made even more difficult in some patients because of brief exposure many years previous to this diagnosis. A tissue specimen is necessary for the diagnosis, and open pleural biopsy often is necessary to differentiate mesothelioma from poorly differentiated adenocarcinoma. Asbestos exposure also is associated with an increased risk of bronchogenic carcinoma, and this risk is enhanced in individuals who also smoke cigarettes. Cigarette smoking does not have this additive effect on the development of pleural mesothelioma. Patients with pleural mesotheliomas may reveal pleural thickening and pleural effusion on chest x-ray.

15. The answer is E (all). (*V E 1*) Tissue oxygenation is a function of cardiac output, hemoglobin concentration, and percent saturation of oxygen in the blood. Even when cardiac output is good, a patient may have local vasoconstriction that can cause inadequate tissue oxygenation to certain organs. A decrease in oxygen affinity and, therefore, an increase in oxygen unloading from hemoglobin can cause tissue anoxia. In this event, the oxygen dissociation curve is said to "shift to the right."

16–20. The answers are: 16-B, 17-C, 18-D, 19-A, 20-A. [*XIV A 1, 4, 5 b (5), B 1, C 1, E 1 a*] Goodpasture's syndrome is a rare, progressive disease of the lungs and kidneys, which is caused by an anti-glomerular basement membrane (anti-GBM) antibody, usually IgG. The anti-GBM antibody reacts with glomerular and alveolar basement membranes to cause alveolar hemorrhage and glomerulonephritis. There is no evidence of necrotizing granuloma in Goodpasture's syndrome, as there is in Wegener's granulomatosis.

Like Goodpasture's syndrome, Wegener's granulomatosis may involve the kidneys and lungs as well as other organs. This disease is characterized by granulomatous inflammation and necrosis of these organs. Wegener's granulomatosis is regarded as a systemic vasculitis; Goodpasture's syndrome is not.

Alveolar proteinosis is characterized by massive accumulations of a phospholipid-rich material in alveoli. The substance, which is closely related in its chemical and physiologic properties to pulmonary surfactant, may well accumulate as a result of impaired clearance. There is no evidence of vasculitis, granuloma, or renal disease in this entity.

The lesion in sarcoidosis classically is a noncaseating granuloma, which occurs in the lungs as well as other organs. Systemic involvement may be demonstrated as uveitis, skin lesions, polyarthritis (bone and joint involvement), Bell's palsy and other cranial neuropathies (neural involvement), and arrhythmias and conduction disturbances (cardiac involvement).

3
Hematologic Diseases
Ronald N. Rubin

I. RED CELL DISORDERS

A. Anemia caused by abnormal hemoglobin synthesis and iron metabolism. Hemoglobin, which represents 95% of the total composition of a red blood cell, is a mixture of globin and the iron-containing heme compound, **protoporphyrin**. Any difficulty in hemoglobin synthesis or iron metabolism will result in hemoglobin-deficient cells. As a rule, such deficient cells exhibit **hypochromia** (i.e., diminished hemoglobin concentration) and **microcytosis** (i.e., diminished size). Both conditions may be detected using the red cell indices available by calculation and the Coulter counter together with an examination of a stained blood smear. Disorders causing such anemia fall into four major classes.

1. Iron deficiency anemia. Iron deficiency is most commonly caused by blood loss when the loss of the iron component exceeds dietary intake of iron. Examples include gastrointestinal blood loss from an ulcer or a tumor and menstrual blood loss. Occasionally in the neonate and young child, new blood formation and subsequent increased iron utilization exceeds iron intake and results in anemia without concomitant blood loss.

  a. Incidence. Iron deficiency anemia is the most common form of anemia in the United States, where 20% of adult women are reported to be iron deficient.

  b. Symptoms. The symptoms of iron deficiency anemia, like all anemias, include fatigue and weakness. Symptoms specific to iron deficiency may include epithelial changes, such as brittle nails and atrophic tongue. In addition, the underlying pathology may dominate the symptoms (e.g., in the case of a peptic ulcer).

  c. Diagnosis. In the appropriate clinical setting, a smear showing hypochromia and microcytosis is adequate (e.g., in a young woman with excessive menstruation and anemia). When more specific tests are needed, a positive diagnosis is made from an absence of marrow iron on bone marrow examination, abnormally low levels of ferritin, and a low serum iron in association with an elevated total iron-binding capacity.

  d. Therapy. Treatment usually is restoration of the body's iron stores to correct the anemia. As a rule, oral iron in the form of ferrous sulfate ($FeSO_4$) suffices, but for patients who do not tolerate this form, liquid forms are available. In difficult cases that are refractory either physiologically or due to an inability to take oral iron, parenteral iron preparations are given. Reticulocytosis occurs 7 days after appropriate treatment; after 3 weeks, the hemoglobin level increases several grams.

2. Anemia of chronic inflammatory disease. This mild to moderate anemia is associated with inflammatory diseases, such as rheumatoid arthritis, serious infections, and carcinoma. This type of anemia is characterized by hemoglobin levels of 8–10 g/dl, although lower levels are possible. It is unusual for the hemoglobin level to be less than 7 g/dl.

  a. Pathophysiology. Patients with this anemia have plentiful iron but have a reticuloendothelial blockade to iron utilization by the bone marrow. Therefore, inadequate amounts of iron are available to the bone marrow for red cell formation in spite of adequate body stores.

  b. Diagnosis. Anemia associated with chronic inflammation is of moderate degree and reveals slight hypochromia and microcytosis. The mean corpuscular volume (MCV) is 80–85 μ^3, and the mean corpuscular hemoglobin concentration (MCHC) is 30%–32%. If stained, the marrow reveals plentiful iron stores. Also, ferritin usually is normal or only slightly elevated. Serum iron is lowered as is the total iron-binding capacity, which is unlike the clinical situation with iron deficiency anemia.

  c. Therapy. Hematinics including iron are not effective treatment for this disorder. If the underlying inflammatory disease is corrected, this anemia usually reverses within 1 month.

3. Sideroblastic anemias. These anemias, caused by disorders in the synthesis of the heme moiety of hemoglobin, are characterized by trapped iron in the mitochondria of nucleated red blood cells. These "ringed" sideroblasts are so-named because the extensive iron deposits in each cell form a ring around the nucleus. The defective heme synthesis causes diminished hemoglobin levels in these cells; as a result, this cell population is hypochromic and microcytic. Often, some normal or slightly macrocytic cells are seen intermingling with the hypochromic, microcytic cells, and a blood smear revealing such a condition is diagnostic of this anemia.

    a. Varieties. There are two types of sideroblastic anemias.

        (1) Hereditary sideroblastic anemia. This X-linked condition is due to an abnormality in pyridoxine (vitamin B_6) metabolism. It is thought to be a congenital defect in the enzyme, δ-**aminolevulinic acid (ALA) synthetase**.

        (2) Acquired sideroblastic anemias are more common than the hereditary type. Drugs such as isoniazid are known to cause sideroblastic anemia, but many cases are idiopathic.

    b. Diagnosis. This anemia may be relatively severe in patients over 60 years old and is characterized by hemoglobin levels of 8–10 g/dl. The Coulter counter reveals normocytic or even macrocytic cells, but examination of the blood smear shows a dimorphous population with some very small cells. The bone marrow reveals erythroid hyperplasia, and iron staining demonstrates the ringed sideroblasts. Iron studies show elevated ferritin levels and high serum irons with high transferrin saturation.

    c. Therapy. All patients should be given a trial of pyridoxine in high doses; in all but the hereditary cases, however, this usually fails. Androgens also are rarely effective. Often these patients are transfusion-dependent. A portion (10%) of acquired idiopathic cases develop acute leukemia. In these instances the sideroblastic anemia was a "preleukemic syndrome." If a drug such as isoniazid or alcohol is involved, the anemia and sideroblastic changes will regress with discontinuation of the drug.

4. Thalassemias are genetic disorders characterized by diminished synthesis of one of the globin chains. These diseases are due to abnormalities in the genes that are responsible for synthesis of the globin portion of the hemoglobin molecule. Thalassemias are named according to the deficient chain.

    a. Varieties

        (1) Alpha-thalassemias. These disorders are characterized by deficient α-chain synthesis usually due to deletion of the α-globin gene from the genome. Ribonucleic acid (RNA) for the α-globin gene is not present in the α-thalassemias. There are four such genes, and, thus, four α-thalassemias; these range from a mild, subclinical, asymptomatic anemia to a severe anemia that is fatal in utero. The α-thalassemias are most prevalent in Oriental populations.

        (2) Beta-thalassemias. These disorders are due to absence or malfunction of the β-globin gene. In the latter case, RNA is present but in reduced amounts or in defective forms. The two β-globin genes in the genome result in two different forms of β-thalassemia. **Beta-thalassemia major** or **Cooley's anemia** is a severe disease that appears in childhood and is fatal by 30 years of age; such patients are transfusion-dependent. Patients with β-**thalassemia minor**, a mild anemia, are not transfusion-dependent and can live full, normal lives. The β-thalassemias are most prevalent in individuals of Mediterranean descent, particularly those from Greece and Italy.

    b. Diagnosis. The thalassemias should be suspected in an anemic patient who reveals marked abnormalities on blood smear. Such abnormalities include microcytosis, hypochromia, and **poikilocytosis** (i.e., the presence of bizarrely shaped red blood cells).

        (1) Alpha-thalassemia is most difficult to diagnose when it exists in the carrier state. Patients with the carrier form present with a mild microcytic hypochromic anemia. There is no excess of the non–β-hemoglobins because all chains have α components. Therefore, detailed and sophisticated chain analysis studies are required for definitive diagnosis. In neonates, however, the diagnosis can be made from cord blood tests that show an increase in **Barts hemoglobin**.

        (2) Beta-thalassemia resembles iron deficiency anemia except that iron is present in the marrow. The diagnosis is confirmed by quantitative globin measurements that reveal an elevation in the non–β-chains (e.g., hemoglobin A_2 and hemoglobin F).

B. Macrocytic anemias are characterized by red blood cells that exceed 100 μ in size. Three major mechanisms are linked to the development of macrocytic anemia.

    1. Accelerated erythropoiesis. Reticulocytes and young erythrocytes are larger than normal; therefore, individuals with large numbers of reticulocytes have a large number of circulating cells of great size. A reticulocyte count confirms the diagnosis.

    2. Increased membrane surface area. Patients with excessive plasma lipids absorb these lipids onto red cell surfaces, which creates an enlarged membrane surface area and a macrocytosis in excess of 100 μ. This condition is most common in patients with liver disease and can be diagnosed by a blood smear that reveals the characteristic **target cell** of liver disease (i.e., a round macrocyte with a redundant membrane).

    3. Defective deoxyribonucleic acid (DNA) synthesis is the main characteristic of the classic **megaloblastic anemias.** In these conditions, red cells cannot produce nucleic acid and so nuclear maturation is arrested. Cytoplasmic maturation proceeds, however, resulting in abnormally large cells. These cells are larger than those seen with accelerated erythropoiesis and with increased membrane surface area. An MCV that exceeds 115 μ^3 is not uncommon.

      a. Etiology. Megaloblastic anemias usually are caused by a deficiency of either vitamin B_{12} or folic acid.

        (1) B_{12} deficiency may result from tapeworm infestation, purely vegetable diets, and intestinal blind loops with bacterial overgrowth. The most common cause, however, is a lack of the intrinsic factor necessary for vitamin B_{12} absorption into the terminal ileum. This condition leads to classic **pernicious anemia.**

        (2) Folic acid deficiency is caused by dietary deficiency due to inadequate intake, absorption, or both.

        (3) Drug-induced disorders of DNA synthesis. Certain chemotherapeutic drugs (e.g., methotrexate) as well as nonchemotherapeutic agents (e.g., phenytoin) interfere with folic acid metabolism and cause megaloblastic anemia and bone marrow changes. These diagnoses can be made easily from patient history.

      b. Clinical manifestations. Patients with these disorders present with varying degrees of anemia associated with large red cells. Because nucleic acid metabolism is necessary for all cellular elements in bone marrow, white cells and platelets are diminished. The ineffective erythropoiesis and intramedullary hemolysis associated with this disorder often result in serum **lactate dehydrogenase (LDH)** levels that exceed 500 units/dl. Both red and white cells in bone marrow reveal the classic megaloblastic sign of immature, open nuclei in association with mature cytoplasmic components. Blood smear shows characteristic oval macrocytes and hypersegmented polymorphonuclear leukocytes.

      c. Differential diagnosis

        (1) Serum levels of both vitamins as well as red cell folic acid levels should be measured to determine whether the deficiency is in folic acid or vitamin B_{12}.

        (2) Vitamin B_{12} has a neurologic function; therefore, when a macrocytic anemia is associated with neurologic symptoms, particularly posterior column signs and symptoms, vitamin B_{12} deficiency should be suspected. The hallmarks of pernicious anemia are macrocytic anemia, neurologic symptoms and signs, and **atrophic glossitis.**

        (3) The **Schilling test** for the presence of intrinsic factor and intestinal function should be performed to differentiate the cause of vitamin B_{12} deficiency.

      d. Therapy. Specific therapy is determined by the vitamin that is missing. Folic acid alone should never be given in an undiagnosed case of macrocytic anemia; folic acid reverses hematologic signs, but neurologic degeneration continues unabated.

        (1) Cases of pernicious anemia due to vitamin B_{12} deficiency require lifelong treatment with parenteral vitamin B_{12}. If reversible causes are found (e.g., intestinal bacterial overgrowth), appropriate measures may reverse the deficiency and obviate the need for permanent vitamin B_{12} therapy.

        (2) Folic acid deficiency is treated with oral preparations of folic acid.

C. Normochromic normocytic anemias represent a vast array of conditions characterized by normal cell size and hemoglobin concentration. These anemias are not related by common pathogenic mechanisms; classification is by the degree of marrow response to the anemia.

    1. Anemia associated with impaired marrow response. The following anemias are characterized by normal or low reticulocyte counts.

      a. Hypoplastic or **aplastic anemia** is an intrinsic marrow disease characterized by an absence of stem cells. Other stem cell lines in marrow are involved, with a resultant **pancytopenia.** Severe cases of this serious disease are associated with a high mortality rate. There is little effective treatment for this disease; patients are supported with blood transfusions. In young patients, bone marrow transplantation techniques have offered hope.

      b. Disorders characterized by infiltration of bone marrow include myeloma, carcinoma, and leukoerythroblastosis. Disruption of bone marrow architecture is common; a blood smear that reveals immature white cells and nucleated red blood cells is a clue to the presence of these conditions. A bone marrow aspirate and biopsy confirm the diagnosis in such cases.

c. **Anemia due to diminished erythropoietin secretion** is the anemia of **chronic renal failure.** Erythropoietin is a protein-lipid molecule required by the marrow for adequate red blood cell formation. With severe kidney disease, the erythropoietin secreted by the kidneys is lost and anemia ensues. The degree of anemia roughly correlates with the degree of renal failure. There is no effective therapy for this anemia, and patients do not respond to dialysis. Proper attention to iron and folic acid stores is important in this group of patients, as deficiencies in these nutrients secondarily complicate the anemia of renal failure.

d. **Other anemias associated with hypoproliferation of bone marrow** include those of hypothyroidism, hypopituitarism, and liver disease.

2. **Anemia associated with appropriately increased red blood cell production.** The following anemias are characterized by increased amounts of reticulocytes.

   a. **Anemia following hemorrhage.** An increased reticulocyte count is the normal marrow response in patients who bleed either overtly (e.g., with surgery) or covertly (e.g., into the gastrointestinal tract) and have adequate iron stores. This condition can be confused with hemolysis; however, the clinical situation of a postoperative patient presenting with a large resolving hematoma confirms the diagnosis of post-hemorrhagic anemia.

   b. **Hemolytic anemias** represent conditions in which the red blood cell survival is shortened. In most cases the marrow is intrinsically normal; thus, adequate new red blood cells can be made, and the patients have elevated reticulocyte counts. Diagnostic of these anemias are signs of increased red cell destruction (e.g., shortened red cell half-life, elevated serum LDH, and reduced serum haptoglobin) combined with signs of accelerated marrow activity (e.g., elevated reticulocyte counts and erythroid hyperplasia in the marrow). The diagnosis of hemolysis should be made first, and the specific cause of the hemolysis should be sought later. Hemolytic anemia exists in hundreds of forms, which are grouped as follows.

      (1) **Hemolytic anemia due to factors extrinsic to the red blood cell**

         (a) **Autoantibodies** can attach to the red cell and cause its destruction by the reticuloendothelial system. A classic example is **Coombs-positive hemolytic anemia** due to either warm (immunoglobulin G) or cold (immunoglobulin M) antibodies. This anemia may be idiopathic or may arise as a complication of collagen disease or lymphoma. In severe cases, steroids and splenectomy may be required to control the anemia.

         (b) **Exogenous agents** such as malarial organisms can render the red blood cell liable to hemolysis.

         (c) **Abnormalities in the circulation** can cause premature destruction of red blood cells. Listed below are examples of such abnormalities; disorders associated with each condition are cited also.

            (i) Lipid abnormalities (spur-cell anemia in advanced liver disease)

            (ii) Fibrin deposition in the microvasculature with shearing of red blood cells (disseminated intravascular coagulation syndrome)

            (iii) Red cell damage due to trauma from prosthetic heart valves

      (2) **Hemolytic anemia due to factors intrinsic to the red blood cell.** These disorders involve congenital abnormalities that render the red blood cell liable to hemolysis.

         (a) **Membrane disorders** include such conditions as **hereditary spherocytosis.** In this disorder, a defect in the membrane sodium-potassium-ATPase pump causes red cell swelling. This results in the characteristic smear finding of small, round, hyperchromic red blood cells without the usual central pallor (i.e., spherocytes). These cells are osmotically fragile and are destroyed in the spleen. Splenectomy usually controls the anemia, although the red cell defect remains.

         (b) **Hemoglobin disorders—hemoglobinopathies.** These diseases, of which more than 250 are known, are caused by point mutations in the DNA code related to variation in a single amino acid in the globin chains. Such amino acid changes cause a variety of structural and functional changes in the red blood cell. The most common hemoglobinopathies cause the hemoglobin to become rigid, and the red cell becomes liable to hemolysis.

            (i) **Examples.** The most common hemoglobinopathy is **hemoglobin S**, which causes **sickle cell anemia.** This disorder occurs in 1% of American blacks and is characterized by repeated painful crises and severe hemolytic anemia. Other common hemoglobinopathies include **hemoglobin C**, **hemoglobin O**, and mixtures such as **hemoglobin SC.**

            (ii) **Diagnosis and therapy.** Diagnoses are confirmed by hemoglobin electrophoresis, which demonstrates the characteristic changes in mobility caused by specific amino acid changes. Therapy involves supportive care with transfusions when indicated (e.g., during hypoplastic crises), analgesics for the pain of microvasculature occlusion, and appropriate treatment of the common and potentially fatal problem of intercurrent infections.

- **(c) Disorders of the cytoplasm and enzymes** occur as congenital hemolytic anemias. A red blood cell lacks a nucleus and mitochondria when it leaves the marrow; therefore, a red cell must survive its 120-day life span with its given complement of enzymes. A deficient red cell is hemolyzed earlier than a normal cell.
  - **(i) Glucose-6-phosphate dehydrogenase (G6PD) deficiency** is an extremely common, X-linked disorder whose 150+ subtypes affect over 100 million individuals worldwide. Deficient individuals are liable to oxidant stress such as occurs with infections or with certain drugs (e.g., sulfa drugs and quinine). A deficiency of G6PD also destroys the reducing capacity of the red blood cells. It is believed that G6PD protects individuals from *falciparum* malaria; this disease is most common in endemic areas.
  - **(ii) Pyruvate kinase (PK) deficiency** is an autosomal recessive example of an enzymopathy. This deficiency is most common in northern European populations. Patients may benefit from splenectomy.

II. HEMATOCRIT DISORDERS.
Increases in hematocrit are caused by either **increased red cell mass** or **decreased plasma volume**. The following discussion deals exclusively with disorders associated with abnormal elevation of hematocrit (i.e., hematocrit of 55% and above).

- **A. Terminology.** The term **polycythemia** often is used to describe an increase in the number of red blood cells, with no reference to fluctuations in leukocytes and platelets. However, this condition is more accurately termed **erythrocytosis**. [There is a condition called **polycythemia vera**, in which leukocytes and platelets also increase in number. See section II C 2 b (2) for a discussion of this disorder.] Erythrocytosis increases hematocrit in two different ways.

  1. **Relative erythrocytosis** refers to an elevation of hematocrit due to diminished plasma volume; red cell mass remains normal in this condition.

  2. **Absolute erythrocytosis** refers to an elevation of hematocrit due to a true increase in red cell mass.

- **B. Pathophysiology.** Blood flow and viscosity are inversely proportional to hematocrit; therefore, an excessively elevated hematocrit can diminish tissue blood flow, decrease tissue oxygen delivery, and increase cardiac work.

- **C. Classification**

  1. **Relative erythrocytosis** exists in two forms.
     - **a. "Stress" erythrocytosis,** or **Gaisbock's syndrome,** occurs predominantly in middle-aged men. This disorder usually is asymptomatic, although it may be associated with increased cardiovascular disease. It is important to differentiate patients with stress erythrocytosis from those with early and subtle manifestations of the much more serious condition, polycythemia vera; the former group requires no treatment.
     - **b. Erythrocytosis occurs secondary to known causes of contracted plasma volume** (e.g., excessive diuresis; nasogastric drainage; severe gastroenteritis, especially in infants; and burns). These conditions are apparent clinically; therapy includes fluid and plasma replacement with treatment of the underlying condition.

  2. **Absolute erythrocytosis** is classified according to the mechanism responsible for increased red cell mass.
     - **a. Hypoxia.** The red cell mass rises secondary to tissue hypoxia, which causes an increase in renal erythropoietin and subsequently a hematocrit elevation.
       - **(1) Etiology.** Causes include severe lung disease, severe heart failure, cyanotic heart disease with right-to-left cardiopulmonary shunts, and abnormal hemoglobins with increased oxygen affinity.
       - **(2) Diagnosis** may be apparent clinically, but blood gas analysis showing arterial oxygen saturation less than 92% and P_{50} analysis (i.e., studies of the oxygen-releasing characteristics of hemoglobin) may be required to confirm the diagnosis.
       - **(3) Therapy** is somewhat conjectural, but phlebotomy is the favored treatment for patients with hematocrits that are persistently greater than 55%.
     - **b. Neoplasia**
       - **(1) Neoplastic erythropoietin sources** cause the red cell mass to increase. This condition would be easily demonstrable if an adequate erythropoietin assay were available; however, this is not the case presently.
         - **(a) Etiology.** Causes include hypernephroma and renal cysts; such renal pathology ac-

counts for more than 90% of this type of erythrocytosis. Other tumors include cerebellar hemangioblastoma, hepatoma, and uterine fibroids.
- **(b) Diagnosis** requires radiologic demonstration of the appropriate tumor, as with intravenous pyelography and liver scanning.
- **(c) Therapy.** Removal of the tumor corrects the hematocrit.

(2) **Autonomous bone marrow.** In the condition **polycythemia vera**, the bone marrow becomes autonomous and synthesizes cells independently of erythropoietin levels. (Theoretically, erythropoietin levels would be near zero if measured accurately.) Polycythemia vera represents a true neoplasm of the marrow stem cells.
- **(a) Diagnosis.** According to the Polycythemia Vera Study Group, diagnosis is confirmed by the presence of all three of the following **major criteria** or by the first two major criteria and any two of the following **minor criteria**.
  - **(i)** The major criteria are elevated red cell mass, arterial oxygen saturation exceeding 92%, and splenomegaly.
  - **(ii)** The minor criteria are leukocytosis, thrombocytosis, elevated leukocyte alkaline phosphatase, and elevated serum vitamin B_{12} level.
- **(b) Therapy** involves removal of red cells, suppression of marrow function, or both.
  - **(i) Phlebotomy** removes red cells and should be performed to lower hematocrit to below 50%. If used alone, this is the safest therapy. Marrow suppression is needed when hematocrit control requires frequent phlebotomy or when other cell lines are elevated.
  - **(ii) Radioactive phosphorus** effectively modulates marrow activity and is well tolerated. This treatment is especially good for elderly patients.
  - **(iii) Chemotherapy** with such agents as chlorambucil is effective but has fallen out of favor due to the leukemogenesis associated with this treatment.
- **(c) Survival** is measured in years and is 7–10 years in most studies. Untreated polycythemia vera, however, has a survival of only 2–3 years. In patients treated with phlebotomy, the major causes of morbidity and mortality are thromboembolic and cardiovascular in nature. Patients treated with chemotherapy succumb to second neoplasms and leukemic transformation.

III. WHITE CELL DISORDERS. The white cells include lymphocytes, monocytes, eosinophils, basophils, and neutrophils (polymorphonuclear leukocytes). Disorders of white blood cells can be considered in terms of excessive or reduced numbers of cells and in terms of functional abnormality.

- **A. Lymphocytes** exist in marrow as well as in the lymphoid tissue of the body. Lymphocyte functions include delayed hypersensitivity, which is performed by T lymphocytes (**T cells**), and antibody production, which is performed by B lymphocytes (**B cells**) and plasma cells.

  1. **Lymphopenia** refers to a diminished number of lymphocytes.
     - **a. Lymphopenia without significant immune deficiency** is seen in many illnesses that cause elevated serum cortisol levels, such as acute infections and inflammatory states. Also, chemotherapy, radiotherapy, and Hodgkin's disease are associated with lymphopenia. In none of these conditions is antibody production severely affected.
     - **b. Lymphopenia with immune deficiency** is associated with the immune deficiency syndromes, most of which are congenital diseases.
       - **(1) Varieties**
         - **(a) B-cell deficiency**
           - **(i) Bruton's agammaglobulinemia** is an X-linked disease characterized by recurrent infections with encapsulated organisms and caused by deficient quantities of opsonizing antibody. Although peripheral lymphocyte counts may be normal, specific counting for B cells shows their absence. Also, lymphoid follicles reveal no germinal centers, which are the B-cell areas. Therapy consists of exogenous gamma globulin and plasma via transfusion.
           - **(ii) Other B-cell deficiency states** include common variable hypogammaglobulinemia and immunoglobin A (IgA) deficiency.
         - **(b) T-cell deficiency. Thymic hypoplasia** (DiGeorge syndrome) is the prototype T-cell deficiency. Patients with this condition have variable total lymphocyte counts but low numbers of T cells with absent T-cell function. Recurrent fungal infections are seen in these patients.
         - **(c) Deficiency of both B and T cells.** Disorders characterized by diminished numbers of both B and T cells include ataxia-telangiectasia syndrome, Wiskott-Aldrich syndrome of immunodeficiency and thrombocytopenia, and severe combined immunodeficiency disease (SCID).
       - **(2) Diagnosis.** For all of the above conditions, diagnosis requires the clinical setting of repeated infections combined with:

(a) Lymphocyte counts of B and T cells

(b) Measurement of specific immunoglobulin levels

(c) Demonstration of the absence of specific B-cell areas (i.e., germinal centers and plasma cells) or T-cell areas (i.e., thymus and lymph node medullary cords)

2. Lymphocytosis is defined as an excessive number of lymphocytes (i.e., > 5000/mm³). The differential diagnosis of absolute lymphocytosis is limited.

   a. Infection. Certain infections cause lymphocytosis. In children, both pertussis and acute infectious lymphocytosis may cause counts that exceed 50,000. In adults, lesser elevations are seen with hepatitis and infectious mononucleosis.

   b. Hematopoietic disorders associated with lymphocytosis include acute lymphoblastic leukemia, chronic lymphocytic leukemia, and other lymphomas.

   (1) Chronic lymphocytic leukemia (CLL). An adult who is over 50 years of age and who manifests a mature lymphocytosis most likely has CLL. The cells associated with CLL are mature lymphocytes that accumulate in the body over time.

   (a) Diagnosis. A peripheral blood smear showing a mature lymphocytosis is adequate. Corroborative findings include marrow infiltration by mature lymphocytes, an enlarged spleen, and lymphadenopathy.

   (b) Staging. CLL tumor burden is related to certain clinical findings; these presentations also have prognostic significance.

   (i) Stage 0 is characterized by peripheral lymphocytosis only. The prognosis for patients with stage 0 CLL is excellent; patients usually survive 10–12 years.

   (ii) Stages 1 and 2. Stage 1 is characterized by peripheral lymphocytosis and lymphadenopathy; **stage 2** is characterized by the presence of splenomegaly. Both stages 1 and 2 have intermediate prognoses, usually 4–7 years.

   (iii) Stages 3 and 4. Stage 3 is characterized by the presence of anemia and **stage 4** by the presence of thrombocytopenia. Both stages 3 and 4 signify marrow failure and have ominous prognoses, about 18 months.

   (c) Therapy for CLL is conservative. The chance of survival is not significantly improved with any known treatment. Excessive therapy can be harmful.

   (i) Early stage CLL. As a rule, stages 1 and 2 CLL should not be treated.

   (ii) Late stage CLL is treated with an alkylating agent (e.g., chlorambucil), with or without steroids. Low-dose total body irradiation also is used.

   (2) Certain well-differentiated **lymphomas** also are characterized by an excessive number of lymphocytes in the blood. These disorders are similar to CLL.

   (3) Acute lymphoblastic leukemia is a disease characterized by maturation arrest in the lymphoid line with tissue infiltration by lymphoblasts. (This disease is discussed in more detail in section IV A.)

B. Basophils, eosinophils, and neutrophils. Disorders in these cells also are classified according to fluctuations in cell numbers and to functional deficiency.

   1. Basophils. An abnormally increased number of basophils is called **basophilia**. This uncommon condition usually is associated with the myeloproliferative syndromes, particularly chronic myeloid leukemia.

   2. Eosinophils. An abnormally increased number of eosinophils is called **eosinophilia**. This condition is more common than basophilia and occurs secondary to other disease processes including:

   a. Neoplasia (e.g., lymphoma and Hodgkin's disease)

   b. Addison's disease

   c. Allergic and atopic disease

   d. Collagen vascular disease (e.g., necrotizing vasculitis)

   e. Parasitic infestation

   3. Neutrophils

   a. Neutrophilia is an excessively increased number of neutrophils in the blood. The following are causes of neutrophilia.

   (1) Most cases of neutrophilia result from such conditions as infection, tumor, stress, collagen disorders, and steroid administration; the underlying disease may not be apparent clinically.

   (2) In unusual cases, more than 50,000 neutrophils appear in the blood. These so-called **leukemoid reactions** can be differentiated from the leukemias by the absence of the circulating blast forms and the finding of elevated leukocyte alkaline phosphatase values.

   (3) Neutrophilia also results from **neoplastic marrow diseases**, such as polycythemia vera and chronic myeloid leukemia (CML).

(a) **Diagnosis of CML.** CML is suspected in patients with excessive white cell counts and splenomegaly. Peripheral blood smears reveal a spectrum of cell forms ranging from mature polymorphonuclear neutrophils to immature blasts. Two findings confirm the diagnosis: the presence of an abnormal marker chromosome (the **Philadelphia chromosome**) in the marrow precursor cells and very low leukocyte alkaline phosphatase levels.

(b) **Prognosis of CML.** The median survival rate for CML patients is 3–4 years. Most patients die during the so-called **blast crisis**, when this chronic disorder converts into a highly malignant variety of acute leukemia.

b. **Neutropenia** is an absolute decrease in the number of circulating neutrophils. Neutropenia occurs rarely as an early manifestation of intrinsic marrow disease (e.g., acute leukemia) but more commonly occurs secondary to exogenous stimuli.

(1) **Infections.** Certain viral infections (e.g., hepatitis and influenza) and bacterial infections (e.g., typhoid fever) cause neutropenia.

(2) **Drugs** are associated with neutropenia and in severe instances can cause agranulocytosis.

(a) **Drug types**

(i) Analgesics and sedatives, including aminopyrines and phenylbutazone, are common offenders.

(ii) Phenothiazines and antithyroid medications also cause neutropenia.

(b) **Agranulocytosis**, which may occur in very severe cases, is characterized by:

(i) Profoundly lowered neutrophil counts (i.e., < 500/mm³)

(ii) Severe prostration, high fever, and often a necrotic pharyngitis

(iii) Bone marrow showing **maturation arrest** (i.e., large numbers of immature white cell forms in an otherwise normal marrow)

(iv) High mortality rates unless treated early and aggressively with support measures and potent bactericidal antibiotics

(3) The **collagen vascular diseases** (e.g., SLE and rheumatoid arthritis) recently have been shown to cause neutropenia via immune destruction of white blood cells.

(4) **Familial forms of neutropenia** include familial benign chronic neutropenia, cyclic neutropenia, and chronic idiopathic neutropenia. These disorders have good prognoses, although they are associated with increased nuisance infections (e.g., boils) when the neutrophil count is less than 500/mm³.

(5) Presently, the most common neutropenia is associated with the **chemotherapeutic agents** used in the therapy of malignant disease. Such agents include alkylating agents (e.g., cyclophosphamide); antimetabolites [e.g., methotrexate, 5-fluorouracil (5-FU), and cytosine arabinoside]; and tumor antibiotics (e.g., doxorubicin).

c. **Functional disorders** of neutrophils involve a compromised ability to fight infection. These conditions are rare; affected individuals present with recurrent infections. The following are prototypical examples.

(1) **Chédiak-Higashi syndrome** is an autosomal recessive disorder characterized by albinism and increased pyogenic infection. Also, neutrophils and other granule-containing cells (e.g., melanosomes) reveal giant, fused, peroxidase-staining granules with decreased ability to kill ingested microbes.

(2) **Chronic granulomatous disease (CGD)** of childhood is an X-linked disorder in neutrophil metabolism characterized by a defect in neutrophil-free radical formation (associated with the oxidative burst and killing activity in neutrophils), resulting in susceptibility to recurrent suppurative infections. This condition often is fatal, and the diagnosis is confirmed by the presence of neutrophils that cannot oxidize nitro blue tetrazolium dye to blue-black from colorless.

IV. **ACUTE LEUKEMIAS.** These disorders in the maturation of hematopoietic tissue are characterized by the presence of immature leukocytes in the marrow and peripheral blood. The immature cells are arrested in the earliest phases of differentiation and are referred to as **blasts**.

A. **Classification.** It is important both prognostically and therapeutically to distinguish the lymphoblastic from the nonlymphoblastic (myeloid) leukemias. Current classification of cells involves special histochemical stains and marker enzymes (e.g., terminal transferase in acute lymphoblastic leukemia); this classification is accurate in more than 95% of cases.

1. **Acute lymphoblastic leukemia (ALL)** is common in children; 85% of cases of ALL occur in children, and 90% of leukemia that occurs in children is ALL.

2. **Acute nonlymphoblastic leukemia (ANLL)** or **acute myeloid leukemia (AML)** is common in adults, and the incidence increases with age. There are several subtypes of AML, three of which are discussed below.

    a. Promyelocytic leukemia is characterized by abnormal promyelocytes with giant granules; this leukemia often is associated with disseminated intravascular coagulation.

    b. Monocytic and myelomonocytic leukemias are characterized by cerebriform monoblast components. Gum and skin infiltration is a common feature of these leukemias, and patient survival is shorter than that associated with other AML varieties.

    c. Erythroleukemia is characterized by abnormal nucleated red cells. Patients with this leukemia typically show poor responsiveness to chemotherapy.

B. Clinical features of acute leukemia represent the effects of marrow infiltration by nonmaturing, functionless blast cells, including subsequent bone marrow failure.

    1. Physical findings include fatigue (due to anemia); fever and infection (due to neutropenia); petechiae and purpura (due to thrombocytopenia); bleeding; and pallor. Infiltrative symptoms may include adenopathy, splenomegaly, and bone pain.

    2. Laboratory findings include pancytopenia, circulating blast forms, and elevated uric acid levels.

C. Diagnosis. The diagnosis of acute leukemia is confirmed by the finding of blast infiltration of the bone marrow. Marrow studies with special stains and enzymes are performed to identify the specific subtype of leukemia involved.

D. Therapy of acute leukemia is complex and carries a 20% early mortality. Treatment, therefore, is best performed by physicians who are experienced in the supportive care needed to maintain the patient through this period and to achieve remissions.

    1. Chemotherapy. Initial therapy consists of chemotherapeutic ablation of the leukemic cell line. In many cases, especially those of AML, it is necessary to ablate all normal marrow as well. Because normal marrow has a shorter generation time than leukemic blasts, recovery with normal marrow tissue is possible. This initial marrow ablation is termed **induction therapy**.

    a. ALL blasts are initially more selectively sensitive to chemotherapy than AML blasts. It often is possible to destroy ALL blasts with some sparing of normal marrow. Thus, induction therapy for ALL is associated with lower morbidity and mortality rates than it is for AML.

    b. Induction therapy for AML usually requires ablation of all marrow elements, both blasts and normal tissue. As a result, a profound **hypoplastic phase** occurs prior to the recovery of normal marrow, and this phase is associated with high morbidity and mortality rates.

    c. Cytosine arabinoside and daunomycin are initial treatment agents for AML.

    2. Radiotherapy is used in ALL to sterilize sanctuary sites of late relapse. Such sites are found in the central nervous system and, possibly, in the testes.

    3. Bone marrow transplantation is being tested as definitive, curative therapy for acute leukemia. Such techniques usually are used after the first remission has been obtained. Marrow transplantation is the treatment of choice, however, for a patient who has an identical twin.

    4. Supportive therapy is extremely important and serves as a prototype for supportive therapy in other forms of neoplasia.

    a. Hemoglobin level should be maintained above 8 g/dl by transfusions of packed red cells.

    b. Hemorrhage is best prevented by prophylactic transfusion of platelet concentrates. Although serious spontaneous bleeding is unusual unless the platelet count falls below 10,000/mm^3, most physicians prefer to maintain platelet counts above 20,000/mm^3. This practice has lowered the incidence of fatal hemorrhage in acute leukemia from 80% to less than 20%.

    c. Control of infection is the major determinant of survival of patients being treated for the acute leukemia that is caused by drug-induced neutropenia.

    (1) Isolation techniques have been tested as means of avoiding infection. Totally protected environments decrease infections but have little impact on remissions and survival. Such environments feature expensive laminar flow rooms, sterilized food, and gut sterilization by nonabsorbable antibiotics. Most physicians do not use these methods but instead maintain strict hand-washing and skin-care techniques, employ long-term central catheters to avoid peripheral indwelling lines, and practice strict rectal care to achieve similar results.

    (2) Infections are treated early and aggressively. Neutropenic patients are susceptible to all organisms, especially gram-negative rods and fungi (e.g., *Candida* and *Aspergillus*).

    (a) Initial temperature elevations require thorough clinical evaluation, vigorous cultures, and treatment with broad-spectrum bactericidal antibiotic combinations of cephalosporins, aminoglycosides (e.g., tobramycin), and semisynthetic penicillins (e.g., ticarcillin).

(b) Secondary temperature elevations that occur after treatment with potent broad-spectrum antibiotics may require the empiric use of antifungal agents (e.g., amphotericin B).

(c) Granulocytopenic patients (i.e., individuals with < 500 cells/mm³) whose infections do not respond to antibiotic therapy after 48 hours may be treated with granulocyte transfusions; however, the exact indications, efficacy, and benefit of this therapy are controversial.

(d) Attention to electrolytes and uric acid is required in those patients with high cell turnover and in those receiving multiple antibiotics.

(i) Treatment with allopurinol and adequate fluids is required for uric acid control.

(ii) Electrolyte levels, especially that of potassium, must be maintained in patients being treated with antibiotics.

E. Prognosis

1. The prognosis for children with ALL is very good; over 95% obtain complete remission. About 50%–60% of cases are disease free at 5 years and are likely cured.

2. The prognosis for patients with AML is poor. Among patients receiving the best care, 75% obtain complete remission and 25% die. Furthermore, the usual duration of remission is only 12–18 months. Although some investigators claim 20% cure rates, there is little common experience with significant cure rates.

V. DISORDERS OF COAGULATION AND HEMOSTASIS

A. General considerations. Hemostasis requires an intact coagulation system of vascular and tissue components, platelets, and coagulation proteins. Deficiency or disease of any of these components may cause either spontaneous or trauma-related hemorrhage.

1. History. A careful history provides clues to the pathogenesis of bleeding. Immediate, mucocutaneous bleeding suggests vascular or platelet disease; delayed deep-tissue bleeding and hemarthrosis suggest coagulation protein deficiency. Genetic transmissions (e.g., the X-linked hemophilias) also are elicited by history, as is ingestion of drugs (e.g., aspirin).

2. Physical findings aid in differentiation of bleeding syndromes. Mucocutaneous petechiae and purpura suggest platelet disorders; hematomas and hemarthrosis suggest coagulopathy.

3. Laboratory testing is vital in the evaluation of bleeding disorders. Single tests rarely provide conclusive results, so various batteries of tests have been developed. The coagulation cascade is shown in Figure 3-1; the interpretation of common tests of hemostasis and blood coagulation is shown in Table 3-1; and the diagnosis of common bleeding disorders based on commonly used tests is shown in Table 3-2.

B. Disorders of blood vessels and vascular tissues. The following bleeding disorders result from pathology in the vessel area itself, with secondary leakage of blood. Most have as their hallmark a visible and usually palpable skin lesion. Testing performed on patients with these bleeding disorders reveals normal coagulation and occasionally increased bleeding times.

1. Autoimmune or allergic purpura (Henoch-Schönlein purpura) occurs most commonly in children and young adults. Its hallmark is a perivascular inflammatory lesion with serosanguineous leakage into the skin and the submucous and serosal areas.

a. The lesions characteristically are symmetrical and on proximal extremities. These are palpable lesions.

b. The syndrome is associated with streptococcal infections and drugs (e.g., penicillin).

c. Lesions in the bowel may cause gastrointestinal symptoms; joint lesions cause arthritis.

d. No specific therapy is uniformly helpful. Prognosis is good except in the 5%–10% of patients who develop glomerulonephritis.

2. Purpura associated with infections may be due to embolic occlusion of the microvasculature (e.g., endocarditis) or to endothelial injury by the infectious agent (e.g., *Rickettsia*). Biopsy and culture of the material may be helpful.

3. Structural malformations of vessels and vascular tissues are associated with the following disorders.

a. Scurvy is a condition caused by vitamin C deficiency; collagen synthesis is impaired as a result of this deficiency. Vessel walls with poor collagen support are pliable and easily ruptured.

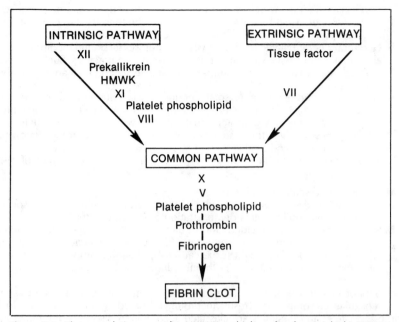

Figure 3-1. The coagulation cascade. *HMWK* = high molecular weight kininogen. (Adapted from Wintrobe MM, et al: *Clinical Hematology,* 8th ed. Philadelphia, Lea and Febiger, 1981, p 418.)

Table 3-1. Interpretation of Common Tests of Hemostasis and Coagulation

Test	Normal Range (±2 SD*)	Causes of Abnormalities
Platelet count	150–450,000/μL	Thrombocytopenia; thrombocytosis
Bleeding time (template method)	2.0–7.5 min	Thrombocytopenia; von Willebrand's disease; platelet dysfunction; vascular disorders
Partial thromboplastin time Standard Activated	 60–90 sec 30–40 sec	Deficiencies or inhibitors of prekallikrein, HMWK[†] factors VIII, IX, XI, XII; lupus inhibitors; heparin
Plasma prothrombin time	11–14 sec	Deficiencies or inhibitors of factors V, VII, X, prothrombin; lupus inhibitors
Plasma thrombin time	12–20 sec	Hypofibrinogenemia; abnormal fibrinogens; heparin
Fibrinogen assay	160–450 mg/dl	Hypofibrinogenemia; abnormal fibrinogens
Fibrin degradation product assay	< 10 μg/ml	DIC[‡]; fibrinogenolysis; liver disease

Note.—Adapted from Wintrobe MM, et al: *Clinical Hematology,* 8th ed. Philadelphia, Lea and Febiger, 1981, p 1051.
*Standard deviation.
[†]High molecular weight kininogen.
[‡]Disseminated intravascular coagulation.

(1) Physical findings associated with scurvy include perifollicular petechiae, gum bleeding, and subperiosteal hemorrhages. Also, bleeding time usually is prolonged.

(2) Therapy with 1 g/day of vitamin C rapidly corrects all bleeding.

b. Hereditary hemorrhagic telangiectasia is an autosomal dominant disorder associated with abnormally thin vessel walls and impaired vascular contractility. Such vessels are markedly friable, liable to burst with trauma, and unable to contract appropriately for primary hemostasis.

(1) Physical findings include small, nodular violaceous lesions on the lips, face, ears, tongue, and gastrointestinal mucosa; these lesions blanch upon pressure. Bleeding is common, especially gastrointestinal bleeding with resultant iron deficiency anemia.

(2) Diagnosis involves the association of three factors: recurrent hemorrhage, multiple telangiectases, and familial occurrence.

c. Steroid therapy diminishes collagen synthesis, resulting in a syndrome of vascular fragility and skin bleeding.

4. Miscellaneous vascular conditions

a. Paraproteinemias, including cryoglobulinemias and amyloidosis, are associated with skin bleeding. Diagnosis requires demonstration of the paraprotein.

b. Senile purpura occurs in elderly individuals as a result of degeneration and loss of dermal collagen, elastin, and subcutaneous fat. This disorder is characterized by benign purpura of the arms, and it is thought to be caused by shearing injury to blood vessels from the hypermobility of the skin on the thinned underlying tissue.

C. Disorders of platelets. Platelets play a role in the primary arrest of bleeding; abnormalities in these coagulation components result in prolonged bleeding times and lead to hemorrhagic diathesis. Platelet abnormalities are classified according to disorders of number and function.

1. Thrombocytopenia (i.e., decreased numbers of platelets) is the most common cause of abnormal bleeding.

a. General considerations

(1) With a platelet count of 100,000/mm³, bleeding time (and clinical bleeding, if the hemostatic system is stressed) begins to prolong. Most individuals experience petechiae or purpura with platelet counts between 50,000 and 20,000/mm³. More

Table 3-2. Presumptive Diagnosis of Common Bleeding Disorders by Primary Screening Tests

Platelet Count	Bleeding Time	PTT*	PT†	Presumptive Diagnosis	Common Etiologies
Decreased	Prolonged	Normal	Normal	Thrombocytopenia	ITP‡; drugs
Normal	Prolonged	Prolonged	Normal	von Willebrand's disease	. . .
Normal	Prolonged	Normal	Normal	Thrombocytopathia	Drugs; uremia
Normal	Normal	Prolonged	Normal	Coagulopathy of intrinsic pathway	Hemophilia A or hemophilia B; factor VIII and lupus-type inhibitors
Normal	Normal	Prolonged	Prolonged	Coagulopathy of common or multiple pathways	Liver disease; vitamin K deficiency; DIC§; heparin
Normal	Normal	Normal	Prolonged	Coagulopathy of extrinsic pathway	Factor VII deficiency
Normal	Normal	Normal	Normal	. . .	Hereditary telangiectasia; scurvy; allergic purpura

Note.—Adapted from Wintrobe MM, et al: *Clinical Hematology*, 8th ed. Philadelphia, Lea and Febiger, 1981, p 1062.
*Partial thromboplastin time.
†Prothrombin time.
‡Idiopathic thrombocytopenic purpura.
§Disseminated intravascular coagulation.

serious spontaneous bleeding may occur with platelet counts less than 20,000/mm³, and such bleeding is a high risk with counts less than 10,000/mm³.

(2) Thrombocytopenia is an indication for a marrow examination, which will reveal either the presence or absence of the platelet precursors, **megakaryocytes**. The presence of megakaryocytes indicates either peripheral destruction or pooling of platelets. The absence of megakaryocytes indicates platelet production problems.

b. **Mechanisms**

  (1) **Impaired platelet production**

    (a) **Etiology.** Megakaryocytes may be selectively suppressed by certain agents (e.g., thiazide diuretics and ethanol). A special case of thrombocytopenia due to impaired platelet production is ineffective thrombopoiesis associated with the megaloblastic hematopoiesis seen in vitamin B_{12} and folate deficiencies. Megakaryocytes are present in marrow but are abnormal (megaloblastic) in morphology and function. Their platelets are abnormal and destroyed in the marrow.

    (b) **Diagnosis** is confirmed by a bone marrow smear that reveals marrow megakaryocytic hypoplasia.

    (c) **Therapy** involves removal of the offending agent, if possible, or treatment of the underlying disease. Patients have essentially normal platelet half-lives and should be transfused with exogenous platelets if they are thrombocytopenic and bleeding. Thrombocytopenia associated with vitamin B_{12} or folate deficiency is rapidly corrected by therapy with the deficient vitamin.

    (d) **Associated conditions.** Impaired platelet production is associated with aplastic anemia, myelophthistic processes with replacement of marrow by tumor or fibrosis, and certain rare congenital syndromes (e.g., rubella infection with absent radii).

  (2) **Abnormal platelet pooling** results when platelets are sequestered from the circulation. **Splenic platelet sequestration** is the most common cause of abnormal platelet pooling.

    (a) **Pathophysiology.** Normally, the spleen holds one-third of the circulating platelet pool. As splenomegaly occurs, higher numbers of platelets are sequestered and, thus, unavailable for hemostasis. In very large spleens, as much as 90% of the platelet pool may be sequestered; however, platelets in the peripheral circulation do have normal survival times.

    (b) **Diagnosis** of hypersplenism is suggested by a moderate thrombocytopenia (platelet counts below 40,000 are unusual), a bone marrow smear that reveals adequate marrow megakaryocytes, and evidence of significant splenic enlargement.

    (c) **Clinical features** in such cases are dominated by the underlying illness causing the splenomegaly (e.g., cirrhosis with portal hypertension).

    (d) **Therapy** usually is not required, although splenectomy may correct the problem. Transfused platelets are sequestered in the same ratio and are less effective than in hypoactive marrow states.

  (3) **Increased peripheral destruction** of platelets is the most common form of thrombocytopenia. Conditions involving increased platelet destruction are characterized by shortened platelet survival and increased numbers of marrow megakaryocytes. These disorders are characterized as either **immune** or **nonimmune thrombocytopenic purpura**.

    (a) **Immune thrombocytopenic purpura**

      (i) **Idiopathic thrombocytopenic purpura** (ITP) is the prototypical immune-mediated thrombocytopenia; no apparent exogenous causes for platelet destruction exist.

        Clinical features. The **acute variant** of ITP occurs in children between the ages of 2 and 6 years and often occurs after a nonspecific viral illness. The **chronic variant** occurs in young adults, more commonly in young women. All ITP patients show varying degrees of thrombocytopenia, which in some acute cases is severe (i.e., associated with platelet counts under 1000/mm³), and all show increased marrow megakaryocytes. Other blood findings and cell lines are normal. Patients present with mucocutaneous bleeding with petechiae, purpura, mucosal bullae, and excessive bleeding after trauma.

        Diagnosis requires exclusion of associated illnesses (e.g., SLE) and thrombocytopenia that is induced by drugs (e.g., quinine). Platelet antibody techniques are available to demonstrate the abnormal presence of such antibody on platelets and in the plasma of these patients.

        Clinical course. The acute childhood variant often runs its course and resolves within 4–8 weeks; the adult form is more chronic and demonstrates relapses and remissions.

        Therapy for the acute childhood form usually involves protection from trauma and, in some cases, a short course of steroids. Treatment of adult ITP is more complex and protracted. Initially, high doses of steroids are given, with complete remission achieved in about 35% of cases. Splenectomy often is necessary and is associated with complete remission in about 65% of cases. Refractory patients may require immunosuppressive therapy. Although platelet transfusions should not be withheld in ITP patients who are bleeding, such exogenous transfusions may be less efficacious than in other thrombocytopenic states due to the same short survival of the platelets.

Prognosis. The overall prognosis is good; only 2%–3% of ITP patients die after 5 years.

(ii) **Other immune-mediated thrombocytopenias** with known eliciting agents for platelet-associated antibody include: post-transfusion thrombocytopenia due to isoantibodies; drug-induced thrombocytopenia (e.g., quinidine-induced); sepsis-associated thrombocytopenia (the incidence of thrombocytopenia with sepsis may be as high as 70%); and SLE.

Therapy involves appropriately addressing the underlying disease. Steroids are of questionable value except in SLE-related thrombocytopenia. Exogenous platelets suffer the same enhanced destruction.

(b) **Nonimmune thrombocytopenic purpura** occurs in the following conditions:
  (i) With infections (e.g., virus and malaria)
  (ii) Following massive blood transfusion with banked blood that is platelet-poor
  (iii) As part of disseminated intravascular coagulation syndrome
  (iv) With cardiac-valve prostheses
  (v) As part of the syndrome of thrombotic thrombocytopenic purpura

2. **Thrombocytopathia** involves platelets that are adequate in number but unable to function properly in hemostasis and in the primary arrest of bleeding.
   a. **Description.** Thrombocytopathia is characterized by:
      (1) Platelet-type mucocutaneous bleeding
      (2) Normal platelet counts but prolonged bleeding times
      (3) Demonstrable abnormalities in platelet function testing (e.g., aggregometry)
   b. **Etiology**
      (1) **Drug-related platelet dysfunction** is the most common cause of abnormal platelet function.
         (a) **Aspirin** permanently acetylates platelet membranes, impairing the platelet prostaglandin synthesis required for proper platelet function. Such impaired platelets may prolong bleeding times and cause bruising and increased hemorrhage with trauma.
         (b) **Other anti-inflammatory drugs** (e.g., indomethacin) cause similar dysfunction but differ from aspirin in that their effects disappear when the agent is withdrawn.
      (2) **Uremia-associated dysfunction**
         (a) The **mechanism** is unclear, although new data implicate uremic toxins in the disaggregation of the high molecular weight polymers of factor VIII that are required for proper platelet function.
         (b) **Therapy.** In bleeding uremic patients, this lesion may respond to dialysis. New data suggest that the administration of high molecular weight forms of factor VIII (e.g., cryoprecipitates) may temporarily correct this lesion.
      (3) **Congenital forms of platelet dysfunction** include Glanzmann's thrombasthenia (an intrinsic platelet disorder) and von Willebrand's disease (a congenital absence of the high molecular weight forms of factor VIII required for platelet aggregation).

D. **Disorders of the coagulation system** can be classified as hereditary or acquired. The hereditary forms usually result from deficiency of a single coagulation protein. Although greatly variable in degree, the clinical manifestations of these disorders are somewhat similar. The acquired forms, which are more complex than the hereditary forms, usually result from multiple and mixed deficiencies in the coagulation proteins.

1. **The hereditary coagulopathies** are best exemplified by the disorders of factor VIII.
   a. **Hemophilia A** is the most common hereditary coagulopathy, accounting for 68%–80% of such conditions.
      (1) **Pathogenesis.** Genetically, hemophilia A is transmitted as a classic X-linked recessive trait—the disorder is carried by females and is manifest in males. Bleeding results from the absence of **VIII^{pro}**, the small molecular weight or **procoagulant portion** of the factor VIII molecule. The large **antigenic portion** of the molecule, **VIII^{ag}**, is present in normal amounts.
      (2) **Clinical features** vary with the degree of deficiency and are summarized in Table 3-3.

The nature of hemorrhage is deep-tissue bleeding with deep hematomas, hemarthrosis, and significant bleeding after stress such as trauma and surgery. Repeated hemarthrosis results in severe disabling arthropathy, which is the clinical hallmark of severe hemophilia A.

(3) **Diagnosis.** The constellation of spontaneous or unexpected hemorrhage, especially hemarthrosis, in a male patient with an appropriate family history is suggestive. Laboratory tests reveal a prolonged **partial thromboplastin time (PTT)**, which is indicative of deficiencies in the intrinsic thromboplastin system; other coagulation tests are normal. The diagnosis is confirmed by factor assay demonstrating low levels of VIII[pro] and normal levels of VIII[ag].

(4) **Therapy** is with VIII[pro] transfusion either in the form of cryoprecipitates or factor VIII concentrates. This form of therapy has markedly lessened the mortality and morbidity rates associated with hemophilia A.

b. **Von Willebrand's disease (VWD)** is a heterogeneous disorder also involving the factor VIII molecule.

(1) **Pathophysiology.** Genetically its transmission is variable, but in its most common form VWD is transmitted as an autosomal dominant trait with variable penetrance. This disorder involves hereditary deficiency of the large antigenic portion of the factor VIII molecule (VIII[ag]) as well as the small procoagulant piece (VIII[pro]). Because VIII[ag] serves as a cofactor for platelet adhesion, patients manifest both coagulopathy and abnormal platelet function.

(2) **Clinical features** include immediate, mucocutaneous (i.e., platelet-type) bleeding due to VIII[ag] deficiency and delayed, deep-tissue, post-trauma (i.e., coagulation-type) bleeding due to VIII[ag] deficiency. As with hemophilia A, the clinical picture for VWD varies with the degree of deficiency.

(3) **Diagnosis** is suggested by abnormal bleeding of a mixed nature in an individual with an appropriate family history. Laboratory tests show prolonged bleeding time, due to decreased platelet function, and a prolonged PTT, due to VIII[pro] deficiency. Measurements of factor VIII demonstrate a combined and equivalent deficiency of VIII[ag] and VIII[pro]. Ristocetin-induced platelet aggregation is abnormal in VWD. Other tests of platelet aggregation are normal.

(4) **Therapy** requires the replacement of both the antigenic and procoagulant portions of factor VIII. Concentrates are rich in VIII[pro] but low in VIII[ag]; therefore, either plasma or cryoprecipitates are the treatment of choice in VWD.

c. **Other hereditary coagulation disorders** are uncommon. Diagnosis requires factor analysis to demonstrate the specific deficiency.

(1) **Hemophilia B (factor IX deficiency)** is identical to hemophilia A in its genetic features

Table 3-3. Clinical and Laboratory Findings in Hemophilia A and Hemophilia B

Severity	Level of Factor VIII or IX (U/dl)	Partial Thromboplastin Time	Clinical Picture
Severe	0–2	Very prolonged	Hemarthrosis and spontaneous bleeding severe and frequent; crippling common
Moderate	2–5	Prolonged	Hemarthrosis and spontaneous bleeding infrequent; disability uncommon; severe bleeding from injuries and surgery
Mild	5–25	Variable	Hemarthrosis and spontaneous bleeding very unusual; unsuspected and severe bleeding from injuries and surgery
Subclinical	25–49	Usually normal	Bleeding after major trauma or surgery possible; diagnosis often missed

Note.—Adapted from Wintrobe MM, et al: *Clinical Hematology*, 8th ed. Philadelphia, Lea and Febiger, 1981, p 1162.

and clinical manifestations. Therapy differs in that either plasma or a purified prothrombin complex (which contains concentrated factors II, VII, IX, and X) is used as a source for factor IX.

(2) Factor XI deficiency is an autosomal recessive coagulopathy with milder clinical manifestations than those of the hemophilias. PTT is prolonged due to low factor XI levels. Plasma serves as adequate replacement therapy.

(3) Factor XII, prekallikrein, and **high molecular weight kininogen deficiencies** are unique in that they cause significant prolongations of PTT yet no predisposition to hemorrhage. Diagnosis is suggested by abnormal PTT with no history of bleeding, even with trauma. Factor analysis is necessary to demonstrate the deficient factor.

(4) Deficiencies for all other factors have been described but are extremely rare and are not discussed here.

2. The acquired coagulation disorders are more complex than the hereditary forms. The acquired coagulopathies usually involve multiple and mixed factor deficiencies and often are complications of other diseases. Coagulation testing shows abnormality in multiple pathways; often the bleeding severity correlates poorly with coagulation abnormalities seen in laboratory testing.

a. Vitamin K-dependent–factor deficiency

(1) Pathophysiology. The liver synthesizes factors II, VII, IX, and X. The final step in their synthesis renders these proteins functional and requires gamma carboxylation of 10 terminal glutamic acid residues, with vitamin K as a cofactor. Interference in this mechanism causes functional deficiency of these clotting proteins. Since many clotting factors are deficient, laboratory testing shows prolonged PTT and **prothrombin time (PT)**. Specific measurements will demonstrate the deficiency of factors II, VII, IX, and X.

(2) Etiology

(a) This coagulopathy occurs with **liver failure** when hepatocyte dysfunction is sufficient to impair synthesis of the above-mentioned factors. In such cases, evidence of liver disease is present (i.e., jaundice and transaminase elevation) in addition to the coagulopathy.

(b) Malabsorption of vitamin K can occur with biliary obstruction as well as with intestinal disease (e.g., sprue). Again, coagulopathy merely complicates the obvious clinical picture.

(c) Particularly in intensive care units, **nutritional deficiency** occurs in patients with poor oral intake of vitamin K and in those in whom antibiotics have removed the gastrointestinal flora that serve as an alternate vitamin K source.

(d) Drugs can interfere with vitamin K metabolism, most specifically the vitamin K antagonist **coumarin**, which is used to treat thrombotic diseases.

(3) Therapy for vitamin K–related coagulopathy varies with the etiology.

(a) In cases of malabsorption and nutritional deficiency, supplemental (often parenteral) vitamin K corrects the coagulopathy.

(b) In cases of excess coumarin, withdrawal of the offending drug with supplemental vitamin K is efficacious.

(c) In bleeding patients or patients who have liver dysfunction and are unable to respond to vitamin K, the deficient factors must be administered in the form of plasma or prothrombin concentrates. It should be noted that the pooled concentrates carry a high risk for hepatitis. They also can cause thrombotic complications in patients with liver disease.

b. Disseminated intravascular coagulation (DIC)

(1) Pathophysiology. DIC is initiated by stimuli in the systemic circulation that activate the coagulation mechanism and cause the abnormal formation of excessive systemic thrombin. The thrombin in turn causes extensive activation of coagulation in the microcirculation, which consumes many coagulation moieties and activates the fibrinolytic system secondarily.

(2) Etiology. DIC is a very common acquired coagulopathy that occurs secondary to other disease processes, such as:

(a) Activation of the intrinsic coagulation pathway by endothelial damage (e.g., in gram-negative sepsis, meningococcemia, and viremia)

(b) Activation of the extrinsic pathway by abnormal entry of tissue thromboplastins into the circulation (e.g., in obstetric complications, carcinomatosis, and massive trauma)

(3) Clinical features vary depending on the balance between intravascular coagulation and fibrinolysis and factor depletion.

(a) In florid acute cases (e.g., amniotic fluid embolism), the coagulopathy is dominant and the major symptoms are bleeding and shock.

(b) In more chronic cases (e.g., carcinomatosis), thrombosis and clotting may predominate.

(c) Many cases of DIC involve abnormal coagulation parameters but no bleeding or clotting, whereas other cases have a mixture of both bleeding and clotting complications.

(4) Diagnosis. Laboratory tests reveal a complicated picture. Many coagulation factors are consumed in the diffuse clotting process; these factor deficiencies prolong both PT and PTT. Platelet consumption results in thrombocytopenia. Fibrinogen deficiency arises from thrombin-mediated clotting as well as plasmin-mediated fibrinolysis. The secondary fibrinolysis is demonstrated by the presence of high titers of fibrin degradation products (FDP).

(5) Therapy is extremely controversial; however, it is unanimously agreed that addressing the underlying "trigger" disease is paramount. The role of both factor replacements and anticoagulants to impair the ongoing thrombin production is less clear. The author's preference is to administer platelets and plasma to bleeding patients with markedly lowered levels and to reserve heparin for patients with thrombotic complications (e.g., skin infarction, acral gangrene, and recognizable vessel thromboses). Many patients require **no** specific coagulation therapy.

c. Liver disease results in a complex coagulopathy involving many aspects of clotting.

(1) Liver disease results in impaired synthesis of vitamin K-dependent–clotting proteins, fibrinogen, antithrombin III, plasminogen, and others.

(2) Impaired clearance of FDP and activated coagulation factors may result in a mild DIC-type condition.

(3) Portal hypertension may result in splenomegaly and excessive platelet pooling with thrombocytopenia.

(4) The accumulation of FDP causes impaired platelet function (thrombocytopathia).

d. Pathologic inhibitors of coagulation

(1) The **lupus-type inhibitor** is the most common coagulation inhibitor. Although first described in patients with SLE, lupus inhibitors most often occur with other conditions or idiopathically.

(a) The inhibitor is poorly characterized but appears to be an inhibitor of the prothrombin–platelet membrane complex (see Fig. 3-1).

(b) Clinical testing reveals prolonged PT and PTT but little evidence of bleeding. The diagnosis is made by demonstrating that patient plasma causes similar abnormalities when mixed with normal plasma, unlike deficiency states where such mixtures correct the abnormality.

(c) Therapy should be directed toward the underlying disease. These patients do not bleed and need not receive coagulation therapy.

(2) Specific inhibitors of coagulation are antibodies with specificity for single coagulation proteins. The most common is factor VIII antibody, which arises in 10% of hemophiliacs who have received factor therapy.

(a) Clinically, such antibodies cause profound bleeding dyscrasias of similar severity to congenital deficiency.

(b) Diagnosis is made by demonstrating a specific factor deficiency that is not corrected by administration of normal plasma.

(c) Therapy is extremely difficult because the antibody also inactivates exogenously administered factors. Steroids and immunosuppressive agents have been used with limited success.

e. Other acquired coagulation disorders. Coagulopathy has been associated with amyloidosis (factor X deficiency); the nephrotic syndrome (due to renal wasting of coagulation proteins, especially factor IX); extracorporeal circulation (thought to activate the coagulation system partially and cause low-grade DIC); and massive transfusions (patient hemorrhages normal blood, but it is replaced with blood bank–derived blood that is poor in coagulation factor and platelet levels).

STUDY QUESTIONS

Directions: Each question below contains five suggested answers. Choose the **one best** response to each question.

1. A 65-year-old white man scheduled for elective surgery is found to have a hematocrit of 67% and an elevated red cell mass when measured isotopically. Additional studies that would be appropriate in this case include all of the following procedures EXCEPT

(A) arterial blood gas test for oxygen saturation
(B) measurement of serum vitamin B_{12} level
(C) platelet count
(D) liver and spleen scanning
(E) lung scanning

2. The presence of hemolysis is indicated by all of the following clinical manifestations EXCEPT

(A) absent or reduced serum haptoglobin
(B) increased number of reticulocytes
(C) elevated serum lactate dehydrogenase (LDH) level
(D) microcytic red blood cell indices
(E) shortened red blood cell survival

3. Absolute erythrocytosis is associated with all of the following conditions EXCEPT

(A) pulmonary arteriovenous fistulae
(B) renal carcinoma
(C) hemoglobin with decreased oxygen affinity
(D) severe pulmonary disease
(E) hepatoma

4. Thrombocytopenia that is caused by increased platelet destruction is most closely associated with which of the following conditions?

(A) Aplastic anemia
(B) Combination chemotherapy
(C) Acute leukemia
(D) Systemic lupus erythematosus
(E) Excessive ethanol intake

Directions: The group of questions below consists of lettered choices followed by several numbered items. For each numbered item select the **one** lettered choice with which it is **most** closely associated. Each lettered choice may be used once, more than once, or not at all.

Questions 5–9

For each description of a clinical situation, select the leukemic state with which it is most closely associated.

(A) Acute lymphoblastic leukemia (ALL)
(B) Acute myeloid leukemia (AML)
(C) Both ALL and AML
(D) Neither ALL nor AML

5. A 4-year-old patient with pancytopenia and circulating blasts

6. A 60-year-old patient with pancytopenia and circulating blasts

7. A 50% long-term survival (? cure)

8. A patient with bleeding and infection

9. A patient with gum and skin infiltration

ANSWERS AND EXPLANATIONS

1. The answer is E. (*II C 2 a, b*) The elevated hematocrit and isotopically confirmed elevated red cell mass indicate the presence of absolute erythrocytosis. Differential diagnosis requires testing for polycythemia vera, which by convention includes demonstration of: a normal arterial oxygen saturation; splenomegaly; elevated vitamin B_{12} level; elevated platelet and leukocyte levels; and elevated leukocyte alkaline phosphatase level. Although severe pulmonary disease can cause absolute erythrocytosis due to chronic hypoxia, lung scanning would not indicate whether the impairment of pulmonary function is sufficient to raise the hematocrit.

2. The answer is D. (*I C 2 b*) The term hemolysis refers to the enhanced destruction of red blood cells before their normal life span of 120 days. In an attempt to compensate for the shortened red cell survival, the bone marrow increases reticulocyte production. Haptoglobin is consumed in the process of binding the excess free hemoglobin released as a result of red cell destruction. Also, lactate dehydrogenase (LDH) is present in excessive amounts due to excessive release during red cell destruction. Red cell indices usually are normal in the hemolytic anemias and so do not aid in the identification of these disorders.

3. The answer is C. (*II C 2 a, b*) A right-shifted P_{50} (i.e., decreased oxygen affinity) means that this hemoglobin variant gives up 50% of its oxygen too easily. In this situation, there is excess oxygen delivery to tissues. Conversely, hemoglobin variants characterized by a left-shifted P_{50} do not appropriately yield oxygen at tissue levels, which results in compensatory secondary absolute erythrocytosis. Pulmonary arteriovenous fistulae and severe pulmonary diseases cause lowered oxygen tension with secondary absolute erythrocytosis. Renal and hepatic tumors may release erythropoietin with secondary absolute erythrocytosis.

4. The answer is D. (*V C 1 b*) Systemic lupus erythematosus triggers the production of an autoimmune antiplatelet antibody that is directly associated with enhanced platelet destruction. Aplastic anemia, combination chemotherapy, ethanol abuse, and acute leukemia are associated with impaired platelet production due to absent or diminished numbers of megakaryocytes.

5–9. The answers are: 5-A, 6-B, 7-A, 8-C, 9-B. (*IV A, B, D*) Acute lymphoblastic leukemia (ALL) is predominantly a disease of childhood. Although induction therapy is much easier and more successful with ALL than with acute myeloid leukemia (AML), ALL often has some component of marrow failure with associated bleeding and infection. With current therapy, remission is obtained in more than 95% of cases; more than 50% of cases have long-term survival and represent possibly cured patients.

AML is most commonly a disease of adults, and its incidence increases with increasing age. Induction therapy is long and difficult to perform, with marrow ablation by chemotherapy associated with almost universal bleeding and infection. Long-term survival is unusual in AML. AML has several subtypes, one of which is characterized by gum and skin infiltration.

4
Oncologic Diseases
Ronald N. Rubin

I. HEAD AND NECK CARCINOMAS

A. Incidence. Head and neck carcinomas account for 5% of the cancers reported each year in the United States. These tumors occur three times more frequently in men than in women and commonly involve the oral cavity (40% of cases), larynx (25%), oropharynx and hypopharynx (15%), and salivary glands (10%).

B. Etiology. The following risk factors have been noted.

1. **Tobacco**, whether smoked or chewed, clearly is associated with an increased incidence of head and neck tumors.

2. **Alcohol** consumption, which alone is a risk factor, works synergistically with tobacco to increase the incidence of these tumors by 10- to 40-fold. (In Mormon societies, which abstain from both alcohol and tobacco, head and neck carcinomas are extremely unusual.)

3. **Epstein-Barr virus** has been linked to the unusual nasopharyngeal carcinoma that is unique to Orientals.

C. Pathology. Most (95%) of these tumors involve squamous cell carcinoma. Exceptions are **mixed tumors** of the salivary glands and nasopharyngeal lymphomas, which are adenocarcinomas and lymphoid neoplasms, respectively. The squamous cell tumors vary from well-differentiated, exophytic varieties to more invasive, poorly differentiated, infiltrating endophytic varieties.

D. Clinical features and diagnosis. Common symptoms include dysphagia, hoarseness, and swellings in the neck. In addition, mass lesions or white patches are evident on physical examination. To confirm the diagnosis, these suspicious lesions must be biopsied.

E. Staging involves careful evaluation of the degree of local involvement and node status, which provides a basis for therapy strategy. Head and neck tumors usually are squamous cell lesions that are more locally invasive than blood-borne. However, at presentation, only 30% of these cancers involve disease that is localized enough to allow cure by radiotherapy or surgery. The remaining majority relapse both locally and systemically after initial therapy.

F. Therapy

1. Small, localized lesions are treated with curative surgery or radiotherapy.

2. Patients with advanced, nonresectable, relapsing, or metastatic lesions benefit significantly from palliative radio- or chemotherapy. Agents that induce a response in 40%–50% of cases include bleomycin, cisplatin, and methotrexate.

3. The role of combined modality therapy (i.e., chemotherapy plus radiotherapy) and the role of combination chemotherapy are limited by increased toxicity and remain to be defined by successful clinical trials.

G. Prognosis. Local recurrences result in 70% of the cases of head and neck tumors, and distant metastases result in 20%–30% of the cases. Once the disease has recurred or metastasis has begun, the chance of survival is poor. The mean survival for such patients is 3–9 months.

II. CARCINOMA OF UNKNOWN PRIMARY ORIGIN

A. Incidence. Neoplasms that show evidence of metastasis but no obvious primary disease origin account for 1% of the cancers that occur in the United States.

B. Etiology remains controversial as the characteristics of primary lesions have not been defined by clinical trials. However, most studies at autopsy agree that common sites of primary disease are the lung, pancreas, stomach, and head and neck region.

C. Pathology. To evaluate a patient with undifferentiated carcinoma, it is imperative that the neoplasm be distinguished from amelanotic melanoma, round cell sarcoma, and lymphoma. Carcinomas often can be separated into epidermoid and adenoid varieties using mucin staining and electron microscopy.

D. Diagnosis is suggested by the failure to find a primary disease origin despite endoscopic and radiologic investigation. The extent of such investigation is controversial and ranges from no evaluation (in cases in which such studies would have no bearing on therapy, which usually would be ineffective anyway) to extensive and costly evaluation (in cases in which a specific diagnosis is sought). There is agreement, however, on the following issues.

1. Tumors for which there is somewhat effective therapy should be investigated.
   a. Breast carcinoma in women should be sought using estrogen-receptor values of biopsy specimens and mammography.
   b. Prostatic carcinoma in men should be sought using bone biopsy, serum acid phosphatase, and prostate biopsy.
   c. Other tumors that respond to systemic therapy include thyroid carcinoma and germ cell carcinoma; the latter can be sought using serum α-fetoprotein and human chorionic gonadotropin.

2. Low-yield studies include brain scanning in solid tumors in the absence of neurologic signs and symptoms and liver scanning in the absence of hepatomegaly and serum enzyme elevations.

3. Before considerable time and money are spent and undue suffering is experienced, the value of obtaining a diagnosis should be weighed against the fact that, in most cases, therapy is not effective and patient survival is brief.

E. Therapy also is controversial and, therefore, varied. Some investigators empirically treat tumors of unknown primary origin as they would tumors of known origin that are at least somewhat responsive to therapy. For example, in women, breast cancer regimens may be used, such as cyclophosphamide, methotrexate, and 5-fluorouracil [5-FU] (CMF) and cyclophosphamide, doxorubicin (Adriamycin), and 5-FU (CAF).

F. Prognosis overall is poor, with a mean survival of less than 9 months. The occasional tumor that turns out to be breast carcinoma or lymphoma may respond well to therapy and extend patient survival.

III. RENAL AND BLADDER CARCINOMAS

A. Incidence. These tumors account for roughly 3% of the cancers that occur in the United States. Renal and bladder carcinomas are more common in men than in women and usually occur in patients who are 40–70 years of age.

B. Etiology

1. **Renal cancers** have been associated with **tobacco**, but no clear occupational carcinogens have been defined.

2. **Bladder cancers** have been related to **tobacco** as well as certain chemical and biologic carcinogens.
   a. **Occupational carcinogens** in the rubber, dye, printing, and chemical industries have been implicated in bladder carcinoma.
   b. **Saccharin** has been proven to cause bladder tumors in animals, but its role in humans is less clear.
   c. **Schistosomiasis** of the bladder has been strongly correlated with squamous cell carcinoma.

C. Pathology

1. Renal tumors are classic clear cell carcinomas (adenocarcinomas), which originate in the proximal convoluted tubule.

2. Bladder tumors are transitional cell in origin. (An exception is the oriental schistosome-related variant, which is squamous cell.)

D. Diagnosis

1. Most renal cancer patients (80%) present with some combination of the following symptoms: flank pain, hematuria, abdominal mass, and systemic symptoms including fatigue, anemia, and weight loss. Renal cancers usually are advanced at diagnosis. Specific diagnostic techniques include intravenous pyelography, ultrasonography of the mass, angiography, cyst puncture for chemical analysis with cytology of cyst fluid, and eventual surgical exploration.

2. Bladder cancer patients present with hematuria in 75% of cases. In the remaining cases, bladder irritability and infection are reported. Most bladder tumors are localized at diagnosis. The diagnostic method is cystoscopy, which is nearly 100% accurate and is followed by biopsy.

E. Therapy and prognosis depend on the extent of disease.

1. Renal carcinoma is treated primarily with surgery. Radical nephrectomy yields a 5-year survival in 75% of cases involving localized tumors but in only 35% of more advanced cases. Metastatic disease has a poor prognosis, and the outlook for the palliative effects of radio- and chemotherapy is dreary at best.

2. Bladder carcinoma is managed according to the degree of invasion.
   a. Superficial, low-grade lesions are best managed by cystoscopic surgery. Although most cases involve local recurrences and serial surgery, more than 75% of cases have long survival. Intrabladder chemotherapy, namely mitomycin, is being evaluated as a means of diminishing the local recurrence rate.
   b. High-stage, high-grade lesions occur in as many as 50% of cases and require total cystectomy with urinary diversion.
   c. Metastatic bladder cancer has a dismal prognosis. Local bleeding and obstructive problems may be palliated with radiotherapy. Up to 25% of patients respond to single-agent chemotherapy with such agents as cyclophosphamide, doxorubicin, 5-FU, methotrexate, and cisplatin. Again, drug combinations clearly enhance toxicity, but, to date, their ability to enhance survival remains unclear.

IV. PROSTATIC CARCINOMA

A. Incidence

1. This tumor accounts for 18% of all cancers that occur in the United States. Of the approximately 50,000 new cases reported each year, only 30% are potentially curable at the time of diagnosis; unfortunately, the remaining majority of cases, when discovered, are characterized by widespread disease.

2. The incidence of prostatic carcinoma increases with age and is uncommon before age 50. There is no race predilection, and benign prostatic hypertrophy does not seem to be a premalignant lesion.

B. Pathology. Nearly all prostatic cancers are adenocarcinomas.

C. Diagnosis remains difficult for early prostatic lesions.

1. **Screening and early diagnosis** involve frequent rectal examinations as part of routine physicals. However, only 10% of prostatic tumors found as nodules on rectal examination are sufficiently localized for cure.

2. **Pathologic examination** of tissue removed for treatment of obstructive prostatic hypertrophy reveals that 10% of cases have malignant pathology.

3. The remaining cases, when found, are in advanced stages; often these cancers are revealed in investigations for metastatic disease in bone.

D. Staging techniques are crucial to the investigation and proper treatment of prostatic carcinoma.

1. **Staging system.** The currently used staging system is as follows.
   a. **Stage A** tumors are tumors that are unsuspected clinically and are found at autopsy or by examining tissue removed for alleged benign disease. The incidence of these tumors ranges from 4% to 21% of tissue removed for alleged benign obstructive disease, depending on the center. These **A1** (well-differentiated) tumors have better prognoses than **A2** (poorly differentiated) tumors.
   b. **Stage B** tumors are neoplasms that are confined to the prostate gland. These are the classic nodules found on rectal examination, which theoretically are curable by surgery. Unfor-

tunately, only 10% of prostate cancers are in this category. Many of these nodules already have pelvic node metastases when discovered on rectal examination.

  c. **Stage C** tumors are cancers that have spread beyond the prostate capsule into the pelvis (e.g., to the seminal vesicles) but not to distant sites. These cannot be cured by surgery and account for 40% of new cases.

  d. **Stage D** tumors are cancers that have spread from the prostate area to pelvic lymph nodes, bone, or beyond. About 50% of new cases are stage D on presentation.

2. **Staging techniques.** All early-stage clinical presentations must be staged accurately to determine the true extent of disease before curative treatment with surgery or radiotherapy is attempted. Useful staging techniques include:

  a. **Computed tomography (CT)** of the pelvis to detect neoplasms in the pelvic organs and lymph nodes

  b. **Acid phosphatase measurements** as a tumor marker for disease outside the prostate capsule*

  c. **Skeletal x-ray** studies

  d. **Surgical exploration and dissection** of pelvic lymph nodes, which are required for cases still in doubt after employing the above techniques

E. **Therapy and prognosis** are determined by the stage of disease at diagnosis.

1. **Stage A1** tumors are associated with a low morbidity, and most physicians believe that, aside from follow-up examinations, therapy is unnecessary. **Stage A2** tumors, if appropriately staged and truly confined to the prostate gland, should be treated with radical radiotherapy (i.e., 7000 rads) with curative intent.†

2. **Stage B** tumors can be cured with radical prostatectomy.†

3. **Stage C** tumors can be cured with radical radiotherapy to the pelvis with boost doses to the prostate gland.

4. **Stage D** tumors cannot be cured and so only palliative treatment is available. Timing of therapy is controversial, although survival seems equivalent whether therapy is offered at the initial diagnosis of stage D disease or at the onset of symptoms.

  a. The following treatment modalities are used commonly.

  (1) **Endocrine therapy** is the initial mode of treatment. Orchiectomy and exogenous estrogens are equivalent. The former has fewer side effects and compliance problems; however, the specific choice of treatment should be individualized.

  (2) **Radiotherapy** to local areas of bone pain offers relief.

  (3) **Chemotherapy** is disappointing, with only 25% of cases responding to single agents (i.e., cyclophosphamide or 5-FU). Cisplatin may be more effective, but further trials are required. Whether combination chemotherapy offers any advantage in return for its enhanced toxicity remains unclear.

  b. Properly applied therapy for stage D disease can improve 5-year survival rates from 6%–20% to 40%.

V. GASTRIC CARCINOMA

A. **Incidence.** Once a very common tumor, gastric cancer is decreasing in frequency for reasons that are poorly understood. This tumor accounts for 2% of all cancers in the United States and occurs most frequently in older men.

B. **Etiology.** The cause of this disease has been well studied, and the following relationships have been found.

1. **Blood group.** The incidence of gastric cancer is slightly higher among individuals with **blood group A** and is somewhat lower among those with **blood group O**.

2. **Certain diets,** such as those rich in additives (e.g., smoked foods and highly spiced oriental foods), are associated with an increased incidence of gastric cancer.

3. In addition, an increased incidence occurs in patients with **achlorhydria**, atrophic gastritis, and pernicious anemia and in those who have undergone surgery for peptic ulcer disease. A unifying factor for these associations may be an increased concentration of **nitrosamine** compounds in gastric juice.

---

*Only 67% of these carcinomas are associated with an increased acid phosphatase level.
†It should be noted that radical radiotherapy and surgery both cause permanent impotence as well as sphincter problems in many cases.

C. **Pathology.** More than 90% of all gastric cancers are adenocarcinomas; sarcomas and lymphomas are less common.

   1. Ulcerative gastric carcinomas are most common, accounting for about 75% of cases.

   2. Polypoid carcinomas account for about 10% of cases, and diffuse, infiltrative scirrhous (linitis plastica) carcinomas comprise the remaining 15%.

D. **Clinical features** include epigastric pain and discomfort, anorexia, early satiety, weight loss, and iron deficiency anemia due to blood loss.

E. **Diagnosis.** Specific diagnostic methods include:

   1. Traditional **x-ray** studies using barium

   2. **Endoscopy** along with direct visualization, cytology, and biopsy, which are 95%–99% accurate when performed in combination

F. **Therapy**

   1. **Surgery** remains the mainstay of therapy. Surgery offers a 50%–60% chance for 5-year survival to patients with tumors confined to the stomach; however, few patients fall into this category. Most patients have positive nodes or tumors at resection margins, for which the cure rate is less than 5%.

   2. **Radiotherapy** is used frequently in nonresectable cases but has little impact on survival.

   3. There is recent enthusiasm for a **palliative combination chemotherapy** regimen of 5-FU, doxorubicin (Adriamycin), and mitomycin. Abbreviated FAM, this regimen may prolong survival in advanced cases and is reasonably tolerated with acceptable short-term toxicity. However, the enthusiasm for FAM has been tempered somewhat by the appearance of a virulent microangiopathic hemolytic syndrome after long-term use of this regimen.

VI. CARCINOMA OF THE EXOCRINE PANCREAS

A. **Incidence.** The incidence of pancreatic carcinoma is increasing. This tumor accounts for 1% of all cancers that occur in the United States and is most common in nonwhite men.

B. **Etiology.** Pancreatic carcinoma shows an increased incidence among cigarette smokers, alcoholics, and patients with chronic pancreatitis. A controversial study also has linked this tumor to excess coffee ingestion.

C. **Pathology.** These tumors are almost exclusively scirrhous adenocarcinomas. Two major syndromes occur and are related to tumor site.

   1. **Tumors in the head** of the pancreas cause obstructive jaundice and account for roughly 67% of pancreatic cancers.

   2. **Tumors in the body and tail** grow to a larger size than those of the head. These tumors cause pain, weight loss, and diabetes mellitus in 25%–50% of cases.

D. **Diagnosis.** The following techniques are used to confirm pancreatic disease and to obtain tissue diagnoses in appropriate clinical settings.

   1. **Disease identification.** Ultrasonography reveals pancreatic abnormality in 90% of cases, and CT identifies pancreatic disease in more than 95% of cases. Angiography is used to determine the extent and operability of the disease.

   2. **Tissue diagnosis** is accurate in 95% of cases using percutaneous needle biopsy of the pancreas with ultrasonographic guidance. Endoscopic retrograde cholangiopancreatography with aspiration cytology also may be diagnostic in up to 95% of cases and may eliminate the need for surgery. However, a significant number of cases still require diagnostic laparotomy.

E. **Therapy and prognosis.** The outlook for pancreatic cancer victims is poor. The few patients who are cured often have small cancers detected by chance during surgery for another illness.

   1. **Curative surgery** (i.e., radical pancreatic surgery) is associated with high mortality rates.

   2. **Palliative surgery** has a large role in the treatment of this disease. A major procedure is bypass of the biliary obstruction with a bile duct–intestinal anastomosis, which relieves jaundice and improves the quality of life. Bypass surgery now is accompanied by a new technique for relief of obstruction. A stent is placed in the dilated bile duct to allow percutaneous drainage—a procedure that obviates the need for laparotomy.

3. Radiotherapy with an external beam in the 3000 rad range offers some palliation but overall does not provide impressive symptom relief or increased survival. Newer techniques of radiotherapy employ **intraoperative radiation** with 8000–10,000 rads delivered locally to spare sensitive nearby structures from exposure. Early studies show increased patient survival rates (20% at 2 years), but such therapy is technically difficult and not widely available.

4. Chemotherapy, to date, has been even more disappointing, with only sporadic response to standard single agents.
  a. 5-FU is easy to use, well tolerated, and the most commonly used chemotherapeutic agent.
  b. A regimen similar to that used in the treatment of gastric carcinoma (i.e., FAM) has been tried, but early results show that this regimen is not as successful in treating pancreatic tumors as FAM is in treating gastric carcinoma.

VII. COLORECTAL CARCINOMA

A. Incidence. Colorectal carcinoma is exceeded only by skin, lung, and breast cancers as the most common malignancy in the United States. This tumor occurs most frequently in patients who are 60–70 years of age.

B. Etiology

  1. Several precancerous lesions are known and include:
    a. Familial polyposis
    b. Ulcerative colitis
    c. Villous adenomas and pedunculated polyps that exceed 1–2 cm in diameter

  2. Etiologic factors that have been suggested but remain controversial include:*
    a. Diet low in fiber
    b. Diet high in animal fat
    c. Excess nitrosamines reaching the colon (as with gallbladder disease)

C. Pathology. Most colorectal carcinomas are adenocarcinomas, which often are mucinous. Classic teaching has maintained that roughly 66% of colorectal cancers are in the rectosigmoid areas, but the advent of colonoscopy is changing this concept to that of a more uniform distribution of cancers throughout the colon. Favored metastatic sites are the liver and peritoneal nodes and serosas.

D. Clinical features vary according to the site of tumor origin.

  1. Right-sided lesions have a greater capacity to enlarge without obstructing; these lesions classically present as occult blood in the stool with iron deficiency anemia.

  2. Left-sided lesions more often have an obstructive component and present with pain, cramps, and narrow stool.

  3. Weight loss and anorexia may occur at any time and regardless of tumor origin.

E. Diagnosis. Colorectal carcinoma must be considered in any patient who is over the age of 50 and shows a change in bowel habit, blood in the stool, or occult blood loss with iron deficiency. The following diagnostic methods are available to evaluate such patients.

  1. Proctosigmoidoscopy can detect and enable the biopsy of lesions located up to 25 cm from the anus.

  2. Colonoscopy, when employed by an expert physician, allows inspection and biopsy of the entire colon.

  3. Air contrast barium enema remains a valuable study.

  4. Carcinoembryonic antigen (CEA) is a tumor-associated antigen that is found in the majority of patients with colorectal carcinoma. However, CEA also is found in the serum of many patients with benign colon diseases. Due to its nonspecificity, CEA should not be used diagnostically but can be used to follow patients known to have colorectal cancers.

F. Therapy is dependent on the depth of tumor invasion into the bowel wall.

  1. Surgery and the Dukes staging system. Surgery is the initial therapy of choice in patients without known metastatic disease (i.e., metastasis usually to the liver, which is suggested by

*These etiologic factors have an underlying theme of cancer development based on the inverse relation between the bulk of the stool and the colon transit time.

abnormal alkaline phosphatase levels and liver scanning). Surgery also serves to stage the disease for prognostic purposes according to the Dukes classification.
   a. **Dukes A** lesions (10% of colorectal cancers) are confined to the mucosa and submucosa and have an 80% 5-year survival rate with surgery alone.
   b. **Dukes B** lesions (35% of colorectal cancers) involve the entire colon wall but have no lymph node metastases. Stage B lesions traditionally have been reported to have a 50% 5-year survival rate with surgery. A more recent study, however, noted a 75% 5-year survivorship with surgery alone.
   c. **Dukes C** lesions (30% of colorectal cancers) involve regional nodes and have a 20% 5-year survival rate with surgery.
   d. **Dukes D** lesions (25% of colorectal cancers) have distant metastases and cannot be cured with surgery.

2. **Radiotherapy** can offer palliation for bleeding, pelvic pain, and related local complications. When used as an adjunct to surgery, however, radiotherapy enhances morbidity without prolonging survival. Adjuvant radiotherapy does offer effective palliation for rectal tumors, in that it seems to lessen the very morbid local recurrence rate.

3. **Chemotherapy** is very disappointing. When used alone, 5-FU offers a 20% response rate with acceptable toxicity. The addition of nitrosoureas [e.g., lomustine (CCNU)] has added to the response rate in some studies but has not increased survival. In patients with symptomatic and predominant hepatic metastases, the infusion of 5-FU using direct intrahepatic artery catheterization has caused tumor shrinkage with palliation of pain and jaundice in more than 50% of cases. The effect on survival is less clear, however.

VIII. BREAST CARCINOMA

A. **Incidence.** Breast carcinoma is the most common malignancy and the number one cause of cancer deaths among women in the United States. As many as 8% of women will suffer from breast cancer in their lifetime.

B. **Etiology.** The following risk factors have been associated with an increased incidence of breast cancer.

   1. **Menstrual function and history** correlate with the incidence of breast cancer. Castration markedly lowers the risk, whereas early menarche and late menopause increase the risk of breast carcinoma.

   2. **Reproductive history** seems to play a role. A first pregnancy before age 18 seems protective, whereas nulliparity or initial pregnancy after age 30 enhances the risk.

   3. A **hereditary influence** is suspected. The risk for breast carcinoma is increased in immediate family members of breast cancer patients and may be higher for a sister than for a daughter.

   4. **Radiation exposure and exogenous estrogens** have been associated with an increased incidence of breast cancer.

   5. **Excess dietary and body fat** have been implicated, but studies making these claims are controversial.

C. **Pathology.** Breast cancers are adenocarcinomas.

   1. **Classification**
      a. **Papillary carcinomas** (1% of breast cancers) are low-grade, noninvasive intraductal lesions.
      b. **Medullary carcinomas** (5%–10% of breast cancers) are large bulky tumors that have a low-grade infiltrating tendency and are surrounded by lymphocytes. These tumors have a better 5-year survival rate.
      c. **Inflammatory carcinomas** (5%–10% of breast cancers) invade the dermal lymphatics and cause skin redness, induration warmth, and an erysipeloid margin. These cancers are very high-grade in malignancy with almost universal lymph node and distant metastases at presentation.
      d. **Infiltrating ductal scirrhous carcinomas** (70% of breast cancers) are characterized by nests and cords of tumor cells surrounded by a dense collagenous stroma.

   2. **Metastasis.** All breast carcinomas are likely to travel first to the axillary and internal mammary nodes and then to the rest of the body, especially bone.

   3. **Tumor sensitivity.** An important biologic determinant of tumor response is the presence or absence of **estrogen receptor (ER)**.

      a. ER-positive tumors are associated with a higher survival rate than **ER-negative** tumors, when ER status is measured as an independent prognostic variable.

      b. ER positivity increases with age. Most premenopausal women are ER negative, while 60%–80% of postmenopausal breast cancer patients have ER-positive tumors.

D. Diagnosis. Classically, the disease presents as a mass or lump in the breast. Today, most physicians perform a biopsy to confirm that the lump is malignant and then proceed with therapy directed to the local disease (see section VIII F below). Although tissue diagnosis ultimately is required, adjuvant studies often are performed to help predict the nature of a breast lesion.

  1. Thermography demonstrates enhanced heat due to increased vasculature in the region of the cancer.

  2. Aspiration of cystic lesions with cytology may confirm the presence of a carcinoma.

  3. Mammography reveals very small (< 1 cm) lesions such as punctate calcifications, which correlate highly with malignancy.

E. Staging according to the extent of disease provides useful prognostic and therapeutic information.

  1. Primary tumor status

    a. Stage I tumors are less than 2 cm in size. There is no node involvement and no distant metastases with these tumors, which are associated with an 80% 5-year survival rate with therapy directed exclusively at the primary lesion.

    b. Stage II tumors usually are 2–5 cm and involve the axillary nodes but no distant sites. These tumors are associated with a 50% 5-year survival rate with therapy directed at the primary lesion.

    c. Stage III tumors usually exceed 5 cm and are associated with extensive chest wall involvement with fixation and growth into contiguous structures.

    d. Stage IV tumors are associated with distant metastases.

  2. Lymph node metastases

    a. Patients with histologically negative axillary nodes have a 10-year survival rate of 75%.

    b. Patients with 1–3 nodes involved have a 10-year survival rate of 35%–65%.

    c. Patients with more than 4 nodes involved have a 10-year survival rate of 20%.

F. Therapy. As discussed above, the evaluation of ER status, tumor size and status, and lymph node involvement provides important information for therapy.

  1. Therapy for local and regional disease

    a. Surgery

      (1) Traditionally, local breast cancer has been controlled with surgical removal of the breast. In recent years, the **modified radical mastectomy** (pectoralis major not removed) has supplanted the **Halsted radical mastectomy**. Axillary node sampling and ER status evaluation should be performed with this newer procedure.

      (2) Even more recently, there has been enthusiasm for lesser surgery (i.e., **lumpectomy**) in combination **with local or regional high-dose irradiation** using an implant technique. Early results indicate that, in competent hands, this therapeutic combination yields local control and survival rates equivalent to those achieved with more extensive surgical procedures.

    b. Adjuvant therapy is designed to remove micrometastases remaining after surgery but in small enough amounts to allow sterilization.

      (1) Adjuvant radiotherapy to the chest wall prevents local recurrence but does not enhance survival. Since most tumors do not recur in the chest wall, the author and many others no longer routinely offer chest wall radiotherapy after definitive surgery.

      (2) Adjuvant chemotherapy in patients with lymph node metastases has been extensively studied yet remains controversial. However, there is overall agreement on the following principles.

        (a) Premenopausal women benefit in terms of an increased disease-free interval and possibly increased survival rates, but postmenopausal women show less impressive benefits from this therapy.

        (b) Adjuvant chemotherapy benefits patients with positive lymph nodes but usually should not be offered to patients with negative nodes.

        (c) Adjuvant chemotherapy should be started as soon as possible and no later than 1 month after surgery.

        (d) The benefits of adjuvant chemotherapy at 6 months appear equivalent to those at 12 months.

(e) Specific therapeutic agents remain controversial, but accepted regimens are CAF, CMF, and cyclophosphamide and doxorubicin (Adriamycin) alone (CA).

(f) The role of hormone therapy (e.g., with tamoxifen) in postmenopausal patients and ER-positive patients is being investigated.

2. Therapy for advanced disease

a. Radiotherapy offers significant palliation for recurrent chest wall tumors and metastatic bone disease.

b. Hormone therapy is efficacious in 70% of ER-positive patients but in less than 5% of ER-negative patients, which emphasizes the importance of determining ER status.

(1) **Surgical hormone manipulations.** In premenopausal women, castration is the initial hormone manipulation, followed by adrenalectomy and hypophysectomy.

(2) **Medical hormone manipulations**

(a) **Aminoglutethimide** inhibits adrenal cortical secretions. This treatment has been proven to be as effective as adrenalectomy.

(b) **Tamoxifen**, an estrogen antagonist, has become the hormone therapy of choice in postmenopausal women.

(c) Oral **diethylstilbestrol** and **progesterone** also are useful in treating postmenopausal patients.

c. Chemotherapy also offers effective palliation and tumor regression. Specific regimens remain controversial, but active agents include doxorubicin (probably the most effective single agent), cyclophosphamide, 5-FU, methotrexate, and mitomycin. Widely used regimens include doxorubicin alone, CMF, and CAF. Response rates vary from 40% to 65% but are not different enough to favor any one regimen distinctly.

IX. CARCINOMA OF THE LUNG

A. Incidence. The frequency of lung cancer is markedly accelerating and has been for the past few decades. Lung cancer traditionally was a disease of men over age 60. However, the male to female preponderance, which once was 10–20 to 1, is decreasing rapidly with the increasing number of women who smoke cigarettes. Today, lung cancer is the leading cause of cancer-related deaths in men in the United States. In women, the mortality rate for lung cancer is approaching that for breast cancer and likely will overtake it in this decade.

B. Etiology. Etiologic studies have linked lung cancer to the following factors.

1. Cigarette smoking. Several studies have demonstrated a correlation between smoking and lung cancer, with increases in daily cigarette usage causing parallel increases in the incidence of lung cancer. Smoking seems to lead to squamous cell and small cell undifferentiated (oat cell) varieties of lung cancer more than to adenocarcinomas. However, new data have shown a relationship between cigarette smoking and adenocarcinomas as well.

2. Exposure to industrial carcinogens has been linked to lung cancer. Although widely publicized as a cause of the less common **mesothelioma**, exposure to asbestos correlates strongly with classic lung cancer as well. Exposure to beryllium also has been linked to lung cancer.

3. Preexisting lung damage. Lung cancer, specifically adenocarcinoma, has been known to develop in areas of tuberculous scars. These tumors are the so-called **scar carcinomas**.

4. A recently recognized syndrome is that of lung cancer complicating head and neck carcinomas as a **second malignancy**. This is not unexpected in light of the association of cigarette smoking and alcohol abuse with squamous cell cancers of both the head and neck region and the lung.

C. Pathology. Four major varieties of lung cancers are encountered, and the pathology of each is important in determining therapy and prognosis.

1. Squamous cell (epidermoid) carcinomas account for about 35%–40% of lung cancers and nearly always are related to cigarette smoking.

a. These tumors usually arise in large airways and are centrally located.

b. Squamous cell carcinomas display high potential for metastasis to the brain and bone but also have marked local invasiveness and cause death in 50% of cases via invasion of mediastinal areas.

2. Adenocarcinomas (mucinous type) account for 30% of lung cancers, and their incidence is increasing. These tumors have been increasingly associated with cigarette smoking, and there is more balance in the number of men and women who are affected. Usually, adenocarcinomas are peripheral lesions, occurring in more distal airways.

    a. Classic adenocarcinomas have extensive metastatic potential and more often kill by metastasis to the brain, bone, and liver than by local invasion.

    b. A variant is the **alveolar cell carcinoma**, which occurs in the alveoli and terminal bronchioles. These cancers cause lobular consolidations visible on chest x-ray, and they classically manifest as bronchorrhea.

3. Small cell undifferentiated (oat cell) carcinomas account for 25% of lung cancers. The cell of origin seems to be the neural crest **amine precursor uptake and decarboxylation (APUD)** cell, as these tumors reveal neurosecretory granules with electron microscopy.

    a. These tumors, which are highly related to cigarette smoking, arise centrally and proximally.

    b. In 10% of cases these tumors manifest as paraneoplastic syndromes such as those of ectopic hormone production [e.g., the syndrome of inappropriate antidiuretic hormone (SIADH) and the ectopic adrenocorticotropic hormone (ACTH) syndrome] and the Eaton-Lambert (myasthenic) syndrome.

    c. Oat cell cancers have an extremely high potential for metastasis to the brain, bone, and liver. Most cases reveal blood-borne micrometastases at diagnosis.

4. Large cell undifferentiated carcinomas account for 5% of lung cancers. Their specific embryologic and histologic relationships to the other three tumor varieties remain controversial at this time. Large cell undifferentiated lesions are questionably related to smoking and usually are found centrally in the mediastinum.

D. Clinical features

1. Local manifestations common to most lung cancers include:
    a. Cough
    b. Hemoptysis
    c. Nonresolving pneumonia due to bronchial obstruction
    d. Chest pain due to thoracic invasion
    e. Pleural effusions and hoarseness due to recurrent laryngeal (mediastinal) invasion

2. Systemic manifestations include:
    a. Weight loss
    b. Anorexia
    c. Bone pain from metastases
    d. Central nervous system (CNS) symptoms and seizures from brain metastases
    e. Syndromes of ectopic hormone production (see section IX C 3 b)

3. On occasion, a routine chest x-ray reveals a lesion. Almost all lung cancer patients have an abnormal chest x-ray.

E. Diagnosis of lung cancers involves a multidisciplinary approach.

1. Sputum cytology confirms the diagnosis in 70% of cases.

2. Bronchoscopy with brushing and biopsy of lesions with cytology confirms the diagnosis in about 95% of cases.

3. Thoracotomy is required for diagnosis in about 5% of cases, especially those involving peripheral **coin lesions**. (Some physicians use **transthoracic needle biopsy** to obtain diagnostic tissues in such cases.)

4. Mediastinoscopy is another helpful technique, which not only obtains a tissue diagnosis but also assesses the resectability of the hilar and mediastinal nodes.

F. Staging

1. Non–oat cell cancers have surgery as primary therapy. The staging of these tumors is designed to determine whether the patient is a candidate for surgery.
    a. Contraindications to surgery
      (1) Local contraindications include: pleural involvement (effusion); lesions that are less than 2 cm from the carina; invasion of mediastinal structures (e.g., the laryngeal nerve); and involvement of contralateral hilar and mediastinal nodes. Techniques used to determine such data include chest x-ray with tomography, bronchoscopy, mediastinoscopy, and, lately, CT of the thorax.
      (2) Distant metastases also are contraindications to surgery. Brain, bone, and liver scanning is indicated in such evaluations.
      (3) Medical contraindications to thoracotomy (e.g., heart disease) must be considered in patients with non–oat cell tumors.

    (4) Detailed **evaluation of pulmonary function** is needed to determine whether the patient can tolerate removal of the diseased lobe or lung.

  b. Of 100 patients presenting with the non–oat cell variety of lung cancer, 70 are not candidates for surgery by at least one of the above criteria. Of the remaining 30 patients, 15 have tumors found to be locally nonresectable at thoracotomy. Thus, only 15 of 100 patients with non–oat cell lung cancers are eligible for an attempt at curative surgery.

 2. Oat cell cancers are treated primarily with chemotherapy. The staging of these tumors does not affect treatment so much as prognosis and response to therapy.

  a. Limited-extent disease (i.e., cancer that is confined to one hemithorax) responds well to aggressive chemotherapy and is curable in perhaps 20% of cases.

  b. Extensive disease (i.e., cancer that has spread beyond one hemithorax) is almost uniformly fatal within 1 year despite its responsiveness to therapy.

G. Therapy

 1. Non–oat cell lung cancers should first be evaluated for resection. As discussed above, curative surgery can be attempted in only 15 of 100 cases. However, these special cases have a 40% 5-year survival rate.

  a. Radiotherapy usually is used palliatively and occasionally is employed for long-term control of disease. Traditionally, radiotherapy has been used to treat cough, hemoptysis, obstructive pneumonia, bone pain, and CNS metastases. Currently, it is suggested that early use of high-dose radiotherapy (6600 rads), even in asymptomatic cases, may enhance patient survival beyond 1–2 years. Squamous cell carcinoma is more radiosensitive than the other non–oat cell lung cancers.

  b. Chemotherapy has been extremely disappointing. With the exception of yet unconfirmed studies using vindesine and cisplatin, few regimens show significant response rates. Furthermore, most regimens are rather toxic and fail to improve survival.

 2. Oat cell lung cancer is treated with aggressive, toxic chemotherapy using **induction regimens** of cyclophosphamide, vincristine, and doxorubicin. Such therapies induce tumor regression in more than 90% of cases. Also, in limited-extent disease, prophylactic radiotherapy to the brain is given. The optimal therapy for the primary tumor remains controversial. High doses of radiation and adjuvant surgical resection are being studied.

  a. In patients with limited-extent disease, therapy may afford prolonged survival in 20% of cases; these cases may represent cures.

  b. Even in patients with extensive disease, therapy can prolong survival from 3 to 12 months and should be offered if clinical performance allows.

X. MULTIPLE MYELOMA

 A. Incidence. Myeloma is a neoplasm of the plasma cells that are derived from B lymphocytes. It is an uncommon neoplasm, accounting for less than 1% of the adult cancers in the United States. The incidence of myeloma increases with advancing age.

 B. Etiology. Although no specific underlying causes have been proven, chronic stimulation to the immune system may play a role in the pathogenesis of myeloma.

 C. Clinical features. With the advent of automated laboratory blood testing, myeloma is found earlier and is a less clinically significant illness than it was 20 years ago.

 1. The major feature of myeloma is the demonstration of an abnormal monoclonal protein **(M protein)** in the blood, urine, or both. This M protein usually consists of any one or a combination of the heavy chains, immunoglobulin G (IgG) and IgA, and the light chains, kappa and lambda.

  a. M proteins consisting of the whole immunoglobulin molecules IgG and IgA account for 50% and 25% of the cases, respectively.

  b. M proteins consisting of only light chains account for 25% of cases.*

 2. Complications of myeloma include:

  a. Infiltration of the marrow by large numbers of usually abnormal plasma cells

  b. Weakness and fatigue due to marrow failure

  c. Osteolytic lesions due to myeloma-induced bone resorption with subsequent pain and fracture

  d. Renal abnormalities due to myeloma infiltration of the kidney, hypercalcemia, toxic effects of light chains on tubules, and amyloid deposition

---

*In these cases, the M protein is found only in the urine.

e. Recurrent infections due to acquired hypogammaglobulinemia

f. Hypercalcemia due to myeloma-stimulated osteoclast activity

3. Currently, the most common presentation is the detection of an abnormal M protein with a bone marrow examination showing plasma cell infiltration. The once common **anemia and backpain** syndromes are seen less frequently today but nevertheless occur.

D. Diagnosis of myeloma requires the demonstration of:

1. An abnormal M protein in excess of 3 g/dl in serum, urine, or both, which may require the following procedures:

a. Electrophoresis

b. Immunodiffusion

c. Quantitative immunoglobulin measurement

2. Marrow infiltration by plasma cells

3. Additional supportive findings, including anemia, skeletal lesions, renal abnormalities, and hypercalcemia

E. Staging of myeloma is based on the linear relationship between the easily measured M protein and the cellular tumor burden in myeloma patients.

1. Stage I myeloma (low tumor burden) patients have normal calcium and bone films and reveal the following blood data:

a. Hemoglobin level: > 10 g/dl

b. IgG level: < 5 g/dl

c. IgA level: < 3 g/dl

2. Stage II myeloma (intermediate tumor burden) patients reveal the following blood data:

a. Hemoglobin level: 8.5–10 g/dl

b. IgG level: 5–7 g/dl

c. IgA level: 3–5 g/dl

3. Stage III myeloma (high tumor burden) patients have hypercalcemia and osteolytic lesions and reveal the following blood data:

a. Hemoglobin level: < 8.5 g/dl

b. IgG level: > 7 g/dl

c. IgA level: > 5 g/dl

F. Therapy for myeloma involves several principles.

1. Patients in whom a differential diagnosis of the so-called **monoclonal gammopathy of unknown significance** cannot be excluded and patients with very low-grade **smoldering myeloma** should not be treated but should be examined at 3–6 month intervals for evidence of disease progression.

2. Responses are obtained in roughly two-thirds of patients requiring therapy.

a. Classically, alkylating agents (e.g., melphalan and cyclophosphamide) and prednisone are used, although some physicians advocate more aggressive regimens that also contain doxorubicin and nitrosoureas.

b. When therapy is effective, the M protein levels fall. Therapy can be stopped if the M protein levels become normal or stabilize at 75% below initial levels. It can be restarted in cases in which disease progression occurs, although results with retreatment are not as good as those with initial therapy.

c. Therapy damages marrow and leads to leukemias and excessive secondary marrow diseases in long-term survivors.

3. Supportive therapy is extremely important in the management of myeloma and includes:

a. Radiotherapy for local bone disease

b. Hydration and proper management of hypercalcemia

c. Orthopedic support and care

G. Prognosis clearly depends on the extent of myeloma at presentation. Patients with smoldering or stage I myeloma may go many years without a need for therapy, whereas patients with stage III myeloma and renal and orthopedic complications do very poorly. Mean survival for patients requiring therapy is 2–3 years.

XI. HODGKIN'S DISEASE

A. Incidence. Although Hodgkin's disease has been studied in great detail due to its unique biology and its responsiveness to therapy, it is an uncommon neoplasm, accounting for less than 1% of cancers that occur in the United States.

B. Epidemiology and etiology

1. **Hodgkin's disease has a characteristic bimodal age distribution.**
   a. A **young adult peak** occurs between the ages of 15 and 30 years and is characterized by equal incidence in men and women, a preponderance of nodular sclerosis pathology, and a more benign clinical course.
   b. A **second adult peak** occurs above age 50 and is characterized by high incidence among men, a preponderence of mixed cellularity, and a more aggressive clinical course.

2. **Clustering of cases** in time and place occurs in Hodgkin's disease, suggesting that viruses or environmental factors may play a role. However, this clustering is sporadic and has not been substantiated by firm evidence.

3. Statistical evidence links early-onset Hodgkin's disease with higher socioeconomic class, and an increased incidence of Hodgkin's disease among family members suggests a genetic predisposition.

C. Pathology. Four major histologic variants of Hodgkin's disease are classically described. Of interest, however, is the fact that the precise nature of the truly malignant cell (the binucleate giant cell called the **Reed-Sternberg cell**) remains a point of controversy despite new techniques that indicate this cell is more likely derived from the mononuclear phagocyte system than from transformed lymphocytes. The Rye histologic classification of Hodgkin's disease is summarized in Table 4-1.

D. Clinical features and staging. Hodgkin's disease tends to spread in an orderly fashion from node group to node group. This contiguous nature is in marked contrast to non-Hodgkin's lymphomas, which are multicentric early in their development.

1. The modified **Ann Arbor classification** is used for staging Hodgkin's disease and is summarized in Table 4-2.
   a. Hodgkin's disease patients, especially young ones, usually present with asymptomatic swelling of a lymph node. The B subclassification implies, however, that Hodgkin's disease may present with such systemic symptoms as fever and weight loss. (Systemic symptoms are unusual with non-Hodgkin's lymphomas.)
   b. Workup is based on the principle that early-stage Hodgkin's disease can be treated locally but late-stage Hodgkin's disease requires systemic therapy. Therefore, patients are aggressively staged to include or exclude stage IV disease. (This staging is far more extensive than staging for non-Hodgkin's lymphomas.)

2. **Staging procedures** include:
   a. Thorough history and physical examination
   b. Chest x-ray
   c. Percutaneous bone marrow biopsy
   d. Liver and spleen scanning and gallium scanning

Table 4-1. The Rye Histologic Classification of Hodgkin's Disease

Subtype	Pattern	Histologic Description	Incidence, Staging, and Prognosis
Lymphocyte predominance	Diffuse	Occasional Reed-Sternberg cells among abundant lymphocytes	More common in young adults; early tumor stage; good prognosis
Mixed cellularity	Diffuse	Moderate numbers of lymphocytes, plasma cells, and Reed-Sternberg cells	Intermediate tumor stage; fair prognosis
Lymphocyte depletion	Diffuse	Abundant Reed-Sternberg cells among scanty stroma	More common in adults over age 50; advanced tumor stage; poor prognosis
Nodular sclerosis	Nodular	Node divided into nodules by fibrous bands; lacunar Reed-Sternberg cells	More common in young women; fair prognosis

Table 4-2. Ann Arbor Classification of Hodgkin's Disease

Stage	Characteristics
I	Involvement of a single lymph node region or a single extralymphatic site
II	Involvement of two or more lymph node regions on the same side of the diaphragm
III	Involvement of two or more lymph node regions on both sides of the diaphragm
IV	Diffuse or disseminated involvement in extralymphatic organs
Subclassifications	
A	Asymptomatic
B	Unexplained loss of 10% of body weight; unexplained fever of greater than 38° C; night sweats

   e. Laparoscopy with liver biopsy
   f. Lymphangiography, which is gradually being replaced by CT in cases involving abdominal nodes

3. Laparotomy, combined with node sampling, splenectomy, and liver biopsy, is recommended for most patients with stages I, II, and III A disease. These procedures probably are not needed for patients with stages III B and IV disease.

E. Therapy for Hodgkin's disease continues to evolve. However, certain principles have been established and should be firmly adhered to, since even advanced disease is curable. Individual variations in treatment should be avoided and, if used, should be limited to well-controlled clinical trials.

   1. Patients with stage I or stage II disease are treated with extended-field radiotherapy.

   2. Patients with stage III A disease are treated with total nodal radiotherapy. Patients who relapse after radiotherapy can be treated successfully with chemotherapy. More than 50% of such patients have long disease-free survival when such techniques are used.

   3. Patients with stage III B or stage IV disease require systemic chemotherapy. Many regimens are available, but the classic is the **MOPP** regimen [i.e., mechlorethamine, vincristine (Oncovin), procarbazine, and prednisone], which is given for at least six cycles plus two additional cycles after complete remission is documented.
   a. Alternative regimens have not been proven to be more efficacious than MOPP and should be reserved for patients who do not respond to MOPP or until clinical trials prove their superiority. However, an extremely promising regimen is BCVPP [i.e., carmustine (BCNU), cyclophosphamide, vincristine, procarbazine, and prednisone].
   b. Combined chemotherapy and radiotherapy also should not be used routinely until further clinical trials prove the effectiveness of such a regimen.
   c. Unless chemotherapeutic agents are given in full doses and according to prescribed schedules, their effectiveness can be significantly compromised.
   d. Both chemotherapy and total nodal irradiation are difficult, toxic, and have many side effects, including severe nausea and vomiting, hypothyroidism, sterility (in some cases), and development of secondary marrow problems including acute leukemia.

F. Prognosis varies mainly with the stage of disease and to a lesser extent with histology. Overall, there is a 55%–60% 5-year survival rate with all cases of Hodgkin's disease.

   1. Patients with stage I or stage II disease have a 5-year disease-free survival rate exceeding 80%.

   2. Patients with stage III A disease have roughly a 67% rate of 5-year disease-free survival.

   3. Patients with stage III B or stage IV disease, if treated with chemotherapy, obtain remissions in 70%–80% of cases, with approximately half of these patients achieving prolonged (i.e., > 5 years) disease-free survival.

XII. NON-HODGKIN'S LYMPHOMAS

A. Incidence. Non-Hodgkin's lymphomas represent a heterogeneous group of lymphoreticular neoplasms. These tumors are uncommon, accounting for about 2% of all new cancers in the United States. Non-Hodgkin's lymphomas are most common among white men, and their incidence rises logarithmically with age.

B. Etiology. Although the cause of these tumors is unknown, several etiologic factors have been uncovered.

    1. Familial aggregation. Multiple instances of affected sibling pairs have been noted, which suggests an underlying genetically altered immune responsiveness (see section XII B 3).

    2. Primary immunodeficiency syndromes have been strongly associated with the development of non-Hodgkin's lymphomas.

    3. Acquired and therapeutic immunosuppression has been shown to enhance 100-fold the incidence of these tumors. A classic example is the increased incidence of lymphoma among renal transplant patients who are treated chronically with immunosuppressive agents. Also, patients with acquired immune deficiency syndrome (AIDS) are at risk for developing non-Hodgkin's lymphomas.

    4. Infectious agents have been implicated in the development of non-Hodgkin's lymphomas by studies that show clustered cases. Specifically, **Epstein-Barr virus** has been linked to Burkitt's lymphoma, a disease usually found in Africa.

C. Pathology. Due to extensive research done in the last decade, it is possible to define the difference in the natural history and prognosis of each non-Hodgkin's lymphoma in terms of pathology. Most are derived from B lymphoid tissue, but the specific nodal area of origin and the specific cell type involved are critical to clinical behavior. The two most commonly used classifications of non-Hodgkin's lymphomas are shown in Tables 4-3 and 4-4.

D. Clinical features of non-Hodgkin's lymphomas are rather nonstriking and insidious.

    1. Painless adenopathy is the most common presentation. Any node area may be involved, and multiple areas of involvement are characteristic. Specific areas of node involvement may elicit localized symptom complexes. The following are examples.
        a. Inguinal node involvement that causes vein compression may lead to deep venous thrombosis.
        b. Retroperitoneal node involvement may lead to increased girth and abdominal pain.

    2. Systemic signs and symptoms such as weight loss and fever are less common in non-Hodgkin's lymphomas than in Hodgkin's disease.

E. Staging and diagnosis first require surgical biopsy of an involved node with careful pathologic examination. Although some physicians vigorously stage patients according to the Ann Arbor classification of Hodgkin's disease (see Table 4-2), more than 90% of non-Hodgkin's lymphomas are multicentric at diagnosis, and many investigators, therefore, choose to perform less ag-

---

Table 4-3. The United States National Cancer Institute Classification of the Morphological Subgroups of Non-Hodgkin's Lymphomas

Low-grade malignant lymphoma
    Small lymphocytic
    Follicular—predominantly small cleaved cell
    Follicular—mixed (small cleaved and large cell)

Intermediate-grade malignant lymphoma
    Follicular—predominantly large cell
    Diffuse—small cleaved cell
    Diffuse—mixed (small and large cell)
    Diffuse—large cell

High-grade malignant lymphoma
    Large cell
    Convoluted lymphoblastic
    Small noncleaved cell (Burkitt's)

Table 4-4. The Rappaport Classification of Non-Hodgkin's Lymphomas

Predominant Malignant Cell	Relative Frequency (%)	Median Survival (years)
Nodular lymphomas		
Histiocytic	7	3.0
Mixed (lymphocytes and histiocytes)	19	7.5
Lymphocytic (poorly differentiated)	18	7.5
Lymphocytic (well differentiated)	1	> 7.5
Total	45	
Diffuse lymphomas		
Histiocytic	32	1.1
Mixed (lymphocytes and histiocytes)	10	1.5
Lymphocytic (poorly differentiated)	10	2.0
Lymphocytic (well differentiated)	3	> 7.5
Total	55	

Note.—This system is based on the specific cell type involved and the presence or absence of nodularity.

gressive staging maneuvers. Unlike the situation in Hodgkin's disease, most investigators refrain from laparotomy and splenectomy.

1. Valuable information regarding the extent of disease can be obtained from bone marrow biopsy, chest x-ray, CT of the mediastinum and retroperitoneum, routine complete blood count and laboratory studies, liver and spleen scanning, and, possibly, gallium scanning.

2. The majority of patients present with extensive nodal disease (stage III) or parenchymal disease (stage IV) at diagnosis (see section XII E).

F. **Therapy and prognosis** for non-Hodgkin's lymphomas vary with the specific pathologic subtype.

1. **Diseases with favorable histologies** (see Table 4-4) may not require treatment for many years.
   a. When therapy is indicated, **nonaggressive chemotherapy** with single alkylating agents (e.g., chlorambucil) is as effective as more aggressive combination regimens and is far less toxic.
   b. **Radiotherapy** may be useful for treating localized disease.
   c. A paradox exists in that although diseases with favorable histologies grow slowly and have prognoses measured in years (see Table 4-4), they are not curable and ultimately relapse even if complete remission is obtained with therapy. Recent data indicate that more than 10% of diseases with favorable histologies degenerate into more aggressive subtypes later in the course of the disease.

2. **Diseases with aggressive and unfavorable histologies** require immediate and intensive treatment.
   a. **Aggressive combination chemotherapy** is used most commonly. Regimens usually contain doxorubicin and are given monthly for at least 6–12 months. About 75% of patients respond to such regimens, and long-term survival has been documented.
   b. A paradox exists in that although diseases with aggressive histologies have median survivals of about 2 years, in those patients who achieve complete remission with therapy, long-term survival is obtained in 40%–50% of cases without further therapy.

STUDY QUESTIONS

Directions: Each question below contains five suggested answers. Choose the **one best** response to each question.

1. Hodgkin's disease is associated with all of the following treatment-related complications EXCEPT

(A) severe gastrointestinal toxicity
(B) sterility
(C) hypothyroidism
(D) microangiopathic hemolytic anemia
(E) acute leukemia

2. All of the following conditions are associated with carcinoma of the colon EXCEPT

(A) familial polyposis
(B) ulcerative colitis
(C) villous adenoma
(D) pedunculated polyps of large size
(E) peptic ulcer disease

3. All of the following statements about gastric carcinoma are true EXCEPT

(A) the incidence of gastric cancer has been decreasing in recent decades
(B) the incidence of gastric cancer is increased in patients with pernicious anemia
(C) the incidence of gastric cancer is increased in individuals with blood group A
(D) most patients with gastric cancer have regional lymph node metastases
(E) gastric cancer responds well to radiotherapy

4. A patient with nodular lymphoma involving the neck, mediastinum, and retroperitoneum would be expected to require all of the following staging procedures EXCEPT

(A) laparotomy with splenectomy
(B) bone marrow biopsy
(C) computed tomography of the mediastinum and abdomen
(D) complete blood count
(E) liver and spleen scanning

5. Bladder carcinoma in the United States has all of the following characteristics EXCEPT

(A) a higher incidence among men than women
(B) a classic presentation of painless hematuria
(C) a high rate of local recurrences
(D) a squamous cell origin in 90% of cases
(E) an association with occupational carcinogens such as aniline dyes

6. Patients with renal cell carcinoma may commonly present with all of the following symptoms EXCEPT

(A) a palpable mass in the flank area
(B) hematuria, either gross or microscopic
(C) pain in the costovertebral area
(D) anemia and systemic symptoms
(E) renal failure requiring dialysis

7. All of the following statements about carcinoembryonic antigen (CEA) are true EXCEPT

(A) CEA level is elevated in most patients with colorectal cancer
(B) CEA level is elevated in patients with benign colon diseases
(C) CEA level is elevated in patients with malignancies other than colorectal cancer
(D) CEA is important as a diagnostic test for colorectal cancer
(E) CEA is most useful in detecting recurrences of colorectal cancer

Directions: Each question below contains four suggested answers of which **one or more** is correct. Choose the answer

A if **1, 2, and 3** are correct
B if **1 and 3** are correct
C if **2 and 4** are correct
D if **4** is correct
E if **1, 2, 3, and 4** are correct

8. Complications of multiple myeloma include

(1) osteolytic lesions
(2) renal failure
(3) hypercalcemia
(4) infections

9. True statements concerning adjuvant therapy for breast cancer after initial surgery or radiotherapy include

(1) premenopausal women show the greatest benefit from adjuvant therapy
(2) adjuvant therapy is effective if started within 6 months of surgery
(3) 6 months and 12 months of adjuvant therapy appear equivalent
(4) hormone therapy routinely is included in adjuvant therapy

10. Diffuse lymphomas are characterized by

(1) an increased incidence among patients with immunodeficiency syndromes
(2) a need for aggressive therapy early in the course of disease
(3) occasional cures with appropriate therapy
(4) a tendency to evolve into acute leukemia

11. A medically fit patient with non–oat cell cancer is being evaluated for tumor resectability. Factors that must be considered include

(1) distance of lesion from the carina
(2) mediastinal node involvement
(3) distant metastases
(4) involvement of lobar fissures

Directions: The group of questions below consists of lettered choices followed by several numbered items. For each numbered item select the **one** lettered choice with which it is **most** closely associated. Each lettered choice may be used once, more than once, or not at all.

Questions 12–17

Match each of the following tumors with its associated risk factor.

(A) Pernicious anemia
(B) Dye and printing chemicals
(C) Asbestos
(D) Ulcerative colitis
(E) Epstein-Barr virus

12. Non-Hodgkin's lymphoma

13. Bladder carcinoma

14. Gastric carcinoma

15. Colorectal carcinoma

16. Lung carcinoma

17. Head and neck carcinoma

ANSWERS AND EXPLANATIONS

1. The answer is D. (*V F 3; XI E 3 d*) Therapy for Hodgkin's disease is difficult and morbid. Chemotherapeutic agents have significant gastrointestinal toxicity. This is especially true for the combination of mechlorethamine, vincristine (Oncovin), procarbazine, and prednisone (i.e., the MOPP regimen), which is the most widely used form of chemotherapy for Hodgkin's disease. Radiotherapy to the neck area can result in hypothyroidism. Chemotherapy and radiotherapy both can cause sterility as well as damage marrow stem cells, resulting in secondary acute leukemia. Microangiopathic hemolytic anemia can occur after long-term use of 5-fluorouracil (5-FU), doxorubicin (Adriamycin), and mitomycin (i.e., the FAM regimen), a palliative combination chemotherapy for gastric carcinoma.

2. The answer is E. (*VII B 1*) Familial polyposis and ulcerative colitis have a clear association with the later development of colon cancer. Villous adenomas and large (i.e., > 1–2 cm) pedunculated polyps of the colon also have been shown to cause a statistical increase in the frequency of colon cancer. Peptic ulcer disease does not result in an increase in the incidence of colon tumors.

3. The answer is E. (*V A, B 1, 3, F*) For poorly understood reasons, the incidence of gastric cancer has been decreasing in recent decades. The incidence of this tumor is increased in certain groups of individuals, such as those with blood group A and individuals with achlorhydria from chronic atrophic gastritis or pernicious anemia. The tumor often has local metastases to regional nodes at the time of surgery. For the most part, gastric carcinoma responds poorly to radiotherapy due to the poor sensitivity of the cells to radiation and to the difficulty in delivering high doses of radiation to the abdomen.

4. The answer is A. (*XII E 1*) More than 90% of nodular lymphomas are widely disseminated at diagnosis. Because this patient has disease on both sides of the diaphragm, the therapeutic decision likely would not be affected by laparotomy, regardless of further findings with this procedure. A complete blood count and bone marrow examination are needed to determine the degree of marrow involvement and reserve if chemo- and radiotherapy are required. Computed tomography (CT) is an excellent method of evaluating the extent of disease and the patient response to therapy. Liver and spleen scanning also are used to document the extent of disease and response to therapy, but these techniques are being replaced by CT.

5. The answer is D. (*III A, B 2, C 2, D 2, E 2*) Bladder cancer occurs more commonly in men than in women and is associated with exposure to certain occupational carcinogens (e.g., those found in the rubber, dye, and printing industries). Patients with bladder tumors classically present with painless hematuria, although other symptoms such as bladder infection and irritability may be seen in about 25% of patients. The main pathologic type found in the United States is that of transitional cell cancer. In the Middle East, infestation by schistosomes results in a unique squamous cell bladder cancer, but this is rare in the United States. The tumor sometimes can be managed in the early stages by local removal. However, bladder cancers tend to recur and, therefore, require aggressive follow-up with intravenous pyelography and cystoscopy.

6. The answer is E. (*III D 1*) The classic triad of symptoms that occur in patients with renal cancer consists of anemia, hematuria, and a palpable mass. Although it is uncommon for all three of these to occur simultaneously, most patients (85% or more) have at least one of these symptoms. Anemia and systemic symptoms (e.g., fevers that have no obvious source) also are characteristic of renal cell cancers.

7. The answer is D. (*VII E 4*) Carcinoembryonic antigen (CEA) level is raised in about 60% of patients with proven colorectal cancer. However, many nonmalignant colon diseases (e.g., colitis) as well as certain noncolon malignant diseases (e.g., lung cancer and breast cancer) also can result in CEA elevations. CEA is most useful as a monitor for recurrent disease in known colorectal cancer patients. Its nonspecificity makes CEA a poor diagnostic tool in the initial diagnosis of colon cancer.

8. The answer is E (all). (*X C 2*) Patients with multiple myeloma most frequently present with an abnormal monoclonal protein (M protein), which is detected in the blood, urine, or both. In addition, myeloma cell–induced bone resorption results in weakened bone, osteolytic lesions, and fractures. The M protein exists in high concentrations in the kidney and acts as a nephrotoxin, contributing (along with hyperuricemia, dehydration, and hypercalcemia) to renal failure in many patients. The myeloma cells also secrete an osteoclast-stimulating factor, which causes hypercalcemia due to calcium resorption from bone. Finally, myeloma leads to acquired hypogammaglobulinemia, which predisposes patients to infections.

9. The answer is B (1, 3). [*VIII F 1 a (2), b (2) (a)–(f)*] Among breast cancer patients, the most significant benefit from adjuvant chemotherapy occurs in premenopausal women. Although dosage effects have been postulated as the cause of the lesser benefit in postmenopausal women, the precise cause of the difference is unclear. Multiple studies have shown that adjuvant chemotherapy is most effective when begun as soon as possible and no later than 1 month after surgery. In addition, several studies have demonstrated that, if started immediately, 6 months of full-dose adjuvant chemotherapy is as effective as longer regimens. Although the role of hormone therapy is being investigated, the data are not sufficient to support the decision to add hormonal agents routinely to adjuvant therapeutic regimens.

10. The answer is A (1, 2, 3). (*XII B 2–3, F 2 b*) Diffuse lymphomas are complications of congenital as well as acquired immunodeficiencies. For this reason, patients with acquired immune deficiency syndrome (AIDS) are at a greater than normal risk for developing diffuse lymphomas. Also, an increased incidence of lymphoma is seen in renal patients who have received long-term immunosuppressive agents.

Diffuse lymphomas have aggressive and unfavorable histologies; these diseases require immediate and intensive therapy if responses and cures are expected. With proper therapy, some of the complete responders have prolonged disease-free survival and represent probable cures.

11. The answer is A (1, 2, 3). (*IX F 1 a*) Involvement of more than one lobe should not preclude surgery in a patient who otherwise is an acceptable medical candidate for lung resection. However, invasion of mediastinal structures does preclude adequate surgical removal. Distant metastases eliminate the possibility of cure with local resection. Inadequate resection margins result after surgery for tumors that are less than 2 cm from the carina.

12–17. The answers are: 12-E, 13-B, 14-A, 15-D, 16-C, 17-E. (*I B 3; III B 2 a; V B 3; VII B 1 b; IX B 2; XII B 4*) Studies have shown clustering of cases of non-Hodgkin's lymphomas, which suggests that infectious agents may play a causative role. In particular, Epstein-Barr virus has been implicated in the development of Burkitt's lymphoma, a disease commonly found in Africa.

Bladder carcinoma has been linked to tobacco as well as certain chemical and biologic carcinogens. For example, there is a well-documented association between occupational exposure to dye and printing chemicals and the development of bladder tumors.

Several relationships have been noted in the etiology of gastric carcinoma. Up to 10% of patients with achlorhydria, atrophic gastritis, and pernicious anemia develop gastric cancer. An increased concentration of nitrosamine compounds in gastric juice has been suggested as an underlying factor in these relationships.

Colorectal carcinoma is a common malignancy in the United States, for which several precancerous lesions are known. Chronic ulcerative colitis of long duration has a documented and statistically significant association with the incidence of colorectal cancer.

In the United States, lung cancer is the number-one cause of cancer-related deaths in men and is second only to breast cancer as the leading cause of cancer deaths in women. Cigarette smoking largely is implicated as a cause of lung cancer, but other etiologic factors have been noted, such as exposure to industrial carcinogens. One of these, asbestos, classically has been linked to the more rare mesothelioma; however, asbestos exposure also has a clear and strong association with lung cancer.

Head and neck tumors are highly unusual in Mormon societies, which abstain from both alcohol and tobacco. This fact exemplifies the statistically based claims that the use of tobacco and alcohol is associated with an increased risk of head and neck cancers. Another noted risk factor is the Epstein-Barr virus, which has been linked to the unusual nasopharyngeal carcinoma that is unique to Orientals.

5
Gastrointestinal Diseases

Anthony J. DiMarino, Jr.
Marta A. Dabezies

I. DISEASES OF THE ESOPHAGUS. The esophagus basically is an organ of transport, with no significant absorptive or secretory function.

A. Common clinical features

1. **Dysphagia**, or difficulty in swallowing, is a symptom often described as a **sticking sensation**.
   a. **Dysphagia for solids** indicates an esophageal obstruction due to:
      (1) Carcinoma
      (2) An esophageal web or ring
      (3) Benign esophageal stricture
   b. **Dysphagia for solids and liquids** indicates an esophageal abnormality due to a motor dysfunction, such as:
      (1) Scleroderma
      (2) Achalasia
      (3) Symptomatic diffuse esophageal spasm

2. **Odynophagia**, or pain on swallowing, may be due to:
   a. **Motor disorders** of the esophagus, especially achalasia and diffuse esophageal spasm
   b. **Mucosal disruption** caused by ingestion of lye or other caustic agents, severe peptic esophagitis, severe infections of the esophagus (e.g., candidal esophagitis and esophagitis due to viruses such as herpes simplex), drug-induced esophagitis (e.g., drugs including potassium chloride tablets, tetracycline preparations, clindamycin, quinidine, and ascorbic acid tablets), and radiation esophagitis

3. **Heartburn** is a substernal burning sensation, which radiates in an orad direction and may be initiated by bending forward. This is a specific symptom of gastroesophageal reflux.

B. Specific disorders

1. **Reflux esophagitis** is caused by the recurrent reflux of gastric contents into the distal esophagus.
   a. **Etiology and pathogenesis**
      (1) Normally, the **lower esophageal sphincter (LES)** blocks reflux of gastric juice into the esophagus. Reflux esophagitis is thought to stem from a defect in this LES mechanism, such as:
         (a) Decreased resting LES pressure
         (b) Prolonged or repeated intermittent relaxation of the LES
         (c) Transient increase in abdominal pressure
      (2) **Secondary causes** of reflux esophagitis should always be suspected and corrected if possible. The following conditions appear to decrease LES pressure.
         (a) **Pregnancy.** Especially during the last trimester, heartburn may be severe and probably is due to progesterone effects on the LES.
         (b) **Drugs** that may decrease the LES pressure as a side effect of smooth muscle relaxation include:
            (i) Anticholinergic agents
            (ii) Beta$_2$-adrenergic agonists used to treat asthma and chronic bronchitis
            (iii) Calcium channel blocking agents
         (c) **Scleroderma** that weakens the esophageal smooth muscle and the LES region may be a cause of severe reflux esophagitis.
         (d) **Surgical vagotomy** also may produce anatomic alterations that lead to reflux esophagitis.

b. Clinical features
  (1) Heartburn is a very specific symptom of regurgitation that is brought on by bending over or lying down. If advanced, this regurgitation may be associated with pulmonary aspiration.
  (2) Dysphagia in the esophagitis patient generally is for solids and may indicate a developing stricture.
  (3) Anemia may occur if recurrent bleeding is present.
c. Diagnosis. Several tests have been proposed for the diagnosis of reflux esophagitis.
  (1) Barium swallow and upper gastrointestinal series. This may be the least sensitive test. Generally, it is positive only in severe gastroesophageal reflux with a very weakened LES or in the presence of esophageal ulceration.
  (2) Acid-reflux test. This test involves monitoring intraesophageal pH after instilling 300 ml of 0.1 *N* hydrochloric acid (HCl) into the stomach. The acid-reflux test probably is a very sensitive test; however, it is an invasive test that requires positioning a pH tube in the distal esophagus.
  (3) Acid-perfusion test (Bernstein test). This test is intended to reproduce the pain associated with reflux and involves esophageal perfusion of 0.1 *N* HCl alternately with normal saline solution.
  (4) Scintigraphy involves the introduction of technetium 99 (^{99}Tc) into the stomach followed by abdominal compression and radiographic counting over the esophagus. This technique can demonstrate reflux as well as provide a useful quantitative measure of its presence, and it has the added advantage of being noninvasive.
  (5) Endoscopy with biopsy is a helpful procedure, especially to rule out associated peptic ulcer disease.
  (6) Esophageal manometry is useful to evaluate the LES pressure. Pressures consistently measured at less than one-third the lower limit of normal usually are associated with significant reflux. This technique is especially useful in the preoperative evaluation of esophageal reflux when a fundoplication is contemplated.
d. Therapy
  (1) Increasing the reflux barrier may be accomplished by:
    (a) Measures such as elevating the head of the bed 2–4 inches and avoiding eating for 3 hours before bedtime
    (b) Alginic acid and antacid combinations
    (c) Drugs that increase LES tone (e.g., bethanecol and metoclopramide)
    (d) Antireflux surgery, especially Nissen fundoplication
  (2) Decreasing gastric acid effects may be accomplished by:
    (a) Antacids
    (b) Histamine$_2$ (H$_2$)-receptor antagonists (e.g., cimetidine and ranitidine)
  (3) Avoiding agents that decrease LES pressure, such as:
    (a) Anticholinergic agents
    (b) Beta-adrenergic drugs
    (c) Calcium channel blocking agents
    (d) Chocolate
    (e) Fats
    (f) Nicotine (smoking)
    (g) Xanthine and its derivatives (e.g., caffeine)
e. Complications
  (1) Benign esophageal stricture probably occurs in a small portion of all reflux esophagitis cases and is best diagnosed by a **bolus barium swallow** or endoscopy with biopsy.
  (2) Esophageal ulceration may be accompanied by hemorrhage; but the primary symptom is severe and unrelenting pain on swallowing.
  (3) Pulmonary aspiration is a serious but rare sequela of reflux esophagitis. Patients over age 30 years who develop repeated pneumonia or asthma should be evaluated for esophageal reflux.
  (4) Barrett's esophagus refers to a condition in which columnar epithelium replaces the normal squamous epithelium of the esophagus, possibly as a result of continuous inflammation. This is considered a premalignant state.

2. Obstructive esophageal conditions
a. Carcinoma. Esophageal cancer most often is squamous cell in type; cases of adenocarcinoma are rare. Carcinoma occurs with varying incidence throughout the world and predominantly in men. The population of the United States is considered at low risk; esophageal cancer strikes only 4 of 100,000 individuals.
  (1) Etiology. Certain factors appear to increase the risk of esophageal cancer.
    (a) Tobacco smoking may increase the risk two to four times.

        (b) Alcohol consumption has been shown to increase the risk up to 12 times in France. Alcohol and tobacco appear to have an additive effect.

        (c) Geographic factors. Incidence levels were found to be 40 times greater in certain regions in China and Iran and may be due to a diet that includes high amounts of nitrosamines, molds, or both.

        (d) Vitamin deficiency, especially of vitamins A and C, may be associated with an increased risk for esophageal cancer.

        (e) Lye ingestion is associated with the development of esophageal cancer many years after exposure.

        (f) Achalasia may be associated with a 10% risk of subsequent carcinomas.

        (g) Barrett's esophagus [see section I B 1 e (4)]. Adenocarcinoma eventually may develop in 10%–15% of cases of Barrett's esophagus.

    (2) Clinical features

        (a) Progressive dysphagia for solids indicates the presence of an ongoing obstructive lesion. Usually, when the esophageal lumen has narrowed to 1.2 cm or less, a **persistent dysphagia** for solid food is noted.

        (b) Pain usually signifies extension of the tumor beyond the wall of the esophagus.

        (c) Dysphagia for liquids, cough, hoarseness, and weight loss generally are symptoms of advanced esophageal carcinoma.

    (3) Diagnosis

        (a) Barium x-ray with a barium-coated bolus (e.g., bread or a marshmallow) should be done when **obstructive dysphagia** is suspected.

        (b) Endoscopy with biopsy and cytology, if performed together, establish a diagnosis in about 90% of cases.

        (c) Computed tomography (CT) and **bronchoscopy** should be used to evaluate the presence and extent of nodal metastases and bronchial invasion.

    (4) Therapy

        (a) Surgery generally is performed if the lesion is in the lower one-third or in the distal portion of the middle one-third of the esophagus. Surgery has the advantage of restoring esophageal patency, but 5-year cure rates average only 5%–10%.

        (b) Radiotherapy is prescribed for lesions located in the proximal part of the middle one-third or in the upper one-third of the esophagus. Approximately 6000 rads usually are administered.

        (c) Esophageal bougienage or stent therapy with silastic tubes may be used in certain cases to maintain esophageal patency.

        (d) Lasers are being used in some centers to vaporize tumors to the extent that a lumen is established.

        (e) Chemotherapy has not been shown to prolong life significantly in controlled trials, but new regimens combining radio- and chemotherapy have shown encouraging results in initial studies.

  b. Benign esophageal stricture may be a sequela of prolonged reflux esophagitis. Heartburn may lessen as solid-food dysphagia worsens due to progression of the stricture. Diagnosis is established by a bolus barium swallow and endoscopy. Treatment generally is with tapered rubber bougies weighted with a mercury core or with balloon dilatation catheters.

  c. Esophageal webs seen in the upper one-third of the esophagus may be due to a failure of complete embryologic recanalization. Webs in this area also may be associated with iron deficiency anemia in the **Plummer-Vinson (Patterson-Kelly) syndrome**. Effective treatment of this syndrome includes administration of iron for the anemia and fracture of the web with an esophageal bougie.

  d. Esophageal rings most commonly occur at the squamocolumnar junction and are called **Schatzki's rings**. Dysphagia for solids often is intermittent in this condition, especially if the narrowest point of the esophagus measures between 1.2 cm and 2 cm. Esophageal bougienage often is effective therapy.

3. Esophageal motor disorders

  a. Oropharyngeal dysphagia is a descriptive term applied to a disorder of the neuromuscular apparatus of the distal pharynx and upper esophagus. Symptoms include difficulty in initiating swallowing, nasal regurgitation, and pulmonary aspiration. The types of disorders associated with oropharyngeal dysphagia include:

    (1) Cerebrovascular accident (CVA), which may be the most common of these disorders and usually is due to transient brain stem edema

    (2) Myasthenia gravis

    (3) Myotonic dystrophy

    (4) Polymyositis

    (5) Bulbar poliomyelitis

(6) Parkinson's disease
(7) Multiple sclerosis
(8) Amyotrophic lateral sclerosis
b. Symptomatic diffuse esophageal spasm (SDES)
(1) Pathology. While occasional reports have described an esophageal muscular hypertrophy, these are not consistent. Most investigators feel that a neural defect exists. LES abnormalities, with incomplete relaxation, that are similar to achalasia have been described in 30% of cases, and documented progression to classic achalasia lends credence to a neural pathogenesis.
(2) Clinical features
(a) **Dysphagia** for both solids and liquids occurs.
(b) **Odynophagia** can occur, especially after ingestion of solids or liquids of extremely hot or cold temperature.
(c) **Spontaneous chest pain** similar to angina pectoris may be noted. Nocturnal pain often is described, with relief afforded by the smooth muscle relaxant, nitroglycerin (the same treatment prescribed for anginal pain). This may further confuse the diagnosis.
(3) Diagnosis is based on clinical evidence. A **corkscrew esophagus** on x-ray is helpful, but esophageal manometry should reveal:
(a) High-amplitude, repetitive, simultaneous contractions in about 30% of the basal state or after ergonovine or edrophonium stimulation (not a routinely performed test)
(b) Several **normal peristaltic sequences** to differentiate SDES from achalasia
(c) Incomplete relaxation of the LES in about 30% of patients
(4) Therapy is successful in about 50% of cases and includes:
(a) Anticholinergic agents
(b) Nitrates (short- or long-acting)
(c) Calcium channel blocking agents
(d) Esophageal bougienage
(e) Hydralazine to decrease peristaltic amplitude
(f) Surgery with a longitudinal esophageal myotomy (in severe, incapacitating cases only)
c. Achalasia
(1) Incidence. Achalasia occurs in approximately 1 in 100,000 individuals in the United States and equally in both sexes. The most common age of onset is between 20 and 40 years.
(2) Pathology. A neural defect is suggested by decreased ganglion cells with fibrosis and scarring in Auerbach's plexus. A **wallerian degeneration** is suggested by examination of vagal esophageal fibers. The dorsal vagal nucleus also is abnormal. A supersensitivity to cholinergic stimulation and exogenous gastrin is described.
(3) Clinical features include:
(a) Dysphagia for solids and liquids in 95%–100% of patients
(b) Weight loss in 90% of patients
(c) Chest pain, which is severe in about 60% of patients
(d) Nocturnal cough in about 30% of patients, indicating possible **overflow aspiration** of unemptied esophageal contents and, in such cases, the need for immediate treatment
(e) Recurrent bronchitis or pneumonia, both of which are serious complications, in about 7%–8% of patients
(4) Diagnosis is made by excluding malignancy (i.e., carcinoma and lymphoma) at the esophagogastric junction, which may mimic achalasia.
(a) **Radiography** may reveal a flaccid, dilated, fluid-filled esophagus with a beak-like tapering over the LES region.
(b) **Manometry** is the most sensitive diagnostic method and should reveal:
(i) Absence of normal peristalsis in the entire esophagus
(ii) Elevated LES pressure
(iii) Incomplete relaxation of the LES, which probably accounts for the major clinical findings because of a persistent obstructing barrier after swallowing
(5) Therapy
(a) **Drugs.** Nitrates, anticholinergic agents, β-adrenergic agonists, and calcium channel blocking agents are effective in less than 50% of patients. Prostaglandins may hold promise as future forms of therapy.
(b) **Pneumatic dilatation** is effective in 70%–90% of cases, has a mortality rate of about 0.2%, and has a perforation rate of about 2%–3%.
(c) **Surgical therapy.** The favored procedure is a **Heller myotomy**, which has a 65%–90% success rate and a rate of surgical complications that averages 3%–4%. The

rate of postoperative reflux may increase to 25%–30% after several years for operations that did not incorporate an antireflux procedure.

    (d) Endoscopic myotomy presently is undergoing clinical trials.

  d. Systemic sclerosis (scleroderma) is a systemic collagen vascular disease involving the skin in 98% of cases. The esophagus is found to be abnormal in 75% of autopsies and in 80% of cases studied manometrically.

    (1) Pathology. The early esophageal effects are felt to be neural since no anatomic abnormality of the smooth muscle can be identified at a time when marked weakness of the esophagus is noted. The strong association with Raynaud's phenomenon, which is believed to have a neural basis, is consistent with this theory. A late defect may include a disuse type of atrophy of smooth muscle elements.

    (2) Clinical features include:

      (a) Dysphagia for solids and liquids

      (b) Severe heartburn in about 50% of patients

      (c) Esophageal stricture in about 25% of long-term survivors

    (3) Diagnosis

      (a) Radiography. A supine esophagogram may reveal poor esophageal emptying due to an absence of peristalsis.

      (b) Manometry, the most reliable diagnostic technique, reveals:

        (i) Decreased LES pressure

        (ii) Initially very weak, low-amplitude peristaltic contractions in the distal smooth muscle portion (lower two-thirds) of the esophagus, which later progress to the absence of distal peristalsis.

    (4) Therapy. Specific treatment for systemic sclerosis is controversial and has included D-penicillamine and colchicine. The esophageal effects are treated with antireflux measures (see section I B 1 f).

  4. Other esophageal disorders

    a. Diverticula

      (1) Zenker's diverticulum is a mucosal herniation (not a true diverticulum) above the cricopharyneal region; obstructive symptoms may occur if there is incomplete emptying of this diverticulum. Large diverticula are treated surgically.

      (2) Traction diverticula occur in the body of the esophagus and in the distal region and at one time were thought to be secondary to an adjacent inflammatory process, such as tuberculosis.

      (3) Epiphrenic diverticula occur in the distal esophagus, above the LES, and often are asymptomatic.

    b. Infections. Bacterial and viral sources of esophageal infection are common, but two agents are of major importance.

      (1) Candidal esophagitis usually occurs in diabetic patients, immunocompromised hosts (e.g., patients on cancer chemotherapy or steroid treatment), and in those with poor esophageal emptying (e.g., patients with achalasia or severe stricture). Major symptoms include odynophagia, and diagnosis is made by endoscopy and cytology. Treatment is with nystatin, ketoconazole, or, in resistant cases, with low doses of amphotericin B.

      (2) Herpes simplex virus (HSV). Esophagitis due to HSV also occurs in immunocompromised hosts and produces isolated ulcers. Biopsy of the ulcerating edges may show characteristic nuclear inclusions. Treatment may depend on individual symptoms, but vidarabine or acyclovir can be tried.

    c. Esophageal burns. Ingestion of caustic agents (i.e., strong alkali or acid) can cause serious esophageal burns. Ingestion of lye or detergents such as chlorine bleach is a common suicidal gesture in adults and a common accident in children. Emergency endoscopy should be performed to assess the extent of damage. Steroids and broad-spectrum antibiotics are recommended initially in management of esophageal burns. Long-term sequelae in survivors may include an esophageal stricture and esophageal carcinoma.

    d. Esophageal tears are seen most commonly after vomiting (75% of cases), straining, and coughing. A mucosal tear (Mallory-Weiss syndrome) produces a significant hematemesis after an initial nonbloody vomitus. Surgery is required in less than 10% of these cases. A rupture of the esophagus (Boerhaave's syndrome) usually occurs above the esophagogastric junction. Air in the left mediastinal region suggests the diagnosis, and immediate surgical intervention is necessary for any chance of survival.

II. DISEASES OF THE STOMACH

A. Gastritis

  1. Acute gastritis is an inflammation of the gastric mucosa, which may be diffuse or localized and usually is self-limited.

a. **Etiology**
   (1) **Drugs** that can damage the mucosal barrier and lead to back-diffusion of acid and pepsin include:
      (a) Aspirin and similar nonsteroidal anti-inflammatory agents
      (b) Alcohol, which may produce an additive effect with aspirin
   (2) **Caustic substances.** Accidental ingestion of strong alkali (e.g., lye), strong acid [e.g., sulfuric acid (H_2SO_4) and HCl], or fixatives [e.g., formaldehyde and trinitrophenol (picric acid)] can be fatal. Patients who survive the ingestion of such corrosives sustain injuries that leave considerable scars with subsequent antral narrowing.
   (3) **Stress** related to severe illness, especially illness involving many organ systems, causes acute gastritis. Ischemia and gastric acid, even at normal levels, may be involved. Antacids, H_2-receptor antagonists, and cytoprotective agents such as sucralfate and prostaglandins may be effective as prophylactic or therapeutic agents in cases of stress-induced gastritis.
   (4) **Infections. Phlegmonous gastritis** (bacterial invasion of the stomach wall) is a rare but fatal condition most commonly caused by streptococci; however, it also has been traced to staphylococci, *Escherichia coli*, and *Proteus* species.
b. **Clinical features**, which are absent in about 30% of patients, include:
   (1) Epigastric burning and pain, nausea, and vomiting
   (2) Gastrointestinal bleeding, which may be severe and associated with hematemesis and shock
c. **Diagnosis** is made on the basis of endoscopic visualization with or without biopsy in most cases. Congestion, friability, superficial ulceration, and petechiae frequently are noted in the gastric mucosa.
d. **Therapy** should begin with removal of offending agents. Antacids, H_2-receptor antagonists, and surface-acting agents (e.g., sucralfate) also are useful. Patients with acute hemorrhagic gastritis usually respond to fluid or blood replacement combined with a regimen of antacids or H_2-receptor antagonists, which keep the gastric pH above 3.5. Surgery rarely is necessary for these patients and is associated with high morbidity and mortality rates.

2. **Chronic gastritis** is characterized by a superficial lymphocyte infiltrate in the lamina propria.
   a. **Etiology.** Chronic gastritis can be caused by:
      (1) Prolonged use of alcohol, aspirin, and other irritating drugs
      (2) Radiation or thermal injury
      (3) Immunologic factors
   b. **Types**
      (1) **Chronic type A gastritis** involves the fundus and body of the stomach, with sparing of the antrum. This type of gastritis is associated with parietal cell antibodies, high serum gastrin levels, and pernicious anemia.
      (2) **Chronic type B gastritis** involves the antrum of the stomach, with relative sparing of the body and fundus. Recently, gastrin cell antibodies have been detected in some patients with this gastritis. More commonly, reflux of duodenal or biliary secretions is linked etiologically to type B gastritis.
   c. **Clinical features** may be few in patients with chronic gastritis. Type A gastritis is associated with hypo- or achlorhydria, whereas type B gastritis is associated with normal acid levels. Hypothyroidism, diabetes mellitus, and vitiligo occur more frequently with type A than with type B gastritis.
   d. **Clinical course.** Data suggest that these lesions may remain unchanged for several years. Approximately 50% of patients with superficial gastritis develop gastric atrophy over a 10- to 20-year period. An increased association with gastric polyps, gastric ulcer, and gastric cancer has been seen in both types of chronic gastritis, with type B showing a higher incidence of gastric cancer than type A.
   e. **Therapy** usually is unnecessary. However, conditions associated with gastritis (e.g., pernicious anemia, hypothyroidism, and diabetes) should be treated accordingly. Some authors suggest yearly gastric cytologic analysis as a means of diagnosing an early cancer in these patients.

3. **Special types of gastritis**
   a. **Eosinophilic gastroenteritis** refers to the infiltration of eosinophils into the gastric antrum, small bowel, or both. This infiltration, which is believed to be immunologically mediated, causes thickening of the intestinal wall with subsequent antral obstruction. Peripheral eosinophilia may occur. Differentiation from other infiltrative diseases (e.g., tuberculosis, sarcoidosis, syphilis, histoplasmosis, Crohn's disease, and carcinoma) may be difficult and depends on endoscopic biopsy. Corticosteroid therapy has been successful in providing a prolonged remission.
   b. **Hypertrophic gastritis** is an uncommon condition associated with massive enlargement of

the gastric folds. On biopsy, gastric mucous cells are hyperplastic, and inflammatory cells are present in some patients.

(1) **Clinical features.** In its most extreme form (i.e., Ménétrier's disease), there is hyposecretion of gastric acid, protein loss from the stomach, peripheral edema, weight loss, and abdominal pain.

(2) **Diagnosis** is made by endoscopy and biopsy, often with a suction apparatus. Lymphoma, amyloid infiltration, carcinoma, and Zollinger-Ellison syndrome also can cause large rugal folds and should be excluded. A type of hypersecretory hypertrophic gastritis is similar to Ménétrier's disease but is associated with high acid output and hyperplasia of parietal gastric cells.

(3) **Therapy** includes anticholinergic agents, which appear to close the tight junctions between cells and decrease protein loss, H_2-receptor antagonists, and steroids. Surgery (gastric resection) is reserved for intractable cases.

B. Gastric neoplasms

1. Gastric carcinoma

a. Incidence. The most common cancer in the United States 60 years ago, gastric carcinoma continues to decline in incidence in this country. The incidence of gastric cancer remains high, however, in Japan and eastern Europe and appears to be inversely related to the incidence of carcinoma of the colon. Gastric carcinoma is twice as common in men as it is in women and usually occurs in patients who are 50–75 years of age. The incidence is highest among individuals of low socioeconomic classes.

b. Pathogenesis. Although the cause of gastric carcinoma is unknown, certain relationships have been noted. A 20% higher incidence of gastric cancer among family members as well as a higher incidence among individuals with blood group A suggest a genetic component. Vitamin C deficiency, food preservatives, and nitrosamines also are thought to play etiologic roles. Premalignant conditions include:

(1) Pernicious anemia

(2) Atrophic gastritis

(3) Postgastrectomy, especially 10–20 years after Billroth II resection

(4) Gastric polyps, which have about a 40% incidence of malignancy if they are adenomatous and larger than 2 cm in diameter*

(5) Immunodeficiency disorders, especially common variable immunodeficiency[†]

c. Clinical features

(1) **Weight loss** and **anorexia** are noted in about 70%–80% of patients.

(2) **Epigastric pain** is described by about 70% of patients.

(3) Several other symptoms may be noted, including early satiety, vomiting, and weakness and fatigue secondary to chronic blood loss and anemia.

(a) Early satiety is particularly common in patients with **linitis plastica**, because the gastric wall does not distend normally.

(b) Vomiting often is a result of pyloric obstruction by the tumor mass but also can result from impaired gastric motility.

(c) Gross gastrointestinal bleeding is rare in gastric carcinomas, occurring in less than 10% of patients. Dysphagia can occur if the lesion is near the esophagogastric junction.

(d) A palpable, left supraclavicular (Virchow's) node may indicate metastatic disease.

d. Diagnosis may be established by the following procedures.

(1) **Upper gastrointestinal series** can reveal a mass, ulcer, or thickened "leather bottle" stomach (**linitis plastica**). The simultaneous use of air contrast techniques enhances the diagnostic accuracy of x-ray.

(2) **Endoscopy** with biopsy and brush cytology has a 95%–99% accuracy in diagnosing gastric cancer.

(3) **Increased serum carcinoembryonic antigen (CEA)** levels as well as elevated 2-glucuronidase levels in gastric secretions may be seen in gastric carcinoma patients. Achlorhydria in response to maximum stimulation and in the presence of a gastric ulcer almost always indicates malignant ulceration.

e. Therapy

(1) **Surgery** is the treatment of choice but is associated with a 5-year survival rate of only about 12%. If the disease is superficial, as it often is in Japan, the survival rate may be as high as 70%. Cancer in a gastric ulcer has a slightly better prognosis, with approximately a 30% 5-year survival rate.

---

*Most gastric polyps are hyperplastic and not thought to be premalignant.

[†]In one series, 33% of such patients developed gastric cancer.

(2) **Chemotherapy** has been noted to have a 25%–40% response rate, but little improvement in survival rate is described at this time.

2. **Gastric lymphoma** usually presents as a bulky mass associated with large, thickened gastric folds. Pain is the most common presenting symptom. Histologic examination usually shows diffuse histiocytic non-Hodgkin's lymphoma, but non-Hodgkin's lymphomas of all types are more common than Hodgkin's disease in the stomach. Gastric lymphoma should be differentiated from Ménétrier's disease, Zollinger-Ellison syndrome, and hypertrophic gastritis. Diagnosis is confirmed by biopsy, either at endoscopy with a suction apparatus or at surgery. Surgery and localized radiotherapy are the generally accepted forms of therapy, with 5-year survival rates approaching 50% in non-Hodgkin's lymphoma patients whose lymphoma is confined to the stomach. Chemotherapy is valuable in patients with systemic disease.

3. **Other gastric tumors**
   a. **Leiomyosarcomas**, which account for about 1% of all gastric malignancies, are similar to gastric lymphomas in treatment procedures and 5-year survival rates.
   b. **Rare gastric malignancies** such as fibrosarcomas, neurogenic sarcomas, and metastatic carcinomas (especially from breast and lung carcinomas and melanoma) must be differentiated from primary gastric carcinoma.
   c. **Benign leiomyomas** usually are less than 4 cm in diameter and occur in the distal antrum. A central ulceration occasionally occurs and may necessitate excision for recurrent upper gastrointestinal bleeding.

C. **Disorders of gastric emptying**

1. **Pyloric stenosis**
   a. **Acquired pyloric stenosis** occurs transiently due to edema from peptic ulcer disease or chronically due to pyloric scarring from recurrent ulcer disease or neoplasm.
   b. **Congenital pyloric stenosis** usually presents in infancy.
      (1) **Incidence.** Congenital pyloric stenosis occurs in about 2–4 of 1000 births and usually is seen in firstborn male children. A familial incidence is noted.
      (2) **Clinical features** include postprandial projectile vomiting of nonbilious material, dehydration, and weight loss. Visible peristalsis may be noted, with a mass palpated in the epigastrium.
      (3) **Diagnosis** is based on radiographic demonstration. A plain film reveals air in the stomach, and a barium swallow confirms the diagnosis.
      (4) **Therapy** is by surgery (Ramstedt operation) and consists of a myotomy of the circular muscle of the pylorus.

2. **Gastric bezoars.** Collections of nondigestible substances sometimes form, which cannot pass through the pylorus. **Trichobezoars** are composed of hair, and **phytobezoars** are composed of plant fibers. Bezoars generally are seen in patients who have undergone previous gastric surgery or in mentally retarded individuals who consume nondigestible substances. The symptoms include those of gastric-outlet obstruction and bleeding from superficial ulcerations. It is important to exclude a gastric mass or cancer, and the diagnosis can be established endoscopically. Bezoars sometimes can be enzymatically dissolved with papain, acetylcysteine, or cellulase; otherwise, surgical removal is necessary.

3. **Gastric diverticula** occur on the posterior wall of the stomach in about 75% of cases and usually are within 2 cm of the esophagogastric junction. Unless they bleed or perforate, these congenital lesions are asymptomatic. **Pseudodiverticula**, seen most commonly in the antrum, are scarred remnants of previous peptic disease.

4. **Gastric volvulus** may occur due to weak ligamentous attachments or may be secondary to a paraesophageal hernia, an intrinsic gastric lesion, or an adjacent mass. Diagnosis is supported by the finding of two separate fluid levels in the left upper quadrant and by a lack of barium passage into the pylorous. Therapy consists of temporary nasogastric suction. Recurrent or acute volvulus with gastric vascular compromise may require surgery.

5. **Gastroparesis.** This disorder of gastric emptying is not due to an obstruction, and the diagnosis should not be made until mechanical obstruction has been ruled out by an upper gastrointestinal series or by endoscopy. Gastroparesis most frequently is caused by insulin-dependent diabetes mellitus of longer than 10 years' duration. However, other conditions associated with gastroparesis include systemic sclerosis , postvagotomy states, and therapy with anticholinergic agents. In diabetes, loss of gastric phase III activity is noted on electric recordings, with other signs of diabetic visceral neuropathy often seen. Treatment with metoclopramide has been effective.

III. PEPTIC ULCER DISEASE

A. Introduction. Peptic ulcer disease refers to a group of disorders of the gastrointestinal tract, which are similar in that they all involve areas of discrete tissue destruction caused by acid and pepsin. Peptic ulcers occur most commonly in the stomach or proximal duodenum, less frequently in the distal esophagus, and rarely in the small intestine.* In general, the clinical features and treatment of peptic ulcer disease are similar regardless of location, although peptic esophagitis caused by reflux of gastric contents has some unique features (see section I B 1). The Zollinger-Ellison syndrome, which is considered a form of peptic ulcer disease, is discussed in detail in section III I.

B. Incidence. Peptic ulcer disease occurs more commonly in men than in women. Duodenal ulcers are three times more common than gastric ulcers and occur about 10 years earlier; the peak of incidence for duodenal ulcers is at about 40 years of age as opposed to 50 years of age for gastric ulcers. The relapse rate at 1 year is about 80% for patients with a duodenal ulcer; patients with a gastric ulcer have a 33% chance of developing a subsequent duodenal ulcer.

C. Pathogenesis. Acid and pepsin are necessary for an ulcer to develop. However, several factors are thought to contribute to the pathogenesis.

1. Social factors
   a. Tobacco smoking increases the risk of developing peptic ulcer disease. Smoking also increases the morbidity and mortality and decreases the healing rate for peptic ulcers. The mechanism may be a decrease in pancreatic bicarbonate secretion and, therefore, a lowered alkaline level in the duodenum, an increase in gastric emptying with a lowered duodenal pH, an increase in serum **pepsinogen I** secretion, or a decrease in pyloric sphincter pressure with an increased reflux into the stomach.
   b. Drugs. Ulcers develop in about 30% of arthritis patients who take high doses of aspirin. Other nonsteroidal anti-inflammatory drugs have been incriminated, with an antiprostaglandin effect suggested as an underlying factor in this group of drugs. Steroids also are thought to break the mucosal barrier and may double the risk of peptic ulcer disease.
   c. Alcohol also compromises the mucosal barrier and increases gastric acid secretion.

2. Physiologic factors
   a. Gastric acid, while essential for ulcer production, generally is measured at normal or decreased levels in gastric ulcer patients and at slightly elevated levels in the basal and stimulated states in duodenal ulcer patients. Many investigators attribute this to an increase in the back-diffusion of hydrogen ion (H^+) into the mucosa and submucosa.
   b. Serum gastrin. In duodenal ulcer patients, serum gastrin levels are normal during fasting and increased in the postprandial state. In gastric ulcer patients, both fasting and postprandial levels of serum gastrin are higher than normal.

3. Genetic factors
   a. First-degree relatives of gastric ulcer patients have three times the risk of developing gastric ulcers when compared to the general population. Similarly, the risk of duodenal ulcer is increased in the first-degree relatives of duodenal ulcer patients.
   b. An increased incidence of duodenal ulcer also has been documented among individuals with **blood group O**, individuals who demonstrate elevated serum pepsinogen I, and those who are nonsecretors of blood group substances.

4. Associated diseases
   a. Some patients with **multiple endocrine adenomatosis, type I (MEA I)** present with gastrin-secreting tumors. This probably accounts for the reported association of duodenal ulcer disease with hyperparathyroidism.
   b. Antral **atrophic gastritis** may be caused by back-diffusion of bile through the pylorus and is associated with a high incidence of gastric ulcers.
   c. Patients with **rheumatoid arthritis** have an increased risk of ulcer disease, which probably is secondary to the drugs used for treatment.
   d. Chronic obstructive pulmonary disease has been found in a significant number of gastric ulcer patients; **cirrhosis of the liver** and **chronic renal failure** are demonstrated in a significant number of duodenal ulcer patients.

5. Psychosomatic factors again are the focus of increasing attention and include chronic anxiety and personality type.

---

*Peptic ulcers in the distal small intestine usually are associated with a **Meckel's diverticulum** that contains gastric mucosa.

D. Clinical features

1. **Pain** is the predominant symptom, although it may be absent in 25% of gastric ulcer patients. The pain characteristically is described as an epigastric burning sensation and may be accompanied by bloating or nausea. Eating may exacerbate the pain in gastric ulcer patients, whereas in duodenal ulcer patients the pain usually is diminished by eating, only to recur 2–3 hours later. Pain may awaken patients from sleep, especially those with duodenal ulcers.

2. Upper gastrointestinal **hemorrhage** may be the presenting sign of peptic ulcer disease, and **anemia** from chronic blood loss also may be seen.

3. Less common symptoms include:
   a. Repeated vomiting, which may indicate gastric-outlet obstruction
   b. Weight loss, which is somewhat more common with gastric ulcer

E. Diagnosis. Since the patient may complain of only vague symptoms, a high index of suspicion is needed.

1. **Radiography** is a useful screening tool. However, an upper gastrointestinal series may miss up to 30% of gastric ulcers, and scarring of the duodenal bulb from chronic or recurrent ulcer disease may make x-ray interpretation difficult. Double contrast techniques may improve diagnostic accuracy. Duodenal ulcers always are benign; however, gastric ulcers may be benign or malignant. Radiographic criteria for benign gastric ulcers include:
   a. Ulcer crater extending beyond the gastric wall
   b. Gastric folds radiating into the base of the ulcer
   c. Thick radiolucent collar of edema (Hampton's line) surrounding the ulcer base
   d. Smooth, regular, round or ovoid ulcer crater
   e. Pliable and normally distensible gastric wall in the area of the ulcer

2. **Endoscopy** may be used as the primary diagnostic maneuver or to confirm a radiographic diagnosis. Since 5% of gastric ulcers that occur in the United States are malignant, many authors advise using endoscopy with multiple biopsies at the margin of the ulcer and simultaneous cytologic brushings for the evaluation of all gastric ulcers.

3. **Gastric acid analysis** may be helpful in individual cases to distinguish benign from malignant gastric ulcers. Since benign ulcers rarely exist in the setting of achlorhydria, the absence of acid should prompt further work-up with gastric biopsies and cytologies. Although gastric ulcers in the presence of achlorhydria nearly always are malignant, most malignant ulcers are found in stomachs with normal acid secretion.

F. Therapy is virtually the same for esophageal, gastric, and duodenal ulcers.

1. **Intensive antacids** have been shown to promote the healing of gastric and duodenal ulcers. The healing rates, which are about 70%–80% at 4 weeks, appear equal to those of the H_2-receptor antagonists and are considerably better than the healing rates with placebo (45%). The timing of antacids is important, and dosage varies according to the neutralizing capacity of the specific antacid. Calcium-containing antacids are no longer recommended as they produce an **acid rebound** due to calcium-stimulated gastrin release. Magnesium may accumulate to toxic levels in renal failure patients taking magnesium-containing antacids. In all patients, the most common side effect of these medications is diarrhea, which can be avoided by placing patients on alternating doses of magnesium- and aluminum-containing antacids.

2. **H_2-receptor antagonists** are the mainstay of treatment because of patient convenience, sustained acid reduction, and increased healing rates with diminished relapse rates.
   a. In a study performed over 1 year, a 400-mg dose of **cimetidine** decreased relapse rates in duodenal ulcers to 20% as compared to a placebo relapse rate of about 80%. Side effects occur in 15%–20% of patients treated with cimetidine and include central nervous system (CNS) effects such as confusion and tremor. Antiandrogenic effects (e.g., gynecomastia and decreased sperm count) also have been reported. Because it is excreted by the kidneys, cimetidine should be given in a reduced dosage to patients with renal failure to minimize side effects. Cimetidine prolongs clearance of such drugs as warfarin, diazepam, and phenobarbital due to its effect on the cytochrome P-450 system.
   b. **Ranitidine**, which is thought to have fewer side effects than cimetidine, is four to five times more potent. It has less effect on the cytochrome P-450 system, and, therefore, drug interactions are fewer. The incidence of CNS effects and gynecomastia also may be lower with ranitidine than with cimetidine.

3. **Anticholinergic agents** have a limited therapeutic role as they decrease meal-stimulated acid secretion by only about 30%. These agents may be used to delay gastric emptying of antacids,

especially at night. More selective anticholinergic agents such as pirenzepine may be more useful.

4. Diet. There is no proof that bland diets promote healing in peptic ulcer disease. In fact, milk may be harmful as it increases acid secretion, probably by calcium- and protein-stimulated gastrin release. Caffeine and alcohol stimulate gastric acid secretion and, therefore, should be restricted in acute cases. Decaffinated coffee also may stimulate acid release. Ulcer patients who smoke should be urged to decrease or stop smoking.

5. Other therapeutic agents

    a. Sucralfate is a nonsystemic agent, which, in the presence of an acid pH, coats the ulcer bed and promotes healing. Sucralfate is as effective as H_2-receptor antagonists and antacids and has no significant side effects, making this drug an attractive form of therapy.

    b. Carbenoxolone has been proven to be useful but slightly less effective than H_2-receptor antagonists in healing peptic ulcers. This derivative of the licorice root decreases gastric permeability to H^+, decreases the peptic activity of gastric juice, and increases the life span of gastric epithelial cells with a thickening of the gastric mucosa. The major drawback of carbenoxolone is its aldosterone-like effect of sodium (Na^+) and water retention.

    c. Bismuth has both ulcer-insulating and pepsin-inactivating properties but does not decrease gastric acid production. Healing rates are slightly better in gastric than in duodenal ulcer patients, and the overall rate of adverse reaction is low. Milk and antacids may interfere with its action and should be avoided for 1 hour before and after ingestion of bismuth.

    d. Prostaglandin E_2 (PGE$_2$) and PGF$_{2\alpha}$ have a cytoprotective effect on gastric mucosa. These agents also increase gastric blood flow and decrease gastrin-stimulated acid secretion. A PGE_2 analog has been shown to be effective in treating peptic ulcer disease, but this drug is still under investigation. The major side effects of prostaglandins are diarrhea and nausea.

    e. Tricyclic antidepressants (e.g., doxepin) have been proven effective, probably because of their H_2-receptor antagonist effects.

6. Gastric irradiation decreases acid production for about 1 year and may have a role in treating recurrent disease in elderly patients who cannot tolerate drugs or surgery.

7. Surgery is effective therapy for peptic ulcer disease and reduces recurrence rates to a very low percentage. The most commonly performed operation is distal subtotal gastrectomy, with wedge resection of a gastric ulcer if one is present. **Vagotomy with drainage (V + D)** and **vagotomy with antrectomy (V + A)** are the usual procedures for complicated peptic ulcer disease. V + D has a higher recurrence rate (about 7%–15% as compared to 3% with V + A) but is associated with less postoperative weight loss than is V + A. A proximal selective vagotomy appears to lessen postoperative complications. However, the high incidence of postoperative complications, regardless of the type of procedure, has limited the role of surgery to treatment of complications (including acute emergencies) and intractable cases.

G. Complications of peptic ulcer disease, as noted above, may be indications for surgery.

1. Hemorrhage occurs in 20% of patients and is the most serious complication, having a 10% mortality rate. If blood requirements exceed 3 units/24 hr for longer than 48–72 hours or if **in-hospital** rebleeding occurs, surgical intervention is indicated. Repeated bleeding episodes occur in about 30%–40% of cases and may require surgery.

2. Perforation occurs in about 5%–10% of all peptic ulcers and is far more common with duodenal ulcers than with gastric ulcers. Of ulcers that perforate, 10% bleed simultaneously. Symptoms and signs include intense pain, a rigid abdomen, decreased bowel sounds, and direct or rebound tenderness. This catastrophic complication is confirmed in about 75%–85% of cases by an erect abdominal x-ray showing free air under the diaphragm. Most cases require immediate surgical intervention, but selected patients have been treated successfully with nasogastric suction and antibiotics.

3. Gastric-outlet obstruction occurs in about 5%–10% of ulcer patients. Of these, 80% of the cases are due to recurrent duodenal ulcer disease, with prepyloric or pyloric channel ulcers less common causes. Early satiety, epigastric fullness, nausea, and vomiting of undigested food (frequently ingested several hours earlier) suggest the diagnosis. Weight loss is common. Physical examination may reveal a succussion splash. The diagnosis is confirmed by aspiration of greater than 300 ml of gastric contents more than 3 hours after a meal or by a positive saline load test. Treatment consists of nasogastric aspiration for at least 72 hours, with close attention to replacement of H^+, Na^+, chloride ion (Cl^-), and potassium ion (K^+). About 25%–40% of patients require surgery since 20%–40% of medically treated patients have recurrent obstruction.

4. Penetration into an adjacent organ usually is a complication of posterior duodenal ulcers, with penetration into the pancreas. Pain usually is sudden in onset and radiates to the back. Serum amylase and lipase levels frequently are elevated. Treatment is with surgery.

H. Postsurgical complications

1. Stomal ulceration after surgery may indicate an unrecognized hypersecretory state (e.g., Zollinger-Ellison syndrome, retained gastric antrum, or incomplete vagotomy). The diagnosis of a stomal ulcer is best made by endoscopy. Treatment is with long-term H_2-receptor antagonists, and repeat surgery may be necessary.

2. Afferent loop obstruction is a rare complication. The patient usually complains of bloating and vomiting of a clear or bilious material about 30–60 minutes after eating. The diagnosis is suggested by the failure of orally ingested barium to enter the loop or by the retention inside the loop of technetium-iminodiacetic acid (tech-HIDA), which is cleared by the liver and biliary system after intravenous injection but does not enter the gastrointestinal tract. Bacterial overgrowth can occur, and surgical revision of the afferent loop may be necessary.

3. Gastritis often is noted endoscopically in patients who have undergone antrectomy or subtotal gastrectomy. Gastritis often is asymptomatic but may cause nausea, vomiting, weight loss, and epigastric pain. Since the gastritis is secondary to constant reflux of duodenal secretions into the stomach, patients may require surgery (a Roux-en-Y anastomosis) to divert these secretions further down the gastrointestinal tract. Some patients may be treated effectively with substances that bind bile acids (e.g., aluminum-containing antacids and cholestyramine) or with sucralfate.

4. Dumping syndrome is a nonspecific term that refers to a variety of postprandial symptoms.
   a. Early dumping syndrome occurs about 30 minutes after a meal and is associated with dizziness, flushing, diaphoresis, and palpitations. These symptoms have been ascribed to osmotic shifts of fluid or release of massive amounts of intestinal hormones as food empties rapidly from the stomach. The early dumping syndrome can be minimized by decreasing the carbohydrate content of meals and by avoiding liquids with meals.
   b. Late dumping syndrome occurs several hours after a meal and is characterized by dizziness, weakness, and drowsiness. This syndrome may be due to reactive hypoglycemia.

5. Nutritional problems
   a. Anemia occurs in approximately 25% of patients after surgery for peptic ulcer disease. Factors that may contribute to iron deficiency include low-grade blood loss from **alkaline pouch gastritis**, diversion of iron away from its preferential absorption site (i.e., the duodenum), and lack of gastric acid needed for conversion of iron to the preferred form for absorption (i.e., Fe^{3+}). A lack of intrinsic factor leads to vitamin B_{12} deficiency in patients who have undergone a substantial gastric resection.
   b. Weight loss occurs in about 50% of postoperative patients but is not severe unless a large gastric resection has been performed. Significant steatorrhea usually indicates a secondary problem (e.g., bacterial overgrowth and unmasked celiac disease), although 50% of patients have an increase in stool fat secondary to rapid transit and poor mixing of food with bile salts and pancreatic enzymes.
   c. Bone thinning may be due to decreased absorption of vitamin D and calcium.

6. Gastric pouch cancer rates have been noted to be two to four times greater in surgically treated ulcer patients than in medically treated patients, especially 10–20 years after Billroth II gastric resection.

I. Zollinger-Ellison syndrome refers to a nonbeta islet cell tumor that produces gastrin and is associated with gastric acid hypersecretion and peptic ulcer disease. The tumors are biologically malignant in 60% of cases and most commonly involve the pancreas. Other tumor sites include the stomach, duodenum, spleen, and lymph nodes. Tumor size varies from 2 mm to 20 cm. About 10% of the patients with Zollinger-Ellison syndrome have a resectable lesion.

1. Clinical features
   a. Pain from peptic ulcer disease is common in Zollinger-Ellison syndrome. In about 75% of cases the ulcers are located in the duodenal bulb. The remaining number of cases involve ulcers that are noted in the distal duodenum or jejunum or are multiple.
   b. Diarrhea is noted in about 50% of cases due to gastric acid hypersecretion. The high acid levels may damage the small intestinal mucosa, inactivate pancreatic lipase, and precipitate bile acids, causing steatorrhea. The high gastrin levels cause incomplete Na^+ and water absorption and increase intestinal motility. In addition, the volume of gastric secretion alone may cause diarrhea.

c. **Endocrine abnormalities.** Zollinger-Ellison syndrome commonly is associated with other endocrinopathies. About 20% of these patients have hyperparathyroidism. Pituitary, adrenal, ovarian, and thyroid tumors also have been reported with Zollinger-Ellison syndrome. A distinct syndrome of pancreatic, pituitary, and parathyroid tumors (i.e., MEA I) shows an autosomal dominant pattern of inheritance.

2. **Diagnosis** is made on the basis of the following findings.
   a. These patients demonstrate elevated gastrin levels in the basal state, which do not increase 1 hour after a meal. Gastrin levels rise by 200 units rather than fall after intravenous secretin administration, and there is an exaggerated response to intravenous calcium administration, which normally causes only a modest rise in gastrin levels.
   b. Patients with Zollinger-Ellison syndrome often have basal gastric acid output rates of more than 10 mEq/hr and basal-to-peak output ratios of greater than 0.6.

3. **Therapy** traditionally has been total gastrectomy. The 10-year survival rate of 50% with this procedure is thought to be due mainly to the slow-growing nature of this lesion since most of the late deaths are due to metastatic disease. Recently, H_2-receptor antagonists combined with anticholinergic agents have been used, especially in conjunction with a V + D procedure. Patients who have been unresponsive to H_2-receptor blockade may become responsive as a result of surgery. A newly described technique of tumor localization involves sampling gastrin levels through cannulation of multiple pancreatic and abdominal veins. This technique offers the hope of surgical cure in cases of multiple primaries and in cases involving a tumor that is too small to be visualized by ordinary means.

IV. DISEASES OF THE SMALL INTESTINE

A. **Intestinal obstruction** is a term used to denote failure of passage of intestinal contents and may be due to **mechanical obstruction** or **adynamic ileus**.

1. **Mechanical obstruction**
   a. **Etiology**
      (1) **Extrinsic causes** include:
         (a) Adhesions from prior surgery
         (b) Incarcerated hernia
         (c) Metastatic tumors
         (d) Volvulus
         (e) Endometriosis
      (2) **Intramural causes** include:
         (a) Hematomas from trauma
         (b) Strictures
         (c) Intramural tumors
      (3) **Intraluminal causes** include:
         (a) Epithelial tumors (especially colonic)
         (b) Intussusception
         (c) Foreign bodies
   b. **Clinical features** include:
      (1) Crampy pain that waxes and wanes in intensity
      (2) High-pitched bowel sounds with rushes and tinkles
      (3) Constipation and obstipation
      (4) Vomiting, which is more prominent in proximal intestinal obstruction
      (5) Distension, which is more prominent in distal intestinal obstruction
      (6) Intestinal ischemia leading first to edema, then to petechial hemorrhages, and finally to necrosis and gangrene*
   c. **Diagnosis** usually is made with plain and upright abdominal x-rays. Characteristic air-fluid levels exist above the area of obstruction, and no air is seen in the rectum. A barium enema may be useful in colonic obstruction. Reflux of barium into the small bowel also may be helpful in the diagnosis of low, small bowel obstructions.
   d. **Therapy** includes:
      (1) Replacement of fluid and electrolytes
      (2) Intestinal decompression with nasogastric suction or small bowel intubation
      (3) Surgery, which usually is required for definitive treatment of the underlying problem

2. **Adynamic** or **paralytic ileus** is a nonobstructive lack of propulsion through the intestinal tract.

---

*This is secondary to increased intraluminal pressure occurring after 6–12 hours of obstruction, when absorption ceases and secretion commences.

    a. Etiology. Adynamic ileus commonly is linked to the following conditions:

        (1) Recent abdominal surgery, which results in ileus that usually is transient (lasting 2–3 days)

        (2) Electrolyte imbalance, especially hypokalemia

        (3) Chemical or bacterial peritonitis

        (4) Severe intra-abdominal inflammation, such as pancreatitis and cholecystitis

        (5) Systemic illness, such as pneumonia

    b. Clinical features. Physical examination shows a distended abdomen with diminished bowel sounds.

    c. Diagnosis. X-ray shows diffuse intestinal gas and air in the rectum.

    d. Therapy includes:

        (1) Bowel rest with a nasogastric tube

        (2) Correction of underlying causes

B. Intestinal pseudo-obstruction is a rare but important entity characterized by what appear to be recurrent episodes of mechanical obstruction but with no demonstrable source of obstruction.

  1. Classification. Pseudo-obstruction can exist with or without an underlying condition.

    a. Pseudo-obstruction occurs secondary to many conditions that affect either the smooth muscle of the gastrointestinal tract or the neurologic and hormonal control of intestinal motility.

        (1) Underlying diseases that involve the smooth muscle include collagen vascular disease (especially scleroderma), amyloidosis, and myotonic dystrophy.

        (2) Underlying neurologic diseases include Chagas' disease, Parkinson's disease, and Hirschsprung's disease.

        (3) Underlying endocrine disorders include hypothyroidism, diabetes mellitus, hypoparathyroidism, and pheochromocytoma.

        (4) Drugs that depress intestinal smooth muscle function include phenothiazines, tricyclic antidepressants, ganglionic blockers, and clonidine.

        (5) Nontropical sprue and ceroid deposits in the bowel are very rare causes of pseudo-obstruction.

    b. Primary pseudo-obstruction occurs in two forms.

        (1) Hereditary **hollow visceral myopathy** is a vacuolization and atrophy of intestinal smooth muscle. This disorder, which is transmitted as an autosomal dominant trait, also affects esophageal and urinary smooth muscle.

        (2) An **autonomic nervous system abnormality** has been described in some families with primary pseudo-obstruction. There may be a decrease in total myenteric plexus neurons or neuronal eosinophilic intranuclear inclusions. Possible symptoms include orthostatic hypotension, ataxic gait, dysarthria, and absent deep tendon reflexes.

  2. Diagnosis is made by rigorously excluding causes of mechanical obstruction while documenting abnormal motility.

    a. Esophageal manometry showing normal or low LES pressure with decreased amplitude of peristalsis distally indicates the smooth muscle vacuolization type of pseudo-obstruction. Incomplete relaxation of the LES with absent peristalsis and repetitive esophageal contractions may indicate an autonomic nervous system abnormality.

    b. Radionuclide gastric emptying scans may show delayed emptying.

    c. Findings on barium studies are nonspecific. Most patients show dilated areas of the intestine.

  3. Therapy is supportive during acute exacerbations. Cholinergic agents and metoclopramide have been used with limited success, and surgery should be avoided. Home parenteral hyperalimentation may be required for nutritional support. Intestinal stasis with bacterial overgrowth may be treated with antibiotics.

C. Small bowel diverticula

  1. Duodenal diverticula usually are found incidentally during an upper gastrointestinal series, at endoscopy, or at autopsy. They occur most frequently in the proximal duodenum, within 1–2 cm of the papilla of Vater, and are asymptomatic in most patients, although duodenal diverticula may rarely cause upper gastrointestinal bleeding. In some cases the common bile duct empties directly into the diverticulum, and common bile duct obstruction may occur due to anatomic interference with emptying.

  2. Jejunal diverticula probably are acquired rather than congenital and usually are asymptomatic. Jejunal diverticula may lead to malabsorption secondary to bile salt deconjugation when stasis is sufficient to allow an increase in small bowel bacteria. This leads to diarrhea, steatorrhea, weight loss, and anemia. Hypo- or achlorhydria also may be present. Continuous or alternating antimicrobial therapy often corrects malabsorption, although surgical removal of multiple diverticula or of a single large diverticulum may be necessary in refractory cases.

3. Meckel's diverticulum is a common congenital structural defect in the intestine, which represents the remnant of the vitelline duct. It is found in about 2% of autopsies and usually is noted in the terminal ileum within 60 cm of the ileocecal valve. Meckel's diverticula average 5–7 cm in length and may be quite large. About one-third of Meckel's diverticula contain gastric mucosa, which may produce acid. Diverticulitis, ulceration, bleeding, perforation, and obstruction are complications requiring surgical intervention and frequently mimicking the symptoms of acute appendicitis. Because of the presence of gastric mucosa, the diagnosis sometimes can be made by means of pertechnetate scanning.

D. Diarrhea is defined as an increase in **stool frequency** and **volume**. The stool usually is liquid, and 24-hour output exceeds 250 g. The patient may experience lower abdominal crampy pain and fecal urgency.

1. Classification. Pathophysiologic criteria are used to classify diarrhea as one of three distinct types.

a. Secretory diarrhea

(1) Pathophysiology. Secretory diarrhea occurs when the secretion of fluid and electrolytes is increased or when the normal absorptive capacity of the bowel is decreased. In some cases, increased secretion is due to activation of the **adenyl cyclase–cyclic adenosine 3′,5′-monophosphate (cAMP) system** in mucosal cells.

(a) Agents that activate the adenyl cyclase–cAMP system include cholera toxin, **heat-labile** *E. coli* toxin, *Salmonella* enterotoxin, and vasoactive intestinal polypeptide (VIP).

(b) Agents that probably do not activate the adenyl cyclase–cAMP system include **heat-stable** *E. coli* toxin, a variety of other bacterial enterotoxins (e.g., those produced by *Clostridium perfringens*, *Pseudomonas aeruginosa*, and *Klebsiella pneumoniae*), castor oil, and phenolphthalein.

(c) Chronic secretory diarrhea is seen in the pancreatic cholera syndrome with VIP secretion, in medullary carcinoma of the thyroid gland with calcitonin secretion, in carcinoid syndrome with serotonin secretion, and in villous adenoma of the rectum.

(2) Diagnosis of secretory diarrhea is based on the demonstration of persistent diarrhea in the absence of food intake and by the lack of a gap between total stool osmolarity and two times the sum of stool Na^+ and K^+ concentrations.

(3) Therapy includes fluid and electrolyte support while the cause of the diarrhea is being determined. In general, diarrhea secondary to bacterial enterotoxin is self-limited. Any contributing exogenous agent (e.g., phenolphthalein and castor oil) must be withdrawn.

b. Osmotic diarrhea is caused by the presence of nonabsorbable substances in the intestine, with the secondary accumulation of fluid and electrolytes. Such nonabsorbable substances include lactose in the patient with lactase deficiency, laxatives (e.g., magnesium citrate and sodium phosphate), and foodstuffs in a patient with malabsorption. The diagnosis is suggested by the absence of diarrhea after a 48- to 72-hour fast (with concurrent intravenous fluid replacement). There is a gap between total stool osmolarity and two times the sum of stool Na^+ and K^+ concentrations.

c. Abnormal intestinal motility may cause diarrhea by several mechanisms.

(1) If small bowel peristalsis is too rapid, an abnormally large amount of fluid and partially digested foodstuffs may be delivered to the colon.

(2) Extremely slow peristalsis may allow bacterial overgrowth to occur and bile salt deconjugation to cause secondary malabsorption.

(3) Rapid colonic motility may not allow adequate time for the colon to absorb fluid delivered to the cecum. (Normally, 90% of the fluid is absorbed.)

(4) Abnormal motility causes or contributes to the diarrhea seen in diabetes, irritable bowel syndrome, postvagotomy states, carcinoid syndrome, and hyperthyroidism.

2. Diagnosis

a. Tests performed on stool samples include:

(1) Culture and sensitivity testing to detect a pathogenic bacterial strain

(2) Microscopic examination to identify ova and parasites (three samples should be sent to increase yield)

(3) Guaiac testing to detect occult blood

(4) Sudan staining to detect fat droplets

(5) Wright or methylene blue staining to detect white blood cells, which indicate invasive infectious causes of diarrhea*

b. **Proctosigmoidoscopy** also is performed, especially to exclude or confirm a diagnosis of inflammatory bowel disease.

3. **Special causes of persistent diarrhea**

  a. **Irritable bowel syndrome** is an intestinal motor disorder of unknown cause.

    (1) Pathophysiology. Studies of colonic myoelectric activity show an increased incidence of 3 cycle per minute slow-wave activity among patients with irritable bowel syndrome (i.e., 40% as compared to 10% in normal individuals). Intestinal contractions after a meal or a cholecystokinin (CCK) injection are more likely to be in the 3 cycle per minute range when compared to the intestinal contractions of normal individuals. The colonic spike activity is delayed from 40 minutes to 70–90 minutes postprandially. The abnormal slow-wave activity may indicate an intrinsic myogenic defect, and the prolonged postprandial spike and contractile activity may indicate a neural or hormonal abnormality.

    (2) Clinical features include alternating diarrhea and constipation with postprandial pain but usually no weight loss, gastrointestinal bleeding, protracted nausea, vomiting, or fever. Diarrhea, if present, generally is characterized by a 24-hour output of less than 500 ml. Neither pain nor diarrhea awakens the patient from sleep.

    (3) Diagnosis is made on the basis of excluding other gastrointestinal pathology with appropriate tests, including stool culture, guaiac testing, and x-ray. The value of colonic myoelectric testing to establish a diagnosis of irritable bowel syndrome is controversial.

    (4) Therapy includes stool bulking agents, antispasmodics, and patient reassurance.

  b. **Disaccharidase deficiency** (i.e., deficiency of the enzymes required to split nonabsorbable disaccharides into absorbable monosaccharides) is a cause of osmotic diarrhea.

    (1) Sucrase and **isomaltase** deficiencies are rare, occurring in 0.2% of the population, and usually present as watery diarrhea in infancy.

    (2) Lactase deficiency usually is not complete (i.e., patients have some enzyme activity) and presents after puberty. It is very common in blacks, affecting 60%–80%, and occurs to a lesser extent in Oriental and Mediterranean populations. Symptoms of lactase deficiency include abdominal bloating, cramping, and watery diarrhea following milk ingestion. Diagnosis can be made by measuring the rise of serum glucose in response to orally administered lactose, with a rise of 20 mg/dl expected after an oral lactose intake of 50–100 mg. Lactose breath tests measure increased H^+ excretion from colonic bacterial digestion of lactose. A relative lactase deficiency may occur after an acute episode of viral enteritis or in association with celiac disease, Whipple's disease, or cystic fibrosis.

  c. **Incontinence** is a disturbing symptom that patients may find difficult to discuss with a physician. Often not true diarrhea, incontinence is associated with inflammatory diseases of the anal canal (e.g., acute gonococcal proctitis, Crohn's disease, and ulcerative colitis) or with systemic neuromuscular diseases (e.g., diabetes mellitus and scleroderma). Incontinence also may be a complication of anal surgery (e.g., fistulectomy and hemorrhoidectomy).

  d. **Laxative abuse** is an increasing cause of diarrhea, which may be associated with psychiatric problems and a desire to lose weight. The type of laxative ingested determines the clinical features. Osmotic diarrhea is caused by magnesium sulfate, nonabsorbable sugars (e.g., lactulose), and sodium phosphate. Dihydroxy bile salts, castor oil, and dioctyl sodium sulfosuccinate (docusate sodium) cause secretory diarrhea. (These secretory agents as well as bisacodyl and phenolphthalein may increase PGE synthesis, thereby reducing or reversing water flux from the intestinal lumen into the blood.) Surreptitious laxative use is difficult to document except in the case of phenolphthalein, where alkalinization of a stool sample by the addition of sodium hydroxide (NaOH) causes the stool to turn pink.

4. **Infectious causes of diarrhea** include the bacteria listed in Table 5-1, which cause food poisoning. Some organisms, such as *Clostridium difficile* and *Entamoeba histolytica*, primarily attach to the colon and rectum, respectively; these organisms are discussed in sections V G and VI B 2. Organisms that most commonly cause diarrhea are discussed below.

  a. *E. coli* is the most common cause of **traveler's diarrhea**, which is the often severe diarrhea that occurs within 2 weeks of a visit to a tropical area. Traveler's diarrhea usually is self-limited.

    (1) A toxogenic, heat-labile or heat-stable *E. coli* can activate cAMP or cyclic guanosine

---

*Toxogenic *E. coli*, viruses, and *Giardia lamblia* are not invasive. Irritable bowel syndrome, malabsorption syndrome, and laxative abuse also do not cause pus in the stool.

Table 5-1. Bacterial Food Poisoning Syndromes

Organism	Incubation Period	Symptoms	Sources of Contamination	Pathogenic Mechanisms	Comments
Staphylococcus aureus	2–8 hours	SP, SV, D	Meat and dairy food handlers	Toxin	Sudden onset; intense vomiting; no therapy needed in most cases
Bacillus cereus	2–8 hours	SP, SV, SD	Reheated fried rice	Tissue invasion	Early vomiting, later diarrhea; recovery within 24 hours
Clostridium perfringens	8–14 hours	V, SD	Reheated meat	Toxin	Profuse diarrhea
Vibrio parahaemolyticus	6 hours–4 days	V, SD, F	Saltwater seafood	Toxin; tissue invasion	Outbreaks usually associated with ingestion of oysters, clams, and crabs
Salmonella species	8–48 hours	V, SD, F, H, systemic disease	Food	Mild tissue invasion; possible toxin	Diarrhea with low-grade fever; carrier state possible; should not be treated
Pathogenic *Escherichia coli*	1–3 days	SD	Food and water	Toxin; tissue invasion	Traveler's diarrhea; prophylaxis or therapy with trimethoprim-sulfa combinations, Pepto-Bismol, or doxycycline
Vibrio cholera	1–3 days	V, SD	Poor hygiene	Toxin	Life-threatening diarrhea; therapy is intravenous replacement of fluid and electrolytes; epidemic occurrence
Shigella species (mild cases)	1–3 days	SD, F, B	Fecal-oral spread; flies	Toxin; tissue invasion	Therapy with ampicillin, trimethoprim, sulfamethizole, or chloramphenicol
Clostridium botulinum	1–4 days	V, H, RE	Canned foods	Toxin	Severe CNS symptoms; ventilatory support needed; high mortality rate
Campylobacter fetus	2–10 days	SD, B	Fecal-oral spread; pets	Tissue invasion	Bloody diarrhea, especially in children; therapy with erythromycin
Clostridium difficile	?	SD, F, B	· · ·	Toxin	Postantibiotic diarrhea; therapy with vancomycin or metronidazole
Yersinia enterocolitica	?	SP, SD, B	Fecal-oral spread; pets	Tissue invasion; possible toxin	May be seen with polyarthritis in children; therapy with tetracycline

Note.—S = severe; P = abdominal pain; V = vomiting; D = diarrhea; F = fever; B = blood in stool; H = headache; and RE = respiratory embarrassment.

3′,5′-monophosphate (cGMP), respectively, to cause this secretory diarrhea. Species of *Shigella, Salmonella,* and *Campylobacter* as well as *E. histolytica* and *Giardia lamblia* are other known causes of traveler's diarrhea.

    (2) Trimethoprim-sulfonamide combinations, Pepto-Bismol, and oxytetracycline preparations recently have been shown to be effective in prevention and treatment.

b. *G. lamblia*, a flagellate protozoan, is the most common cause of **water-borne infectious diarrhea** in the United States. It also is common in developing nations because of sewage contamination of drinking water. Infected patients may be asymptomatic, have mild diarrhea, or develop a prolonged illness characterized by malabsorption, diarrhea, bloating, and crampy abdominal pain. Since the organism preferentially resides in the upper small intestine, the diagnosis can be made by demonstration of trophozoites in duodenal aspirates, although examination of stools for cysts and trophozoites is a good screening test. Treatment with metronidazole or quinacrine usually is successful.

c. Viruses commonly cause acute self-limited diarrhea. Although many different viruses may cause gastroenteritis, the only causes of viral gastroenteritis that can be identified with certainty are the **Norwalk agent** (probably a parvovirus) and the **rotavirus.**

d. *Salmonella*. Salmonellosis can be highly variable in its presentation. Gastroenteritis, the most common form of salmonellosis, is an acute self-limited diarrheal syndrome with crampy abdominal pain and fever. **Enteric fever** is a severe illness primarily caused by *Salmonella typhi* or *Salmonella paratyphi* but also seen with infection by other types of salmonella. Clinical manifestations include prolonged fever, abdominal pain, rash, and diarrhea. Salmonellal **septicemia** may be seen in patients with osteomyelitis, mycotic aneurysms, or abscesses with no evidence or history of gastrointestinal disease. Salmonellosis is diagnosed using stool and blood culturing techniques. Since a prolonged carrier state may be induced, patients with gastroenteritis are not treated with antibiotics. In severe infection, ampicillin, trimethoprim-sulfamethoxasole, or chloramphenicol is used.

e. *Shigella*. Shigellosis is characterized by acute diarrhea with fever and crampy abdominal pain. If left untreated, the disease progresses to a chronic bloody diarrhea without fever but with weight loss and debilitation, which may last for weeks. Diagnosis is made by positive stool culture. In contrast to salmonellosis, antibiotic therapy for shigellosis offers symptomatic improvement, with decreased duration of excretion of the organism.

f. *Campylobacter* infection is the most common cause of **bacterial diarrhea** in the United States. Symptoms include diarrhea, which may be bloody, and fever. Diagnosis is made by positive stool culture but requires special media and handling. Treatment is erythromycin as the organism is resistant to most other commonly used antibiotics.

g. Cryptosporidiosis is a protozoal infection, which is seen commonly in immunocompromised patients such as those with acquired immune deficiency syndrome (AIDS). This diarrheal syndrome rarely occurs in normal individuals except in a self-limited fashion, particularly in animal (calf) handlers. The diarrhea is watery, profuse, and debilitating. Diagnosis is made by a modified acid-fast stain of stool. No effective therapy is available, although spiramycin may provide temporary relief.

h. *Isospora belli* infection presents similarly to cryptosporidiosis.

5. Nonbacterial food poisoning

    a. Fish poisoning is due to ichthyosarcotoxins (toxins found in the flesh of poisonous fish).

        (1) Ciguatera poisoning is acquired from certain bottom-dwelling fish found in temperate and tropical coastal zones. Ingestion of such fish is followed in 30 minutes to 30 hours by nausea, vomiting, diarrhea, and paresthesia or numbness of the lips, tongue, and limbs. Treatment is supportive.

        (2) Scombroid poisoning is acquired from certain fish species (usually tuna, mackerel, and bonito) that are susceptible to the production of a toxin by the action of *Proteus morgani*. Symptoms resemble those of a histamine reaction and include flushing, headache, dizziness, abdominal cramping, vomiting, and diarrhea. The symptoms appear soon after ingestion and last 4–6 hours. Antihistamines may be used for symptomatic relief.

        (3) Tetraodon poisoning. Puffer fish produce a neurotoxin termed **tetrodotoxin,** which may cause paresthesia of the face and extremities with nausea, vomiting, and diarrhea. Ventilator support may be necessary.

    b. Mushroom poisoning occurs after ingestion of any of the 50 species of mushrooms known to be toxic to man. *Amanita verna, Amanita virosa,* and *Amanita phalloides* account for most cases of mushroom poisoning. Patients develop nausea, vomiting, fever, diarrhea, and abdominal pain 6–24 hours after injection; 1–4 days later, hepatic and renal insufficiency may develop with subsequent coagulopathy, heart failure, convulsions, and coma. Mushroom poisoning has a mortality rate of 40%–90%. Diagnosis is made by history of ingestion or by detection of mushroom toxins in the gastric aspirate. Treatment is supportive. Thioctic acid may be curative and should be administered promptly.

E. Malabsorption of food or nutrients results from a defect at any step of the digestive process or in any of the organs that participate in normal digestion. The clinical features vary widely, since malabsorption may involve a single nutrient or multiple nutrients.

1. **Etiology**
   a. **Maldigestion** refers to a defect either in intraluminal hydrolysis of triglycerides or in micelle formation, which results from the following conditions:
      (1) Pancreatic insufficiency due to chronic pancreatitis, pancreatic carcinoma, or cystic fibrosis
      (2) Deficiency of conjugated bile salts due to cholestatic or obstructive liver disease (e.g., cholangiocarcinoma)
      (3) Bile salt deconjugation due to bacterial overgrowth in blind loops (after Billroth II gastrectomy) or in jejunal diverticula or in association with enterocolonic fistulae or motility disorders (e.g., scleroderma and pseudo-obstruction)
      (4) Inadequate mixing of gastric contents with bile salts and pancreatic enzymes as a result of previous gastric surgery, especially Billroth II gastrectomy
   b. **Intrinsic small bowel diseases that cause malabsorption**
      (1) **Celiac disease** causes flattening of the villi and inflammatory cell infiltration in the lamina propria (see section IV E 4 c).
      (2) **Whipple's disease** is a systemic disease, which may be infectious in origin and causes mucosal damage and lymphatic obstruction (see section IV E 4 d).
      (3) **Collagenous sprue** refers to the deposition of a collagenous substance in the lamina propria in a patient who otherwise presents with the clinical and histologic features of celiac disease. Fifty percent of patients with collagenous sprue are steroid responsive.
      (4) **Nongranulomatous ulcerative ileojejunitis** is a rare condition of unknown etiology characterized by fever, weight loss, crampy abdominal pain, bloating, and diarrhea. Intestinal ulcerations may occur, and splenomegaly is noted in 20% of cases. Despite therapeutic attempts with steroids and immunosuppressive drugs, the clinical course often is relentless and the prognosis poor.
      (5) **Eosinophilic gastroenteritis** is characterized by peripheral eosinophilia and infiltration of the wall of the stomach, small intestine, or colon by mature eosinophils. Many patients present with a specific food allergy and other allergic disorders such as asthma, eczema, and allergic rhinitis, and some patients show symptoms of gastritis. Diagnosis is made by biopsy of the gastric antrum or small bowel, which reveals the eosinophilic infiltration. Steroid therapy may induce a prolonged remission. Elimination diets to remove possible allergens have been successful in some patients.
      (6) **Amyloidosis** (either primary or secondary) may affect the small intestine by amyloid infiltration of the submucosa. Altered motility that allows bacterial overgrowth also may contribute to malabsorption. Diagnosis is made by biopsy (usually of a rectal valve) with special stains such as Congo red. Treatment primarily is supportive. A trial of antibiotics for bacterial overgrowth may be given.
      (7) **Crohn's disease** may cause malabsorption by mucosal damage, by multiple strictures with bacterial overgrowth, or as a result of the need for multiple bowel resections (see section IV G).
   c. **Inadequate absorptive surface** results from extensive small bowel resection, usually for Crohn's disease or vascular compromise of the small intestine. Resection of up to 50% of the small intestine is well tolerated if the remaining bowel is normal, and survival is possible following more extensive resection but requires careful management. If the proximal small bowel is resected, calcium, folic acid, and iron may not be absorbed. If the ileum is removed, bile acid and vitamin B_{12} absorption is impaired greatly. Hepatic dysfunction, oxalate kidney stones, and increased gastric acid secretion are common complications of extensive bowel resection. Initial therapy includes intravenous fluid and electrolyte administration or parenteral hyperalimentation. Oral feedings should include medium-chain triglycerides (MCT oil), fat-soluble vitamins, and iron. Intramuscular vitamin B_{12} and antidiarrheal agents (to slow the transit time) may be needed. Cholestyramine resin may bind nonabsorbed bile salts and lessen the diarrhea; however, this drug also depletes the total body bile salt pool and usually is not used if more than 100 cm of distal ileum has been resected.
   d. **Lymphatic obstruction** is present in the following disorders that cause malabsorption.
      (1) **Intestinal lymphangiectasia** may be primary (congenital) or secondary to intestinal tuberculosis, Whipple's disease, trauma, neoplasia, or retroperitoneal fibrosis.
      (2) **Intestinal lymphoma** may mimic Crohn's disease or adult celiac disease both clinically and radiographically. Clues to the differential diagnosis include persistent fevers and a short duration of symptoms. Enlarged lymph nodes or hepatosplenomegaly may be found on physical examination, and CT may reveal enlarged retroperitoneal nodes.

Diagnosis often is made only after surgical biopsy. Therapy includes local resection and radiotherapy. Chemotherapy is used for disseminated disease.

e. Multiple defects contribute to malabsorption in the following settings.

    (1) Post gastrectomy. Malabsorption can result following Billroth II gastrectomy, when poor mixing of gastric contents with pancreatic enzymes and stasis in the afferent loop with bacterial overgrowth both are present. Therapy includes surgical correction of the afferent loop and broad-spectrum antibiotics.

    (2) Radiation enteritis interferes with blood supply to the intestine. However, bacterial overgrowth also may occur secondary to a radiation-induced intestinal stricture. Lymphatic obstruction due to edema or fibrosis also may be a part of the syndrome.

    (3) Diabetes mellitus. Altered gut motility from diabetic neuropathy, bacterial overgrowth, and exocrine pancreatic insufficiency all have been implicated as mechanisms of diabetes mellitus–induced malabsorption.

f. Other causes of malabsorption

    (1) Abetalipoproteinemia is a rare disease with neurologic manifestations (e.g., ataxia, nystagmus, incoordination, and retinitis pigmentosa), morphologically abnormal ''spiny'' red blood cells, and low serum cholesterol and triglyceride levels. Steatorrhea occurs because apoprotein B, which is necessary for normal chylomicron formation, is lacking in intestinal cells. Fat is found in the epithelial cells at small bowel biopsy. Treatment with medium-chain triglycerides bypasses the absorption defect. Fat-soluble vitamin supplementation also may be required.

    (2) Infections can cause malabsorption and may be viral, bacterial, or parasitic. **Viral and bacterial enteritis** may cause temporary malabsorption secondary to disaccharidase deficiency, mucosal damage, or both. **Tropical sprue** is an endemic malabsorption disorder occurring in the tropics, which is felt to have an infectious etiology because travelers are susceptible to the disease, and treatment with tetracycline usually is effective. Other infectious causes of malabsorption include hookworm, tapeworm, strongyloidiasis, and *Capillaria philippinensis* (roundworm) infection, which are common outside the United States, and giardiasis, which is relatively common in the United States.

    (3) Chronic intestinal ischemia may cause malabsorption when two of the three major intestinal vessels are occluded (as can be shown angiographically). Presenting symptoms usually are weight loss and crampy postprandial pain, with bloody diarrhea occasionally present. Vascular surgery has resulted in improvement in several reported series.

    (4) Hypogammaglobulinemia may cause malabsorption, especially if it is associated with serum immunoglobulin A (IgA), serum IgG, or intestinal IgA deficiency. Intestinal and serum IgM also may be increased. Small bowel biopsy shows absence of plasma cells. Nodular lymph hyperplasia may be noted in the distal small bowel on x-ray, and *G. lamblia* may be detected in stool or duodenal aspirate. Treatment of the giardiasis with metronidazole or quinacrine may improve absorption.

    (5) Metastatic carcinoid syndrome is associated with an increased production of 5-hydroxytryptamine (serotonin), which causes increased gastrointestinal motility. Methysergide or cyproheptadine may be used for therapy.

    (6) Hypoparathyroidism may present as steatorrhea. The mechanism by which parathormone affects fat absorption is unknown, but vitamin D–dependent calcium absorption may play a role.

    (7) Drugs that may cause malabsorption include neomycin, kanamycin, bacitracin, and polymyxin. Phenytoin causes a selective folic acid malabsorption.

2. Clinical features are extremely variable; patients may present with some or all of the following clinical manifestations.

    a. Passage of abnormal stools, which are greasy, soft, bulky, and foul smelling and may float in the toilet because of their increased gas content; a film of grease or oil droplets may be seen on the surface of the water

    b. Weight loss, which may be severe and involve marked muscle wasting

    c. Edema and ascites secondary to hypoalbuminemia

    d. Anemia secondary to altered absorption of iron, vitamin B_{12}, folate, or a combination of these

    e. Bone pain or fractures from vitamin D deficiency

    f. Paresthesias or tetany from calcium deficiency

    g. Bleeding from vitamin K deficiency

3. Diagnosis is based on clinical evidence, with confirmation by laboratory tests.

    a. Stool fat analysis may be qualitative or quantitative. A positive Sudan stain indicates excretion of greater than 15 g of fat per day in the stool. A 72-hour fecal fat collection can be used to quantify the amount of fat absorption. Normally, an individual absorbs 93%–95%

of all dietary fat ingested. Pancreatic disease often is associated with fecal fat excretion in excess of 20–30 g/day on a 100 g/day fat diet.

b. d-Xylose absorption testing. Since d-xylose, a five-carbon sugar, does not require enzymatic degradation or micelle formation for absorption, it can be used to measure intestinal mucosal integrity. After a 25-g oral dose, a 5-hour urine collection should contain at least 4–5 g of d-xylose.

c. Testing for unabsorbed carbohydrate. Lowered stool pH is noted when unabsorbed carbohydrates reach the colon and bacterial fermentation occurs. This is particularly common in lactase deficiency but also may be seen in celiac disease and short bowel syndrome.

d. Pancreatic function testing involves measuring the bicarbonate and total fluid output from the duodenum after secretin stimulation. In pancreatic insufficiency, these are low.

e. Measurement of serum carotene levels. Since vitamin A is fat soluble and serum carotene level is a reflection of vitamin A metabolism, a low serum carotene level with normal vitamin A intake may be a useful screening test for fat malabsorption.

f. Bacterial overgrowth testing

   (1) Direct culture of jejunal aspirates yielding greater than 10^4 organisms/ml of aspirate is considered abnormal. The diagnosis is strongly suggested by the presence of fastidious anaerobes (clostridia and bacteroides), facultative anaerobes (lactobacilli and enterococci), or coliforms.

   (2) Bile acid breath tests are becoming more popular. The tests are based on the fact that bacteria will deconjugate **^{14}C-labeled glycine-cholate** before it can be absorbed. ^{14}C glycine then is metabolized to $^{14}CO_2$, which is exhaled and measured in the breath of patients with bacterial overgrowth.

   (3) Measurement of tryptophan metabolites. Elevated urinary levels of **indican** and **5-hydroxyindoleacetic acid (5-HIAA)** are due to increased metabolism of tryptophan. This test is not specific, however, since abnormal levels of tryptophan metabolites also are obtained in carcinoid syndrome and Whipple's disease.

g. Small bowel x-ray, especially by the intubated air contrast technique, may be useful. Pooling or flocculation of barium does not occur as frequently as with previous barium techniques but, if noted, suggests celiac disease. Thick folds may be seen in Whipple's disease, lymphoma, amyloidosis, radiation enteritis, Zollinger-Ellison syndrome, and eosinophilic enteritis.

h. The **Schilling test** is used to diagnose vitamin B_{12} malabsorption. An abnormal first-stage Schilling test (administration of labeled vitamin B_{12} only) with a normal second-stage Schilling test (administration of a complex of vitamin B_{12} and intrinsic factor) indicates gastric defects such as pernicious anemia and lack of intrinsic factor due to gastric resection. The second-stage test may be abnormal due to bacterial overgrowth or to resection or inflammation of the terminal ileum, which is the site of absorption. Severe celiac disease also may cause an abnormal second-stage test.

i. Small bowel biopsy is essential for the diagnosis of many cases of malabsorption. In properly prepared specimens, normal villous crypt ratios are 3:1 or 4:1. Flattening of the villi with inflammatory cell infiltration is characteristic of celiac disease, but flattened villi alone may be seen in infectious enteritis, giardiasis, lymphoma, and bacterial overgrowth.

4. Characteristics and management of specific causes of malabsorption

a. Pancreatic insufficiency may be due to chronic pancreatitis, pancreatic carcinoma, or cystic fibrosis. The pancreatic-secretin test shows low fluid and bicarbonate output. Treatment is pancreatic enzyme replacement. H_2-receptor antagonists may increase the potency of enzymes when given 1 hour before meals since acid may inactivate the exogenous enzymes.

b. Bacterial overgrowth may be due to altered motility (e.g., in diabetes and amyloidosis), small bowel diverticula, strictures (e.g., in lymphoma and Crohn's disease), or to blind loops after Billroth II gastrectomy. Surgical correction of the anatomic problems may be considered, but treatment with antibiotics frequently is successful. Ampicillin or tetracycline may be used. Some patients require continuous therapy, and in these cases antibiotics should be rotated.

c. Celiac disease (nontropical sprue)

   (1) Although the **etiology and pathogenesis** are not fully understood, it is clear that an abnormal sensitivity to gluten, a component of wheat, causes damage to the intestinal mucosa of these patients. The importance of genetic factors is demonstrated by the presence of abnormal small bowel biopsies in 10%–15% of first-degree relatives of patients. In addition, 60%–90% of celiac patients have human leukocyte antigen B8 (HLA-B8) and HLA-Dw3 compared to 20%–30% of the general population. An additional B lymphocyte antigen is present in 70%–80% of celiac patients as compared to 15% of the general population. Together, these factors may contribute to a binding of gluten to intestinal epithelial cells and, hence, to the immunogenicity of the bound product.

(2) **Clinical features** include diarrhea, steatorrhea, weight loss, and abdominal bloating. Symptoms may begin at childhood and then lessen, only to reappear in the third to sixth decade.

(3) **Diagnosis** requires small bowel biopsy, which shows villous atrophy, crypt hypertrophy, and cuboidal change in the epithelial cells with inflammatory cell infiltration in the lamina propria.

(4) **Therapy** is based on withdrawal of gluten from the diet by eliminating wheat, rye, barley, and oat. Only corn and rice flour are permitted. Although clinical response to gluten withdrawal often is dramatic and may be seen in a few days, histologic recovery demonstrated on repeat small bowel biopsy may be delayed for months and, in up to 50% of patients, may never be demonstrated. In severely ill patients, steroids may be of short-term benefit.

(5) **Complications**

(a) **Lymphoma and carcinoma** occur in about 10%–15% of cases, with lymphoma twice as common as carcinoma.

(b) **Intestinal ulcers or strictures** may be late complications in some patients with celiac disease.

(c) **Dermatitis herpetiformis** is a skin lesion characterized by papular vesicular eruptions and pruritus. Most patients have an abnormal intestinal biopsy showing villous atrophy, and the skin lesions may respond to gluten withdrawal.

d. **Whipple's disease** is a systemic disorder most common in middle-aged men.

(1) **Etiology and pathogenesis** of Whipple's disease are not completely understood. Numerous small gram-positive cocci are noted in macrophages in individual organs, and an L-form streptococcus has been postulated as the infectious agent.

(2) **Clinical features** depend on organ involvement. In the intestine, periodic acid–Schiff (PAS)-positive macrophages (i.e., macrophages that contain bacilli) are found in the lamina propria. The mesenteric lymph nodes, heart, spleen, lungs, and CNS also may be involved. Malabsorption is caused by mucosal damage and lymphatic obstruction. Fever is noted in one-third to one-half of patients. Arthralgia and arthritis are present in 60% of patients and may precede the gastrointestinal symptoms.

(3) **Diagnosis** is made by intestinal biopsy with a PAS stain. A small bowel x-ray may reveal thickened folds. In rare cases, the disease is focal and the biopsy is normal.

(4) **Therapy** with penicillin, ampicillin, or tetracycline is required for at least 4–6 months and may be continued intermittently (i.e., every other day) thereafter. The relapse rate is approximately 10%.

F. **Protein-losing enteropathy (PLE)** refers to the excessive loss of serum proteins into the gastrointestinal tract. Three types of disorders may cause PLE.

1. **Mucosal ulceration** causes leakage of protein at the ulcer site and results from the following conditions:
   a. Malignant disease involving the gastrointestinal tract
   b. Multiple peptic ulcers
   c. Nongranulomatous ileojejunitis

2. **Mucosal disease** without ulceration but with altered metabolism or cell turnover leads to increased permeability to protein. Such diseases include:
   a. Ménétrier's disease
   b. Celiac disease
   c. Whipple's disease
   d. Infectious enteritis

3. **Lymph flow obstruction** causes increased lymphatic pressure and protein leakage. Lymphatic obstruction results from the following conditions:
   a. Lymphoma
   b. Lymphangiectasia
   c. Cardiac disease, such as constrictive pericarditis and tricuspid valve disease
   d. *C. philippinensis* infection

G. **Crohn's disease (regional enteritis)** is a chronic granulomatous disease, which may occur anywhere in the gastrointestinal tract from the mouth to the anus. The ileum most often is involved, with more than 50% of Crohn's disease patients having ileocolitis. The first peak of incidence occurs between the ages of 12 and 30 years; a secondary peak occurs at age 50 years.

1. **Etiology**
   a. **Genetic factors** appear to play a role, with an increased incidence of disease noted in

monozygotic twins and siblings. Men are affected more often than women, and the disease is more common among Jews. In comparison to the general population, Jewish men have six times the risk of developing Crohn's disease.

  b. Infectious agents have been postulated but never identified as a cause of Crohn's disease. An inflammatory response can be induced in the foot pads and intestinal walls of mice by injecting an extract of Crohn's disease tissue, and this may reflect a small transmissible agent, such as an RNA virus or a cell wall–defective bacteria. Recently, a mycobacterium has been proposed as an etiologic agent.

  c. An **immunologic mechanism** presently is the most prominent theory. Abnormal numbers, subsets, and functions of T cells have been identified.

  2. Pathology includes:

  a. Marked thickening of the involved intestinal wall with transmural inflammation

  b. Enlarged and matted mesenteric lymph nodes

  c. Focal granulomas in 50% of specimens

  d. Deep serpiginous or linear ulcerations leading to cobblestoning and fistula formation

  e. Stricture formation secondary to scarring

  f. Alternating areas of normal and involved mucosa

  3. Clinical features are characterized by periodic exacerbations and remissions.

  a. Pain often is colicky, especially in the lower abdomen, and may be increased after meals due to the obstructive nature of the pathologic process.

  b. Systemic symptoms are common and include fever, weight loss, malaise, and anorexia.

  c. Diarrhea is the usual presenting symptom.

  d. Extraintestinal manifestations are numerous.

   (1) Anemia as well as growth or sexual retardation probably are due to inadequate caloric intake.

   (2) Hepatobiliary disorders include fatty liver, pericholangitis, nonspecific hepatitis, cirrhosis, and sclerosing cholangitis. There is an increased risk of gallstones. Liver enzyme or liver biopsy abnormalities are noted in 50%–70% of Crohn's disease patients.

   (3) Renal disorders include right ureteral obstruction secondary to contiguous bowel involvement and nephrolithiasis. An increase in calcium oxalate stones is due to increased oxalate absorption, and an increase in uric acid stones is ascribed to increased cell turnover and a concentrated acid urine.

   (4) Peripheral arthritis is noted in 10%–12% of patients and ankylosing spondylitis in 2%–10%.

   (5) Skin problems include erythema nodosum and, rarely, pyoderma gangrenosum.

   (6) Episcleritis or uveitis may occur in 3%–10% of patients.

  e. Fistulae to the skin or other organs occur in about 20% of patients. **Perianal fistulae** or abscesses are especially common in Crohn's colitis.

  4. Diagnosis is made on the basis of clinical signs and symptoms combined with characteristic x-ray findings, including deep (collar button) ulcerations, long strictured segments (string sign), and skip areas. Colonoscopy may be helpful when there is colonic involvement, and biopsies may show granuloma formation. Laboratory studies are not specific for Crohn's disease but may show multifactorial anemia, leukocytosis, an increased sedimentation rate, and evidence of malabsorption or protein loss. The differential diagnosis includes lymphoma, tuberculosis, radiation enteritis, and *Yersinia* infection (especially in acute enteritis).

  5. Therapy is symptomatic. No specific therapy or cure exists.

  a. Supportive measures include short-term, broad-spectrum antibiotics, antidiarrheal agents, bowel rest with intravenous fluid support, total parenteral nutrition, and vitamin supplementation.

  b. Sulfasalazine in doses of 3–4 g/day may be used alone or in combination with corticosteroids to treat acute disease. This may be more effective in Crohn's ileitis.

  c. Vitamin B$_{12}$ injections are indicated when ileal disease causes malabsorption of this nutrient.

  d. Increased oral calcium, vitamin D, or both may be helpful in patients with calcium oxalate stones by binding oxalate in the bowel and decreasing urinary oxalate.

  e. Metronidazole is effective in treatment of perineal and perianal fistulae.

  f. Corticosteroids have been proven effective by the National Cooperative Crohn's Disease Study, especially in patients with small bowel disease. When remission is obtained, the dose should be tapered gradually.

  g. Surgery may be necessary for recurrent intestinal obstruction, enterocutaneous fistulae, and perforation and for growth retardation that does not respond to increased caloric intake. The recurrence rate after initial resection may be as high as 80% within 15 years.

H. Small bowel tumors

1. **Malignant tumors** of the small intestine are rare and include adenocarcinomas, carcinoid tumors, lymphomas, and leiomyosarcomas.
   a. **Etiology and pathogenesis.** Some small bowel malignancies arise de novo, but many are related to underlying conditions such as Crohn's disease and celiac disease. Rarely, these malignancies arise from the polyps of Peutz-Jeghers syndrome, familial polyposis, and Gardner's syndrome. A particular type of lymphoma called **Mediterranean lymphoma** is endemic in the Middle East. Patients with celiac disease may have a 10%–15% incidence of small bowel malignancy, usually lymphoma.
   b. **Pathology.** Adenocarcinoma is especially common in the proximal small bowel; lymphomas and carcinoid tumors primarily occur in the appendix and ileum. The most common primary small bowel tumor is asymptomatic carcinoid, which usually is found in the appendix. However, small bowel tumors of clinical significance most commonly are metastatic from the breast, kidney, ovary, and testis as well as from melanoma.
   c. **Clinical features** include bleeding, obstruction, and malabsorption. Carcinoid tumors of the appendix may present as acute appendicitis but usually are asymptomatic. Rarely, appendiceal carcinoid tumors are metastatic to the liver and in such cases may cause **carcinoid syndrome**, which is characterized by flushing and diarrhea.
   d. **Therapy and prognosis.** Surgery is the treatment of choice but the prognosis is poor, especially for adenocarcinomas. Lymphomas and leiomyosarcomas have a better prognosis if they are localized to a small segment of the bowel. Radio- and chemotherapy are used postoperatively to treat systemic lymphomas. Carcinoid tumors grow slowly, and patients may survive for many years even if the disease is metastatic.

2. **Benign tumors** of the small intestine include adenomas, lipomas, and leiomyomas, which may present with obstruction or bleeding but usually are asymptomatic.

I. Acute appendicitis is a common and curable cause of an acute abdomen, which occurs at any age and in both sexes but most often occurs in males between 10 and 30 years of age.

1. **Pathogenesis.** It is believed that the primary event is an obstruction of the appendiceal lumen by a fecalith, inflammation, foreign body, or neoplasm. After obstruction of the lumen, increased intraluminal pressure and infection may cause appendiceal necrosis and perforation.

2. **Clinical features** include pain in the right lower quadrant, which initially is vague but becomes localized to McBurney's point, peritoneal signs, fever, and leukocytosis in the 10,000 to 20,000 range. Rectal tenderness is common in **pelvic appendicitis**, and **retrocecal appendicitis** causes psoas muscle pain on hip extension. Patients at the extremes of age, greatly obese patients, and patients on corticosteroids may present with nonspecific complaints and a relatively benign physical examination. Thus, a high index of clinical suspicion must be maintained in these cases.

3. **Differential diagnosis** includes acute gastroenteritis, mesenteric adenitis, Meckel's diverticulitis, and Crohn's disease. In young women, ovarian torsion, ruptured ovarian cyst, and pelvic inflammatory disease should be considered. In elderly patients, diverticulitis, cholecystitis, incarcerated hernia, and mesenteric thrombosis should be ruled out.

4. **Therapy** is surgery, which should be performed as early as possible to prevent perforation.

V. DISEASES OF THE COLON

A. Constipation

1. **Simple constipation** is the result of delayed transit of intestinal contents. The highly refined, low-fiber diets of Western nations probably contribute to this problem. Although the epidemiologic definition of constipation is less than three stools per week, individual differences do exist. Treatment of simple constipation is directed toward increasing intestinal bulk by increasing dietary fiber content with fruits, vegetables, and bulking agents such as psyllium hydrophilic colloids, which trap water and electrolytes within the bowel lumen. Long-term use of potent laxatives should be avoided as they may result in destruction of colonic intramural nerve plexuses and **cathartic colon**.

2. **Constipation may occur with a variety of diseases**, including ulcerative proctitis, rectal fissures or abscesses, and rectal strictures as well as the varied causes of diffusely decreased intestinal activity discussed in section IV A and B. Irritable bowel syndrome, which may present as either constipation or diarrhea, is discussed in section IV D 3 a.

B. Colonic diverticula are outpouchings of the mucosa only and, therefore, are not true diverticula. In the United States, colonic diverticula occur in about 50% of individuals over age 60.

1. Pathogenesis. In Western nations, colonic diverticula have been linked to low-fiber diets. Diets low in fiber and bulk are thought to cause an increased intraluminal pressure, particularly in the narrow sigmoid colon. (This belief is based on LaPlace's law, which states that the smaller the radius of a cylinder the greater the pressure generated at a given tension.) Eventually, the increased intraluminal pressure causes a mucosal herniation at the site of a perforating arteriole carrying blood from the serosal surface to the mucosa.

2. Clinical features often are absent in uncomplicated colonic diverticula. However, patients may complain of crampy abdominal pain in the left lower quadrant, with alternating diarrhea and constipation. Relief of these symptoms after bowel movement often is noted.

3. Therapy is aimed at increasing stool bulk and, thereby, decreasing intraluminal pressure with high-fiber foods and hydrophilic colloids. Often this results in symptomatic improvement, probably by regulating bowel frequency. Anticholinergic agents sometimes are used but have not been proven effective.

4. Complications
a. Diverticulitis occurs in about 25% of patients with diverticulosis. Generally, there is a microperforation (rarely a free perforation) with peridiverticular abscess. Symptoms include left lower abdominal pain, fever, and constipation. Because of the characteristic leukocytosis and left lower abdominal tenderness on physical examination, this condition sometimes is called **left-sided appendicitis**. Treatment with antibiotics, intravenous fluids, and bowel rest (i.e., nothing by mouth) is effective in most cases. Ampicillin is used most commonly. Severely ill or toxic patients, however, may require additional antibiotics for adequate coverage of *Pseudomonas* and anaerobes.
b. Bleeding occurs in about 20%–25% of cases and usually is brisk, painless, and not associated with straining. Blood transfusion may be necessary. In most cases, bleeding stops spontaneously with only supportive therapy. Arteriography or rapid sequence nuclear scanning using technetium sulfur colloid or technetium-labeled erythrocytes may localize the bleeding portion of the colon and allow segmental surgical resection if necessary.

C. Hirschsprung's disease is a congenital cause of megacolon, which occurs in 1 of 5000 live births and is more common in males.

1. Etiology. Hirschsprung's disease is caused by incomplete caudad migration of neural crest cells, which renders the internal anal sphincter and a variable segment of the rectum and sigmoid without innervation. The involved segment constitutes a functional obstruction, and the normal proximal colon becomes dilated.

2. Clinical features. The disease may present in infancy as meconium ileus, intestinal obstruction, or severe constipation, or it may present in later life with milder symptoms.

3. Diagnosis. Physical examination reveals the absence of stool in the rectum, and barium enema shows a narrowed (diseased) segment with a dilatated proximal colon (normal segment) in about 75% of cases. Anal manometry is a good screening test for this disease and reveals a lack of reflex relaxation in the internal anal sphincter upon rectal distension. The absence of ganglion cells on a full-thickness rectal biopsy is diagnostic.

4. Therapy. Treatment is surgical.

D. Ulcerative colitis is a chronic inflammatory disease of the colonic mucosa and submucosa. Ulcerative colitis and Crohn's disease share some features and, despite some dissimilarities, often are placed together under the generic heading of **inflammatory bowel disease**. Ulcerative colitis occurs in 2–7 of 100,000 individuals, and females are affected more commonly than males. The major peak of incidence occurs between the ages of 15 and 30 years, with a lesser peak between the ages of 50 and 65 years.

1. Etiology and pathogenesis are similar to those of Crohn's disease. Family members have an increased risk for the development of inflammatory bowel disease; about 15%–17% of patients have a first-degree relative with inflammatory bowel disease. Viral, bacterial, and immunologic theories (similar to Crohn's disease) have been proposed, and a two- to four-fold increased incidence is noted in Jews.

2. Pathology. The hallmarks of ulcerative colitis are the microabscesses of the crypts of Lieberkühn, which are seen in about 70% of cases. The inflammatory response generally is limited to the mucosa. Macroscopic ulcerations are noted with confluence of the inflammatory response. Pseudopolyps occur when normal mucosa is isolated by severe ulcerations, but there are no skip areas. The rectum and distal colon most commonly are involved. Pancolitis is seen in 25% of cases. Ulcerative colitis with rectal sparing is extremely uncommon.

3. Clinical features are mild when the disease is limited to the rectum (**ulcerative proctitis**). Moderate-to-severe symptoms may occur with extensive disease, particularly pancolitis, and include bloody diarrhea, weight loss, fever, left lower abdominal cramping pain, and nocturnal passage of a small volume of blood and mucus. Fulminant disease occurs in 15% of cases.

4. Diagnosis is based on clinical presentations along with the exclusion of infectious, parasitic, and neoplastic etiologies.

   a. Stool examination reveals mucus, blood, and white blood cells without parasites or bacterial pathogens.

   b. Proctoscopy reveals friability, edema, and hyperemia of the mucosa. Ulcerations and a mucopurulent exudate may be present. Islands of normal tissue may have the appearance of pseudopolyps. Numerous biopsies should be taken.

   c. Barium enema should not be performed in a severely ill or toxic patient. If the symptoms are subacute, a barium x-ray after minimal preparation may reveal lack of haustral markings, fine serrations (compatible with small ulcerations), large ulcerations, and pseudopolyps.

5. Therapy varies with the severity and extent of disease.

   a. In acute flares, bowel rest with intravenous fluids may be useful for short periods. Total parenteral nutrition allows prolonged bowel rest with repletion of vitamins, minerals, electrolytes, and calories in the form of carbohydrate, protein, and fat.

   b. Sulfasalazine has been shown to induce remission and decrease relapse rates in ulcerative colitis patients. The active moiety may be the antiprostaglandin substance, 5-aminosalicylic acid, which is released in the colon by bacteria. Side effects include headache, nausea, rash, and agranulocytosis.

   c. Corticosteroids, which are administered by enema (especially in distal disease such as ulcerative proctitis) or systemically, may be effective in inducing remission. Prednisone is given in doses of 20–60 mg/day, and adrenocorticotropic hormone (ACTH) is administered in doses of 40–80 units/24 hr.

   d. In mild-to-moderate cases without evidence of toxic megacolon, antidiarrheal agents, anticholinergic agents, and sedation may be used cautiously.

   e. Surgery (total colectomy) is reserved for:

   (1) Toxic megacolon that is unresponsive to 24–72 hours of intensive conservative medical measures

   (2) Perforation

   (3) Massive hemorrhage that is unresponsive to conservative treatment (rare)

   (4) Carcinoma

   (5) Suspected carcinoma in colonic strictures

   (6) Growth failure in adolescents, which is unresponsive to conservative treatment

   (7) Dysplasia noted on biopsy at the time of sigmoidoscopy or colonoscopy, which should be done routinely for screening in long-standing diseases

   (8) Cure, especially after 10 years of disease because of the increased risk of cancer

6. Complications. The systemic complications noted for Crohn's disease (see section IV G 3 d) occur in ulcerative colitis with equal frequency. Additional complications of ulcerative colitis, which usually are not seen in Crohn's disease, are noted below.

   a. Toxic megacolon refers to an acute dilatation of the colon (usually the transverse portion) to a diameter in excess of 6 cm. This complication of ulcerative colitis probably is due to severe inflammation, which affects large segments of the colonic musculature as well as neural control of the colon. Anticholinergic and antidiarrheal medications also may contribute. Patients usually are severely ill, with high fever, abdominal pain, and a marked leukocytosis. Treatment is intensive medical therapy for 48–72 hours. Patients who do not respond should undergo an emergency total colectomy.

   b. Carcinoma of the colon is associated with long-standing disease of great extent (usually pancolitis). At 10 years, the risk of carcinoma is 10% and may increase to 25% at 20 years and 40% at 25 years. The malignancies often are multicentric and aggressive. Strictured areas of the colon present a particularly difficult problem because of the difficulty in differentiating intensive inflammatory disease from ischemic narrowing or carcinoma. Yearly colonoscopic examinations with biopsies every 10–20 cm should be performed in patients who have had ulcerative colitis for longer than 8–10 years. If high-grade dysplasia is noted, a prophylactic total colectomy should be seriously considered.

7. Prognosis. Mortality rates are about 20% in toxic megacolon, with higher rates noted in patients over 60 years of age. About 10% of patients do not experience a recurrent attack after the initial onset of disease. Continuous symptoms occur in 10% of patients. About 70%–80%

of patients have recurrent remissions and relapses, and about 20% of patients eventually require total colectomy.

E. Angiodysplasia refers to small vascular abnormalities, which usually are seen in the ascending colon or cecum in patients over 60 years of age. Angiodysplasia is believed to result from obstruction of intestinal capillaries and venules as these vessels pass through the muscularis. Most patients are asymptomatic, but the abnormal vessels are a common cause of painless lower gastrointestinal bleeding in older individuals. Diagnosis may be made by angiographic or colonoscopic demonstration of intraluminal extravasation of blood during the acute episode. Bleeding usually can be managed conservatively, but a right colon resection occasionally is needed for recurrent or massive bleeding. Involvement of the small bowel or stomach also has been reported but is less common. An association with aortic stenosis has been reported, and some authors suggest that correction of the aortic valvular disease may palliate the gastrointestinal bleeding.

F. Tumors of the colon

    1. Benign tumors. There are several histologic types of benign colonic polyps. **Adenomatous polyps** are considered to be precursors of adenocarcinoma, and the risks for adenocarcinoma increase when the polyps are larger than 2 cm, villous rather than tubular, and sessile rather than pedunculated. About 5%–10% of individuals over age 40 have colonic polyps, but most of these are small hyperplastic lesions that carry no malignant potential. Other benign tumors include leiomyomas, lipomas, and fibromas.

        a. Clinical features. Rectal bleeding occurs and may be microscopic or macroscopic. Large polyps may cause symptoms of an incomplete intestinal obstruction with occasional crampy abdominal pain.

        b. Diagnosis is made using an air contrast barium enema, endoscopic visualization of the colon, or both procedures.

        c. Therapy for pedunculated lesions is colonoscopic removal with snare electrocautery. Sessile lesions may require surgical excision. Because carcinoma occurring in an adenomatous polyp may be focal, careful histologic sectioning of the entire polyp, not just a biopsy, is necessary to exclude carcinoma. If malignancy invades the stalk of a polyp, a segmental resection of the colon is indicated to rule out lymphatic spread. Synchronous polyps occur in 20% of cases and metachronous lesions in about 30% of cases. Therefore, an air contrast barium enema, full colonoscopy, or both should be performed at the time a polyp is first identified and every 2 years thereafter. Yearly stool Hemoccult testing also should be performed. First-degree relatives of a patient with colonic polyps or carcinoma have approximately a four- to five-fold increased risk of developing a similar lesion.

    2. Inherited polyposis syndromes

        a. Familial polyposis is an autosomal dominant syndrome characterized by adenomas of the colon. When osteomas or soft tissue tumors are present, this condition is called **Gardner's syndrome.** Colonic malignancy often develops by age 40. A subtotal resection of the colon with close subsequent observation should be performed by age 30.

        b. Peutz-Jeghers syndrome is an autosomal dominant polyposis syndrome with mucocutaneous pigmentation, particularly of the buccal mucosa. The polyps are hamartomas, not adenomas, which carry a low risk for malignant transformation and may be present in the stomach and small bowel as well as in the colon. Patients may have recurrent gastrointestinal bleeding.

        c. Turcot syndrome refers to colonic adenomas with CNS tumors. This polyposis syndrome has a high risk of malignancy, and its pattern of inheritance has not been established.

        d. Juvenile polyposis is an autosomal dominant syndrome with gastrointestinal bleeding from juvenile polyps of the colon, small bowel, and stomach. The risk of malignancy is slightly increased in later life.

        e. Cronkhite-Canada syndrome is a very rare association of intestinal polyps with alopecia, hyperpigmentation, and a lack of fingernails.

    3. Adenocarcinoma of the colon has been steadily increasing in frequency in the United States and now ranks second to lung cancer in men and to breast cancer in women as the major life-threatening malignancy.

        a. Epidemiology. The incidence of colorectal carcinomas is increased in developed countries, especially those with a diet high in red meat and low in fiber. In the United States, the incidence is decreased in Seventh-Day Adventists who practice strict vegetarianism, which also suggests an association with diet. In addition, asbestos workers, machinists, and factory woodworkers have a higher incidence of colorectal carcinomas than the general population.

        b. Etiology

            (1) Diet has been the focus of most etiologic studies. The high red meat and animal fat diet in the United States promotes the growth of bacterial strains that produce carcinogens in the colonic lumen. Bile salts also may contribute to this process. Vitamins A, C, and E in certain foods may inactivate the carcinogens, and broccoli, turnips, and cauliflower induce benzpyrene hydroxylase, which also may inactivate ingested carcinogens.

    (2) The role of **genetic factors** is demonstrated by familial polyposis syndromes and by the fact that first-degree relatives of patients with carcinoma or polyps have a three- to five-fold increased risk of developing colorectal carcinoma.

    (3) Other risk factors include:

        (a) Ulcerative colitis, especially pancolitis and disease of greater than 10 years' duration (10% risk)

        (b) Prior history of colon cancer or adenoma (10% risk)

        (c) Familial polyposis syndrome

        (d) History of female genital or breast cancer

        (e) History of juvenile polyps

        (f) Family cancer syndromes

        (g) Immunodeficiency diseases

  c. Clinical features vary depending on the location and size of the tumor. Tumors in the left colon, especially those in the distal 25 cm, may present as obstruction. Right colon tumors frequently present as iron deficiency anemia and fatigue. Other common symptoms include a change in bowel habit, a decrease in stool size, obvious blood in the stool, and crampy abdominal pain. Metastatic disease usually involves the liver; however, the bone, lung, and brain also may be affected.

  d. Diagnosis is made by barium enema demonstration of polyps or tumors followed by endoscopic visualization with biopsy and cytology. The air contrast barium enema is far more sensitive than the single contrast examination and is the diagnostic procedure of choice. Despite these techniques, it can be difficult to differentiate the tumor from diverticulitis, benign stricture, and Crohn's disease. High-risk patients should have frequent stool guaiac testing and thorough evaluation of unexplained blood loss. CEA determinations, while not useful for screening purposes, may be used for periodic follow-up in patients with a prior history of carcinoma of the colon, with a rising titer indicative of recurrent or metastatic disease.

  e. Therapy is excision of the tumor. Although focal carcinoma without stalk invasion in a polyp can be cured by colonoscopic snare cautery, most tumors require segmental resection of the bowel along with the omentum and regional lymph nodes. Radiation may be used preoperatively and in patients with recurrent disease. Rectal tumors traditionally have been treated with abdominal perineal resections, but recent studies suggest that local excision, radiotherapy, and fulguration may offer excellent results with a decreased risk. Chemotherapy has been disappointing, with only a 15%–20% response rate. When administered by intrahepatic artery perfusion, however, chemotherapy may be useful for decreasing pain in patients with liver metastasis.

  f. Prognosis. The overall 10-year survival rate is 45% and has not changed significantly over the past several years. Cancer confined to the mucosa (often detected by Hemoccult testing or sigmoidoscopy) is associated with an 80%–90% survival rate, while cancer that is limited to the regional lymph nodes is associated with a 50%–60% survival rate.

G. Pseudomembranous colitis is an acute, potentially severe disease of the colon characterized by exudative plaques that cover the intestinal mucosa.

  1. Pathogenesis. The disease is caused by an enterotoxin produced by *C. difficile*, an anaerobic bacterium. It is thought that antibiotic therapy may "select out" the *C. difficile* organism, allowing proliferation and toxin production. Symptoms begin 3 days to 4 weeks after initiating antibiotic therapy. Virtually all antibiotics have been associated with this disease, but clindamycin, ampicillin, and the cephalosporins are the most common offenders.

  2. Clinical features include watery diarrhea, crampy abdominal pain, lower abdominal tenderness, and fever. Leukocytosis is common. Severely ill patients may develop dehydration and electrolyte disturbances. Toxic megacolon and colonic perforation are rare but serious complications that may require surgical intervention.

  3. Diagnosis is made by demonstration of *C. difficile* toxin in the stool or by sigmoidoscopic visualization of the characteristic yellow-white plaques on an erythematous and edematous mucosa. Biopsy of the plaques shows a mucinous, fibrinous, polymorphonuclear exudate. Most patients have disease throughout the colon; however, the disease may be confined to the right colon, and in such cases sigmoidoscopy is negative.

  4. Therapy. The first step in treatment is to discontinue unnecessary antibiotics, which results in improvement in most patients. Cholestyramine may be used to bind the toxin. The organism is sensitive to vancomycin, bacitracin, and metronidazole.

VI. DISEASES OF THE RECTUM AND ANUS

A. Ulcerative proctitis is a localized form of ulcerative colitis, which has a better prognosis and a greatly decreased risk of malignancy as compared with ulcerative colitis. Symptoms include diarrhea, rectal bleeding, and tenesmus; only rarely do fever, weight loss, and the systemic complications of ulcerative colitis occur. Diagnosis is made by ruling out other causes of proctitis, especially infection, and by documenting the absence of inflammation above the rectum by sigmoidoscopy. Sulfasalazine and rectal corticosteroids often are effective treatment. In about 15%–20% of cases, ulcerative proctitis progresses to diffuse ulcerative colitis.

B. Infectious proctitis

1. **Venereal diseases** that cause infectious proctitis include syphilis, gonorrhea, lymphogranuloma venereum, and herpes simplex. These diseases are especially common in homosexual men who may have multiple simultaneous infections.

   a. **Syphilis** of the rectum almost always is primary syphilis. The chancre, which is painless, appears 10–90 days after exposure. Diagnosis is made by dark-field examination of discharge from the chancre and by serologies, although it should be kept in mind that the Venereal Disease Research Laboratory (VDRL) test does not become positive until 1–2 weeks after the appearance of the chancre.

   b. **Gonorrhea** may be asymptomatic or may cause rectal bleeding and diarrhea. Diagnosis is made by culturing the organism.

   c. **Lymphogranuloma venereum** is caused by one strain of *Chlamydia trachomatis*, a gram-negative obligate intracellular bacterium. When left untreated, the acute proctitis may develop into a chronic destructive inflammation with late stricture formation. The organism is difficult to culture, although culture in yolk sacs and tissue cultures are possible. Serologic diagnosis generally is more available. Titers of greater than or equal to 1:16 are highly suggestive of current infection.

   d. **Herpes simplex** may cause constipation, hematochezia, severe anorectal pain, tenesmus, and mucopurulent discharge from the rectum. Bladder dysfunction with impotence may be present. Rectal biopsy demonstrates intranuclear inclusions. The symptoms subside spontaneously but may recur.

2. **Amebiasis** (i.e., infection by *E. histolytica*) may present as a diffuse colitis or extraintestinal disease (e.g., meningitis and liver abscess), or it may be confined to the rectosigmoid, especially in homosexual men. Symptoms are extremely variable, ranging from mild diarrhea to bloody dysentery. Diagnosis is made by demonstrating the organism in the stool or in biopsies obtained at the time of sigmoidoscopy of the characteristic flask-shaped ulcers.

C. Solitary rectal ulcer is a syndrome consisting of a superficial ulceration of unknown etiology combined with passage of mucus or blood and dull rectal pain. The ulcers usually are 2 cm in diameter and located 7–10 cm from the anal verge. They are multiple in 25% of patients. Recent evidence suggests that a weakness in the rectal sling musculature may be a contributing cause. Diagnosis is made by excluding other causes of rectal ulcers, including infections, inflammatory bowel disease, and carcinoma. Treatment is supportive.

D. Hemorrhoids are dilatated internal or external veins of the hemorrhoidal plexus located in the lower rectum. In the United States, 60%–70% of the population experiences symptoms of hemorrhoids at some time. Signs and symptoms include perianal pruritus, rectal bleeding (especially small amounts on the toilet tissue or bright droplets into the toilet bowl), anal pain, and a palpable mass in the anal region. The diagnosis is made by anoscopy or sigmoidoscopy. Treatment is with stool softeners, supportive care with heat or antiedema measures, or surgery. Internal hemorrhoids may be tied with rubber banding.

E. Anal fissures, abscesses, and **fistulae** refer to tears, infections, and hollow channels from the rectum to the perianal skin, respectively. Locally applied heat, sitz baths, and antibiotics may be effective. Occasionally, however, it is necessary to drain surgically or to excise an abscess or a fistulous tract.

F. Pruritus of the perianal skin has many causes, including infection (bacterial, fungal, or parasitic), localized anorectal disease (e.g., fistulae and fissures), dermatologic diseases (e.g., psoriasis and eczema), poor hygiene, diarrhea, and systemic diseases such as diabetes mellitus. The underlying condition should be treated. In addition, local care with careful cleaning following defecation and nightly application of hydrocortisone cream may be helpful in controlling symptoms.

    G. Squamous cell carcinoma of the anus is a rare malignancy that presents as bleeding, pain, a mass, and change in bowel habits. Treatment is surgical, and the 5-year survival rate is 60%.

VII. DISEASES OF THE PANCREAS

  A. Acute pancreatitis

    1. Etiology

      a. Common causes. About 70% of cases of acute pancreatitis that occur in the United States are due to either alcohol abuse or gallstones.

        (1) In **alcoholic pancreatitis**, proteinaceous plugs develop in the pancreatic ducts and calcify in the body of the pancreas, leading to stasis and atrophy of distal segments. Alcoholic pancreatitis is most common in men who have ingested large amounts of alcohol over a period of at least 10 years.

        (b) In **gallstone pancreatitis**, the passage of a common duct stone may initiate reflux of biliary or intestinal contents into the pancreatic gland.

      b. Less common causes of acute pancreatitis include:

        (1) Postoperative pancreatitis, which may be quite severe and is especially common after hepatobiliary tract surgery

        (2) Abdominal trauma

        (3) Hyperlipidemia, which is an associated finding in 15% of cases but also may be causative since dietary and medical treatment of hypertriglyceridemia reduces recurrences

        (4) Drugs such as azathioprine, thiazides, sulfonamides, and corticosteroids

        (5) Hypercalcemia

        (6) Uremia

        (7) Peptic ulcer disease, with penetration into the pancreas

        (8) Cystic fibrosis (in rare cases)

        (9) Endoscopic retrograde cholangiopancreatography (ERCP)

        (10) Viral infections, especially mumps

        (11) Vascular insufficiency

        (12) Pancreatic cancer, probably by localized ductal obstruction

        (13) Hereditary pancreatitis, which may be inherited in an autosomal dominant pattern and carries an increased risk for development of pancreatic carcinoma

        (14) Ampullary lesions or duodenal disease involving the ampulla and periampullary regions

        (15) Idiopathic causes

    2. Clinical features include:

      a. Abdominal pain, which often is a steady or severe pain in the periumbilical region and may radiate to the back

      b. Nausea and vomiting, which occur in 70% of cases

      c. Abdominal tenderness, usually without guarding or rebound

      d. Diminished or absent bowel sounds

      e. Epigastric fullness or mass, which usually is found late in the course of the disease

      f. Retroperitoneal bleeding, causing a hematoma at the umbilicus (**Cullen's sign**) or flank (**Turner's sign**), which is seen in hemorrhagic pancreatitis

    3. Diagnosis usually is based on characteristic clinical presentations, especially in a patient with a history of previous pancreatitis.

      a. Elevated serum amylase levels almost always exist during an acute attack but also may be due to perforated ulcer, intestinal infarction obstruction, ruptured ectopic pregnancy, amylase-producing tumors, salivary gland disease, and decreased amylase clearance due to amylase-globulin complexes (macroamylase) or renal disease.

      b. Elevated serum lipase levels also are found in acute attacks.

      c. The amylase-to-creatinine clearance ratio may be elevated above the normal range of 1%–4% in acute pancreatitis. However, this ratio also is elevated postoperatively, in diabetic ketoacidosis, and in burn patients.

      d. Abdominal x-ray may reveal a localized ileus (sentinel loop) in the small bowel region adjacent to the pancreas.

    4. Therapy is supportive and includes intravenous administration of fluids and analgesics and bowel rest. Morphine may cause sphincter of Oddi spasm and should be avoided. Nasogastric suction often is used to drain gastric secretions and thereby limit pancreatic stimulation; however, the effectiveness of this procedure has not been proven.

    5. Complications account for the 10% mortality rate associated with acute pancreatitis and include the following conditions.

      a. Hemorrhagic pancreatitis. This condition is considered an extension of edematous pancreatitis due to chemical mediators (e.g., elastase), which leads to retroperitoneal hemorrhage and widespread tissue necrosis. Hemorrhagic pancreatitis is more common after trauma, postoperative pancreatitis, and the initial attack of acute pancreatitis and may require peritoneal lavage or surgical intervention for placement of drains. Blood may be present in the peritoneal cavity. The diagnosis is suggested by a falling hematocrit in a severely ill patient. An elevated methemalbumin level also may be noted.

      b. Adult respiratory distress syndrome is due to increased alveolar capillary permeability and may cause severe hypoxia requiring mechanical ventilation.

      c. Pancreatic abscess is suggested when high fever, elevated serum amylase levels, and leukocytosis persist beyond 7–10 days. Gas shadows in the region of the pancreas may be revealed by an abdominal flat plate or by CT. Treatment includes surgical drainage and antibiotics.

      d. Pancreatic pseudocyst refers to a collection of fluid and debris within the pancreas or in a space lined by the pancreas and other adjacent structures. Diagnosis is made by ultrasonography. About 50% of pseudocysts (usually smaller ones) resolve spontaneously. Those persisting beyond 6–10 weeks require drainage to avoid potentially serious complications such as hemorrhage and rupture.

      e. Pancreatic ascites may occur due to a leaking pseudocyst with pancreatic ductal destruction. The diagnosis is suggested by very high serum amylase levels in peritoneal fluid. Conservative therapy with total parenteral nutrition and repeated paracentesis may lead to resolution, but pancreatic resection may be necessary in intractable cases.

B. Chronic pancreatitis results in permanent structural damage of pancreatic tissue.

    1. Etiology. Most of the causes of acute pancreatitis in the United States also can result in chronic pancreatitis. A notable exception is gallstones, which cause only recurrent acute attacks of pancreatitis. Alcohol abuse accounts for 90% of cases of chronic pancreatitis in adults. Cystic fibrosis is the most common cause of chronic disease in children.

    2. Clinical features
      a. Pain, the usual presenting symptom, typically occurs in the epigastrium after eating and radiates to the back.
      b. Malabsorption occurs in association with steatorrhea and weight loss.
      c. Jaundice occurs due to edema and fibrosis in the pancreatic head and causes obstruction of the pancreatic portion of the common bile duct.
      d. Diabetes is common; however, ketoacidosis, nephropathy, and diabetic vascular disease rarely occur.

    3. Diagnosis is suggested by the development of continuous pain and signs of pancreatic insufficiency in a patient with known recurrent pancreatitis, especially when due to alcohol ingestion. Specific tests include:
      a. Abdominal x-ray, which reveals pancreatic calcification in 30%–40% of cases
      b. Secretin-stimulation testing with duodenal intubation and aspiration, which reveals a low bicarbonate concentration in the pancreatic secretion and low enzyme output
      c. ERCP, which shows diffuse ductal dilatation with an irregular, beaded ("chain of lakes") appearance

    4. Therapy is aimed at controlling the manifestations of the disease since the underlying damage to the gland is permanent. In addition, agents that may promote further damage (e.g., alcohol) should be withdrawn.
      a. Control of pain may require narcotic analgesics, but care must be taken to avoid addiction. With abstinence from alcohol over a period of time, some patients experience a lessening of pain.
      b. Replacement of pancreatic enzymes is indicated if steatorrhea is documented. Antacids or cimetidine may increase the effectiveness of oral enzyme preparations.
      c. Insulin may be needed in advanced cases.
      d. Surgery is a last resort and generally is employed for severe pain or recurrent, severe attacks. Subtotal (80%) pancreatectomy and the Puestow procedure (i.e., anastomosis of the pancreatic duct lengthwise to a loop of the jejunum) are used most commonly.

C. Adenocarcinoma of the pancreas accounts for more than 90% of pancreatic malignancies. This tumor has been increasing in incidence during the twentieth century and now is second only to colon carcinoma as the number-one cause of gastrointestinal cancer-related death. Men are affected more commonly than women, and the average age at presentation is 55–65 years.

    1. Etiology. The risk of pancreatic carcinoma is significantly increased in patients with hereditary pancreatitis and in smokers, and the risk is slightly increased in diabetics. A recent study has shown that the risk of this cancer is doubled in individuals who drink coffee, but this finding awaits confirmation.

2. Clinical features
   a. Common symptoms. About 75% of patients have pain that has been present for 3–4 months by the time of diagnosis. The pain typically is postprandial epigastric or periumbilical discomfort, which radiates to the back and is relieved by sitting up or bending both knees. Jaundice is present in about 65% of patients, and weight loss is described in 60% of patients. Diarrhea and steatorrhea also are somewhat common. The gallbladder may be palpable (**Courvoisier's sign**) in some patients. A palpable epigastric mass may be found on physical examination.
   b. Less common symptoms include unexplained thrombophlebitis, depression, and the new onset of diabetes mellitus.

3. Diagnosis often requires a high index of suspicion in the patient with constant epigastric or periumbilical distress.
   a. Laboratory tests reveal an elevated serum alkaline phosphatase level in 80% of patients, which often is due to hepatic metastasis but may be due to compression of the pancreatic portion of the common bile duct. Elevated levels of CEA, lactate dehydrogenase (LDH), and serum glutamic-oxaloacetic transaminase (SGOT) also are common. Jaundice is found in 65% of patients, and 25% of patients have high serum amylase levels.
   b. An upper gastrointestinal series may reveal a widened loop or an "inverted 3 sign" due to indentation by the pancreas along the medial aspect of the duodenum.
   c. CT and ultrasonography of the pancreas demonstrate a mass in 75%–80% of the cases.
   d. ERCP is abnormal in approximately 85%–90% of patients and generally shows a discrete stricture in the main pancreatic duct with proximal dilatation.
   e. Angiography may reveal displacement or encasement of the pancreatic or duodenal arteries. The venous phase may be especially useful if the superior mesenteric vein or splenic vein is occluded.
   f. Secretin-stimulation testing may reveal a decrease in the volume of pancreatic secretion but normal enzyme and bicarbonate concentrations.
   g. Chiba (skinny) needle biopsy under the guidance of CT or ultrasonography may be used to obtain cytology, which is positive for malignancy in 80%–90% of cases.

4. Therapy and prognosis. The overall 5-year survival rate for patients with pancreatic carcinoma is less than 5%.
   a. Surgery is the mainstay of therapy, but only 15% of patients are candidates for curative resection. The **Whipple procedure** (resection of the pancreas with excision of the common bile duct and duodenum) has a 20% surgical mortality rate and a 5% 5-year survival rate. Palliative biliary and gastrointestinal bypass surgery may provide relief of pruritus, jaundice, and symptoms of gastric-outlet obstruction.
   b. Chemotherapy has a 15%–20% response rate but does not prolong survival.
   c. Radiotherapy decreases the size of the tumor mass in about 60%–70% of patients and can be used for palliation.

5. Islet cell tumors account for 50% of pancreatic adenocarcinomas. They may be multicentric and tend to grow slower than tumors of ductular origin. Islet cell tumors frequently are associated with endocrine adenomas in the pituitary and parathyroid glands (e.g., in MEA I syndrome).
   a. Gastrinoma causes the Zollinger-Ellison syndrome and is discussed in detail in section III I.
   b. Insulinoma is characterized by inappropriately high insulin levels in the presence of hypoglycemia. Since only 10%–15% of insulinomas are malignant, surgical resection is the treatment of choice.
   c. Glucagonoma is found in patients with a syndrome of diabetes mellitus, weight loss, anemia, and a characteristic rash (migratory necrolytic erythema). Most glucagonomas are malignant, but surgical debulking may provide symptomatic improvement. Streptozotocin is the most commonly employed chemotherapeutic agent.
   d. Somatostatinoma usually occurs in association with the triad of diabetes, steatorrhea, and gallstones. About 50% of patients have a positive family history of islet cell tumors. The diagnosis usually is made either incidentally at surgery for another problem (e.g., cholecystitis) or late in the course of the disease when metastatic disease is present. Streptozotocin therapy has been effective in a small number of patients.
   e. VIPoma (also called pancreatic cholera, Verner-Morrison syndrome, and the watery diarrhea, hypokalemia, and achlorhydria [WDHA] syndrome) is a tumor of nonalpha, nonbeta islet cells that secrete vasoactive intestinal polypeptide (VIP), which causes watery diarrhea. Solitary lesions may be cured by surgical resection. Some patients are responsive to corticosteroids, and streptozotocin has been used successfully in patients with metastatic disease.

VIII. DISEASES OF THE BILIARY TRACT

A. Gallstones are extremely common, occurring in 20% of the population of the United States. Most gallstones that occur in Western populations are composed primarily of **cholesterol**, which is thought to precipitate from supersaturated bile, especially at night when bile is concentrated in the gallbladder. **Pigment gallstones**, composed primarily of calcium bilirubinate, are found in patients with chronic hemolysis as well as in Oriental populations. In the Orient, biliary infection with β-glucuronidase–producing organisms leads to increased amounts of poorly soluble deconjugated bilirubin in bile. One-third to one-half of patients with gallstones are asymptomatic and should be treated expectantly. Surgical removal of asymptomatic gallstones is unnecessary except for diabetic patients in whom the risk of acute cholecystitis with complications is high.

B. Acute cholecystitis

1. **Etiology.** In 90%–95% of cases, acute cholecystitis is caused by obstruction of the cystic duct by an impacted gallstone, which leads to edema of the gallbladder wall with submucosal hemorrhage and mucosal ulceration. Polymorphonuclear infiltration is a later event and probably is due to the low bacterial count of the obstructed gallbladder. **Acalculous cholecystitis** may occur secondary to salmonellosis, polyarteritis nodosa, sepsis, and trauma.

2. **Clinical features.** An attack of acute cholecystitis starts with crampy pain in the epigastrium or right upper quadrant, which may radiate to the back near the right scapular tip (biliary colic). The pain is thought to be generated by ductal obstruction and often is postprandial, typically subsiding within several hours. An elevated temperature or white blood count, fever, nausea, vomiting, and ileus also may be present. Right upper quadrant tenderness on deep inspiration is known as **Murphy's sign**. Jaundice occurs in 20% of patients and is thought to be due to common duct stones or edema of the common bile duct.

3. **Diagnosis** is suggested by the characteristic clinical picture, especially in a patient known to have gallstones. Most gallstones consist of cholesterol and are radiolucent; 10%–15% of gallstones contain enough calcium to appear radiopaque. Although gallbladder ultrasonography can show the presence of stones (i.e., the fluid-filled gallbladder appears lucent, while the stones within it are sono-opaque and cast shadows), this test cannot be used to demonstrate cystic duct obstruction. Failure to visualize the gallbladder during radionuclide scanning following an intravenous injection of iminodiacetic acid (HIDA scanning) strongly suggests cystic duct obstruction. Oral cholecystography also fails to visualize the gallbladder but is not as reliable as HIDA scanning.

4. **Therapy** initially is supportive with intravenous fluid replacement and nasogastric suction for 24–48 hours. Later, the gallbladder may be removed surgically. Cholesterol stones in patients who are not operative risks may be treated with chenodeoxycholic acid to dissolve the stones. If several small stones are present and floating, a 50%–70% chance of dissolving the stones may be expected over a period of 12–24 months.

5. **Complications** generally require early surgical intervention.
   a. **Empyema** refers to a pus-filled gallbladder. Patients may be toxic and are at high risk for perforation.
   b. **Perforation**
      (1) Localized perforation occurs several days to 1 week after the onset of acute cholecystitis and leads to a pericholecystic abscess.
      (2) Free perforation into the abdominal cavity, which has a 25% mortality rate, occurs early in the clinical course, probably because inflammation in the early stages is insufficient to wall off the abscess.
      (3) Perforation into an adjacent organ may involve the duodenum, jejunum, colon, or stomach. If a large stone is passed into the lumen, intestinal obstruction (**gallstone ileus**) may result.
   c. **Emphysematous cholecystitis** is due to gas-forming bacteria (often clostridia, *E. coli*, or streptococci) in the gallbladder lumen and wall. Men are affected more commonly than women, and 20%–30% of patients have diabetes mellitus. Early surgical intervention is indicated to prevent perforation.

6. **Postcholecystectomy syndrome** refers to abdominal pain that persists after cholecystectomy. The usual cause is an initially mistaken diagnosis, with pain persisting from the underlying process (e.g., pancreatic disease and irritable bowel syndrome). Some patients may have common duct stones.

C. Chronic cholecystitis is a clinical term used to describe a condition of recurrent subacute symptoms due to gallstones. Patients with chronic cholecystitis show wide variability in the thickening and fibrosis of the gallbladder wall and in the inflammatory infiltrate. The diagnosis is based on failure to visualize the gallbladder with oral cholecystography. After ruling out other sources of chronic abdominal pain (e.g., peptic ulcer disease, pancreatitis, and irritable bowel syndrome), a cholecystectomy may be performed to relieve symptoms.

D. **Choledocholithiasis** usually occurs due to a gallstone being passed into the common duct from the gallbladder or to a retained gallstone that was missed during operative cholangiography or common duct exploration. Occasionally, a stone forms de novo in the common duct, especially when there is stasis from ductal obstruction. Symptoms frequently are intermittent and include colicky pain in the right upper quadrant, fever, chills, and jaundice accompanied by elevated serum levels of alkaline phosphatase and the transaminases. Sepsis may result from **ascending cholangitis**, which is a closed space infection. Antibiotics are given as needed to control infection, but definitive treatment consists of surgical removal of the stone or endoscopic sphincterotomy and stone extraction. Patients who are poor surgical risks and in whom there is access to the biliary tree (i.e., with a **T tube**) may be treated with an infusion of mono-octanoin to dissolve the stones.

E. **Biliary dyskinesia** is a clinical syndrome of right upper quadrant symptoms, which is similar to chronic calculous cholecystitis but shows no abnormality of the biliary tree. An abnormality of biliary motor function is proposed, and manometric findings in patients with biliary dyskinesia are being studied in an effort to define this entity better. Patients may respond to smooth muscle relaxants (e.g., nitrates and calcium channel blocking agents) or to sphincterotomy.

F. **Biliary stricture** is a narrowing of the common bile duct generally due to a surgical injury or scarring subsequent to exploration of the common bile duct. Rarely, trauma or choledocholithiasis may result in a biliary stricture. Patients usually present with intermittent obstructive jaundice several weeks to months after biliary tract surgery. Cholangiography demonstrates the presence of a smooth concentric narrowing of the duct, with proximal dilatation a frequent finding. The usual treatment is surgical anastomosis of the dilatated proximal end of the bile duct to the intestine, but some patients may be treated with percutaneous transhepatic or endoscopic balloon dilation.

G. **Sclerosing cholangitis**, a rare disease that causes progressive narrowing of the bile ducts, generally is diagnosed in the third or fourth decade of life and is three times more common in men than in women. About 30% of patients have inflammatory bowel disease, but the biliary and intestinal diseases have independent clinical courses. The usual presenting symptom is pruritus. However, early diagnosis now is possible in asymptomatic patients who show marked elevation of the serum alkaline phosphatase levels on routine biochemical screening. ERCP or percutaneous cholangiography should establish the diagnosis. Treatment with corticosteroids, long-term antibiotics, or both has been used with varying success. Surgical anastomosis of the diseased duct to the intestine may be difficult or impossible. Endoscopic or percutaneous dilation of strictures is possible in some cases.

H. **Cystic malformations of the bile ducts**

1. **Choledochal cysts** present as jaundice, cholangitis, or a large cyst filled with numerous stones. Diagnosis may be made by cholangiography. Surgery is used to excise the cyst or to anastomose the cyst to the intestine.

2. **Caroli's disease** is characterized by saccular dilatation of the intrahepatic ducts, which may be associated with right upper quadrant pain, cholangitis, or both due to ductal stone formation. Hepatic fibrosis with portal hypertension may develop, especially in patients with medullary sponge kidney. Surgical decompression occasionally is helpful, and antibiotics are used during acute episodes of cholangitis.

I. **Tumors of the gallbladder**

1. **Adenocarcinoma** of the gallbladder is a disease of older women. The tumor affects three times as many women as it does men, and the average age at diagnosis is 65–75 years. Although most patients have associated gallstones, cancer develops in less than 1% of all patients with stones. Symptoms generally mimic those of acute or chronic cholecystitis. On physical examination, a mass may be palpable in the right upper quadrant, and obstructive jaundice may be seen secondary to local spread of the tumor to the common bile duct. A calcified gallbladder may be noted on abdominal x-ray. An operation consisting of cholecystectomy, lymph node dissection, and removal of a small portion of the adjacent liver is indicated if no obvious metastatic disease is found, but prognosis generally is poor.

2. **Benign tumors** of the gallbladder include abnormalities of the mucosal lining (e.g., adenoma-

tous hyperplasia, cholesterolosis, and cholesterol polyps), cystic changes in the glands, and papillary adenomas. These lesions usually are asymptomatic. However, in some patients with no other demonstrable causes for abdominal pain, cholecystectomy has provided relief of symptoms.

J. Tumors of the bile duct. Adenocarcinoma of the bile duct (**cholangiocarcinoma**) is a disease of older men and is not associated with gallstones.

1. **Etiology.** An increased risk is noted in patients with ulcerative colitis and in those exposed to benzene or toluene derivatives. Parasitic infection of the biliary system has been linked to the high rate of cholangiocarcinoma in Oriental populations.

2. **Pathology.** Most tumors are of the scirrhous or papillary type. An extensive desmoplastic reaction may make diagnosis difficult. Two-thirds of the tumors are located in the common bile duct or at the bifurcation of the common hepatic duct (**Klatskin tumors**).

3. **Clinical features.** Jaundice, with or without pain, is present in most patients, and weight loss also is common. Pruritus may be severe. Common duct tumors causing obstruction distal to the cystic duct result in a palpable gallbladder that is not tender.

4. **Laboratory data.** Serum alkaline phosphatase levels are markedly increased as are direct and total bilirubin levels. Serum transaminase levels show smaller increases and generally are less than 200 mg/dl.

5. **Diagnosis.** Dilatation of the intrahepatic ducts is revealed by ultrasonography or CT, and percutaneous cholangiography or ERCP generally suggests the diagnosis. The differential diagnosis includes pancreatic carcinoma, choledocholithiasis, biliary stricture, and sclerosing cholangitis.

6. **Therapy.** Surgery is the treatment of choice for approachable lesions; however, most hepatic duct tumors are not surgically resectable. A pancreaticoduodenectomy (Whipple procedure) may be used to treat distal lesions that have no obvious tumor extension. Palliative procedures include biliary bypass surgery and stenting tubes left in at the time of the percutaneous cholangiography. Frequent replacement of these tubes may be necessary as they are prone to blockage. Cure is rare and is achieved in only 10% of patients, but because the tumors are slow growing, palliative bypass surgery or stenting may offer patients several years of symptomatic relief.

IX. DISEASES OF THE LIVER

A. Acute liver disease (Table 5-2)

1. **Acute viral hepatitis**, one of the most common health problems in the world, is caused by any one of several viruses.
   a. **Etiology**
      (1) **Hepatitis A** is an RNA virus transmitted primarily by the fecal-oral route. The incubation period is 2–6 weeks. Acute infection is anicteric in 50% of cases. Hepatitis A does not lead to chronic disease or a carrier state.
      (2) **Hepatitis B** is a DNA virus transmitted parenterally. Individuals at high risk include intravenous drug abusers, homosexual men, and those exposed to blood and blood products (e.g., patients and health professionals in dialysis units). The incubation period ranges from 1 to 6 months. About 10% of patients develop chronic disease or a persistent carrier state.
      (3) **Non-A, non-B hepatitis** probably is caused by more than one virus and usually is transmitted by blood transfusions. The incubation period may be as short as 2 weeks or as long as 6 months. Up to 20%–30% of patients develop chronic hepatitis. Of these, about 50% have chronic active hepatitis and many go on to develop cirrhosis.
      (4) **Delta agent** is a small, defective RNA virus that is infectious only in the presence of hepatitis B infection because it relies on hepatitis B proteins for replication. It can, therefore, complicate acute hepatitis B infection but is seen more commonly as a "super infection" with a rise in liver function tests in a patient with chronic hepatitis B. Delta hepatitis generally has a chronic, severe clinical course.
      (5) **Other viruses** that can cause acute hepatitis include the Epstein-Barr virus, cytomegalovirus, herpes simplex virus, and those causing yellow fever and rubella.
   b. **Pathology.** The lesions of acute viral hepatitis are similar regardless of etiology and include mononuclear cell infiltration, cellular ballooning and necrosis, and condensed cytoplasm with pyknotic nuclei (**acidophilic bodies**).

Table 5-2. Comparison of Viral Hepatitis Types A, B, Non-A, Non-B, and Delta

	Hepatitis A	Hepatitis B	Non-A, Non-B Hepatitis	Delta Hepatitis
Type of Virus	RNA	DNA	? (clinical syndrome similar to hepatitis B)	RNA (hepatitis B required for replication)
Incidence in the United States (%)	41	11	?	?
Incidence after Blood Transfusion (%)	0 to extremely rare	10–20	60–70 (?)	?
Incubation Period	2–6 weeks	1–6 months	2–20 weeks (?)	1–6 months
Infectivity Stage	Last 3 weeks of inoculation to 1–2 weeks after jaundice occurs	During hepatitis B surface antigen positivity	?	?
Complications	Fulminant hepatitis (rare)	Fulminant hepatitis (rare but more common than with hepatitis A); chronic active hepatitis	Fulminant hepatitis (rare but more common than with hepatitis A); chronic active hepatitis	Present in 20%–50% of cases of fulminant hepatitis and/or chronic active hepatitis
Mechanism of Spread	Fecal-oral	Parenteral	Parenteral	Parenteral
Prevention	Pooled immune serum globulin	Hepatitis B immune globulin; vaccination	Pooled immune serum globulin	?
Carrier State	Rare, if ever	Rare	?	?

   c. Clinical features of viral hepatitis include:
     (1) Malaise, anorexia, and fatigue
     (2) Arthritis and urticaria, which are especially common in hepatitis B and ascribed to circulating immune complexes
     (3) Influenza-like syndrome, which is especially common in hepatitis A
     (4) Jaundice (with dark urine or light stools), which is seen in 50% of cases
     (5) Hepatic enlargement or tenderness
     (6) Splenomegaly, which occurs in 20% of patients
   d. Diagnosis of acute viral hepatitis is based on the above clinical features as well as such laboratory findings as elevated levels of the transaminases [i.e., SGOT and serum glutamic-pyruvic transaminase (SGPT)], serum bilirubin, and serum alkaline phosphatase. In addition, the rise in bilirubin exceeds the increase in alkaline phosphatase.
     (1) In hepatitis A, the IgM antibody is elevated early in the course followed by an elevation of the IgG antibody in 2–3 months.
     (2) In hepatitis B, a positive surface antigen usually is diagnostic. However, since this is an early finding, it may be necessary to follow the rise of anti-core and later of anti-surface antibodies to document acute infection (Fig. 5-1).
     (3) There is no specific test for non-A, non-B hepatitis.
     (4) Delta hepatitis may be diagnosed by a rising delta antibody titer. A persistently high or slowly falling hepatitis delta antibody is seen in chronic states.
   e. Therapy is supportive and includes intravenous fluids for hydration, for correction of electrolyte abnormalities, and to provide caloric intake if nausea and vomiting are present. Vitamin K should be given if the protime is elevated.
   f. Clinical course and complications. Nearly all cases of acute viral hepatitis are benign, with most patients demonstrating normal results on liver function testing by 8–10 weeks. Complications may occur, however, and include the following conditions.
     (1) Fulminant hepatitis is a rare complication of hepatitis A but occurs in 1%–2% of patients with hepatitis B and non-A, non-B hepatitis. It is an especially common complication of delta hepatitis super infection in patients with chronic hepatitis B antigenemia. Patients usually present with progressive jaundice, hepatic encephalopathy, and ascites. Hepatorenal syndrome is common. Elevated prothrombin time is an early sign. The initially elevated serum transaminases later fall, and liver size decreases as a result of necrosis of the liver parenchyma. The mortality rate varies with age and approaches 90%–100%, especially in patients over age 60.
     (2) Chronic persistent hepatitis may follow hepatitis B or non-A, non-B hepatitis and is defined as an elevation of serum transaminases for a period of more than 6 months. Liver biopsy shows a periportal lymphocytic infiltrate but no extension beyond the portal limiting triad and no fibrosis. Most patients are asymptomatic, although some report

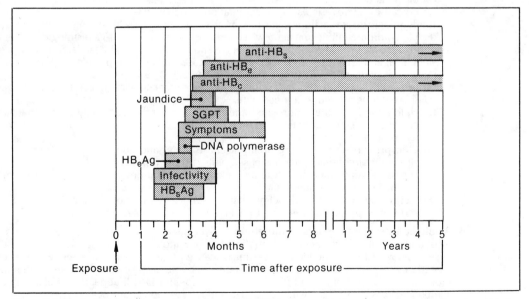

Figure 5-1. Typical clinical course of acute hepatitis B. HB_sAg = hepatitis B surface antigen; HB_eAg = hepatitis B e antigen; *SGPT* = serum glutamic-pyruvic transaminase; *anti-HB$_c$* = hepatitis B core antibody; *anti-HB$_e$* = hepatitis B e antibody; and *anti-HB$_s$* = hepatitis B surface antibody.

fatigue, anorexia, and abdominal pain. Results of liver function testing are only mildly abnormal. The clinical course is benign.

  (3) **Chronic active hepatitis** is another complication of hepatitis B and non-A, non-B hepatitis, in which serum transaminase levels are raised for a period of more than 6 months. The pathology shows inflammation, necrosis, and fibrosis bridging portal areas or between portal areas and central veins. Patients may progress to cirrhosis, and on physical examination may have splenomegaly, spider angiomata, caput medusae, and other signs of chronic liver disease. There is no effective treatment, but recent trials of interferon and other antiviral agents have produced promising results. Liver biopsy is necessary for diagnosis.

  (4) A **chronic carrier state** for hepatitis B surface antigen exists in 0.2% of the population of the United States. A carrier state also may exist for non-A, non-B hepatitis since blood donated by apparently normal individuals may transmit this disease when transfused. Carriers of hepatitis B virus may have an increased risk of hepatoma.

  (5) **Cholestatic hepatitis** may occur and is characterized by the alkaline phosphatase level being elevated disproportionately to the transaminase level. The clinical course is typical of acute viral hepatitis, but this presentation must be differentiated from biliary tract obstruction.

  (6) **Aplastic anemia** is seen rarely after acute viral hepatitis. The mortality rate is high, and no treatment has been proven effective.

  (7) **Pancreatitis** is noted in 10%–40% of cases.

g. Prevention

  (1) Immune serum globulin is effective when administered after exposure to hepatitis A and also may be partially protective against hepatitis B and non-A, non-B hepatitis.

  (2) Hepatitis B immune globulin, which is immune globulin containing high titers of antibody to hepatitis B, conveys passive immunity and is recommended after confirmed exposure to hepatitis B (e.g., from skin puncture by a contaminated needle).

  (3) Hepatitis B vaccine, a preparation of the surface antigen, conveys active immunity and is recommended for individuals at high risk, such as dialysis patients and medical personnel with frequent exposure to blood products.

2. Drug-induced liver disease may follow exposure to virtually any drug and presents as a variety of clinical syndromes and histologic findings. Any given drug may induce liver disease that overlaps two or more categories of disease mechanisms (Table 5-3).

  a. Direct toxicity by a chemical (e.g., carbon tetrachloride) or a metabolite (e.g., acetaminophen) usually represents a dose-related injury. Acetaminophen overdose can be treated with N-acetylcysteine, which binds to the toxic metabolite and provides cysteine for glutathione synthesis.

  b. Liver disease may result from **interference with** the **metabolism** of bilirubin (e.g., by estrogens and androgens) or with protein synthesis (e.g., by intravenous tetracycline, which causes microvesicular fat accumulation in hepatocytes).

  c. Immunologic drug reactions can cause a variety of syndromes, including cholestatic jaundice (a syndrome mimicking acute viral hepatitis), a condition with a histologic picture indistinguishable from chronic active hepatitis, and granulomatous hepatitis. Skin rashes, eosinophilia, and fever may be present. In some cases, it has been postulated that a drug or metabolite binds to the liver cell membrane and acts as a **hapten**.

  (1) **Isoniazid** causes a clinical condition that is similar to viral hepatitis and has been shown to be related to a metabolite.

  (2) **Halothane** and other fluorinated anesthetics frequently cause only mild hepatitis or postoperative fever after first exposure but may cause fulminant hepatitis and death on reexposure.

  (3) **Chlorpromazine** and **chlorpropamide** cause cholestatic jaundice. An inflammatory infiltrate that frequently includes eosinophils is shown on liver biopsy.

  (4) **Diphenylhydantoin** causes a serum sickness–like syndrome, which may result in massive hepatic necrosis and death.

  (5) **Methyldopa** may cause the clinical and histologic findings of chronic active hepatitis, and some authors believe that a metabolite is responsible.

3. Alcoholic liver disease refers to the group of liver disorders caused by acute and chronic alcoholism. Acute effects include **alcoholic fatty liver** and **alcoholic hepatitis**, which are discussed below. Chronic alcoholism is a major cause of **cirrhosis of the liver**, which is discussed in section IX B 2 b. In the United States, alcoholic liver disease represents the fourth most common cause of death of individuals aged 35–55 years. It appears that alcohol consumption of less than 80 g/day in men and 40 g/day in (nonpregnant) women generally is not associated with alcoholic liver disease.

  a. Alcoholic fatty liver occurs because alcohol alters normal lipid metabolism. Most patients

Table 5-3. Agents of Drug-Induced Liver Disease

Drugs Causing Direct Toxicity	Drugs Causing Altered Metabolism	Drugs Causing Immune-Mediated Reactions			
		Viral Hepatitis-like	Granulomatous Hepatitis	Inflammatory Cholestasis	Chronic Active Hepatitis
Acetaminophen	Androgens	Halothane	Allopurinol	Chlorpromazine	Acetaminophen
Aspirin	Corticosteroids (?)	Isoniazid	Hydralazine	Chlorpropamide	Aspirin
Alcohol	Estrogens	Oxacillin	Phenylbutazone	Erythromycin	Isoniazid
Carbon tetrachloride	Ethanol	Phenytoin	Phenytoin	estolate	Methyldopa
Heavy metals	Intravenous	Sulfonamides	Quinidine	Propylthiouracil	Nitrofurantoin
Methotrexate	tetracycline	Valproic acid	Sulfa drugs	Thiazides	Oxyphenisatin
Mushroom toxins (phalloidin and phallin)					
Phosphorus					

present with hepatomegaly but otherwise are asymptomatic unless they have other systemic problems related to alcohol use (e.g., pancreatitis and delirium tremens). Laboratory abnormalities include increases in gamma glutamyl transpeptidase (GGPT), serum transaminases, and alkaline phosphatase. Histologic examination shows large droplet fatty change in the liver. The prognosis is excellent for patients who completely abstain from alcohol consumption.

   b. Alcoholic hepatitis is an acute syndrome that generally occurs in the setting of heavy alcohol consumption. Many patients are reported to have ingested in excess of 100 g of alcohol daily for more than 1 year. (Approximately 100 g of alcohol are contained in 8 oz of 100-proof whiskey, in 30 oz of wine, and in eight 12-oz cans of beer.) The role of decreased vitamin and protein intake is controversial.

   (1) Clinical features include fever, jaundice, hepatomegaly, and liver tenderness. Ascites, encephalopathy, and variceal bleeding occasionally are present.

   (2) Laboratory data include leukocytosis, increased SGOT (usually less than 350 IU/ml), elevated serum bilirubin, decreased serum albumin, and a modest increase in serum alkaline phosphatase. Occasionally, a cholestatic phase is present with marked elevations in the alkaline phosphatase and direct bilirubin. The SGPT almost always is lower than the SGOT. Alcohol-induced thrombocytopenia is present in 10% of patients.

   (3) Diagnosis is based on liver biopsy that reveals large droplet fatty liver, polymorphonuclear infiltration, alcoholic hyaline (Mallory bodies), hepatocyte necrosis, and, occasionally, sclerosis of central veins.

   (4) Therapy is supportive and includes a daily diet of 2500–3000 kcal with supplemental B vitamins (especially thiamine) and folate. Absolute abstinence from alcohol is crucial. Corticosteroids have a controversial therapeutic role but may be useful in very severe cases.

B. Chronic liver disease

   1. Chronic active hepatitis most commonly is caused by viral infection or drugs. When associated with neither of these etiologies, chronic active hepatitis generally is thought to be immunologically mediated, although an immunologic mechanism has not been proven. This form of chronic active hepatitis sometimes is called **lupoid hepatitis** because the typical patient is a young woman with elevated antinuclear antibody.

   a. Clinical features include malaise, fatigue, and vasculitis. As the disease progresses, the clinical picture is dominated by manifestations of chronic liver disease, including ascites, encephalopathy, and variceal bleeding.

   b. Diagnosis is based on liver biopsy that shows piecemeal necrosis and bridging fibrosis. The serum transaminases are persistently elevated to levels that often are 10 times the normal levels. Elevated antinuclear antibody is present in 50% of patients, and anti–smooth muscle antibody is found in 75%.

   c. Therapy with high-dose corticosteroids, azathioprine, or both is beneficial in the immune-mediated type of chronic active hepatitis but usually not in the drug- and virus-associated diseases. Treatment is continued until the serum transaminases fall to less than twice the normal levels and a repeat liver biopsy shows resolution of the inflammation (generally after a period of more than 1 year).

   2. Cirrhosis of the liver

   a. Overview of pathology. Two basic types of liver cirrhosis occur, but the sine qua non of all cirrhotic liver disease is the presence of fibrosis with the formation of nodules that lack a central vein.

   (1) Chronic sclerosing cirrhosis is characterized by minimal regenerative activity of the hepatocytes, resulting in fibrosis without substantial nodule formation. The liver is small and hard.

   (2) Nodular cirrhosis is characterized by regenerative activity and the appearance of numerous fine nodules. The liver initially may be quite large.

   b. Alcohol-induced cirrhosis. Chronic alcohol abuse causes cirrhosis of the liver (**Laennec's cirrhosis**), which in most cases is thought to be a sequela of alcoholic hepatitis. The **clinical features** of alcohol-induced cirrhosis reflect impaired blood flow through the liver due to obstruction by fibrotic bands, resulting in portal hypertension, and to a decrease in hepatocytes available for metabolic functions. Long-term alcohol use also may be directly toxic to the testis, resulting in testicular atrophy and impotence. These effects are compounded in men by increased circulating estrogens, which cause spider angiomata, gynecomastia, and palmar erythema. **Complications** of alcohol-induced cirrhosis are described below.

   (1) Ascites

   (a) Pathogenesis. Increased back pressure into capillaries as well as decreased oncotic pressure because of decreased albumin synthesis allow accumulation of a transudative fluid in the peritoneal cavity. In addition, increased circulating aldosterone (possibly secondary to altered liver metabolism) contributes to Na^+ and water retention.

(b) Diagnosis may be obvious on physical examination if fluid accumulation is large. Ultrasonography is effective for detecting small amounts of fluid. Paracentesis, which may require guidance through ultrasonography, yields a straw-colored fluid with less than 2.5 g/dl of protein, a white blood cell count of less than $300/mm^3$ (usually mononuclear), a normal glucose level, and a low serum amylase level.

(c) Therapy is based on Na^+ restriction (usually 500 mg/24 hr) and bed rest (to decrease endogenous aldosterone production). Fluid restriction may be necessary if hyponatremia develops. Aldosterone antagonists (e.g., spironolactone) and mild diuretics are used if initial measures fail. Because peritoneal lymphatics have a limited ability to mobilize ascites, weight loss should be limited to 2 lb/day unless peripheral edema exists.

(d) Complications include respiratory compromise and rupture of the umbilicus in cases of massive ascites. Infection of even a small amount of fluid (e.g., due to spontaneous bacterial peritonitis) can be fatal.

(2) Varices occur due to the development of collateral vessels that bypass the obstructed liver and are common in the esophagus and hemorrhoidal plexus.

(a) Diagnosis of esophagogastric varices may be suggested by an upper gastrointestinal series but is best made by endoscopy. Endoscopy is essential in the acutely bleeding patient since mortality is high (40%–50% for each episode of bleeding) and early treatment can be lifesaving.

(b) Short-term therapy with vasopressin by continuous intravenous infusion is effective in 60% of patients. Balloon tamponade with a **Sengstaken-Blakemore tube** controls bleeding in 80% of patients but carries a risk of aspiration and esophageal rupture. Emergency surgery has a 50% mortality rate. Endoscopic sclerotherapy also may be used in acute cases.

(c) Long-term therapy to reduce the chance of rebleeding includes multiple sclerotherapy procedures until all varices are obliterated and propranolol to reduce portal pressure. Surgical portal decompression decreases the frequency of bleeding but does not increase survival rates because of increased encephalopathy and liver failure. In Japan, devascularization of the distal esophagus and proximal stomach (Sugiura procedure) has been effective.

(3) Portosystemic encephalopathy is a reversible neurologic syndrome characterized by mood changes, confusion, drowsiness, disorientation, and coma.

(a) Etiology. The **primary cause** of hepatic encephalopathy is unclear. Elevated ammonia levels are found in the blood. More recently implicated, however, are false neurotransmitters and elevated levels of mercaptans and fatty acids. In addition, increased levels of aromatic amino acids and decreased levels of branched-chain amino acids are noted in the blood, brain, and urine. **Secondary causes** of hepatic encephalopathy are thought to include:

(i) Azotemia, due to increased nitrogen load

(ii) Constipation, which causes increased ammonia production and absorption due to prolonged contact of intestinal contents with the gastrointestinal tract

(iii) Increased dietary protein, which causes increased production of ammonia and other nitrogenous wastes

(iv) Gastrointestinal bleeding, which delivers a protein load to the gastrointestinal tract

(v) Hypokalemia

(vi) Alkalosis, which together with hypokalemia leads to impaired renal excretion of ammonia and to increased transfer of ammonia across the blood-brain barrier

(vii) Infection, which leads to increased tissue catabolism and increased protein load

(viii) Sedatives, whose direct depressant effect on the brain is compounded by decreased hepatic catabolism of the drugs

(b) Therapy includes reversal of any of the secondary causes noted above. In addition:

(i) Lactulose effectively decreases colonic pH and traps ammonium ion (NH_4^+) in the gastrointestinal tract. It also is an effective cathartic.

(ii) Neomycin decreases intestinal flora, which convert gastrointestinal proteins into ammonia.

(iii) Dietary protein should be limited to less than 40 g/day.

(4) Hepatorenal syndrome is a progressive renal failure that occurs in patients with severe liver disease. It is a **functional** renal failure because the kidneys are morphologically normal and function well when transplanted into normal recipients. The mortality rate in hepatorenal syndrome is 90%–100%.

    (a) Etiology. Although the exact mechanism of hepatorenal syndrome is not known, several factors are implicated, including:
        (i) Afferent arteriolar vasoconstriction, which leads to increased renal vascular constriction
        (ii) Relative shunting of blood from the cortex to the medulla of the kidney
        (iii) Decreased glomerular filtration rate
        (iv) Decreased renal blood flow
    (b) Diagnosis is suggested by the combination of oliguria (i.e., urine output of less than 300 ml/24 hr) with rising blood urea nitrogen (BUN) and creatinine concentrations in a patient with severe liver disease. Additional laboratory findings include urinary Na^+ concentration of less than 10 mEq/L, concentrated urine, and benign urine sediment. It is important to rule out other causes of oliguria (e.g., acute tubular necrosis, hypovolemia, and urinary tract obstruction).
    (c) Therapy generally is unsuccessful. No drugs have been shown to be beneficial. Success occasionally is reported with LeVeen shunts, portacaval shunts, and liver transplantation.
  (5) Coagulation defects usually are due to decreased hepatic synthesis of clotting factors. In addition, splenomegaly may contribute to thrombocytopenia.
c. Nonalcoholic cirrhosis may be caused by a variety of disease processes and toxins but, in general, has clinical features that are similar to those of alcohol-induced cirrhosis.
  (1) Primary biliary cirrhosis is a disease of unknown etiology. The usual patient age at diagnosis is 40–60 years, and 90% of patients are women.
    (a) Pathogenesis. The mechanism of primary biliary cirrhosis is thought to be immunologic and involves inflammatory destruction of small intrahepatic biliary ducts. Early histologic changes include lymphocytic infiltration and periductal granuloma formation. Later in the disease process, the portal areas may show an absence of ducts.
    (b) Clinical features
        (i) There is a lack of symptoms early in the course of this disease. However, an early diagnosis often is suspected on the basis of a marked increase in the alkaline phosphatase level noted on routine biochemical screening.
        (ii) The first symptom usually is pruritus, which may be devastatingly severe, especially at night.
        (iii) Jaundice occurs in later stages of the disease, as do osteopenia (in 25% of patients) and xanthomas (in about 10% of patients).
        (iv) In addition, primary biliary cirrhosis is associated with such conditions as Sjögren's syndrome (in 75% of patients), the presence of antithyroid antibody (in 25% of patients), rheumatoid arthritis (in 5% of patients), and the syndrome of calcinosis, Raynaud's phenomenon, esophageal motility dysfunction, sclerodactyly, and telangiectasia—**CREST syndrome**—(in 3% of patients).
    (c) Diagnosis is made by the constellation of increased serum cholesterol, markedly increased alkaline phosphatase (four to six times the normal level), increased direct bilirubin, and the presence of a positive antimitochondrial antibody, which is found in over 90% of patients. The liver biopsy shows characteristic changes. Extrahepatic biliary obstruction must be ruled out.
    (d) Therapy is supportive and includes administration of antipruritic agents and supplementation of vitamins D and K and calcium. Medium-chain triglycerides, which do not require bile salt micelles for adsorption, may be used as a dietary supplement. The pruritus may respond to cholestyramine, which binds bile salts in the intestine. Effective results recently have been achieved with certain drugs (azathioprine, colchicine, and chlorambucil) and with hepatic transplantation.
  (2) Secondary biliary cirrhosis usually occurs after several years of biliary tract obstruction.
    (a) Etiology includes common bile duct stones, common duct strictures, cholangiocarcinoma, ampullar carcinoma, sclerosing cholangitis, and chronic pancreatitis with compression of the common duct as it traverses the pancreatic head.
    (b) Clinical features are similar to those of primary biliary cirrhosis but may be superceded by manifestations of the underlying disease. In addition, patients may develop cholangitis with shaking chills, fever, leukocytosis, and jaundice. Antimitochondrial antibodies usually are not present.
    (c) Therapy is aimed at relieving the obstruction and includes surgery, external drainage, and placement of an indwelling stent.
d. Cardiac cirrhosis is a rare, late manifestation of severe prolonged right ventricular failure, which is most often seen with rheumatic heart disease (either mitral or aortic stenosis with tricuspid regurgitation). Constrictive pericarditis and severe cardiomyopathy also may be associated with cardiac cirrhosis. Clinical features include an enlarged liver, ascites, and

splenomegaly. Prothrombin time often is prolonged and precludes the use of anti-coagulants in treatment of the valvular lesion. Prognosis depends on the course of the cardiac disease.

  e. Other causes of cirrhosis include Wilson's disease, α_1-antitrypsin deficiency, hemochromatosis, drug-induced liver disease, and virus-induced cirrhosis of the liver.

  f. Vascular problems mimicking cirrhosis

    (1) Budd-Chiari syndrome or **hepatic vein thrombosis** is due to hypercoagulable states, abdominal trauma, and birth control pills. Patients usually present with ascites, and liver biopsy shows centrilobular congestion. Attempts to catheterize the hepatic vein are unsuccessful, and the mortality rate is 50%–90%. Portacaval shunts may prolong survival.

    (2) Splenic vein thrombosis is due to abdominal trauma, pancreatitis, and tumor. Although the portal vein remains patent, esophagogastric varices develop as splenic vein collaterals. Diagnosis is made by angiography, and therapy with splenectomy is curative.

  g. Nodular transformation of the liver is a noncirrhotic cause of portal hypertension characterized by the unexplained development of small nodules, especially in the perihilar area. Recurrent variceal bleeding may occur.

3. Liver abscess

  a. Amebic liver abscess. Of the six *Entamoeba* species found in the human colon, *E. histolytica* is the only true pathogen. In the United States, homosexual men and institutionalized individuals are at greatest risk for amebic liver abscess. This disease also is common where diarrheal disease due to *E. histolytica* is endemic.

    (1) Clinical features include right upper quadrant pain and fever. Pleuritic pain, chills, and night sweats also may be noted. There is a history of intestinal amebiasis in 50% of patients.

    (2) Laboratory data. More than 50% of patients reveal elevations in the white cell count (> 20,000/mm³), serum transaminases, and serum bilirubin. The serum alkaline phosphatase level is abnormal in approximately 80% of affected individuals.

    (3) Diagnosis is suggested by a filling defect demonstrated in the liver through the use of gallium scanning. Ultrasonography and CT also may be helpful in the diagnosis of amebic liver abscess. Aspiration of a cystic cavity may reveal "anchovy paste" fluid with trophozoites. Serologic tests (e.g., the indirect hemagglutination and gel diffusion tests) are positive in 95% of cases.

    (4) Therapy with amebicides (e.g., metronidazole, choloroquine, and diiodohydroxyquin) may be effective alone or may be combined with CT-directed aspiration of the abscess cavity. Liver scanning should be continued until healing occurs.

    (5) Complications include rupture of the cyst into the pleural space, lung, bowel, and retroperitoneum. Rarely, a cyst will extend to the body surface.

  b. Pyogenic liver abscess usually is due to biliary tract disease, including acute cholecystitis and cholangitis. Other infections (e.g., appendicitis and diverticulitis) as well as intrinsic hepatic lesions also are important causes. In 10% of cases, the etiology cannot be determined. About 70% of abscesses contain mixed flora, with the most commonly found organisms being anaerobes, *E. coli, Klebsiella* species, *Staphylococcus aureus*, and streptococci.

    (1) Clinical features include fever, chills, right upper quadrant pain, anorexia, and nausea. Pleuritic pain occasionally is seen, and weight loss is common. Tender hepatomegaly is present in 50% of cases. The alkaline phosphatase is elevated in about 80% of patients, jaundice is present in about 33%, and blood cultures are positive in 40%. CT combined with liver scanning, ultrasonography, or both can be used to detect an abscess greater than 2 cm.

    (2) Diagnosis is suggested by the clinical presentations and can be confirmed by CT- or ultrasonography-guided aspiration.

    (3) Therapy. Antibiotics, with or without external drainage, frequently are successful and necessary for multiple small abscesses. Treatment usually is continued for 4–6 weeks. Occasionally, surgical drainage may be required.

  c. Focal hepatic candidiasis is a recently described entity consisting of hepatic and splenic granulomas containing *Candida albicans* hyphae in immunocompromised hosts. Most patients have previously received cytosine arabinoside for acute leukemia.

    (1) Clinical features include a fever of unknown origin in an immunocompromised host. Signs of oropharyngeal candidiasis are seen in patients, and right upper quadrant pain or tenderness may be present.

    (2) Diagnosis is made by liver biopsy. At laparotomy or laparoscopy, small white nodules less than 5 mm in width are noted. Liver function abnormalities include modest bilirubin and enzyme elevation with an increase in alkaline phosphatase.

(3) **Therapy** consists of systemic amphotericin B, often in conjunction with 5-fluorocyto-sine.

4. Hepatic cysts
  a. Solitary cysts, generally found in the right lobe of the liver, usually are asymptomatic but may cause pain and fever secondary to bleeding, infection, or rupture.
  b. Polycystic liver disease is the presence of multiple cysts that range from several millimeters to greater than 10–15 centimeters in diameter. Like solitary cysts, most cysts in polycystic liver disease are asymptomatic except in cases involving hemorrhage, infection, or rupture. Renal cysts are found in 50% of patients; cysts also may be noted in the pancreas, spleen, and lungs. Results of liver function testing usually are normal, although mild elevation of the serum alkaline phosphatase may be seen. Surgical aspiration or decompression occasionally is necessary.
  c. Hydatid cysts are formed when the infecting organism (i.e., *Echinococcus granulosus* or *Echinococcus multilocularis*) is ingested and travels via the portal circulation to the liver. The cyst usually enlarges for 10–20 years after the initial infection before it becomes symptomatic. This disease is most common in Greece, France, Italy, South America, and Iceland and may be seen elsewhere in the descendants of individuals from these regions. Complications include rupture, infection, hemorrhage, and slow leakage causing allergic manifestations. The clinical features include calcification of a solitary cyst (seen in 50% of patients) and the presence of daughter cysts within a larger cyst. Diagnosis is made by a positive complement fixation or indirect hemagglutination test. Liver biopsy and aspiration are not suggested because leakage may cause fatal anaphylaxis. Treatment is surgical.
  d. Peliosis hepatitis is due to blood-filled multiple hepatic cysts. The liver often has a mottled blue appearance. Rupture with bleeding may be fatal. There is an association with tuberculosis, therapy with androgenic steroids, and the use of oral contraceptives. Progressive hepatomegaly with liver failure may result. CT may reveal multiple defects. A percutaneous liver biopsy reveals characteristic changes but is dangerous because of the vascular nature of the lesions.

5. Granulomatous hepatitis most often is secondary to systemic infections (e.g., tuberculosis and sarcoidosis), fungal infections, syphilis, and viral infections (e.g., infectious mononucleosis, cytomegalovirus infection, and varicella). Q fever, parasitic diseases, Hodgkin's disease, and beryllium toxicity also may cause granulomatous hepatitis. In addition, granulomatous hepatitis may be a manifestation of drug reactions involving phenylbutazone, sulfa drugs, hydralazine, or allopurinol. Occasionally, no cause can be found. Symptoms include weakness, fatigue, markedly increased erythrocyte sedimentation rate, and fever. Diagnosis is made by liver biopsy. Therapy for the secondary form of granulomatous hepatitis includes withdrawal of the offending agent and treatment of the underlying lesion. The idiopathic form may respond to corticosteroid therapy.

C. Systemic diseases with prominent liver involvement

1. Alpha$_1$-antitrypsin deficiency is a genetic defect of the glycoprotein that normally inhibits proteolytic enzymes such as trypsin, chymotrypsin, and elastase. There are 24 alleles in the **protease inhibitor (Pi) system**. Ninety percent of the population of the United States is phenotype PiMM. The ZZ genotype is homozygous for the disease state, and patients have less than 20% of normal serum levels of α_1-antitrypsin. Individuals with phenotype PiMZ have about 50%–60% of normal levels. Homozygotes (PiZZ) usually present with liver disease in childhood. PiMZ heterozygotes, especially those who smoke, may develop liver disease and chronic obstructive pulmonary disease as adults (see also Chapter 2, section I B 3). Not all individuals with the abnormal genotypes develop disease. Diagnosis is made on the basis of a decreased α_1-globulin level on a protein electrophoresis, a decreased α_1-antitrypsin level in the serum, and by Pi typing. Liver biopsy reveals PAS-positive globules in portal areas. There is no effective therapy. Liver transplantation may be used in advanced cases.

2. Amyloidosis involves the liver in 50% of cases. Patients have hepatomegaly on physical examination but usually are asymptomatic. Results of liver function testing often are normal but may reveal a marked elevation of serum alkaline phosphatase.

3. Hemochromatosis is an inherited disorder (thought to be autosomal recessive), in which increased adsorption of iron leads to iron deposition in the liver, heart, pancreas, and other organs. Men are more commonly affected than women.
  a. Clinical features include hepatomegaly, hyperpigmentation, and abnormalities of the cardiac conduction system, testes, and joints. Cirrhosis and diabetes also may develop.
  b. Laboratory findings include elevated serum transaminases, increased serum iron with elevated percent saturation, and high serum ferritin. Liver biopsy shows iron deposits in both hepatocytes and Kupffer cells. This finding rules out secondary iron overload (hemo-

siderosis), in which iron is deposited in Kupffer cells alone. A skin or intestinal biopsy as well as an analysis of family members for elevated ferritin levels also may be helpful in the differential diagnosis.

    c. Therapy. Repeated phlebotomy (usually once or twice weekly for several months or years) decreases total body iron stores, which may be at 10 times the normal level. Phlebotomy is continued until anemia develops or serum iron and ferritin levels normalize. Untreated patients have an increased risk of hepatoma.

4. Sarcoidosis. About 70% of patients with sarcoidosis have granulomas in the liver. Patients usually do not have symptoms referable to the liver, but an increase in serum alkaline phosphatase may be noted. Forty percent of patients have hepatomegaly. A liver biopsy showing noncaseating granulomas may aid in the diagnosis.

5. Wilson's disease is an autosomal recessive disease characterized by excessive copper deposition, which, if untreated, may lead to fulminant hepatic failure. Copper also is deposited in the brain, kidney, and cornea, which causes Kayser-Fleischer rings. CNS disease may be prominent if the diagnosis is made in adulthood. Diagnosis is suggested by decreased serum ceruloplasmin levels and is confirmed by an increased hepatic copper concentration in a liver biopsy sample. Treatment with D-penicillamine still is controversial.

6. Liver disease of pregnancy

    a. Cholestasis usually is noted in the last trimester of pregnancy and is benign. Patients may complain of pruritus and jaundice, and all symptoms disappear rapidly following delivery. The syndrome is thought to be mediated by estrogens, progesterone, or both, and subsequent use of oral contraceptives or pregnancy may cause a recurrence of symptoms.

    b. Acute fatty liver is a severe disease usually occurring in a primagravida in the last trimester of pregnancy. Fulminant liver failure may develop, and an association with toxemia has been reported. Prognosis is poor but is improved by prompt delivery. Pathologic changes in the liver include small droplet fatty change similar to that seen in fatty liver induced by tetracycline and valproic acid.

D. Inherited disorders of bilirubin metabolism

1. Gilbert's syndrome occurs in 7% of the population of the United States. Decreased uridine diphosphate (UDP) glucuronyl transferase activity leads to mild unconjugated hyperbilirubinemia usually less than 3 mg/dl, which increases after fasting.

2. Crigler-Najjar syndrome exists in two forms. **Type I** is very rare and is characterized by an absence of hepatic UDP glucuronyl transferase activity. Patients usually die in infancy. **Type II** also is rare and is characterized by markedly diminished hepatic UDP glucuronyl transferase, leading to unconjugated hyperbilirubinemia in the range of 5–25 mg/dl. Phenobarbitol may be used to induce microsomal enzyme activity. In most cases, there are no clinical sequellae.

3. Rotor's syndrome is a rare autosomal recessive condition. Impaired transport of conjugated bilirubin out of the hepatocyte leads to conjugated hyperbilirubinemia in the range of 2–10 mg/dl. The liver biopsy is normal, and the clinical course is benign.

4. Dubin-Johnson syndrome is similar to Rotor's syndrome, except that liver biopsy shows the accumulation of a dark pigment within hepatocytes. The elevated serum bilirubin may respond somewhat to phenobarbitol therapy.

E. Tumors of the liver

1. Benign tumors

    a. Hepatic adenomas usually occur in women of childbearing age and are more common in those who use birth control pills.

        (1) Clinical features may be completely absent. Some patients report right upper quadrant fullness. Occasionally, spontaneous rupture of the adenoma leads to intra-abdominal hemorrhage, which is fatal in 25% of patients.

        (2) Diagnosis is made by demonstration of a hepatic mass by CT and a **cold spot** through liver scanning. Results of liver function testing are normal, and serum α-fetoprotein is normal. Because the tumors are hypervascular, liver biopsy is not suggested.

        (3) Therapy includes cessation of birth control pill usage and monitoring of tumor size to document regression. If regression does not occur, the tumor should be removed surgically to prevent rupture.

    b. Focal nodular hyperplasia also occurs primarily in women; the theory that this lesion is associated with oral contraceptives is controversial. The lesion is composed of central connective tissue with radiating septa, which divide the mass into nodules. Liver scanning may not reveal an abnormality because all elements of liver tissue, including Kupffer cells, are present. However, CT and angiography demonstrate a hypervascular mass. The clinical course is benign. There is no potential for malignant transformation, and hemorrhage, rupture, and necrosis are rare.

    c. Hemangiomas are the most common benign tumors of the liver and are found at autopsy in 5%–7% of patients. Women are affected more commonly than men.

        (1) Clinical features usually are absent. Large lesions may be associated with thrombocytopenia and hypofibrinogenemia, especially in infants. Hemangiomas also may be associated with telangiectasias of other organs.

        (2) Diagnosis is made by angiography or rapid-sequence CT. Abdominal x-rays may show calcification. Liver scanning shows a **cold spot**, which ultrasonography reveals as a solid mass. Hemangiomas usually are single but may be multiple.

        (3) Therapy usually is not necessary. However, corticosteroid therapy, radiotherapy, and embolization all have been shown to be effective in decreasing the size of the hemangiomas.

2. Malignant tumors

    a. Primary hepatocellular carcinoma (hepatoma) occurs five times more frequently in men than in women and accounts for about 2.5% of all malignancies in the United States. In parts of South Africa and Asia, hepatoma may account for 50% of all carcinomas. The peak age of incidence is 40–60 years.

        (1) Etiology is not known, but the following **risk factors** are noted.

            (a) Cirrhosis is present in 75%–90% of patients. Patients with a history of postnecrotic or alcohol-induced cirrhosis, hemachromatosis, or α_1-antitrypsin deficiency are at higher risk than patients with a history of primary biliary cirrhosis, cardiac cirrhosis, or Wilson's disease. Children with **hereditary tyrosinemia** have a 40% risk of hepatoma.

            (b) Previous infection with hepatitis B. Serologic markers are found in a high percentage of patients with hepatoma. It is thought that the risk of hepatoma is increased 20-fold by infection with hepatitis B.

            (c) Aflatoxin, which is produced by the mold *Aspergillus flavus*, is a common contaminant of grain and peanuts in parts of Africa where there is a high incidence of hepatoma.

            (d) Long-term androgen therapy has been linked to the incidence of hepatoma.

            (e) Schistosomiasis and **clonorchiasis** are endemic in parts of the world where hepatoma is common (i.e., Africa and Japan).

        (2) Clinical features include:

            (a) Hepatomegaly

            (b) Hepatic bruit or friction rub

            (c) Ascites, which may be bloody (50% of patients)

            (d) Nonspecific symptoms such as malaise, anorexia, weight loss, and abdominal pain (about 33% of patients)

            (e) Clinical deterioration or sudden rise in the serum alkaline phosphatase in an otherwise stable cirrhotic patient

        (3) Diagnosis

            (a) Liver function testing shows an elevated serum alkaline phosphatase with only a modest elevation of the serum transaminases.

            (b) Gallium scanning reveals focal **filling defects**.

            (c) The α-fetoprotein is elevated in 75% of patients in the United States and in 85%–90% of patients in Africa and Japan.

            (d) Angiography reveals a hypervascular mass with a **tumor blush**.

            (e) Liver biopsy can be used to confirm the diagnosis but should be performed with caution because of the vascular nature of the lesions.

        (4) Therapy. No effective treatment exists, and average survival is less than 6 months following the time of diagnosis.

            (a) Surgery can be attempted if a tumor is confined to one lobe of the liver and is associated with a 5-year survival rate of less than 10%.

            (b) Patients only rarely respond to radiotherapy or chemotherapy.

    b. Angiosarcoma is a rare vascular tumor, which accounts for 2% of hepatic malignancies. Angiosarcoma generally is seen in men aged 50–70 years.

        (1) Etiology. There is a strong correlation between the incidence of angiosarcoma and a history of exposure to vinyl chloride, arsenic, or Thorotrast (a radiologic contrast medium no longer in use). The tumor may be discovered as late as 10–25 years following exposure.

        (2) Clinical features are nonspecific. This tumor has a tendency to rupture or bleed spontaneously, and hemoperitoneum is noted in 15% of patients.

(3) Diagnosis is based on liver function tests showing an elevated serum alkaline phosphatase, liver scanning showing a defect, and arteriography showing a vascular tumor. Since fatal hemorrhage has been reported following closed liver biopsy, an open procedure always should be used to obtain tissue for definitive diagnosis.

c. Metastatic disease is much more common than primary hepatic malignancy. Only lymph nodes are more commonly involved by metastatic disease than the liver. Up to 50% of patients dying from malignant disease have liver involvement. The most common primary tumors showing spread to the liver are carcinomas of the gastrointestinal tract, malignant melanoma, and carcinomas of the pancreas, lung, breast, kidney, and ovary. In addition, lymphoma commonly involves the liver.

(1) Clinical features include fever, right upper quadrant pain, and hepatomegaly. A friction rub may be present over the liver. Jaundice may be directly due to hepatic involvement or to nodal compression in the porta hepatis (especially in colonic, breast, and bronchogenic carcinomas and in lymphoma).

(2) Diagnosis is suggested by an elevated serum alkaline phosphatase and by abnormal findings obtained through ultrasonography and liver scanning; the diagnosis is confirmed by liver biopsy. A blind biopsy is positive in 65% of patients, and yield can be increased by making multiple passes and by using guidance by CT or ultrasonography. Aspiration cytology also can be used to establish the diagnosis.

(3) Therapy depends only on the underlying tumor type. Lymphoma may respond to systemic radiation and chemotherapy, and malignancies of the breast and ovary may respond to hormone manipulation. Perfusion of chemotherapeutic agents directly into the hepatic artery may be useful for some tumors. Occasionally, patients with a solitary metastatic lesion may be cured by resection. The outlook for most patients with metastatic disease, however, is grim, with a median survival of 3 months.

X. DISEASES OF THE PERITONEUM, MESENTERY, AND ABDOMINAL VASCULATURE

A. Diseases of the peritoneum

1. Ascites refers to the accumulation of fluid in the peritoneal cavity.

a. Pathogenesis. The following mechanisms lead to ascites formation:

(1) Increased hydrostatic pressure, which may be due to:
  (a) Cirrhosis
  (b) Hepatic vein occlusion (Budd-Chiari syndrome)
  (c) Inferior vena cava obstruction
  (d) Constrictive pericarditis
  (e) Congestive heart failure

(2) Decreased colloid osmotic pressure, which may result from:
  (a) End-stage liver disease with poor protein synthesis
  (b) Nephrotic syndrome with protein loss
  (c) Malnutrition
  (d) Protein-losing enteropathy

(3) Increased permeability of peritoneal capillaries, which may result from:
  (a) Tuberculosis peritonitis
  (b) Bacterial peritonitis
  (c) Malignant disease of the peritoneum

(4) Leakage of fluid into the peritoneal cavity, leading to:
  (a) Bile ascites
  (b) Pancreatic ascites (usually secondary to a leaking pseudocyst)
  (c) Chylous ascites (secondary to lymphatic duct disruption due to lymphoma or trauma)
  (d) Urine ascites

(5) Miscellaneous causes of ascites include:
  (a) Myxedema
  (b) Ovarian disease (Meigs' syndrome)
  (c) Chronic hemodialysis

b. Diagnosis. The presence of ascites usually is indicated on physical examination by abdominal distension, a fluid wave, or shifting dullness. Abdominal ultrasonography can reliably detect small amounts of fluid. Paracentesis can be performed with or without guidance by ultrasonography, and the ascites fluid should be analyzed.

(1) Total protein content greater than 2.5 g/dl is diagnostic of exudative ascites, which usually is seen in tumors, infections, and myxedema.

(2) Amylase concentration is elevated in pancreatic ascites.

(3) Triglyceride concentration is elevated in chylous ascites.

(4) Cytology frequently is positive in malignancy.

(5) White cell count greater than 350/mm³ is suggestive of infection. If most cells are polymorphonuclear, bacterial infection should be suspected. When mononuclear cells predominate, tuberculosis or fungal infection is likely.

(6) Red cell count greater than 50,000/mm³ denotes hemorrhagic ascites, which usually is due to malignancy, tuberculosis, or trauma. Hemorrhagic pancreatitis, ruptured aortic aneurysm, and ruptured hepatic adenoma may cause frank bleeding into the peritoneal cavity.

(7) Gram staining and culture document bacterial infection.

(8) A pH of less than 7 suggests bacterial infection.

c. Therapy depends on the underlying cause. Transudative ascites may be treated by bed rest, Na⁺ restriction, and careful use of diuretics [see section IX B 2 b (1) (c)]. Paracentesis of up to 1 L of fluid may provide relief of acute respiratory embarrassment secondary to tense ascites, but removal of more than 1 L at a time may lead to hypovolemia and shock as fluid reaccumulates in the peritoneal cavity. A LeVeen shunt may be used for intractable or malignant ascites but causes a high risk for development of infection and disseminated intravascular coagulation.

2. Bacterial peritonitis

a. Pathogenesis

(1) Primary or **spontaneous bacterial peritonitis** usually develops in the setting of preexisting ascites.

(2) Secondary or **acute bacterial peritonitis** usually results from a perforated viscus, a ruptured appendix, an intestinal infarction, or ulcerative colitis.

b. Clinical features include:

(1) Abdominal pain, with or without guarding and rebound

(2) Fever

(3) Leukocytosis

(4) Paralytic ileus

c. Diagnosis

(1) Paracentesis aids in determining whether the fluid is exudative or transudative, has an elevated white cell count (a predominance of polymorphonuclear cells is diagnostic), and can be cultured to identify the infecting organism.

(2) X-ray examination reveals free air under the diaphragm in the presence of a perforated viscus, may show a nonspecific ileus, or may show a hazy appearance consistent with ascites.

d. Therapy

(1) Supportive measures include intravenous administration of fluids, correction of electrolyte abnormalities, and nasogastric suction.

(2) Antimicrobial therapy includes ampicillin and an aminoglycoside to cover gram-negative organisms, pneumococcus, and other streptococci. (Anaerobes also are common offenders.)

(3) Surgical intervention is necessary in cases of secondary bacterial peritonitis.

3. Other causes of peritonitis

a. Bile peritonitis

(1) Pathogenesis. Bile spillage into the peritoneal cavity (e.g., from a ruptured gallbladder or gallbladder puncture during liver biopsy) results in a chemical peritonitis.

(2) Clinical features include severe abdominal pain and shock secondary to exudation of fluid from the damaged peritoneum.

(3) Therapy is surgical after patients have been stabilized with intravenous volume replacement and correction of electrolyte abnormalities.

b. Starch peritonitis

(1) Pathogenesis. About 2–4 weeks after abdominal surgery, granulomatous peritonitis develops if the peritoneal cavity has been contaminated with surgical glove powder (starch), lint from surgical drapes, particles of suture material, or talc.

(2) Clinical features include abdominal pain, distension, tenderness, and fullness.

(3) Diagnosis. Examination of the ascites fluid under a polarized microscope shows starch granules termed **maltese crosses**. Laparoscopy reveals studding of the peritoneal surface.

(4) Therapy is with corticosteroids or nonsteroidal anti-inflammatory agents.

c. Gonococcal peritonitis (Fitz-Hugh–Curtis syndrome) usually is seen in young women and is due to an ascending infection originating in the pelvis. *Chlamydia* recently has been reported to cause an identical syndrome.

(1) Clinical features, which mimic those of acute cholecystitis, include abdominal pain, fever, and right upper quadrant peritoneal signs. Occasionally, a hepatic friction rub is present.

(2) **Diagnosis.** Laboratory tests show an elevated white blood cell count and mild abnormalities in liver function. Pelvic examination may reveal adnexal tenderness, and culture of cervical mucus usually is positive. Laparoscopy shows **violin-string adhesions** from the liver to either the right adnexa or the abdominal wall.

(3) **Therapy** is penicillin. If *Chlamydia* also is present, tetracycline is given.

4. **Subphrenic abscess** refers to a collection of pus located inferior to the diaphragm and above the liver, spleen, or stomach.

   a. **Pathogenesis.** Abscess formation usually is a complication of diverticulitis, a ruptured appendix, a perforated ulcer, or an abdominal wound with peritoneal soiling. Occasionally, an abscess is seen after uncomplicated abdominal surgery.

   b. **Clinical features** include fever, leukocytosis, and abdominal and shoulder pain.

   c. **Diagnosis** may be suggested by an x-ray showing elevation of one hemidiaphragm but usually requires demonstration of the abscess cavity by CT or ultrasonography.

   d. **Therapy** is surgical drainage and broad-spectrum antibiotics to combat gram-negative as well as anaerobic organisms.

5. **Tumors of the peritoneum**

   a. **Metastatic lesions** are the most common peritoneal tumors. The primary lesion usually is adenocarcinoma of the gastrointestinal tract, pancreas, or ovary. However, sarcomas, lymphomas, leukemias, and carcinoid tumors all may involve the peritoneum.

      (1) **Diagnosis** is made by paracentesis showing an exudative fluid with a moderately increased lymphocyte count and positive cytology. Needle biopsy of the peritoneum also may be used.

      (2) **Therapy** is directed at the underlying malignancy. Intraperitoneal injection of a sclerosing agent occasionally may be helpful.

   b. **Mesothelioma** is seen most commonly in men over age 50 years and is associated with asbestos exposure.

      (1) **Clinical features** include abdominal distension, abdominal pain, nausea, vomiting, and weight loss.

      (2) **Diagnosis** requires demonstration of malignant cells through paracentesis with cytology, needle biopsy, or laparotomy with biopsy.

      (3) **Therapy** includes radiotherapy, chemotherapy, or both, but patient response usually is poor.

   c. **Pseudomyxoma peritonei** is a rare condition characterized by the presence of thick gelatinous material in the peritoneal cavity.

      (1) **Pathogenesis.** This condition results from the rupture of either an appendiceal mucocele or an ovarian mucinous cystadenoma. Some authors have reported the presence of low-grade malignancy in a high percentage of the underlying tumors.

      (2) **Clinical features** include increasing abdominal girth without shifting dullness in an otherwise healthy individual.

      (3) **Diagnosis** often requires laparotomy.

      (4) **Therapy** is surgical removal of the mucinous material and underlying tumor.

B. **Diseases of the mesentery**

1. **Mesenteric panniculitis** (mesenteric Weber-Christian disease) is a rare condition usually seen in elderly men, which causes inflammation and fibrosis of the mesentery.

   a. **Pathogenesis** is thought to involve overgrowth of normal fat tissue in the mesentery with subsequent degeneration, necrosis, and progression to fibrosis and scar formation. The initiating event may be ischemia, infection, or trauma.

   b. **Clinical features** include crampy abdominal pain, fever, weight loss, nausea, and vomiting. Lymphatic obstruction may develop with resultant ascites, steatorrhea, and protein-losing enteropathy.

   c. **Diagnosis** requires laparotomy, which reveals a thickened fibrotic mesentery with fat necrosis and infiltration by foamy macrophages.

   d. **Therapy** with corticosteroids has varying results. In many patients, the process appears self-limited, and the prognosis is excellent.

2. **Mesenteric cysts** are congenital anomalies of the mesenteric lymphatic system, which present as slowly enlarging, painless, round, smooth, mobile masses. Treatment is drainage or excision. Mesenteric cysts are benign but rarely may cause symptoms due to rupture, bleeding, or torsion.

3. **Mesenteric adenitis** generally is seen in children and young adults and mimics acute appendicitis.

      a. Etiology. Mesenteric adenitis usually is caused by viral infection; however, many cases are due to *Yersinia* infection.

      b. Clinical features are abdominal pain, which may be severe, nausea, vomiting, and fever. Some patients have additional evidence of a viral infection (e.g., pharyngitis and myalgia).

      c. Diagnosis usually is made at laparotomy for presumed appendicitis.

      d. Therapy includes antibiotics, if *Yersinia* is identified, and supportive care.

C. Diseases of the abdominal vasculature

1. Abdominal aortic aneurysm usually presents as an asymptomatic pulsatile mass, but some patients note abdominal pain, back pain, and leg ischemia. The cause usually is atherosclerosis. Leakage of blood into surrounding tissues with associated abdominal, back, or flank pain may precede overt rupture by several weeks. Rupture into the duodenum—presenting as massive gastrointestinal hemorrhage—or into the abdomen may be catastrophic. Treatment is surgical with replacement of the aneurysm with an aortic graft made of Dacron or some other synthetic material. Postoperative aortoenteric fistulae with erosion of the graft into the duodenum (usually in the setting of an infected graft) may be seen several years after aneurysmectomy and may result in fatal bleeding if not recognized early.

2. Mesenteric ischemia usually is seen only when there is significant occlusion of two of the three major splanchnic vessels. The syndrome usually is seen in older patients with a history of cardiovascular disease.

      a. Clinical features include intermittent crampy abdominal pain occurring 15–30 minutes after eating and lasting several hours. Because of the association of pain with eating, patients characteristically develop a fear of eating and decrease their intake to the point of substantial weight loss. Physical examination frequently discloses evidence of peripheral vascular disease, but there are no specific findings indicating intestinal ischemia. The presence or absence of an abdominal bruit is not helpful.

      b. Diagnosis is difficult and must be based on strong clinical suspicion combined with angiographic demonstration of significant narrowing (greater than 50%) in two of the three major splanchnic arteries.

      c. Therapy is surgical vascular reconstruction. Vasodilators have not been shown to be effective.

      d. Ischemic colitis is due to a lack of arterial blood to the colon. While any portion of the colon may be affected, the most common site is the left colon and, in particular, the so-called "watershed area" at the splenic flexure. This area is vulnerable as it is the site where the superior mesenteric arterial supply ends and the inferior mesenteric arterial supply begins. The rectum usually is spared due to its generous blood supply.

        (1) Clinical features include bloody diarrhea, lower abdominal pain, and occasional vomiting. The older adult who has a history of heart disease or has had abdominal aortic aneurysm surgery (with ligation of the inferior mesenteric artery) is particulary susceptible.

        (2) Diagnosis is suggested by negative findings for other causes of bloody diarrhea in the elderly population (i.e., polyp, carcinoma, diverticulosis, and angiodysplasia). The white cell count may be elevated to about 20,000/mm^3. A flat plate x-ray of the abdomen may show "thumb printing" (submucosal hemorrhage and edema). A barium enema is a safe study and may reveal diffuse submucosal change. Generally, sigmoidoscopy reveals only bloody fluid.

        (3) Therapy is supportive with bowel rest, intravenous fluids, blood replacement, and antibiotics to prevent secondary invasion. Infarction rarely occurs.

        (4) Prognosis generally is good. Late strictures may develop, which could require balloon dilatation or surgery.

      e. Vasculitis. Involvement of the mesenteric vessels by polyarthritis nodosa, lupus erythematosus, or rheumatoid vasculitis mimics arterial embolization (causing bowel infarction) or chronic mesenteric ischemia. The diagnosis is suggested by the systemic features of the disease. Surgery is required for acute infarction. Otherwise, medical treatment with corticosteroids, immunosuppressive agents, or both frequently is effective.

STUDY QUESTIONS

Directions: Each question below contains five suggested answers. Choose the **one best** response to each question.

1. Which of the following esophageal disorders is best characterized by dysphagia for both solids and liquids?

(A) Esophageal carcinoma
(B) Achalasia
(C) Schatzki's ring
(D) Benign esophageal stricture
(E) Barrett's esophagus

2. Chronic type A gastritis is associated with all of the following clinical findings EXCEPT

(A) the presence of parietal cell antibody
(B) elevated serum gastrin levels
(C) achlorhydria
(D) antral involvement
(E) pernicious anemia

3. All of the following signs are radiographic criteria for benign gastric ulcers EXCEPT

(A) ulcer crater extending beyond the gastric wall
(B) gastric folds radiating into the ulcer crater
(C) stiff, nonpliable gastric wall near the ulcer crater
(D) ulcer crater that is smooth, regular, and round
(E) collar of edema surrounding the ulcer base

4. All of the following statements concerning ulcerative proctitis are true EXCEPT

(A) the risk of malignancy is lower than that associated with ulcerative colitis
(B) the disease progresses to diffuse ulcerative colitis in 15%–20% of cases
(C) symptoms include diarrhea and rectal bleeding, with systemic symptoms occurring only rarely
(D) other causes of proctitis (e.g., infection) must be ruled out to confirm the diagnosis
(E) proctosigmoidoscopy shows disease extending to the descending colon but not involving the transverse or ascending colon

5. Although irritable bowel syndrome is a disease of unknown cause, pathophysiologic studies suggest that the etiology most likely involves

(A) an underlying indolent infection
(B) an underlying immunologic defect
(C) a neuromuscular defect
(D) a hypersensitivity to certain foods
(E) a premalignant state

6. All of the following statements concerning sclerosing cholangitis are true EXCEPT

(A) 30% of patients have inflammatory bowel disease
(B) endoscopic retrograde cholangiopancreatography or percutaneous cholangiography is used to establish the diagnosis
(C) the disease is more common in men than in women
(D) the treatment usually is surgical anastomosis of the bile ducts to the intestine
(E) early diagnosis can be suspected in asymptomatic patients on the basis of an elevated serum alkaline phosphatase

7. Although most cases of acute viral hepatitis resolve spontaneously, complications may occur. Which of the following statements best describes the complications of hepatitis B infection?

(A) The chronic carrier state is associated with an increased risk of hepatoma
(B) Chronic persistent hepatitis usually leads to progressive deterioration of liver function and must be treated aggressively
(C) Chronic active hepatitis can be diagnosed within 2–4 weeks of the acute infection with hepatitis B virus
(D) Chronic active hepatitis is characterized on liver biopsy by a periportal lymphocytic infiltrate without fibrosis or extra-portal extension
(E) Fulminant hepatitis is characterized by rapidly rising transaminase levels in an enlarging liver

Directions: Each question below contains four suggested answers of which **one or more** is correct. Choose the answer

    A if **1, 2, and 3** are correct
    B if **1 and 3** are correct
    C if **2 and 4** are correct
    D if **4** is correct
    E if **1, 2, 3, and 4** are correct

8. Etiologic agents of odynophagia include

(1) *Candida*
(2) herpes simplex virus
(3) tetracycline
(4) clindamycin

9. Gastroparesis, or disordered gastric emptying not due to an obstruction, may be caused by

(1) anticholinergic drug therapy
(2) diabetes mellitus
(3) postvagotomy states
(4) systemic sclerosis

10. Anemia is one of several complications that may follow Billroth II gastrectomy for peptic ulcer disease. Factors that may contribute to postsurgical anemia include

(1) iron malabsorption
(2) gastritis in the gastric pouch
(3) vitamin B_{12} malabsorption
(4) dumping syndrome

11. Adenomatous polyps of the colon are a premalignant lesion. The risk for adenocarcinoma is increased when the polyps are

(1) located in the right colon
(2) larger than 2 cm
(3) tubular rather than villous
(4) sessile rather than pedunculated

12. Complications of acute cholecystitis that require early surgical intervention include

(1) gallbladder empyema
(2) ileus
(3) emphysematous cholecystitis
(4) jaundice

13. Cirrhosis of the liver is a late manifestation of many diseases other than alcoholic liver disease, including

(1) Wilson's disease
(2) constrictive pericarditis
(3) α_1-antitrypsin deficiency
(4) halothane-induced liver disease

14. Ischemic colitis is due to inadequate arterial blood supply to the colon. True statements concerning ischemic colitis include

(1) the rectum usually is spared because it has a generous blood supply
(2) the most commonly affected site is the hepatic flexure
(3) symptoms include bloody diarrhea and abdominal pain
(4) the diagnosis is suggested by pseudopolyps on abdominal flat plate x-ray

Directions: The group of questions below consists of lettered choices followed by several numbered items. For each numbered item select the **one** lettered choice with which it is **most** closely associated. Each lettered choice may be used once, more than once, or not at all.

Questions 15–18

For each case history involving a patient with diarrhea, select the most likely etiology.

(A) Ulcerative colitis
(B) Laxative abuse
(C) Pseudomembranous colitis
(D) Viral gastroenteritis
(E) *Campylobacter* infection

15. A healthy 20-year-old man has an acute diarrheal disease characterized by bloody stool, crampy abdominal pain, and low-grade fever. His symptoms resolve spontaneously in 5 days and do not recur.

16. A healthy 20-year-old man has an acute onset of bloody diarrhea, crampy abdominal pain, and fever. His symptoms persist for several weeks, after which he consults a physician who notes bleeding, friable mucosa on proctosigmoidoscopy.

17. A 30-year-old woman develops severe, watery diarrhea 2 weeks after undergoing antibiotic therapy for pelvic inflammatory disease. Proctosigmoidoscopy shows plaque-like lesions covering the mucosa.

18. A 30-year-old woman complains of chronic watery diarrhea. Stool examination shows an osmolarity of 300 mEq/dl, a Na^+ concentration of 30 mEq/dl, and a K^+ concentration of 45 mEq/dl. Shortly after she is hospitalized for evaluation and begun on a 48-hour fast, her diarrhea disappears.

ANSWERS AND EXPLANATIONS

1. The answer is B. [*I A b (2), B 2, 3*] Esophageal motor disorders, such as achalasia, are characterized by dysphagia for both solids and liquids. Obstructive esophageal conditions, such as carcinoma, stricture, and Schatzki's ring, cause dysphagia for solids but allow free passage of liquids. The dysphagia associated with Schatzki's ring is intermittent; in carcinoma and stricture, however, the dysphagia is constant. Barrett's esophagus is the replacement of normal squamous epithelium with columnar epithelium; there is no dysphagia in this condition.

2. The answer is D. (*II A 2 b–c*) Chronic type A gastritis probably is immunologically mediated, an assumption that is based on the serologic finding of parietal cell antibody. Parietal cells are gastric acid–producing cells located in the body and fundus (but not the antrum) of the stomach. As a result of parietal cell damage, chronic type A gastritis is characterized by hypo- or achlorhydria, and because there is little or no gastric acid to shut down production of gastrin, serum gastrin levels are very high. Intrinsic factor also is produced by parietal cells and, therefore, is deficient in these patients. This leads to the common finding of pernicious anemia in chronic type A gastritis.

3. The answer is C. (*III E 1*) Although endoscopy and biopsy are required to confirm that a gastric ulcer is either benign or malignant, an upper gastrointestinal series can provide useful diagnostic information. Since a malignant ulcer typically occurs in the middle of a gastric mass, the ulcer crater does not extend outside the gastric wall, the folds cannot radiate all the way to the ulcer base, and there is no edema of the surrounding mucosa. In addition, benign ulcers tend to be smooth and round, whereas malignant ulcers are irregular in shape.

4. The answer is E. (*VI A*) Ulcerative proctitis—a localized form of ulcerative colitis—by definition is confined to the rectum and distal sigmoid colon. If the descending colon or proximal sigmoid colon is involved, the disease is felt to be ulcerative colitis. Ulcerative proctitis has a better prognosis and a lower risk of malignancy than ulcerative colitis and only rarely is associated with the systemic symptoms occurring in ulcerative colitis (e.g., fever and weight loss).

5. The answer is C. (*IV D 3 a*) Irritable bowel syndrome, a common cause of alternating diarrhea and constipation, is a functional disorder of motility, which probably has a neuromuscular or hormonal basis. There is no evidence to suggest the existence of an underlying infection or an immunologic defect. The incidence of carcinoma among patients with irritable bowel syndrome does not exceed that among the general population. Treatment includes high-fiber diet, antispasmodics, and patient reassurance.

6. The answer is D. (*VIII G*) Sclerosing cholangitis is a rare disease that leads to a progressive narrowing of the bile ducts. The disease is more common in men than in women and in patients with inflammatory bowel disease. Visualization of the diseased bile ducts with endoscopic retrograde cholangiopancreatography or percutaneous cholangiography can establish the diagnosis, even in asymptomatic patients with early disease manifested only as elevated serum alkaline phosphatase. Because the ducts are diseased, surgical anastomosis of the ducts is difficult if not impossible. A variety of medical regimens have been tried, but none has been uniformly successful.

7. The answer is A. [*IX A 1 f (1)–(4)*] The chronic carrier state for hepatitis B virus is associated with an increased risk of hepatoma and is found in 0.2% of the population of the United States. Chronic active hepatitis cannot be diagnosed until at least 6 months following the acute infection with hepatitis B. In chronic active hepatitis, the inflammation and fibrosis extend past the portal area and, thus, correlate with profuse deterioration of liver function, which may result in cirrhosis or liver failure. Fulminant hepatitis occurs in about 1%–2% of cases of hepatitis B and non A, non B hepatitis. This rare complication usually is associated with falling transaminase levels as liver tissue is destroyed and the liver decreases in size.

8. The answer is E (all). (*I A 2 b, B 4 b*) Odynophagia, or pain on swallowing, may be caused by motor disorders of the esophagus (e.g., achalasia) or mucosal disruption (e.g., due to infection-related or drug-induced esophagitis). The most important agents of esophageal infection are *Candida* and herpes simplex virus. Infections by these agents are commonly seen in immunocompromised hosts such as patients on cancer chemotherapy. Drugs that may cause mucosal disruption include potassium chloride tablets, tetracycline preparations, clindamycin, quinidine, and ascorbic acid tablets.

9. The answer is E (all). (*II C 5*) Although all of the conditions listed may cause gastroparesis, this disorder usually is seen in patients with insulin-dependent diabetes of longer than 10 years' duration. Electrical recordings show loss of phase III activity as well as other signs of diabetic visceral neuropathy. Many patients respond to metoclopramide. There also is some evidence that rigorous control of serum glucose levels may be helpful.

10. The answer is A (1, 2, 3). (III H 5) Anemia occurs in 25% of patients after surgery for peptic ulcer disease. Several factors may be involved. Iron absorption is poor because of a lack of gastric acid, which is required for conversion of Fe^{2+} to Fe^{3+} (the preferred form for absorption), and because iron is absorbed best in the duodenum. Vitamin B_{12} absorption also is poor after Billroth II gastrectomy. Normally during gastric digestion, vitamin B_{12} is released from food and bound to a glycoprotein called "R binder." In the duodenum, gastric acid causes vitamin B_{12} to separate from the R binder, after which it binds to intrinsic factor. (In patients who have undergone a subtotal gastrectomy, intrinsic factor also may be lacking.) Inflammation in the remaining portion of the stomach is a common postsurgical problem, which may be due to bile in the gastric pouch and may lead to chronic gastritis with chronic, low-grade blood loss. Dumping syndrome causes dizziness and weakness after eating but does not contribute to anemia.

11. The answer is C (2, 4). (V F 1) Although adenomatous polyps of the colon are benign, they are considered to be precursors of adenocarcinoma. An increased risk for malignancy is noted in adenomatous polyps that are larger than 2 cm, villous (not tubular), and sessile (not pedunculated). Location within the colon is not a factor in predicting malignancy. If malignancy is present but is confined to the mucosa, polypectomy is curative.

12. The answer is B (1, 3). (VIII B 2, 5) Gallbladder empyema refers to a pus-filled gallbladder. Patients with gallbladder empyema are toxic and at high risk for gallbladder perforation. Emphysematous cholecystitis refers to infection of the gallbladder with gas-forming organisms. This complication of acute cholecystitis also increases the risk for gallbladder perforation. Jaundice and ileus are common findings in patients with uncomplicated cholecystitis, which may be managed medically.

13. The answer is A (1, 2, 3). [IX A 2 c (2), B 2 d, e] Wilson's disease is a systemic disorder of copper metabolism, which can lead to cirrhosis or fulminant hepatitis. Constrictive pericarditis and other disorders causing prolonged right-sided heart failure also may lead to cirrhosis, although this is a rare manifestation. Alpha$_1$-antitrypsin deficiency causes both lung and liver disease (cirrhosis). Some drugs can cause cirrhosis, but exposure to halothane can result in acute hepatitis that may be fulminant and fatal.

14. The answer is B (1, 3). (X C 2 d) Ischemic colitis is most severe where the arterial blood supply to the colon is most limited (splenic flexure) and least severe where the blood supply is richest (rectum). The symptoms are nonspecific and include bloody diarrhea, lower abdominal pain, and occasional vomiting. Diagnosis is suggested by negative findings for other causes of bloody diarrhea (e.g., polyp, carcinoma, and diverticulitis). Abdominal flat plate x-ray may show thumb-printing, which represents submucosal edema and hemorrhage.

15–18. The answers are: 15-E, 16-A, 17-C, 18-B. (IV D 3 d, 4 f, V D, G) Campylobacter infection is the most common cause of bacterial diarrhea. The diarrhea can be severe and bloody, and proctosigmoidoscopy during the acute phase can show ulcerated, friable mucosa. The disease is self-limited, however, and complete healing of the mucosa takes place.

Ulcerative colitis may present as an acute diarrheal illness that fails to resolve. Proctosigmoidoscopy shows diffuse friability, bleeding, and ulceration of the mucosa. Biopsy of the involved mucosa characteristically shows abscesses in the crypts of Lieberkühn.

Pseudomembranous colitis may arise as a complication of therapy with broad-spectrum antibiotics (e.g., clindamycin). Clindamycin suppresses most anaerobic bacteria of the colon but actually causes an overgrowth of the anaerobe, Clostridium difficile, which produces an enterotoxin that is responsible for the development of pseudomembranous colitis. The characteristic lesion is a white plaque (pseudomembrane), which is seen in the sigmoid of 75%–90% of patients. The diagnosis can be established by measuring the toxin of C. difficile in the stool of patients in whom disease is confined to the right side of the colon.

Laxative abuse is an important cause of both secretory and osmotic diarrhea. Secretory diarrhea, which is diagnosed on the basis of the absence of an osmotic gap on stool electrolyte studies, may be caused by such laxatives as castor oil, bisacodyl, and phenylphthalein. Osmotic diarrhea, which is diagnosed on the basis of the presence of an osmotic gap, may be caused by such laxatives as milk of magnesia, lactulose, sorbital, and magnesium-containing antacids. Since the only other causes of osmotic diarrhea are disaccharidase deficiency and maldigestion, the presence of an osmotic gap on stool electrolyte studies always should raise the suspicion of laxative abuse.

6

Renal Diseases and Fluid and Electrolyte Disorders

Stanley Goldfarb
Carl S. Goldstein

Part I: Renal Diseases

I. CLINICAL ASSESSMENT OF RENAL FUNCTION

A. Urinalysis

1. **Urine color** normally is yellow.
   a. **Darkening on standing** may be seen with some diseases (e.g., porphyria) and with certain drugs (e.g., methyldopa).
   b. **Red-orange-brown urine** may be seen with hematuria, hemoglobinuria, and myoglobinuria and with certain drugs (e.g., phenothiazines).

2. **Urine chemistry.** Qualitative chemical analysis of urine is performed with commercially available **dipsticks**.
   a. **Blood** usually is not present in normal urine. Intact erythrocytes, hemoglobin, and myoglobin all produce positive test results.
   b. **Glucose** usually is not present in normal urine above 0.3 g/24 hr.
   c. **Ketone bodies** are present in the urine of healthy individuals only during fasting. Sodium nitroprusside reagent detects acetoacetate but not β-hydroxybutyrate.
   d. **Protein** usually is not present in normal urine above 150 mg/24 hr. The dipstick detects only albumin, not immunoglobulins or light chain polypeptides, which must be assayed using acid precipitation.
   e. **Bilirubin** is not present in normal urine. If elevated in blood, water-soluble conjugated bilirubin is filtered and present in urine.
   f. **Urine pH** can be maximally acidified below a pH of 5.0 and maximally alkalinized above a pH of 7.5.

3. **Urine concentration and dilution** are measured by either specific gravity (normal = 1.000–1.025) or osmolality (normal = 50–1000 mOsm/kg urine). Many factors can affect urine concentration and dilution.

4. **Urinary sediment** of formed elements is prepared by centrifugation of urine at 2000 RPM for 10 minutes. The sediment from 12 ml of urine is resuspended in 1 ml of supernatant and is examined microscopically.
   a. **Crystals** that are seen in acid urine include cystine and uric acid; those found in alkaline urine include calcium phosphate and calcium oxalate.
   b. **Cells** that are found in various disease states include erythrocytes, leukocytes, and epithelial cells (i.e., renal tubular, transitional, or squamous).
   c. **Bacteria** may be seen and are best confirmed with Gram staining of the sediment.
   d. **Casts** are cylindrical elements formed in disease states associated with low intrarenal urine flow or heavy proteinuria. The cast is a protein coagulum, which is formed in the renal tubule and traps any tubular luminal contents within its matrix. Casts are named for the elements recognized within them, such as:
      (1) Red cell cast
      (2) White cell cast
      (3) Renal tubular cell cast
      (4) Granular cast
      (5) Hyaline cast
      (6) Waxy cast

B. Renal function testing

1. **Glomerular filtration rate (GFR)** is a measure of the amount of plasma ultrafiltrate derived

from blood in a specified time period. (A normal GFR is 115–125 ml/min.) In most kidney diseases, GFR is an accurate index of overall renal function.

2. **Urine concentrating ability** is determined by measuring urine osmolality after 18–24 hours of water deprivation and again after the administration of 5 units of **vasopressin**. Under these conditions, urine reaches an osmolality of 900 mOsm/kg (or a specific gravity of 1.023) in 90% of normal individuals.

3. **Urine diluting ability** is determined by measuring urine osmolality and volume 5 hours after a water load of 20 ml/kg body weight. Urine reaches an osmolality of 100 mOsm/kg (or a specific gravity of 1.003), and urine volume exceeds 80% of the water load in normal individuals.

4. **Renal urine acidification.** Fasting urine pH normally is below 5.5. Acidification can be tested by administering 100 mg ammonium chloride/kg body weight to decrease plasma bicarbonate concentration below 20 mEq/L. Urine normally acidifies (i.e., urine pH drops below 5.5) under these conditions.

C. **Radiography**

1. Plain-film radiography, tomography, ultrasonography, and computed tomography (CT) are useful noninvasive techniques for determining renal size and the presence of obstruction, stones, or mass lesions.

2. Intravenous urography and arteriography may also help to define intrarenal morphology.

D. **Renal biopsy**

1. **Indications** for renal biopsy include acute renal failure of unknown etiology or abnormal course, delayed recovery from acute renal failure, and a poorly functioning or deteriorating renal allograft. Also, renal biopsy occasionally may be indicated in cases of nephrotic syndrome and diabetes and in defining the progression of lupus nephritis.

2. **Contraindications** for renal biopsy include diastolic blood pressure exceeding 100 mm Hg, infection at the biopsy site, and abnormal blood coagulation.

II. **ACUTE RENAL FAILURE** is defined as sudden, rapid, but potentially reversible deterioration in renal function sufficient to cause nitrogenous waste accumulation in body fluids.

A. **Etiology**

1. **Prerenal causes.** Significant decreases in renal vascular perfusion may cause a decrease in GFR and may result from the following conditions with or without preservation of renal tubular function:
   a. A true decrease in arterial blood volume
   b. A decrease in effective renal perfusion (e.g., due to heart failure)
   c. Renal vascular disease (e.g., renal artery stenosis)

2. **Postrenal causes.** Interruption of urine flow at any level of the urinary tract, bilaterally or unilaterally, can result in acute renal failure. Frequent **sites of urinary obstruction** include:
   a. **Renal tubules**, by accumulation of uric acid or oxalate crystals
   b. **Renal pelvis**, by tumor or staghorn calculus
   c. **Ureteropelvic junction**, by obstruction with a calculus or by renal papillary necrosis
   d. **Ureter**, by obstruction with a calculus, thrombus, or tumor or by extrinsic compression by retroperitoneal lymph nodes
   e. **Ureterovesical junction**, by obstruction with a calculus, thrombus, or tumor or by edema of the ureteral orifice
   f. **Bladder outlet**, by obstruction with a calculus, stricture, thrombus, or tumor or by prostatic enlargement
   g. **Urethra**, by the presence of a stricture or foreign body; by prostatic enlargement; or by trauma

3. **Renal parenchymal causes.** Acute renal failure can result from severe injury to any portion of the kidney.
   a. **Acute tubular necrosis (ATN)**
      (1) Nearly 60% of all cases of ATN are **surgery-related**, 38% occur in a medical setting, and 2% are pregnancy-related.
      (2) **Ischemia-related** cases of ATN can arise from any cause of hypotension.
      (3) **Nephrotoxin-related** cases of ATN are caused by aminoglycosides and other antibiotics, radiographic contrast material, heavy metals, certain organic solvents, methoxyflurane, antineoplastic agents (e.g., cisplatin), hemoglobin, and myoglobin.

b. Intrinsic renal diseases include:
   (1) Acute primary or secondary glomerulonephritis
   (2) Tubulointerstitial nephritis
   (3) Radiation nephritis
   (4) Renal vasculitis
   (5) Crystal- or paraprotein-mediated glomerular and tubular disease

B. Clinical features

1. Azotemia. Rising **blood urea nitrogen (BUN)** and **serum creatinine** levels are the most readily available laboratory signs of a decrease in GFR. These biochemical changes may be independent of clinical symptoms. Confounding variables that influence BUN and creatinine must be considered before renal failure is confirmed.
   a. BUN level is affected by the amount of dietary protein, by catabolic drugs (e.g., glucocorticoids and tetracycline), and by resorption of gastrointestinal or soft-tissue hemorrhage.
   b. Creatinine level is affected by endogenous creatinine production (within muscle tissue), by renal creatinine secretion (which is blocked by such drugs as cimetidine and trimethoprim), and by noncreatinine chromogens (usually drugs) that cause measurement errors.

2. Derangement of urine volume
   a. Anuria, or a urine output of less than 100 ml/day, usually is an ominous sign; however, urine volume per se confers very little diagnostic specificity.
   b. Oliguria is defined as a urine output (generally less than 400 ml/day) that is insufficient to excrete the daily osmolar load. Although most patients with acute renal failure are oliguric, 25%–50% of such patients are not and produce more than 800 ml of urine daily.
   c. Polyuria. Patients may have acutely rising BUN and serum creatinine levels yet produce more than 3 L of urine daily. This condition may represent a less severe form of acute renal failure, with preservation of small amounts of glomerular filtration in the presence of tubular damage. Patients with partial urinary tract obstruction frequently present with polyuria.

C. Diagnosis

1. Patient history. Acute renal failure usually results from several, often synergistic renal injuries. A patient history should include information concerning:
   a. Recent surgical and radiographic procedures
   b. Past trauma
   c. Past and present use of medications
   d. Allergies
   e. Past transfusions
   f. Recent infections
   g. Underlying chronic renal disease
   h. Family history of renal disease

2. Physical examination. The physical examination should be organized so as to parallel the differential diagnosis.
   a. Prerenal failure is suggested by clinical signs of:
      (1) Intravascular volume depletion (e.g., orthostatic changes in blood pressure and pulse and poor skin turgor)
      (2) Congestive heart failure (e.g., elevated jugular venous pressure, a third heart sound, dependent edema, and pulmonary rales)
      (3) Pericardial tamponade (e.g., pulsus paradoxus)
      (4) Renal artery stenosis (e.g., abdominal bruit)
   b. Acute allergic interstitial nephritis is suggested by signs of allergy (e.g., periorbital edema, eosinophilia, maculopapular rash, and wheezing).
   c. Lower urinary tract obstruction is suggested by a suprapubic or flank mass.

3. Urinalysis
   a. Microscopic examination of urinary sediment provides information for the differential diagnosis.
      (1) The presence of few formed elements or only **hyaline casts** is suggestive of prerenal or postrenal failure.
      (2) An abundance of **erythrocytes** is uncommon in the absence of calculi, trauma, infection, or tumor.
      (3) An abundance of **leukocytes** may signify infection, immune-mediated inflammation, or an allergic reaction somewhere in the urinary tract.
      (4) **Eosinophiluria** occurs in up to 95% of patients with acute allergic interstitial nephritis.

A special (Hansel's) stain often is needed to distinguish eosinophils from neutrophils in urine.

(5) Brownish pigmented cellular casts and many renal tubular epithelial cells are observed in 75% of patients with ATN. Pigmented casts without erythrocytes in the sediment from urine with a positive dipstick for occult blood indicate either **hemoglobin-uria** or **myoglobinuria**.

b. **Urine culture** should be performed in all patients with acute renal failure.

c. **Urine and blood chemistries.** Several biochemical indices aid in the evaluation of acute renal failure. Mainly, these tests distinguish acute oliguria due to prerenal azotemia from that due to parenchymal renal disease on the basis that renal tubular function is preserved in the former condition and severely disturbed in the latter. All of these biochemical measures have limitations; their value is recognized when they are used adjunctively, not exclusively.

(1) The **renal failure index** is the ratio of the urine sodium concentration to the urine-to-plasma creatinine ratio expressed as a percentage $[U_{Na}/(U_{Cr}/P_{Cr}) \times 100]$. Generally, values below 1% indicate prerenal failure, and values above 1% indicate parenchymal disease.

(2) The **fractional excretion of sodium** is the ratio of the urine-to-plasma sodium ratio to the urine-to-plasma creatinine ratio expressed as a percentage $[(U_{Na}/P_{Na})/(U_{Cr}/P_{Cr}) \times 100]$. Values below 1% suggest prerenal failure, and values above 1% suggest renal parenchymal disease.

(3) **Abnormal blood chemistries** occasionally aid in the diagnosis of renal failure. A ratio of BUN-to–serum creatinine above 20 is common in prerenal azotemia.

4. **Radiography**

a. **Ultrasonography** is the method of choice for identifying the presence of two kidneys, for evaluating kidney size and shape, and for detecting **hydronephrosis** or **hydroureter**. Kidneys measure 20% smaller by ultrasonography than by intravenous urography. Renal calculi, abdominal aneurysms, and renal vein thrombosis sometimes are detected by ultrasonography.

b. **Retrograde pyelography** is performed by injecting contrast material into the ureteral orifice during cystoscopic examination. This method should be performed only after intravenous urography has been attempted. Specific indications for retrograde study include:

(1) Cases of suspected obstructive uropathy, in which the kidneys and collecting system are not visible with urography

(2) Cases in which adequate detail of ureteral and renal pelvic anatomy is not obtained with urography

(3) Cases of unexplained hematuria, in which results of urographic and cystoscopic examination are normal

5. **Biopsy.** The histologic severity and clinical course of acute renal failure usually do not correlate well; therefore, biopsy is relevant in only a selected group of candidates. (Patients who follow a classic laboratory and clinical course of ATN usually do not benefit from renal biopsy.)

6. **Cystoscopy** is indicated in all cases of urethral obstruction and in some cases of ureteral obstruction.

D. **Clinical course**

1. **Stages.** Acute renal failure due to ATN typically occurs in three stages: an **azotemic stage**, a **diuretic stage**, and a **recovery stage**. The initial, azotemic stage can be either oliguric or nonoliguric.

2. **Morbidity and mortality rates** are affected by the presence of oliguria.

a. Gastrointestinal bleeding, septicemia, metabolic acidemia, and neurologic abnormalities are more common in oliguric patients than in nonoliguric patients.

b. The mortality rate for oliguric patients is 50%, whereas that for nonoliguric patients is only 26%.

3. **Prognosis** is affected by both the severity of the underlying disease and the clinical setting in which acute renal failure occurs. For example, the mortality rate among cases of ATN is 60% for those following surgery or trauma, 30% for those occurring as complications of medical illness, and 10%–15% for those involving pregnancy. Patients with no complicating illness who survive an episode of acute renal failure have a 90% chance of complete recovery of kidney function.

E. **Therapy**

1. **Preliminary measures**

a. **Exclusion of reversible causes.** Obstruction should be relieved, nephrotoxic drugs should

be withdrawn, infection should be treated, and electrolyte derangements should be corrected.
   b. **Correction of prerenal factors.** Intravascular volume and cardiac performance should be optimized.
   c. **Maintenance of urine output.** Although the prognostic importance of oliguria is debated, management of the nonoliguric patient is clearly easier than that of the oliguric patient. Hemodynamic parameters and intravascular volume should be optimized. Loop diuretics may be useful to convert the oliguric form of ATN to the nonoliguric form.

2. **Conservative measures**
   a. **Fluid and electrolyte management.** Patients with acute renal failure are catabolic and usually lose 0.3 kg of body weight daily. Weight gain or stability usually indicates salt and water retention.
      (1) Total oral and intravenous water administration should equal daily **sensible losses** (via urine, stool, and nasogastric or surgical tube drainage) plus estimated **insensible** (i.e., respiratory and dermal) **losses**, which usually equal 400–500 ml/day.
      (2) Combined dietary and intravenous sodium and potassium intake should not exceed the measured 24-hour urinary losses of these electrolytes.
      (3) Sodium bicarbonate should be administered if acidemia becomes severe (i.e., if serum bicarbonate concentration drops below 16 mEq/L).
      (4) Oral phosphate-binding antacids (e.g., aluminum hydroxide) should be given if the serum phosphate concentration exceeds 6.0 mg/dl.
      (5) Magnesium-containing drugs (e.g., magnesium citrate and magnesium hydroxide–containing antacids) should be withheld.
   b. **Dietary management.** Adequate caloric intake is essential for patients with renal failure. Generally, this means a diet that provides 40–60 g of protein and 35–50 kcal/kg lean body weight.

3. **Drug usage.** A patient who develops renal failure abruptly shows only a 1.0 mg/dl/day increase in serum creatinine since endogenous creatinine production remains constant. Therefore, it is impossible to calculate appropriate drug doses based on a patient's serum creatinine level. Pharmacokinetic measurement of serum drug levels often is necessary for safe drug use.

4. **Dialysis** is indicated in the management of progressive renal failure that leads to severe uremia, intractable acidemia, hyperkalemia, or volume overload.

F. Complications

1. **Intravascular volume overload** is recognized by weight gain, hypertension, elevated central venous pressure (as indicated by internal jugular vein distension), and pulmonary or peripheral edema.

2. **Hyperkalemia** (i.e., serum potassium concentration > 5.5 mEq/L) develops due to excessive potassium intake, tissue necrosis, or hemolysis.

3. **Hyponatremia** (i.e., serum sodium concentration < 135 mEq/L) results from excessive water intake relative to sensible, insensible, and dialytic losses.

4. **Hyperphosphatemia** (i.e., serum phosphate concentration > 5.5 mg/dl) results from excessive phosphorus intake (e.g., due to hyperalimentation solutions) or tissue necrosis.

5. **Hypocalcemia** (i.e., serum calcium concentration < 8.5 mg/dl) usually is due to hyperphosphatemia or hypoalbuminemia.

6. **Hypercalcemia** (i.e., serum calcium concentration > 10.5 mg/dl) occurs during the recovery phase and is most common following rhabdomyolysis-induced acute renal failure.

7. **Acidemia** (i.e., arterial blood pH < 7.35) is seen most commonly with low cardiac output states or infection.

8. **Hyperuricemia** [i.e., serum uric acid concentration > 6.5 mg/dl (in women) and > 7.0 mg/dl (in men)] is a common finding in acute renal failure. This condition usually does not require therapy unless the serum uric acid concentration exceeds 15.0 mg/dl.

9. **Bleeding** may develop secondary to qualitative platelet dysfunction, which may be related to the severity of azotemia.

10. **Seizures.** Major motor or grand mal seizures may develop following early signs of neurologic dysfunction or may be abrupt.

11. Chronic renal failure
   a. Some depression in GFR or impairment of certain tubular functions (e.g., urine concentrating ability and potassium secretion) may persist in up to 10% of patients following recovery from acute renal failure.
   b. Progression to chronic renal failure is more likely with preexisting renal disease, advanced age, and extended length of oliguria.

III. CHRONIC RENAL FAILURE is defined as a substantial and irreversible reduction in renal function to less than 20% of normal.

A. Etiology

   1. Prerenal causes of chronic renal failure include severe, long-standing renal artery stenosis and bilateral renal arterial embolism.

   2. Renal causes include chronic glomerulonephritis, chronic tubulointerstitial nephritis, systemic lupus erythematosus (SLE), diabetes, amyloidosis, hypertension, neoplasia, and radiation nephritis.

   3. Postrenal causes derive from long-standing urinary obstruction.

B. Clinical features are highly variable.

   1. Neurologic signs of lethargy, somnolence, confusion, and neuromuscular irritability develop either gradually or abruptly.

   2. Cardiovascular signs of hypertension, congestive heart failure, and pericarditis also may be precipitous.

   3. Gastrointestinal signs, particularly anorexia, nausea, and vomiting, are very common.

   4. Metabolic signs can either be nonspecific (e.g., fatigue, pruritus, and sleep disturbances) or be referable to a specific defect (e.g., bone pain from secondary hyperparathyroidism).

C. Diagnosis

   1. Patient history should include information concerning past or present illness and drug use, previous surgery, and family history of renal disease.

   2. Physical examination is directed toward identifying the clinical signs described above. Intravascular volume overload and central nervous system (CNS) irritability are urgent concerns.

   3. Urinalysis and urine culture should be performed during the initial evaluation.

   4. Blood chemistries are important for determining management strategy. The severity of renal failure may be approximated using serum creatinine and BUN levels. Low plasma bicarbonate, high plasma inorganic phosphorus, and low plasma hemoglobin may provide insight into the duration of renal failure.

   5. Radiography. Chronic, end-stage kidneys are small (< 8 cm in length) and functionless. Occasionally, solitary cysts form after end-stage renal disease is established.

D. Therapy

   1. Dietary restrictions are vital to the proper care of patients with chronic renal failure. Dietary protein is restricted to 1.0–1.5 g/kg lean body weight, and dietary sodium is restricted to 4 g/day unless residual urine output obligates greater daily losses. (In these cases, urine sodium concentration should be measured and replaced, but not exceeded, in the diet.) Dietary intake of potassium, magnesium, and phosphorus is restricted, and a fluid intake limit is established based on daily losses.

   2. Renal replacement therapy is necessary for the maintenance care of end-stage renal disease.
      a. **Indications** include clinical uremia, severe azotemia (i.e., GFR < 20 ml/min), intractable hyperkalemia or acidemia, and intravascular volume overload.
      b. **Modalities** include hemodialysis, peritoneal dialysis, and renal allograft transplantation.

E. Complications arise in the course of chronic renal failure and during long-term renal replacement therapy. (A more detailed discussion of renal replacement therapy and the complications associated with this treatment appears in Part I: section IV).

   1. Hematologic disorders include severe anemia and bleeding.

2. **Cardiovascular disorders** include hypertension, pericarditis, cardiomyopathy, arrhythmias, congestive heart failure, endocarditis, and shock.

3. **Neuromuscular disorders** include generalized seizures, confusion, lethargy, emotional lability, myopathy, peripheral neuropathy, and syndromes related to nerve compression (e.g., **carpal tunnel syndrome**).

4. **Gastrointestinal disorders** include ulcers, gastroduodenitis, colitis, and hepatitis.

5. **Endocrine disorders** include secondary hyperparathyroidism, clinically euthyroid hypothyroxinemia, hyperprolactinemia, altered pituitary and gonadal function, and gynecomastia.

6. **Immune system disturbances** include lymphocytopenia, anergy, increased serum anticomplement activity, and abnormal monocyte motility. There is no proven increase in vulnerability to infectious diseases.

7. **Metabolic disorders** include renal osteodystrophy (osteitis fibrosa and osteomalacia) and altered drug metabolism.

IV. MEDICAL COMPLICATIONS OF RENAL REPLACEMENT THERAPY

A. **Introduction.** Renal replacement therapy is indicated for uremia; intractable hyperkalemia, acidemia, and congestive heart failure; extracellular fluid volume overload that is unresponsive to diuretics; and certain intoxications and poisonings. The choice of modality (i.e., hemodialysis, peritoneal dialysis, or renal transplantation) is based on patient age, underlying diseases, complicating medical conditions, patient preference and motivation, and the practical considerations relating to donor availability and to available sites of peritoneal or vascular dialysis access.

B. **Hemodialysis** is a renal replacement therapy involving **extracorporeal circulation** of blood through a dialysis membrane–containing unit via a surgically constructed vascular fistula. Percutaneous puncture and cannulation of the vascular access is required at each treatment. Blood and dialysate are separated by the semipermeable membrane, which allows solutes and water to move from blood to dialysate along concentration and osmotic pressure gradients. Complications can develop at any stage of the procedure.

1. **Improper dialyzer preparation** may allow contamination by preservative (formalin), air bubbles, or bacteria, leading to systemic toxicity, embolism, sepsis, or membrane rupture.

2. **Improper water treatment** may fail to remove excess calcium, magnesium, aluminum, fluoride, or copper, leading to elevated blood levels of these substances and possible poisoning.

3. **Equipment failure** may occur with power failure, air leaks in the blood conduits, dialyzer rupture, improper dialysate composition, blood loss from line separation, and hypo- or hyperthermia due to improperly warmed dialysate.

4. **Allergic reactions** to material leached from tubing or dialyzer include eosinophilia, urticaria, anaphylaxis, fever, and hypotension.

5. **Vascular access problems** are extremely common and include bleeding from puncture sites or suture lines, aneurysmal dilatation and rupture, occlusion by stricture or thrombus, infection (e.g., cellulitis, endarteritis, endocarditis, and sepsis), high-output congestive heart failure, and peripheral vascular insufficiency.

6. **Anticoagulant complications** can lead to local access bleeding or distant, occasionally life-threatening, hemorrhage.

7. **Transfusion complications** include secondary hemosiderosis and transfusion-related hepatitis.

8. **Cardiac arrhythmias** frequently complicate hemodialysis, beginning during the last several hours of treatment and persisting for about 6 hours following treatment. Asymptomatic ventricular ectopy exceeding 1000 premature ventricular contractions (PVCs)/hr may be observed.

9. **Dialysis disequilibrium** is a syndrome of headache, nausea, vomiting, muscle aches, and cramps, which develops if a large amount of solute (urea) is removed too quickly during treatment, particularly during the first several dialyses when total body urea load is likely to be high.

C. **Peritoneal dialysis** is a renal replacement therapy involving installation of 1–3 L of sterile dialysate into the peritoneal cavity via a surgically planted catheter and drainage of the dialysate after a specified **dwell period**. Frequent, brief exchanges (i.e., forty-eight 1-hour exchanges) may be done weekly in-center. Longer exchanges (i.e., four 6-hour exchanges) also are effective and may be done at home daily. Maintenance peritoneal dialysis also is associated with specific complications.

1. **Excessive removal of fluid** may result in hypotension, light-headedness, weakness, or syncope.

2. **Catheter-related complications** include occlusion (usually by fibrinous debris), infection, malposition, and, rarely, fracture.

3. **Dialysate-related complications** that develop if dialysate is too rapidly infused or inadequately warmed include abdominal or back pain, nausea, and vomiting.

4. **Peritonitis** is the most serious complication occurring in chronic peritoneal dialysis patients. Infection develops by inoculation through or around the catheter or by contamination of dialysate. Recurrent peritonitis is associated with high morbidity rates, frequent hospital stays, and considerable expense. Sepsis, peritoneal fibrosis, and loss of dialysis efficiency can complicate multiple infections and may constitute criteria for withdrawal from this form of therapy. Treatment of peritonitis is with parenteral and intraperitoneal antibiotics.

D. **Renal allograft transplantation** may be performed from a donor to a recipient if these individuals are **histocompatible**. Histocompatibility is measured by determination of **human leukocyte antigen (HLA)** types, **mixed lymphocyte reactivity (MLR)**, and **blood group** types. Donor kidneys may be from a living relative or from a cadaver in whom there is no evidence of infectious disease, specifically, bacteremia, hepatitis, acquired immune deficiency syndrome (AIDS), cytomegalovirus, syphilis, and malaria. Transplant recipients are given maintenance immunosuppressive agents (e.g., prednisone, azathioprine, cyclosporine, and cyclophosphamide) to prevent graft rejection. Complications of transplantation derive from several sources.

1. **Immunosuppression disorders** include leukopenia (alkylating agents), hepatitis (azathioprine), cystitis (cyclophosphamide), diabetes, obesity, cataracts, and, possibly, peptic ulcer disease and pancreatitis (prednisone).

2. **Secondary hypertension** may develop from extracellular fluid overload (prednisone), high renin secretion from native kidneys, vascular stenosis of the graft from anastomotic stricture or extrinsic compression by lymphocele or urinoma, rejection, recurrent glomerular disease, ureteral obstruction, or hypercalcemia. Coincident primary (essential) hypertension also may develop.

3. **Infection** may occur at any time following transplantation by common pathogens as well as opportunistic organisms. Common infections include urinary tract infection (60% of patients), pneumonia (20% of patients), wound or cannula infection, hepatitis, and sepsis. Uncommon organisms encountered in transplant recipients include cytomegalovirus (frequently asymptomatic but may cause pneumonia, hepatitis, retinitis, encephalitis, or mononucleosis syndrome), *Cryptococcus, Listeria monocytogenes* (meningitis), *Pneumocystis carinii*, and *Legionella pneumophila*.

4. **Rejection** may be **hyperacute** (immediate and intraoperative), **acute** (occurring within 4–60 days following transplantation), or **chronic** (occurring later than 60 days following transplantation).
   a. Acute rejection is associated with fever, decreased creatinine clearance, oliguria, sodium retention, graft enlargement and tenderness, hypertension, and proteinuria.
   b. Chronic rejection is clinically less dramatic, and can be suspected on the basis of decreased creatinine clearance, low-grade fever, increased proteinuria, hyperchloremic metabolic acidosis, hypertension, oliguria, weight gain, and edema. Five percent of allografts are lost due to chronic infection that occurs within 5 years after transplantation. Treatment for rejection may include high-dose corticosteroids, alkylating agents, cyclosporine, antilymphocyte globulin, and, occasionally, transplant (graft) nephrectomy.

5. **Malignancy** develops in 2%–7% of transplant recipients, a rate that is 100 times greater than that in healthy, age-matched individuals. The average time for malignancy to develop is 40 months but may range from 1 to 158 months. Lymphomas develop sooner (within 27 months after transplantation). Cancer of the skin and lips, lymphomas, cervical carcinoma, lung carcinoma, head and neck cancer, and colon carcinoma account for the majority of tumors, in order of frequency.

V. PROTEINURIA

A. **Definition.** Normal adults excrete less than 150 mg of protein in a 24-hour period, the major component of which is **albumin**. Urinary protein excretion exceeding 150 mg/24 hr is termed proteinuria (also called **albuminuria**).

B. Etiology

1. **Prerenal causes** of detectable protein in the urine include conditions in which the nephron is structurally intact.
   a. **Hyperproteinemic states** increase urinary protein excretion by increasing the filtered protein load and overwhelming the intrinsic protein catabolic pathways in the kidney. Such conditions include:
      (1) Rhabdomyolysis (myoglobulin)
      (2) Hemolysis (hemoglobin)
      (3) Plasma cell dyscrasia (immunoglobulin)
      (4) Disseminated intravascular coagulation [DIC] (fibrin split products)
      (5) Pancreatitis (amylase)
   b. **Hemodynamic alterations** may disturb **Starling's forces** in the glomerular capillaries, favoring increased permeability to plasma proteins. This may be seen in congestive heart failure and constrictive pericarditis and occasionally occurs with strenuous exercise or fever.

2. **Renal parenchymal causes** of increased urinary protein excretion include several diseases.
   a. **Glomerulonephritis**, particularly **focal glomerulosclerosis** (both the membranous and nil lesion forms), may increase urinary protein excretion over a large range (2–10 g/24 hr). **Albumin** constitutes the major component of urinary protein in these cases, and the **nephrotic syndrome** (hypoalbuminemia, edema, and hyperlipidemia) usually results.
   b. **Tubulointerstitial nephritis**, which may be idiopathic or secondary to systemic infection or drug ingestion, increases urinary protein excretion less selectively; that is, proteins other than albumin are excreted. **Tamm-Horsfall protein** and β_2-**microglobulin** are two such tubular proteins. **Amyloidosis** is another recognized cause of nonalbuminous proteinuria.

3. **Orthostatic proteinuria** refers to an increase in urinary protein that is detected only when the patient has been standing. The 24-hour urinary protein output tends to remain constant at about 0.5–2.5 g/24 hr, renal function remains normal, and the prognosis is excellent.

C. Diagnosis

1. **Patient history** should include information concerning recent infections, drug exposures, and intensive athletic activity as well as coincident medical illness and family history of renal disease.

2. **Physical examination** should be conducted for signs of underlying infectious, neoplastic, heredofamilial, rheumatologic, or metabolic disease, which may aid in making a specific diagnosis. It is essential to examine for the presence or absence of edema.

3. **Urinalysis**
   a. Screening tests for proteinuria include urine **dipsticks** (albumin only) and **sulfosalicylic acid precipitation** (albumin, paraproteins, immunoglobulins, and amyloid).
   b. Quantitative, 24-hour testing for urinary protein is essential, particularly in low-volume/high-concentration states (e.g., in congestive heart failure).
   c. Lipiduria is suggested by oval fat bodies on microscopic study.

4. **Urine and blood chemistries** should include quantitative protein measurement and protein electrophoresis. Elevated blood lipids and hypoalbuminemia support a diagnosis of nephrotic syndrome.

5. **Biopsy** is indicated in the evaluation of significant proteinuria and nephrotic syndrome when there is no obvious cause identified by noninvasive means. Pathologic study should include electron microscopy, immunofluorescence, and the use of special stains (e.g., Congo red for amyloid).

D. Therapy

1. **Treatment of the primary illness** often leads to resolution of the nephrotic syndrome in patients whose renal disease is secondary to an underlying disease.

2. **Diuretics** may be used for symptomatic treatment of edema, but care must be exercised to prevent intravascular volume depletion, which may predispose to thrombosis.

3. **Antilipemic agents.** The use of **clofibrate** and **cholestyramine** to reduce hyperlipidemia in nephrotic syndrome is controversial.

4. Increased dietary protein. Diets rich in protein of high biologic value may be instituted in the absence of azotemia.

E. **Complications** include consequences of hyperlipidemia (atherosclerosis and coronary artery disease), vitamin D deficiency (bone disease), loss of coagulation proteins (thrombosis), and salt retention (congestive heart failure). It has been suggested that patients with nephrotic syndrome are more susceptible to bacterial infections, particularly spontaneous bacterial peritonitis in children.

VI. HEMATURIA

A. **Definition.** Normal adults excrete 500,000–2,000,000 erythrocytes/24 hr, which amounts to less than 3 erythrocytes per high-power field of resuspended urinary sediment.

B. **Etiology**

1. **Renal parenchymal sources**
   a. **Glomerular diseases** that produce hematuria include primary glomerulonephritis and glomerulonephritis that is associated with SLE, vasculitis, systemic infection, or hereditary disease. In addition, red cell casts usually are seen in the urinary sediment.
   b. **Vascular and tubulointerstitial diseases** produce hematuria by hypersensitivity reactions, renal infarction (due to vascular occlusion), papillary necrosis, and pyelonephritis.
   c. **Trauma**, either blunt or penetrating, causes hematuria in the presence of renal contusion, laceration, or avulsion.
   d. **Renal epithelial or vascular tumors** also produce hematuria.

2. **Lower urinary tract sources** of hematuria include tumors, calculi, varices, infection, drug toxicity (cyclophosphamide), foreign bodies, and prostatic infection or neoplasia.

3. **Systemic coagulation disturbances** of either platelet function or coagulation proteins can lead to hematuria.

C. **Clinical features**

1. **Occult (microscopic) hematuria** refers to grossly normal urine in which numerous erythrocytes are detected microscopically.

2. **Gross (macroscopic) hematuria** refers to bloody or obviously discolored urine.

3. **Intermittent hematuria** refers to periods of gross hematuria separated by periods of occult or no hematuria.

4. **Glomerulonephritis** is suggested by the concurrent findings of hematuria, red cell casts, hypertension, and edema.

D. **Diagnosis**

1. **Urinalysis**
   a. Dipstick testing can differentiate hematuria from **pigmenturia** (i.e., hemoglobinuria or myoglobinuria). A positive **orthotoluidine test** in the absence of microscopically detected erythrocytes practically confirms the diagnosis of pigmenturia.
   b. Microscopic examination with phase-contrast optics often demonstrates dysmorphic erythrocytes in circumstances of hematuria due to glomerular disease.
   c. Urine culture should be performed routinely.
   d. Hematuria that occurs only at the end of urination is characteristic of **urinary schistosomiasis**, for which special studies are indicated.

2. **Radiography** may be extremely important.
   a. Intravenous urography can demonstrate renal masses, cysts, vascular malformations, papillary necrosis, ureteral stricture or obstruction by calculus, bladder tumor, and ureteral deviation.
   b. Special studies (e.g., angiography and nuclear scanning) occasionally are of value in delineating mass lesions.

3. **Biopsy** occasionally may assist in making a diagnosis of **renal hematuria with thin basement membranes** or in characterizing the lesion of a primary glomerular disease.

4. **Cystoscopy** is indicated in the evaluation of hematuria when normal results are obtained with physical examination, urinalysis, and intravenous urography.

E. Therapy

　1. The underlying disorder must be identified and treated.

　2. Urine volume should be maintained to prevent clots and obstruction in the lower urinary tract.

F. Complications

　1. Iron deficiency anemia may rarely complicate chronic, significant hematuria.

　2. Lower urinary tract clots can induce obstruction.

VII. HYPERTENSION

A. Definition. Hypertension is defined as a peripheral arterial blood pressure measurement exceeding 140/95 in men over age 45, 160/95 in women over age 45, and 130/90 in any adult between 20 and 45 years of age. Nomograms must be used in the interpretation of blood pressure in children.

B. Etiology

　1. Primary hypertension (also called **idiopathic** or **essential hypertension**) accounts for 90% of all cases of high blood pressure.

　2. Secondary hypertension
　　a. Renal hypertension may result from primary glomerular and tubulointerstitial disease, renal artery stenosis (renovascular hypertension), renin-producing tumors, and states of sodium retention.
　　b. Endocrine hypertension may result from acromegaly, hyperthyroidism, adrenal cortical disease (Cushing's syndrome, hyperaldosteronism, and congenital adrenal hyperplasia), adrenal medullary disease (pheochromocytoma), hypercalcemia, exogenous estrogens (birth control pills), corticosteroids (both glucocorticoids and mineralocorticoids), and sympathomimetic drugs.
　　c. Coarctation of the aorta is associated with hypertension, but the mechanism is not fully known.
　　d. Pregnancy-related hypertension is discussed in Part I: section XVIII D.
　　e. Neurogenic causes of hypertension include increased intracranial pressure, dysautonomia, encephalitis, and brain tumor.
　　f. Extreme sympathetic nervous system hyperactivity can induce high blood pressure in cases of extensive burns, psychosis, trauma, or stress.
　　g. Hypervolemic states, pathologic or iatrogenic, may be associated with hypertension.
　　h. Systolic hypertension may be seen in cases of high cardiac output (e.g., as occurs with aortic insufficiency, Paget's disease of bone, or arteriovenous fistulae).

C. Clinical features

　1. Occult hypertension may exist for years, identified only by routine or incidental screening.

　2. Accelerated hypertension is characterized by evidence of mild-to-moderate injury to a target organ (e.g., the brain, heart, retina, or kidney). Acceleration may be an asymptomatic increase in blood pressure de novo or may be a complication of chronic stable hypertension.

　3. Malignant hypertension is a rapidly progressive, severe form of accelerated hypertension, which nearly always is complicated by damage to the retina (hemorrhage or papilledema), brain (hemorrhage), heart (myocardial infarction or congestive heart failure), or kidney (hematuria or azotemia).

D. Diagnosis

　1. Patient history must identify age of onset, rate of progression, family history, presence and duration of target-organ symptoms, previous and present dietary habits, drug treatment, and patient compliance. The evaluation may be streamlined by the identification of symptoms associated with underlying disease, such as:
　　a. Nocturia and symptoms of uremia (chronic renal failure)
　　b. Headache, leg cramps with exercise, and cool lower extremities (coarctation)
　　c. Sweating and palpitations (pheochromocytoma)
　　d. Polyuria and weakness (hyperaldosteronism)
　　e. Tremor, diarrhea, and weight loss (hyperthyroidism)

2. **Physical examination** should include inspection of retinal fundi, determination of heart size (by detection of the point of maximal intensity, loudness of heart sounds, evidence of hyperdynamic circulation, and heart failure), a careful search for a systolic and diastolic abdominal or flank bruit, and a detailed neurologic examination. Electrocardiography is routine in older patients.

3. **Blood pressure measurements** should be made in a standard and reproducible manner. A sphygmomanometer of appropriate size should be used, and 3 readings taken 1 minute apart should be made on 3 separate days.

4. **Urinalysis** may identify the presence of target-organ damage (hematuria), the loss of concentrating ability (isosthenuria in the hydropenic patient), and evidence of underlying renal disease (active urinary sediment). Urine culture is not necessary.

5. **Blood and urine chemistries.** Blood analysis should routinely include a blood count and determination of blood sugar and serum electrolytes, creatinine, cholesterol, and fasting triglycerides. If the clinical assessment suggests underlying disease, more specific studies are indicated, including determination of serum thyroxine, calcium, and cortisol. Urine chemistries are helpful in cases of suspected pheochromocytoma (metanephrine), hyperaldosteronism (potassium), or Cushing's syndrome (urinary free cortisol).

6. **Radiography**
   a. **Rapid sequence intravenous urography** shows disparate renal size, delayed nephrogram, and late increase in nephrogram intensity in unilateral renal artery stenosis. Similar information may be obtained by radioisotopic renography in advanced cases. However, this technique is associated with a high rate of false-negative results.
   b. **Renal artery angiography**, with or without renal vein renin measurements, is the most definitive means of identifying renal artery stenosis. A new radiographic technique, **digital subtraction angiography**, may provide equivalent or superior anatomic detail and requires much smaller volumes of radiographic contrast material.

E. **Therapy**

1. **Therapy for underlying and complicating conditions**
   a. Underlying disorders should be identified and treated.
   b. Complicating risk factors should be eliminated, such as obesity, a high-salt diet, cigarette smoking, physical inactivity, use of oral contraceptives, and hyperlipidemia.

2. **Medical therapy** may be carried out in a stepwise fashion as follows:
   a. **Step 1:** Administer a diuretic agent or β-blocker*
   b. **Step 2:** Add a β-blocker, methyldopa, clonidine, or reserpine*
   c. **Step 3:** Add hydralazine or prazosin
   d. **Step 4:** Add minoxidil or an angiotensin-converting enzyme (ACE) inhibitor

3. **Percutaneous transluminal angioplasty** (balloon dilatation) should be tried in patients with non-ostial atherosclerotic lesions who are poor surgical candidates, who have renal insufficiency, or who refuse surgery.

4. **Surgical therapy** is reserved for patients with renovascular hypertension. Vascular reconstruction should be undertaken in good surgical candidates, particularly children with operable fibromuscular hyperplasia, and in patients who have had restenosis following percutaneous transluminal angioplasty.

VIII. NEPHROLITHIASIS

A. **Definition.** Renal calculi or stones arise due to papillary calcification or precipitation in urine of organized crystalline bodies of calcium salts, uric acid, cystine, or struvite.

B. **Etiology.** Certain conditions predispose to the formation of renal calculi.

1. **Calcium phosphate stones** develop in patients with hyperparathyroidism, distal renal tubular acidosis, idiopathic hypercalciuria, and medullary sponge kidney.

2. **Calcium oxalate stones** occur in association with idiopathic hypercalciuria, excessive dietary oxalate, vitamin C abuse, small bowel inflammation or resection, primary hyperoxaluria, and hypercalcemic states.

3. **Uric acid stones** arise as a result of persistently concentrated and acid urine, hyperuricosuria, hyperuricemia (in gout), and excess dietary purine.

---

*Calcium channel blockers may possibly be valuable as step 1 or step 2 agents.

4. **Cystine stones** represent the major clinical manifestation of cystinuria.

5. **Struvite stones.** Struvite is the name given to **triple phosphate** or **magnesium-ammonium-calcium phosphate**. Struvite stones, which consist of struvite with or without hydroxyapatite [$Ca_{10}(PO_4)_6(OH)_2$], result from urinary tract infection (chronic or recurrent) by urease-producing bacteria such as *Proteus, Providencia, Klebsiella, Pseudomonas, Serratia,* and *Enterobacter* species.

C. Clinical features may vary considerably.

1. **Occult passage** of small, asymptomatic stones may occur. More frequently, however, asymptomatic renal stones are identified radiographically during evaluation for other, unrelated conditions.

2. **Hematuria** regularly accompanies stone movement within the urinary tract and may be microscopic or gross. Hematuria may occur with or without pain.

3. **Frequency and dysuria** are common complaints of patients with stones lodged in the intravesical segment of the distal ureter and may be mistaken as the symptoms of **cystitis**. Dysuria also occurs during the passage of grumous or pultaceous **sludge**.

4. **Abdominal pain, tenesmus, and rectal pain** may occur with a stone in the renal pelvis and often are accompanied by nausea and vomiting.

5. **Renal colic**, with flank pain radiating to the inguinal ligament, urethra, labia, testis, or penis, is typical of a stone in the midureter.

6. **Acute obstruction** by a stone may occur, generating renal colic. **Subacute obstruction** may occur with few or no symptoms.

7. **Infection** often complicates stone disease and usually produces flank or back pain, fever, and chills, particularly with urinary obstruction.

D. Diagnosis

1. **Patient history** should identify other family members with stone disease as well as the patient's past and present use of drugs and vitamins (particularly vitamins A, D, and C).

2. **Physical examination.** Acute renal colic must be differentiated from other causes of abdominal, pelvic, and back pain.

3. **Urinalysis** provides data in all cases.
   a. Urine pH is inappropriately high in renal tubular acidosis, favoring calcium phosphate stone formation. Low urine volume with low urine pH is a risk factor for uric acid stones.
   b. Crystals often are found appropriate to urine pH, with **acid urine** containing crystals of uric acid and cystine and **alkaline urine** containing crystals of calcium oxalate, calcium phosphate, and struvite.
   c. Bacteriuria may signal infection-related stones, and in such cases urine culture should be performed.

4. **Urine and blood chemistries** are critical to the metabolic evaluation of the patient with nephrolithiasis.
   a. A blood sample should be examined for levels of electrolytes, creatinine, BUN, calcium, phosphate, and uric acid.
   b. A 24-hour urine collection should be studied for urine volume and pH and levels of calcium phosphate, uric acid, oxalate, creatinine, sodium, potassium, and cystine.

5. **Radiography**
   a. **Plain abdominal films** are useful for identifying the composition of renal stones. Calcium stones are intensely radiopaque; cystine, struvite (infection-induced), and mixed uric acid–calcium stones are moderately radiopaque. Abdominal films also help to localize stones, and serial films indicate disease activity as reflected by increases in stone size and number.
   b. **Intravenous urography** is necessary for evaluating radiolucent stones and obstruction of urine flow.

6. **Cystoscopy** is indicated for the detection and removal of bladder calculi and for the removal of ureteral stones lodged near the ureterovesical junction.

E. Therapy

1. **Medical therapy** is predicated on the identified metabolic disorder. In all circumstances, however, a urine volume of more than 2 L/day should be achieved.

     a. Calcium phosphate stones. Primary hyperparathyroidism should be treated promptly by parathyroidectomy; distal tubular acidosis requires independent evaluation; and idiopathic hypercalciuria is treated with diuretics (thiazides or amiloride) or oral neutral potassium phosphate.

     b. Calcium oxalate stones. Therapy includes dietary restriction of oxalate-rich food, elimination of large doses (i.e., > 500 mg/day) of ascorbic acid, and administration of diuretics (thiazides or amiloride) or oral neutral potassium phosphate.

     c. Uric acid stones. Therapy includes administration of oral sodium bicarbonate to maintain an alkaline urine (i.e., a urine pH above 7) and, in selected patients, restriction of dietary purine or administration of allopurinol.

     d. Cystine stones. Sodium bicarbonate is administered to keep urine pH above 7.5, and acetazolamide is given at bedtime to maintain urine alkalinity during the night. Noncompliant patients and those with severe or refractory stone disease may be candidates for oral D-penicillamine or intrarenal stone dissolution by alkaline or acetylcysteine irrigation.

     e. Struvite stones. Treatment is aimed at maintaining urinary asepsis, which may require antibiotics.

  2. Surgical therapy (removal) is indicated for obstructing stones if there is infection proximal to the stone or if the stone is radiographically determined to be too large to pass spontaneously. **Staghorn calculi** should be removed if renal function is in jeopardy.

  3. Extracorporeal shock wave lithotripsy is a new technique for treating nephrolithiasis. Electrically induced shock waves are generated in a water bath and are focused on the stone, leading to its in situ dissolution. This technique is safe, effective, and does not require surgery.

IX. URINARY TRACT OBSTRUCTION

  A. Introduction. An obstruction in the urinary tract may occur at any point between the renal tubules and the urethra. Urinary obstruction may be acute or chronic, unilateral or bilateral, and partial or complete. Chronic urinary obstruction often is partial and may be asymptomatic, particularly in slowly progressive cases. The consequences of urinary obstruction include structural changes in the lower urinary tract as a result of increases in pressure opposing normal urine flow (**obstructive uropathy**), gross dilatation of the calyces and collecting system of the affected kidney (**hydronephrosis**), and, ultimately, renal parenchymal damage (**obstructive nephropathy**).

  B. Etiology. The causes of urinary obstruction can be divided into **mechanical** causes, which may be intrinsic or extrinsic, and **functional** causes.

    1. Intrinsic mechanical causes

     a. Intrarenal tubular obstruction results from precipitation of uric acid, sulfonamide, or paraprotein crystals.

     b. Extrarenal pelvic or ureteral obstruction is caused by calculus, thrombus, papillary necrosis, or tumor.

     c. Structural lesions of the ureter or bladder include stricture, tumor, urethral valves, ureteroceles, and foreign body.

    2. Extrinsic mechanical causes

     a. Compression. Urinary obstruction can result from compression by:

      (1) Prostatic hypertrophy or carcinoma

      (2) Uterine prolapse or tumor

      (3) Ovarian abscess, cyst, or tumor

      (4) Endometriosis

      (5) Pregnancy

      (6) Enlarged or aneurysmal pelvic vessels

      (7) Retroperitoneal tumor, infection, or fibrosis

     b. Surgical misadventures that result in obstruction include accidental ureteral ligation.

    3. Functional causes. Ureteral or bladder dysfunction results from myelodysplasia, injury or congenital defect of the spinal cord, tabes dorsalis, diabetes mellitus, multiple sclerosis, and autonomic neuropathy including drug-induced neuropathy (e.g., due to disopyramide).

  C. Clinical features vary depending on the site of the obstruction and the speed with which the obstruction develops.

    1. An absence of symptoms often occurs in chronic, slowly advancing obstructive disease. The clinical picture often is overshadowed by signs of the primary disease (e.g., in a case of metastatic tumor or surgical complications) until biochemical evidence of renal impairment develops.

2. Pain and renal enlargement (abdominal or flank mass) usually is the case in acute obstruction. The pain characteristically is a steady crescendo, is most severe in the flank, and radiates toward the ipsilateral testis or labium.

3. Urinary symptoms predominate in obstructive disease of the bladder or urethra. Hesitancy, decreased force of urinary stream, urinary frequency, and dribbling are common in the context of obstruction.

4. Renal functional impairment typically is expressed as tubular defects in acid and potassium transport as well as defective tubular responsiveness to hormone action. Clinically, hyperkalemia, mild acidemia, and polyuria precede azotemia, which may progress to renal failure.

D. Diagnosis

1. Urinalysis varies but may reveal inappropriately dilute urine, hematuria (in cases of obstruction due to calculus or tumor), or bacteriuria. Because infection often complicates obstruction, causing serious detriment to renal function, urine culture is essential. Examination of the urinary sediment often shows no abnormality but may reveal crystals of uric acid or sulfonamide.

2. Blood chemistries usually are not diagnostic.

3. Radiography provides the clinical sine qua non of obstruction. Ultrasonography or CT reliably detects evidence of hydronephrosis, such as calyceal blunting and dilatation of the renal pelvis, ureter, or both. Intravenous urography may fail to visualize the kidneys if the GFR is decreased substantially. Retrograde urography occasionally may help to identify unilateral (particularly partial) ureteral obstruction. Nuclear scanning of the kidney often is specific enough to confirm the diagnosis.

E. Therapy

1. Relief of obstruction is paramount and should be appropriate to the structural nature of the occluding lesion. Methods include surgery, ureteral stent, and nephroscopic stone removal.

2. Medical management following relief of obstruction is aimed at correcting **postobstructive diuresis**. Many factors contribute to this diuresis, including the excretion of solute (urea) that was retained during the period of obstruction and the impaired concentrating ability that usually exists in the recently obstructed kidney. Management during this period involves careful, adequate fluid replacement with frequent assessment of body weight, intravascular volume, and blood and urine electrolyte concentration.

F. Complications

1. Infection, particularly in the context of obstructing calculi, must be detected and promptly treated to prevent extensive pyelonephritis, perirenal abscess, and sepsis.

2. Hypertension may complicate obstruction and occurs secondary to both intravascular volume expansion and ischemic stimulation of renin secretion.

3. Polycythemia has been reported in association with hydronephrosis and is purportedly due to increased erythropoietin release.

4. Persistent tubular defects may continue beyond 1 year following relief of obstruction. Impaired concentrating ability and limited excretion of a potassium load are the most common defects.

5. Chronic renal failure can develop from obstructive disease, most commonly with long-standing obstruction or with complicating urinary tract infection.

X. URINARY TRACT INFECTION

A. Definition. Urinary tract infections are defined in terms of the involved urinary structures, such as:

1. Cystitis (inflammation of the bladder)

2. Urethritis (inflammation of the urethra)

3. Pyelonephritis (inflammation of renal tubules and interstitium)

4. Prostatitis (inflammation of the prostate gland)

B. Etiology. A clinical urinary tract infection occasionally develops from simple inoculation of the lower urinary tract during instrumentation or sexual intercourse. More commonly, however, other risk factors exist, which increase the likelihood that inoculation will progress to clinical infection.

1. **Agents of infection**
   a. **Common agents** of urinary tract infection include *Escherichia coli, Proteus, Klebsiella, Enterobacter, Pseudomonas, Serratia*, enterococcus, *Candida, Neisseria gonorrhoeae, Trichomonas vaginalis*, and herpes simplex virus.
   b. **Uncommon agents** include *Staphylococcus* and mycobacteria that cause tuberculosis.
   c. **Rare agents** include *Nocardia, Actinomyces, Brucella*, adenovirus, and *Torulopsis*.

2. **Routes of inoculation**
   a. **Urethral inoculation** is very common among women, particularly those with vaginal and periurethral colonization by virulent bacteria. Local trauma, either mechanical (e.g., intercourse) or biologic (e.g., vaginitis and intertrigo), can predispose to superinfection of the periurethral mucosa. Surgery, particularly cystoscopy, can contaminate the bladder urine.
   b. **Hematogenous spread.** It is extremely unusual for gram-negative bacterial sepsis to induce pyelonephritis in the absence of other risk factors.

3. **Risk factors**
   a. **Obstruction** that induces urinary stasis and impairs host defenses (i.e., via decreased renal blood flow and decreased delivery of leukocytes and antibodies) is a crucial predisposing factor.
   b. **Vesicoureteral reflux** may promote ascending infection in several ways, including increased delivery of bacteria, increased size of the inoculum, incomplete bladder emptying, altered renal hemodynamics, and, possibly, altered host defenses.
   c. **Instrumentation**, particularly the use of urinary drainage (Foley) catheters, frequently is associated with significant bacteriuria.
   d. **Pregnancy** is clearly associated with altered ureteral smooth muscle function and a higher incidence of asymptomatic bacteriuria. The asymptomatic bacteriuria noted in pregnant women is more likely to progress to pyelonephritis than that which occurs in nonpregnant women.
   e. **Diabetes mellitus** is associated with a high rate of infection. Part of this risk is mediated through neurogenic bladder disturbances, and part is due to other immune disorders in diabetes.
   f. **Immune deficiency**, whether it is congenital, acquired, or drug-induced, increases the risk of urinary infection in concert with the generally increased patient susceptibility.

C. **Clinical features**

1. **Symptoms of lower tract infection** include urinary frequency, dysuria, burning, suprapubic pain, malodorous or cloudy urine, and continence difficulties. These symptoms (in any combination) are most common in urethritis, prostatitis (with or without perineal pain and ejaculatory pain), and cystitis.

2. **Symptoms of acute pyelonephritis** (parenchymal renal infection) include flank pain, fever, malaise, and any symptoms of lower tract infection.

3. **Septic shock** is frequently seen in the elderly or institutionalized patient. Possible presenting signs include hypothermia, mental status alterations, syncope, and coma.

D. **Diagnosis**

1. **Urinalysis** of fresh, unspun urine should be performed. The identification of 1 bacterium per high-power field ($400\times$) is indicative of a colony growth on culture of more than 10^5 colonies/ml. Analysis of the centrifuged sediment usually reveals leukocyturia (neutrophils) and bacteriuria. Gram staining of the urinary sediment is routine and may further characterize the offending organism, allowing more specific therapy before culture results are known. Microscopic hematuria is common.

2. **Routine urine culture** is the definitive method of diagnosis. A clean-catch, midstream specimen should be submitted for plating within 3 hours; the specimen should be refrigerated if any delay is anticipated. Unquestionably, the growth of more than 10^5 colonies/ml in the presence of symptoms signifies infection worthy of treatment. The diagnostic significance of culture growth below this level is debated. However, a growth of less than 10^5 colonies/ml may warrant therapy under appropriate clinical circumstances, such as severe symptoms, history of partial antibiotic treatment, known recurrent infections, suspicion of the accuracy of the laboratory report, and the presence of renal calculi.

3. **Special urine cultures** must be ordered specifically. In cases with typical symptoms but

repeatedly negative routine cultures, infection by *Ureaplasma* or *Chlamydia* (called **urethral syndrome**) should be suspected and the laboratory instructed to search for these organisms. Herpes simplex virus requires special culture methods, and *N. gonorrhoeae* requires immediate inoculation on Thayer-Martin (chocolate agar) media and carbon dioxide incubation. Sterile pyuria, even in the asymptomatic patient, should arouse suspicion of renal tuberculosis. A first morning urine specimen is best for this purpose.

4. **Blood chemistries** provide little information but occasionally demonstrate leukocytosis.

5. **Radiography.** Intravenous urography is helpful in the evaluation of infection complicating chronic vesicoureteral reflux, obstruction, calculi, and chronic pyelonephritis. Voiding cystourethrography and retrograde ureterography occasionally are indicated in the evaluation of recurrent infections, particularly in children.

E. Therapy

1. **Antibiotics.** Initial antibacterial therapy is selected on the basis of the urinalysis and the understanding of the epidemiology and bacteriology of the infection. The appropriateness of this therapy must be confirmed by culture and sensitivity testing in refractory, relapsing, and atypical cases.
   a. **Uncomplicated lower tract infection** may be treated with a single dose of amoxicillin (3.0 g orally), trimethoprim-sulfamethoxazole (320 mg/1.6 g orally), or aminoglycoside (e.g., gentamicin, 10–30 mg intramuscularly). Special recommendations exist for gonorrhea, syphilis, and trichomoniasis.
   b. **Relapsing urinary tract infection and pyelonephritis** should be treated for 14 days. Clinically stable patients may be treated at home with trimethoprim-sulfamethoxazole (80 mg/400 mg orally, twice daily) or ampicillin (250 mg orally, four times daily).
   c. **Prostatitis** must be treated for at least 14 days with antibiotics that penetrate and remain active in prostatic tissue and fluid (e.g., trimethoprim and carbenicillin).
   d. **Recurrent infections.** Antibacterial suppression is indicated in the management of recalcitrant infections without rectifiable underlying causes. Typical regimens include trimethoprim-sulfamethoxazole (40 mg/200 mg orally, once daily), mandelamine (500 mg orally, four times daily), and sulfisoxazole (500 mg orally, once daily).
   e. **Catheter-associated bacteriuria** in the acutely catheterized patient usually resolves following removal of the catheter. Failure to do so or the development of symptoms within 12–24 hours necessitates appropriate antibacterial therapy.

2. **Corrective surgery** is indicated for the removal of calculi and for the repair of obstructing anatomic lesions.

F. Complications

1. **Abscess formation**, in either the kidney parenchyma or the surrounding retroperitoneal space, often complicates infection proximal to unrelieved obstruction. Persistent systemic symptoms and resistant bacteriuria should prompt diagnostic study using ultrasonography or CT.

2. **Xanthogranulomatous pyelonephritis** is a form of chronic bacterial infection characterized by granuloma formation with lipid-laden macrophages. *Proteus mirabilis* is the organism most frequently recovered from renal abscess fluid. There is a history of nephrolithiasis in 73% of patients, and in many cases a staghorn calculus is identified at surgery.

3. **Emphysematous pyelonephritis** is a rare, life-threatening complication of bacterial pyelonephritis. Seen most frequently in diabetics, this disease is characterized by gas-forming bacterial infection.

4. **Chronic renal failure.** Chronic pyelonephritis can lead to end-stage renal disease, particularly if it coexists with renal calculi or obstruction. Most cases of chronic renal failure due to chronic pyelonephritis are not bacterial in origin but represent a broad spectrum of chronic tubulointerstitial disease.

XI. GLOMERULAR DISEASE

A. Hereditary nephritis (Alport's syndrome)

1. **Inheritance and incidence.** Hereditary nephritis is inherited as an autosomal dominant trait with variable penetrance. The actual incidence is unknown, and males and females appear to be affected equally.

2. **Clinical features.** Hematuria, red cell casts, pyuria, proteinuria, and progressive renal failure

occur with variable severity. Renal failure is more common in males. High-frequency sensorineural hearing loss, often without clinically significant deafness, is characteristic. Keratoconus, lenticonus, megalocornea, spherophakia, and macrothrombocytopenia may be associated findings.

3. **Therapy and prognosis.** No treatment is successful in slowing or preventing the renal failure, and prognosis is variable. Males tend to progress to uremia by the fourth decade of life; most females have only microscopic hematuria. The severity of the disease differs among family members.

B. **Minimal change disease** (also called **lipoid nephrosis** or **nil lesion nephrotic syndrome**)

1. **Incidence.** Minimal change disease occurs at an annual rate of 16.1 cases per 1 million children and 2.2 cases per 1 million adults. The male-to-female ratio is 2:1 in children and 1:1 in adults. Minimal change disease accounts for 77% of cases of idiopathic nephrotic syndrome in children but only 23% of cases in adults.

2. **Pathology** is scant and nonspecific.
   a. Fusion of epithelial foot processes is seen with electron microscopy but is common to all proteinuric states.
   b. Normal-appearing capillaries and basement membranes as seen by light, immunofluorescence, and electron microscopy are the rule.
   c. Mesangial prominence and sclerotic glomeruli occasionally are described.

3. **Clinical features and diagnosis**
   a. Nephrotic syndrome is the typical presentation by patients of all ages. Early morning periorbital edema and ascites are more common in children. Proteinuria usually exceeds 100 mg/kg/day.
   b. Hypertension occurs in 10% of children and in 35% of adults.
   c. Hematuria in children is gross in 1.5% of cases and microscopic in 23%; in adults, gross hematuria occurs in 0.8% and microscopic hematuria in 19%.
   d. Azotemia develops in 23% of children and in 34% of adults.

4. **Therapy**
   a. **Glucocorticoids.** The remission rate with adequate steroid treatment (i.e., 1–2 mg/kg/day for 4–8 weeks) is 90% for both children and adults. Prolonged remission is seen in 10%–60% of patients; however, relapse is common and is multiple in 25%–50% of patients. Relapses typically are steroid responsive, with only 5% of initially steroid-responsive patients developing steroid resistance or dependence.
   b. **Cytotoxic agents** (e.g., cyclophosphamide and chlorambucil) have been effective in steroid-resistant and multiple relapsing cases. Occasionally, steroid-resistant patients gain steroid sensitivity following therapy with cytotoxic alkylating agents. Chlorambucil appears to lead to more stable and longer remissions than does cyclophosphamide. The possibility of gonadal (chromosomal) damage caused by these drugs must be carefully considered before they are used in patients who are planning to have children.

5. **Prognosis.** Minimal change disease is associated with low mortality rates (i.e., 10% among adults and 1.5% among children), with only 10% of deaths caused by renal failure. Infection, hypovolemia, and treatment-related complications account for more than 80% of deaths.

C. **Membranous glomerulonephritis**

1. **Etiology**
   a. **Primary (idiopathic) membranous glomerulonephritis** accounts for 30%–50% of cases of idiopathic nephrotic syndrome in adults but less than 1% of cases in children.
   b. **Secondary membranous glomerulonephritis** may occur with a variety of underlying conditions, including:
      (1) **Infection** (e.g., chronic hepatitis B, syphilis, malaria, schistosomiasis, and filariasis)
      (2) **Rheumatic disease** (e.g., SLE)
      (3) **Neoplasm** (e.g., carcinoma of the lung, colon, stomach, breast, and kidney; non-Hodgkin's lymphoma; leukemia; and Wilms' tumor).
      (4) **Drug therapy** (e.g., with mercury, gold, D-penicillamine, and captopril)

2. **Pathology.** The stages of membranous glomerulonephritis are defined by the following characteristic findings.
   a. **Stage I:** Normal appearance by light microscopy; subepithelial electron-dense deposits by electron microscopy
   b. **Stage II:** Spike-like projections of basement membrane material by light microscopy (best visualized with a silver impregnation stain); variable basement membrane thickening

      c. Stage III: Thick glomerular basement membrane, with a "moth-eaten" or "swiss-cheese" appearance due to encirclement of immune deposits by spike-like projections of normal glomerular basement membrane

      d. Stage IV: Thickening of the capillary wall with areas of segmental or global glomerulosclerosis; possible tubulointerstitial fibrosis

3. Clinical features. More than 85% of adults present with proteinuria (> 3.5 g/day/1.73 m² body surface area). The GFR usually is normal at diagnosis and often remains normal for 4–5 years thereafter.

4. Clinical course. Membranous glomerulonephritis has a variable course. About 20%–30% of patients achieve a lasting spontaneous remission, 20%–30% develop variable degrees of persistent proteinuria and nonuremic azotemia, and the remainder advance to end-stage renal disease, usually over a 5-year period.

5. Therapy with glucocorticoids or cytotoxic agents has not been proven effective. The unpredictable outcome of this disease makes the evaluation of therapy very difficult. Some nephrologists advocate the use of short (6-week) courses of high-dose (60–100 mg/day) oral prednisone.

6. Complications may intervene, causing an abrupt decrease in renal function.

      a. A **hypercoagulable state** exists in nephrotic patients. This condition is seemingly more common with membranous glomerulonephritis and may be closely related to the severity of hypoalbuminemia. Renal vein thrombosis is a recognized problem; pulmonary embolism and arterial thrombosis also have been described.

      b. Intravascular volume depletion secondary to vigorous diuretic administration leads to decreased renal blood flow.

      c. Hypertension, obstruction, or infection may impair GFR in patients with this glomerulonephritis.

      d. Superimposed renal disease such as acute allergic interstitial nephritis may occur in response to drugs (e.g., furosemide).

D. Mesangial proliferative glomerulonephritis

1. Etiology is unknown.

2. Pathology

      a. The mesangial proliferative lesion in glomerulonephritis is a global and diffuse increase in the number of mesangial cells and in mesangial matrix. Mesangial deposits are seen in 50% of biopsies using special stains. In progressive disease, the mesangial prominence frequently evolves into focal and segmental sclerosis.

      b. The glomerular basement membrane, the capillary endothelium, and the epithelium lining Bowman's space are normal.

3. Clinical features may include asymptomatic proteinuria or hematuria. Although 24-hour urinary protein excretion can exceed 3.5 g, the complete nephrotic syndrome is inconsistently seen. One-third of patients are hypertensive at the time of diagnosis. Creatinine clearance is reduced in only 25% of patients at presentation. Serum complement component levels are normal.

4. Clinical course. Mesangial proliferative glomerulonephritis has a very variable course. Some patients progress rapidly to renal failure, while many patients have symptoms of fluctuating severity for years.

5. Therapy with high-dose (1–2 mg/kg/day) glucocorticoids has been reported to be effective in remission induction. Some steroid failures respond to treatment with cyclophosphamide or chlorambucil.

E. Membranoproliferative glomerulonephritis is one name given to a group of glomerulonephritic disorders. Historically, this group of disorders has also been referred to as **mesangiocapillary glomerulonephritis, chronic lobular glomerulonephritis**, and **hypocomplementemic nephritis**.

1. Incidence and etiology

      a. Collectively, the disorders in this group account for 41% of cases of idiopathic nephrotic syndrome in children and 30% of cases in adults. Males and females are affected equally.

      b. Membranoproliferative glomerulonephritis may be idiopathic or secondary to SLE, cryoglobulinemia, or chronic viral or bacterial infection.

2. Pathology. There are three pathologic types of membranoproliferative glomerulonephritis, each with distinct features.

      a. Type I is characterized by an intact glomerular basement membrane, subendothelial and mesangial deposits, significant mesangial prominence with matrix interposition, and immunofluorescent positivity for IgG, complement components (C1q, C4, and C2), and properdin.

b. Type II (also called **dense deposit disease**) is characterized by intramembranous and subepithelial deposits (''humps'') in 50% of cases, mesangial deposits, moderate mesangial prominence with interposition, and immunofluorescent positivity for IgG, C3, and properdin.

c. Type III is characterized by features of true membranous glomerulonephritis and features of type I membranoproliferative glomerulonephritis.

3. Clinical features

a. This glomerulonephritis has a highly variable presentation. An indolent, slowly evolving course including hematuria and proteinuria, with or without an active urinary sediment, is common. Nephrotic syndrome also is present in many cases. Rapid progression to renal failure with edema and severe hypertension (acute nephritis) has been described.

b. Hypocomplementemia is the most characteristic laboratory finding but is not universally present. The degree of C3 depression may be used as a rough guide to disease activity.

4. Clinical course. In membranoproliferative glomerulonephritis there is progressive deterioration of renal function. Spontaneous clinical remissions have been reported, but glomerular pathology and immunochemistry remain abnormal. Chronic glomerulonephritis with end-stage renal disease develops in most cases.

5. Therapy rarely is effective, although occasional reports claim some benefit of treatment with steroids, alkylating agents, or anticoagulants.

F. Focal glomerulosclerosis

1. Incidence and etiology

a. Focal glomerulosclerosis accounts for 5%–12% of cases of idiopathic nephrotic syndrome in adults and is the most common cause of steroid-resistant nephrotic syndrome in children. Males are affected slighly more commonly than females. Although it is typically a disease of children and young adults, focal glomerulosclerosis has been recognized in patients over 70 years of age.

b. Focal glomerulosclerosis is of unknown etiology. It is seen occasionally in the context of AIDS, heroin and other intravascular drug use, and with chronic vesicoureteral reflux, but the causal relationships are uncertain.

2. Pathology. The hallmark lesion of focal and segmental glomerulosclerosis evolves through several stages, including mild mesangial prominence, loss of glomerular cellularity, and collapse of capillary loops. Adhesions between sclerotic portions of the glomerular tuft and Bowman's capsule are seen.

3. Clinical features and diagnosis

a. Nephrotic syndrome is the most common clinical presentation. Hypertension and renal failure occur infrequently in childhood but become more prevalent with advancing age.

b. There are no specific laboratory findings. Proteinuria tends to be heavy (i.e., > 15 g/24 hr), and the biochemical derangements of nephrotic syndrome are accordingly severe.

4. Therapy rarely is successful since focal glomerulosclerosis is characteristically steroid resistant. Focal glomerulosclerosis is reported to recur in 30%–40% of renal allografts within 3 weeks to 1 year following transplantation.

G. Goodpasture's syndrome (see also Chapter 2, section XIV B)

1. Definition. Goodpasture's syndrome refers to a group of illnesses defined by the following triad of findings: **glomerulonephritis** (usually crescentic), **pulmonary hemorrhage**, and **anti-glomerular basement membrane (anti-GBM) antibody**. The renal and pulmonary components may be severe or clinically silent. The presence of the anti-GBM antibody, however, has become the sine qua non of the diagnosis. Although many systemic illnesses include renal disease and pulmonary hemorrhage [e.g., SLE (see Part I: section XI M), necrotizing vasculitis (see Part I: section XI N), Wegener's granulomatosis (see Part I: section XI N 3), Henoch-Schönlein purpura (see Part I: section XI K), cryoglobulinemia (see Part I: section XI O), thrombotic thrombocytopenic purpura (see Part I: section XV D), legionnaire's disease, and renal disease complicated by pulmonary embolism or congestive heart failure], **only those illnesses with detectable anti-GBM antibody are considered bona fide Goodpasture's syndrome.**

2. Clinical features and diagnosis

a. Clinical presentation is highly variable.

(1) Generalized, systemic symptoms may precede organ-specific complaints. Fever and myalgia are common; arthritis, lymphadenopathy, and palpable purpura are not seen and, when present, suggest lupus nephritis or necrotizing vasculitis.

    (2) Renal involvement usually is in the form of rapidly progressive renal failure. Proteinuria usually is mild, and the urinary sediment contains erythrocytes and red cell casts. This "nephritic" picture may be mild or severe.

    (3) Pulmonary manifestations include radiographic infiltrates, hemoptysis, cough, and dyspnea. The lung disease usually precedes kidney disease by a period of days to weeks.

  b. Laboratory findings

    (1) The most important finding is evidence of circulating IgG anti-GBM antibody, which is present in more than 90% of patients. Evidence of renal or pulmonary insufficiency reflects the severity of organ involvement. Iron deficiency anemia may be seen in patients with long-standing pulmonary bleeding.

    (2) The pathologic appearance of the kidney is typically that of a crescentic, proliferative glomerulonephritis. Crescents involve 80%–100% of glomeruli and are highly cellular. Vasculitis is not seen.

3. Clinical course. Like the clinical presentation, the course of Goodpasture's syndrome is variable. Some patients with minor recurrent pulmonary hemorrhage may be labeled as having idiopathic pulmonary hemosiderosis for years until an abnormal urinary sediment prompts measurement of anti-GBM antibody. Other patients develop abrupt-onset, fulminating disease and die due to complete renal failure and suffocation by massive pulmonary bleeding over a period of hours to days.

4. Therapy. Several methods of therapy appear to benefit patients with Goodpasture's syndrome.

  a. Short courses of high-dose, intravenous ("pulse") corticosteroids have been reportedly helpful in controlling pulmonary hemorrhage early in the disease.

  b. There has been a variety of clinical trials involving combinations of corticosteroids and alkylating immunosuppressive agents.

  c. A promising approach to rapidly deteriorating renal function has been intensive, daily plasmapheresis combined with chemotherapy.

  d. Nephrectomy should be reserved for extreme and intractable cases.

H. Idiopathic crescentic glomerulonephritis is a pathologically defined entity, which typically presents as a rapidly progressive deterioration of renal function. It is imperative to recognize that other lesions may induce the clinical syndrome of **rapidly progressive glomerulonephritis**. This section considers only the idiopathic cases; that is, those cases not due to other crescentic glomerular diseases.

1. Incidence and etiology

  a. Idiopathic crescentic glomerulonephritis accounts for about one-third of all cases of crescentic glomerulonephritis. Males are affected twice as frequently as females, and the median age at onset is 58 years.

  b. The etiology is unknown.

2. Clinical features. Idiopathic crescentic glomerulonephritis presents as abrupt-onset renal failure, with rapid loss of renal function (in less than 3 months), frequently normal blood pressure, and normal kidney size. About half of patients are oliguric and azotemic at the time of presentation. Transient, mild pulmonary infiltrates or hemoptysis is seen in half of patients. Nonspecific symptoms (e.g., weakness, nausea, cough, weight loss, fever, myalgia, and arthralgia) often announce the disease. With the exception of lung involvement, extrarenal involvement is rare.

3. Diagnosis. There are no diagnostic laboratory findings. The diagnosis is based on the discovery of epithelial crescents in a majority of glomeruli in the renal biopsy specimen. Crescents contain epithelial cells, mononuclear phagocytes, fibrin, and fibrinogen. Extensive involvement is the rule, with crescents often surrounding the glomeruli. Proliferation of glomerular endothelial cells is common, as is focal and segmental necrosis. A mononuclear interstitial infiltrate is typical.

4. Clinical course and prognosis are very bleak. Renal failure requiring renal replacement therapy develops in 3–6 months in more than 50% of patients. Patients who are nonoliguric at the time of presentation and have serum creatinine levels below 6 mg/dl may have a more favorable prognosis, which, for some, includes stabilization or gradual improvement of renal function.

5. Therapy. There are no controlled experimental data to support a standard therapeutic approach to idiopathic crescentic glomerulonephritis. Favorable results have been reported in isolated cases using many different treatments, including pulse corticosteroids, alkylating agents, plasmapheresis, and anticoagulant or antiplatelet drugs.

I. **Postinfectious glomerulonephritis** is an acute glomerulonephritis that occurs with a variety of local or systemic infections. (Glomerulonephritis that is associated with infective endocarditis and visceral abscess is discussed in section XI Q.) Postinfectious glomerulonephritis has been described as a sequela of disease due to viruses (hepatitis B, Epstein-Barr, cytomegalovirus, herpes zoster, mumps, variola, and rubella), fungi (*Coccidioides immitis*), protozoa (*Plasmodium malariae* and *Toxoplasma gondii*), and helminths (schistosomes, *Wuchereria bancrofti*, *Loa loa*, and *Trichinella spiralis*). The prototypical postinfectious glomerulonephritis, however, is **poststreptococcal glomerulonephritis**, which is the subject of the remainder of this section.

1. **Incidence and etiology**
   a. Poststreptococcal glomerulonephritis primarily affects school-aged children. The disease is rare before 2 years of age but has been reported in adults. The male-to-female ratio is 2:1.
   b. Preceding infection with nephritogenic strains of Group A β-hemolytic streptococci (particularly type 12) is the rule, although positive culture of the organism is demonstrated in less than 20% of cases at the time of renal disease. The site of infection (i.e., the skin or pharynx) appears to vary with the geographic area of study. The latent period between infection and clinical glomerular disease is 7–15 days and in rare cases is as long as 3 weeks.

2. **Pathology.** Poststreptococcal glomerulonephritis is a diffuse proliferative disease with mesangial and endothelial hypercellularity. Acute poststreptococcal glomerulonephritis frequently features a polymorphonuclear leukocytic infiltrate and interstitial edema. Electron-dense deposits (subepithelial "humps") and foot process fusion are seen by electron microscopy. Immunofluorescence often identifies granular deposits of C3 along the capillary basement membrane. Occasionally, IgG or IgM also may be found.

3. **Clinical features and diagnosis**
   a. The typical clinical presentation is a sudden onset of hematuria and edema. Associated features include gastrointestinal complaints, lethargy, encephalopathy, oliguria, and intravascular volume overload with pulmonary edema, hypertension, and ascites.
   b. The characteristic, but not diagnostic, laboratory profile is azotemia, hypocomplementemia (CH_{50} or C3), hematuria, leukocyturia, and proteinuria. Nephrotic syndrome develops in less than 15% of patients. Supporting data include elevated titers of antistreptolysin O, antihyaluronidase, and anti-DNase B antibodies, all of which suggest preceding streptococcal infection.

4. **Clinical course and prognosis**
   a. The typical course of acute poststreptococcal glomerulonephritis is recovery, particularly among children. The acute nephritis resolves with amelioration of edema and hypertension 1–3 weeks after onset. Proteinuria may persist for several months, exacerbated by erect posture and exercise. Microscopic hematuria similarly disappears slowly over a period of several months.
   b. The long-term prognosis is controversial. Clearly, some patients advance to end-stage renal disease. Factors associated with this poor prognosis are severe oliguria or anuria, crescents in the biopsy specimen, persistent heavy proteinuria, and relatively older age. Persistence of hypocomplementemia and progressive renal failure may, however, indicate an alternative diagnosis (e.g., membranoproliferative glomerulonephritis).

5. **Therapy.** Hypertension must be treated aggressively, particularly in children, who develop florid hypertensive encephalopathy at normal adult blood pressures. Hydralazine is an effective agent in this setting. Furosemide or bumetanide will likely be required for the fluid retention that occurs secondary to this drug and for the underlying edema-forming disease. Antibiotic use is controversial, although a 10-day course of penicillin in the nonallergic patient is safe enough for routine use. Prophylaxis following poststreptococcal glomerulonephritis is not indicated since recurrences are exceedingly rare.

J. **IgA glomerulonephritis (Berger's disease)**

1. **Definition and incidence.** This clinicopathologic entity was fully defined in 1968, when the routine application of immunofluorescent microscopy identified mesangial deposits of IgA in renal biopsies from patients with recurrent hematuria but normal renal function. The incidence of this disease varies remarkably with geographic location, and males are affected three to four times as frequently as females.

2. **Pathology** is characteristic.
   a. Diffuse, sometimes irregularly distributed IgA deposits are seen in the mesangium. IgM or IgG also may be present.

b. Focal and segmental glomerulonephritis with mesangial proliferation is common. Mesangial prominence may be the only pathologic finding.

c. Electron-dense deposits are routinely identified in the mesangium.

d. Rare cases may have crescents, extensive glomerular sclerosis, or both.

3. Clinical features and diagnosis

a. The patients, who usually are between 20 and 40 years of age, most commonly present with recurrent, often macroscopic hematuria but normal GFR and normal tubular function. A minority of patients present with nephrotic syndrome and, very rarely, acute renal failure.

b. There are several, possibly diagnostic, laboratory findings.

(1) Serum IgA levels may be elevated (in 50% of cases), depressed, or normal.

(2) Biopsies from normal-appearing skin have immunofluorescent positivity for IgA in 50% of cases.

4. Clinical course and prognosis are variable.

a. The 20-year survival rate is about 50%. Although they continue to have intermittent hematuria, many patients maintain normal renal function throughout life.

b. A minority of patients progress to renal failure. Factors that predict a poor prognosis include advanced age at disease onset, heavy proteinuria, hypertension, and the presence of crescents or segmental sclerosis on renal biopsy.

5. Therapy. There is no evidence suggesting that any specific therapy is beneficial.

K. Henoch-Schönlein purpura

1. Definition. Henoch-Schönlein purpura is a systemic disease characterized by purpura, arthritis, abdominal pain, bloody diarrhea, and nephritis. Purpura, although the hallmark of this disease, may be slight and go unnoticed.

2. Incidence. Henoch-Schönlein purpura affects mainly children. The peak incidence of systemic disease is at 4 years of age, and the peak incidence of nephritis is at 8 years of age. In older patients, confusion with polyarteritis nodosa is likely. Males are affected more commonly than females at all ages. Clinical nephritis affects 30% of patients, but almost all patients have abnormal findings at kidney biopsy.

3. Pathology. The histopathology ranges from mild, diffuse mesangial prominence to focal and segmental proliferative glomerulonephritis on a background of diffuse mesangial proliferation. The hallmark of Henoch-Schönlein purpura is the invariable immunofluorescent positivity for IgA in the mesangium.

4. Clinical features and diagnosis

a. The clinical presentation often is preceded by a precipitating event, such as an infection [due to virus (e.g., herpes zoster), mycoplasma, or streptococcus], vaccination, an insect bite, or drug administration. Rash usually develops early and evolves from morbilliform to purpuric. The legs and buttocks are affected most commonly. Arthritis typically is mild and nondeforming. Gastrointestinal bleeding and pain may dominate the presentation.

b. Laboratory findings are exceedingly nonspecific, although elevated serum IgA is reported frequently. Serum complement component levels usually are normal.

5. Clinical course and prognosis

a. The clinical course is variable. Patients with recurrent purpura, heavy proteinuria, and clinically severe nephritis at the time of presentation and patients whose biopsies show epithelial crescent formation tend to do poorly.

b. Among all children with systemic Henoch-Schönlein purpura, the 15-year survival rate is 90%. By 10 years, however, 15% of these patients have persisting disease and 8% have renal impairment. Among adults, 50% heal completely, 15% progress to renal failure, and about 35% have persisting disease.

6. Therapy. Several treatment methods have been attempted in Henoch-Schönlein purpura (e.g., immunosuppression, steroid therapy, and anticoagulation) but without proven benefit.

L. Diabetic nephropathy

1. Incidence. End-stage renal disease develops in 5%–15% of patients with diabetes. Among patients with juvenile-onset diabetes, 50% develop renal disease within 20 years of the onset of diabetes. Among new patients considered for maintenance renal replacement therapy (largely chronic hemodialysis), 25%–50% have chronic renal failure secondary to diabetes.

2. Pathogenesis

a. The evolution of diabetic nephropathy is symptomatically quiet until late in the disease process. Early in diabetes, the GFR often is above normal. This elevated GFR may be due to vascular factors or to changes in growth hormone (GH), cellular metabolic substrates, or membrane permeability. The exact cause is unknown.

b. After 15–20 years of diabetes, proteinuria develops. Although small amounts of protein are lost initially, after 3–5 years of proteinuria, nephrotic syndrome often develops, as does azotemia. End-stage renal disease occurs 18–24 months after the onset of azotemia.

3. Pathology. There are two major pathologic lesions associated with diabetes.

a. Diffuse glomerulosclerosis is characterized by an eosinophilic thickening of the mesangium and basement membrane. This lesion is present in 90% of diabetics and probably is responsible for the proteinuria, nephrotic syndrome, and renal failure seen in these patients. However, diffuse glomerulosclerosis is neither diagnostic of nor exclusive for diabetes.

b. Nodular glomerulosclerosis, also known as **Kimmelstiel-Wilson syndrome,** consists of round nodules that are homogenous at the center and have circumferential layering of nuclei. These nodules often are multiple within a given glomerulus and may be confluent. Nodular glomerulosclerosis is both specific for and diagnostic of diabetes, but it is found in only 50% of patients with diabetic nephropathy. This lesion is not responsible for nephrosis and renal failure.

4. Laboratory findings are indicative of slowly deteriorating GFR and include elevated levels of BUN, creatinine, uric acid, and phosphate and decreased levels of bicarbonate and calcium. Serum complement and immunoglobulin levels are normal.

5. Clinical course. The natural history of diabetic nephropathy is amazingly predictable; it is virtually impossible to slow the rate of progression toward uremia. Factors that accelerate renal deterioration include hypertension, urinary obstruction, infection, the administration of nephrotoxic drugs, and the use of intravenous radiocontrast material.

6. Therapy

a. Treatment of diabetic nephropathy is supportive. There is no unequivocal evidence linking tight control of blood glucose to moderation of renal disease. Restriction of dietary protein (i.e., to 40 g/day) has been advocated recently as a means of preserving remnant nephron integrity in slowly progressive renal diseases such as diabetes. Avoidance of nephrotoxins, treatment of high blood pressure, and surveillance for urinary obstruction (neurogenic bladder) are prudent conservative measures.

b. End-stage renal disease is treated using any established modality. Patients who undergo transplantation of a kidney from a living relative have a better 5-year survival rate than those who undergo chronic hemodialysis. Several dialysis treatment centers have reported good results using continuous ambulatory peritoneal dialysis in diabetes. Insulin may be given intraperitoneally, by which improved diabetic control appears possible.

M. Lupus nephritis refers to a spectrum of renal pathology. Presently, four major lesions and three superimposed lesions are recognized.

1. Major lesions

a. Focal proliferative lupus nephritis develops during the first year of clinical lupus in 50% of patients.

(1) Pathology. The lesion is sharply delineated segmental endothelial and mesangial cell proliferation, which usually affects less than 50% of all glomeruli.

(2) Clinical features and diagnosis

(a) Proteinuria is seen in almost all cases; however, nephrotic syndrome is rare. Hematuria is common, and mild renal insufficiency is seen occasionally. Hypertension is not present.

(b) Serologic findings include positive **fluorescent antinuclear antibody** and modest elevations in anti-DNA antibodies. Complement components (C3 and C4) are at normal or decreased levels.

(3) Clinical course and prognosis

(a) Remission, as measured by cessation of proteinuria, is seen in about 50% of patients. Relapses commonly occur with extrarenal flares of systemic lupus. Transition to other forms of the disease (e.g., diffuse proliferative or membranous lupus nephritis) occurs in at least 20% of patients.

(b) Renal failure is rare unless the disease progresses to diffuse proliferative lupus nephritis.

(c) The 5-year mortality rate is 10%.

b. Diffuse proliferative lupus nephritis most commonly develops within the first year of clinical lupus.

  (1) Pathology. Mesangial and endothelial cell proliferation affect most glomeruli with varying severity. Capillary lumina are obliterated, and crescents affect up to 30% of glomeruli. Deposits of IgG, C3, C4, and C1q are diffuse. IgA and IgM deposits also are seen frequently.

  (2) Clinical features and diagnosis

    (a) Proteinuria and hematuria are universal; more than 50% of patients present with nephrotic syndrome. Eventually, almost all patients become nephrotic. Azotemia is common early in the course of the disease and may be severe. Hypertension occurs in a minority of cases.

    (b) Serologic findings include positive fluorescent antinuclear antibody, highly elevated anti-DNA antibodies, and depressed levels of C3 and C4. Cryoglobulinemia develops in some cases.

  (3) Clinical course and prognosis

    (a) Remission of the nephrotic syndrome is seen in 33% of patients and sometimes is sustained. Transition to mesangial lupus nephritis occurs occasionally in association with clinical remission.

    (b) The 5-year mortality rate is 50%. Death is due to uremia or active systemic lupus, which frequently is complicated by infection. Hypertension and renal failure may occur as sequelae even after long periods of clinical remission.

c. Membranous lupus nephritis develops during the first year of clinical lupus in about 50% of patients.

  (1) Pathology. The histopathologic pattern of membranous lupus nephritis is very similar to that of idiopathic membranous glomerulonephritis (see Part I: section XI C 2).

  (2) Clinical features and diagnosis

    (a) Proteinuria is seen in all patients; hematuria also is common. Nephrotic syndrome is seen at presentation in 50% of patients and ultimately occurs in 80% of patients. Hypertension and renal insufficiency are rare at the outset of membranous lupus nephritis.

    (b) Serologic findings include positive fluorescent antinuclear antibody, normal or only mildly elevated anti-DNA antibodies, and normal or decreased levels of C3 and C4.

  (3) Clinical course and prognosis

    (a) Remission from nephrotic syndrome is seen in 33% of patients, but relapses are common. Transition to focal or diffuse proliferative lupus nephritis has been reported but is rare.

    (b) The 5-year mortality rate is 10% for patients who develop hypertension and renal insufficiency during persistent nephrotic syndrome

d. Mesangial lupus nephritis may occur as the earliest form of lupus nephritis.

  (1) Pathology. Biopsy shows mesangial prominence with an increase in matrix and in the number of mesangial cells.

  (2) Clinical features and diagnosis

    (a) The complete spectrum of clinical findings is not fully known. Many patients are asymptomatic or present with only mild urinary abnormalities.

    (b) Serologic findings include positive fluorescent antinuclear antibody, mild anti-DNA antibody elevations, and normal or mildly decreased C3 and C4 levels.

  (3) Clinical course and prognosis

    (a) Urinary abnormalities may remit, and transition to diffuse proliferative or membranous lupus nephritis occurs in 15% of patients.

    (b) This mesangial lesion is not associated with clinical progression unless there is transition to a less favorable histology.

2. Superimposed lesions

  a. Glomerulosclerosis is a secondary or superimposed lesion that is seen most commonly in diffuse proliferative lupus nephritis with a protracted course. Progressive glomerulosclerosis may be a cause of renal failure in patients whose systemic lupus remits.

  b. Interstitial lupus nephritis usually coexists with glomerular disease but may develop alone.

    (1) Pathologically, this lesion is characterized by intense, mononuclear interstitial infiltration, tubular damage, and interstitial fibrosis.

    (2) IgG and C3 are identified in peritubular capillaries and in tubular basement membranes. Parallel electron-dense deposits are seen.

    (3) Clinical disorders of tubular function (e.g., disorders of potassium excretion, acid excretion, and urine concentration and dilution) are seen in addition to variable, nonselective proteinuria.

    c. Necrotizing vasculitis usually complicates diffuse proliferative lupus nephritis and presents as rapidly accelerating hypertension and renal failure. Histopathologically, an acellular necrosis of vessel walls is seen with proteinaceous occlusive thrombi.

3. Therapy

    a. Criteria for therapy are not rigidly established. Clearly, progressive azotemia and nephrotic syndrome deserve treatment. The response of membranous lupus nephritis to therapy varies among reported series. Due to the poor prognosis associated with diffuse proliferative lupus nephritis, this lesion currently is treated even in cases with few clinical signs or symptoms of renal disease.

    b. Methods of therapy

        (1) Regimens of glucocorticoid therapy vary. Generally, however, high-dose induction therapy is followed by judicious reduction to low daily or alternate-day doses for maintenance therapy. Induction therapy with oral prednisone (1–2 mg/kg/day) and pulse intravenous methylprednisolone (1–2 g/day) has been described.

        (2) Other therapeutic methods (e.g., cytotoxic agents and plasmapheresis) presently are under controlled evaluation.

N. Vasculitis

1. Introduction. The kidney frequently is involved in systemic vasculitis, although the actual incidence is unknown. A spectrum of renal syndromes are associated with vasculitis, ranging from modest "microscopic" involvement of arterioles, venules, and capillaries (a syndrome referred to as **hypersensitivity vasculitis**) to extensive "classic" involvement of medium-sized vessels (a syndrome referred to as **polyarteritis nodosa**).

2. Polyarteritis nodosa

    a. Etiology. This type of vasculitis may be primary (idiopathic) or secondary to drugs, viral infections (e.g., hepatitis B), or rheumatic diseases (e.g., lupus and rheumatoid vasculitis).

    b. Pathology. The kidneys show a focal necrotizing arteritis in vessels ranging in size from the renal artery to the interlobular veins.

    c. Clinical features and diagnosis

        (1) The clinical presentation often is vague, consisting of low-grade fever, myalgia, arthralgia, and weight loss.

        (2) The laboratory findings are numerous and, although nonspecific, frequently suggest the diagnosis of polyarteritis nodosa when considered collectively. Anemia, leukocytosis, and elevated erythrocyte sedimentation rate are seen frequently. Renal involvement is announced by variable combinations of the following findings: hematuria, proteinuria, red cell casts, sterile pyuria, azotemia, and hypertension. Rheumatoid factor may be positive. Hepatitis B surface antigen (HB_sAg) and cryoglobulins sometimes are present in the blood.

        (3) The diagnosis can be confirmed by renal angiography, which shows multiple small aneurysms with segmental infarctions.

    d. Clinical course and prognosis. Progression to organ destruction or death is the expected outcome.

3. Wegener's granulomatosis (see also Chapter 2, section XIV C) is a special case of vasculitis (necrotizing granulomatous vasculitis) with renal involvement. The disease affects patients of all ages but is more common in middle-aged men.

    a. Pathology. The characteristic and diagnostic lesion of necrotizing vasculitis and granulomatous inflammation is most reliably discovered in pulmonary or upper airway biopsy material. Renal involvement occurs in about 50% of cases. Kidney histology, however, usually is not specific. A focal and segmental necrotizing vasculitis and glomerulitis often are found.

    b. Clinical features and diagnosis

        (1) Wegener's granulomatosis affects the kidney and upper respiratory tract, including the nose, throat, and bronchi. Saddle nose deformity may occur. Less frequently involved are the orbit, skin, peripheral nerves, CNS, gastrointestinal tract, and heart. Ulcerative vasculitic lesions, including nasal septal perforation, are the most recognizable presenting signs.

        (2) The hematologic and serologic features of Wegener's granulomatosis extensively overlap those of polyarteritis nodosa. Radiographically, however, renal arterial aneurysms are rare.

    c. Clinical course. Wegener's granulomatosis has a variable course. Long-term remissions are seen occasionally with therapy. Death usually results from renal failure, sepsis, hemorrhage, or DIC.

    d. Therapy with daily high-dose glucocorticoids and daily cyclophosphamide (1–3 mg/kg/day) has increased the 1-year survival rate from less than 20% to greater than 80%.

O. Cryoglobulins and cryoglobulinemia

1. **Cryoglobulins** are proteins that precipitate at low temperatures and dissolve on rewarming. Three types of cryoglobulins are defined:
   a. **Type I:** Monoclonal cryoglobulins
   b. **Type II:** Mixed cryoglobulins that include a monoclonal component with antibody activity against polyclonal IgG
   c. **Type III:** Mixed cryoglobulins in which both components are polyclonal

2. **Cryoglobulinemia** (i.e., the presence of cryoglobulins in the blood) occurs in a variety of clinically dissimilar conditions. Renal disease is associated primarily with types I and II and probably has an immune complex–mediated pathophysiology.
   a. **Clinical features**
      (1) **Type I cryoglobulinemia** is associated with hematologic malignancies. Heavy proteinuria, hematuria, and, occasionally, anuria are seen. The histologic lesion usually is a membranoproliferative glomerulonephritis. Serum complement (C4 and C1q) levels are depressed. Immunoglobulin and complement are identified in the glomerulus by means of immunofluorescence.
      (2) **Type II cryoglobulinemia** is associated with a syndrome of immune-complex vasculitis; about 50% of patients have renal disease. There is a wide spectrum of clinical signs, which vary greatly in severity. Hypertension, azotemia, and anuria are poor prognostic signs. Endocapillary proliferation and mesangial prominence are common pathologic features. Immunoglobulin is found by means of immunofluorescence, and typical cryoglobulin deposits are seen with electron microscopy.
      (3) **Type III cryoglobulinemia** may be associated with a variety of other diseases, with or without renal disease, including systemic lupus erythematosus, hepatitis B, and systemic infections. Although they are common, type III cryoglobulins occur in smaller quantities than type I and type II.
   b. **Diagnosis** involves the detection, characterization, and quantitation of cryoglobulins in serum.
   c. **Therapy** in idiopathic cases is not standardized. Encouraging results have been obtained with plasmapheresis.

P. Multiple myeloma

1. **Definition.** Multiple myeloma represents a neoplastic transformation of a monoclonal B lymphocyte into a plasma cell, which produces excessive quantities of immunoglobulin or immunoglobulin fragment (**paraprotein**). More than 50% of patients with multiple myeloma die due to complications of renal failure, and a much higher percentage of multiple myeloma patients have some form of renal involvement.

2. **Pathology.** Although there is no "myeloma glomerulonephritis," there are many mechanisms of renal injury in multiple myeloma.
   a. **Bence Jones proteinuria** is extremely toxic to the tubular epithelium and may lead to ATN.
   b. **Myeloma kidney** refers to extensive intratubular deposition of eosinophilic, homogeneous proteinaceous material. This condition occurs with or without plasma cell infiltration of the renal interstitium.
   c. **Amyloidosis** may develop from myeloma, leading to amyloid nephropathy.
   d. **Renal tubular syndromes**, including Fanconi's syndrome, renal tubular acidosis, and nephrogenic diabetes insipidus, often complicate light-chain disease. These tubular disorders may precede myeloma by many years. Patients with minimally decreased GFR but prominent tubular dysfunction tend to excrete predominantly kappa light chains.
   e. **Hypercalcemia** may complicate multiple myeloma and induce acute renal failure.
   f. Severely hyperuricemic and hyperuricosuric patients may develop **acute urate nephropathy**, specifically the variety termed **tumor lysis syndrome**, which develops as a result of chemotherapy that is not preceded by allopurinol administration.
   g. Hyperviscosity and intravascular volume depletion predispose to acute renal failure in multiple myeloma, particularly with the administration of contrast media for radiographic study.

3. **Clinical features and diagnosis**
   a. The clinical presentation of renal disease in multiple myeloma often is subtle. Anemia and bone pain in the presence of any form of abnormal urinary finding should prompt evaluation for myeloma. Slowly progressive renal insufficiency is typical; however, acute renal failure may be seen in certain circumstances (e.g., in the presence of hypercalcemia).
   b. Many chemical abnormalities are seen commonly in multiple myeloma. Pseudohyponatremia develops secondary to the presence of large quantities of paraprotein, altering the nonaqueous phase of plasma. The anion gap is low and occasionally is negative due to the

positive charges on the immunoglobulin molecules. This is not seen in IgA myeloma. Urine protein concentration is increased, reflecting excretion of the huge paraprotein burden. As mentioned earlier, dipstick measurement for protein is insensitive to immunoglobulin and often gives false-negative results. Thus, acid precipitation with sulfosalicylic acid is required.

   4. Therapy and prognosis. Although no specific therapy exists for the renal disease, chemotherapy for the malignancy, meticulous regulation of intravascular volume and electrolyte status, and dialysis (when necessary) may prolong life.

Q. Glomerulonephritis in infective endocarditis represents the prototypical bacterial illness, which may lead to the induction of glomerulonephritis, presumably through an immune-complex mechanism. Glomerulonephritis is thought to occur by similar means in visceral abscess and in infections arising from extracorporeal circulation devices (**shunt nephritis**). It is possible that any endovascular infection can produce this glomerulonephritis.

   1. Pathology. The histologic severity ranges from mild mesangial proliferation to severe membranoproliferative glomerulonephritis.

   2. Clinical features. About 15% of patients with infective endocarditis develop renal involvement. Nonimmune mechanisms of injury include septic emboli, ischemic ATN with severe congestive heart failure, and, indirectly, antibiotic nephrotoxicities. Immune-complex glomerulonephritis presents with hematuria, red cell casts in the urine, and azotemia.

   3. Therapy. There is no specific therapy for the renal disease. Except in fairly advanced cases, successful treatment of the underlying infection usually leads to resolution of the renal disease.

XII. RENAL CYSTIC DISEASE

A. Adult polycystic kidney disease

   1. Definition and incidence. Adult polycystic kidney disease represents the most common cause of renal failure and death in adults with renal cystic disease. Inherited as an autosomal dominant trait, adult polycystic kidney disease achieves 100% gene penetrance by the time that the patient is 80 years of age. Males and females are affected equally. Adult polycystic kidney disease must be distinguished from **childhood** (autosomal recessive) **polycystic kidney disease**, which is universally fatal by the third decade of life, and the **congenital multicystic variant of renal dysplasia**.

   2. Clinical features
   a. The typical presentation of enlarging flank or abdominal masses, abdominal pain, and slowly progressive renal failure becomes clinically evident by about the fourth decade of life, and renal replacement therapy becomes necessary within 10 years of the onset of symptoms. Family history is positive in more than 75% of cases. Associated clinical findings may include hypertension, polyuria and nocturia, erythrocytosis, and nephrolithiasis.
   b. Hepatic cysts are demonstrated in 33% of cases; however, liver insufficiency is rare, unlike in the childhood form.
   c. Intracranial (**berry**) **aneurysms** occur in 12% of patients. In some series, 6% of all patients with berry aneurysms have adult polycystic kidney disease.

   3. Diagnosis. Adult polycystic kidney disease must be distinguished from multicystic diseases of other origins, and the diagnosis is made most easily on the basis of specific ultrasonographic findings. Coincident findings include hematuria, impaired urine concentrating ability, and low-grade proteinuria. Heavy proteinuria, persistent hematuria, and pyuria should be investigated since they rarely occur in uncomplicated adult polycystic kidney disease.

   4. Therapy is restricted to the treatment of end-stage renal disease as it develops. Genetic counseling is important since 50% of offspring are affected. Women with adult polycystic kidney disease are not at an increased risk for fetal demise or hypertension during pregnancy except as contributed by existing renal insufficiency.

B. Nephronophthisis (medullary cystic disease)

   1. Definition and incidence. Medullary cystic disease is the most common cause of end-stage renal disease in children and adolescents. Four variants are recognized based on the patient age at onset and the pattern of inheritance.
   a. Sporadic nephronophthisis accounts for about 20% of cases and has no familial occurrence.

     b. Juvenile nephronophthisis accounts for 50% of cases and is recessively inherited.

     c. Renal-retinal dysplasia accounts for about 15% of cases, is recessively inherited, and is associated with retinitis pigmentosa.

     d. Adult-onset medullary cystic disease accounts for about 15% of cases and is characterized by dominant inheritance.

   2. Pathology. The kidney is small in medullary cystic disease, which distinguishes this disease from polycystic and multicystic diseases. Cysts may be located at the corticomedullary junction or in the medulla. Acystic forms have been described. Interstitial fibrosis is prominent, but calcification does not occur.

   3. Clinical features. Loss of urine concentrating ability and failure to conserve sodium appropriately are almost invariable early signs of disease. The initial presentation often includes polyuria, polydipsia, and enuresis, although an azotemic presentation also is common. Progression to renal failure is a constant clinical feature.

   4. Therapy is aimed at maintaining sodium and water homeostasis during the evolution of disease. Genetic counseling may be appropriate in clearly familial disease. The possibility of subclinical disease in siblings must be considered when a donor is being selected for transplantation.

C. Medullary sponge kidney

   1. Definition and incidence. Medullary sponge kidney is not a true cystic disease but rather a renal collecting tubule ectasia. It is a common problem, which is identified in 1 of every 200 urograms in large series.

   2. Prognosis is excellent; many patients have no detectable impairment of renal function. Hypercalciuria is common, as are subtle defects in the ability to concentrate and acidify the urine. Nephrocalcinosis, of variable severity, is found in 50% of cases.

D. Simple renal cyst

   1. Definition and incidence. The simple cyst is the most common renal cystic disease; at least half of all individuals older than 50 years of age have one or more macroscopic renal cysts. Renal cysts may be solitary or multiple and unilateral or bilateral. They usually are located in the cortex and bulge through the renal capsule, but they may occur in the medulla. Large renal cysts are more common among adults, and multilocular cysts are rare.

   2. Clinical features. Symptoms are rare; simple cysts usually are diagnosed during patient evaluation for other problems. Bleeding and infection stimulate the cyst wall to thicken, and calcareous plaques often form within the cyst wall.

   3. Clinical course. Simple cysts usually are static, although regression may occur from one radiographic assessment to the next. Solitary cysts may undergo malignant degeneration, although this is rare. Hemorrhagic cysts are more likely to contain a neoplasm than nonhemorrhagic cysts (i.e., in up to 30% of cases as compared to less than 1% of cases). Multiple simple cysts may develop in end-stage renal disease in patients who have undergone long-term (> 7 years) hemodialysis.

   4. Diagnosis may be made by CT, ultrasonography, urography, or angiography. Large cysts with abnormal ultrasonographic appearance should undergo cyst puncture for fluid aspiration and cytology and for contrast radiology.

   5. Therapy. In the absence of infection or tumor, no specific therapy is indicated for this benign disease.

XIII. TUBULOINTERSTITIAL DISEASE

A. Acute interstitial nephritis

   1. Definition. Acute interstitial nephritis appears to be a kidney-based hypersensitivity reaction, usually to a drug. Although the true incidence of acute interstitial nephritis is not known, several hundred cases have been formally reported, and there is an increasing awareness of this disease with increased case recognition.

   2. Etiology. Drugs implicated in the pathogenesis of acute interstitial nephritis include **β-lactam antibiotics** (e.g., methicillin, oxacillin, and cephalothin) and **other antibiotics** (e.g., sulfonomides, tetracyclines, and vancomycin); **nonsteroidal anti-inflammatory drugs** (e.g., ibuprofen, indomethacin, fenoprofen, and tolmetin); **diuretics** (e.g., thiazides and furosemide); and many **other unrelated drugs** (e.g., phenytoin, cimetidine, sulfinpyrazone, methyl-dopa, and phenobarbital).

3. Clinical features. The typical presentation is the development of acute renal failure with fever, rash, and eosinophilia.

4. Diagnosis
   a. Urinalysis classically shows mild or no proteinuria, microscopic hematuria, pyuria, and eosinophiluria. Some patients with acute interstitial nephritis due to nonsteroidal anti-in-flammatory drugs present with nephrotic syndrome characterized by urinary protein ex-cretion exceeding 3.0 g/24 hr.
   b. Biopsy shows patchy, irregular interstitial infiltration with inflammatory cells. Monocytes and lymphocytes are constant findings. Eosinophils may be abundant or completely ab-sent. Fibrosis is extremely unusual and should suggest underlying or preexisting renal dis-ease. Rarely, acute interstitial nephritis may progress to a chronic interstitial nephritis, and fibrosis may be prominent. Glomeruli are normal or show only mild mesangial prom-inence.

5. Therapy includes discontinuation of the etiologic drug and initiation of supportive measures (e.g., dietary restrictions, blood pressure management, and acute dialysis). The value of glucocorticoid therapy is unclear; however, the use of steroids may be justified in patients with severe or rapidly progressive renal insufficiency.

6. Prognosis is excellent provided that the offending drug is promptly withdrawn. Recovery time varies and may be prolonged in oliguric patients and in patients with extensive intersti-tial cellular infiltrates. Temporary dialysis may be needed. Rarely, patients progress to end-stage renal disease.

B. Chronic interstitial nephritis. In general, the clinical features common to these interstitial dis-eases include a relative **preservation of glomerular function** until late in the disease but an **im-pairment of tubular functions** (e.g., urine concentration, dilution, and acidification and potas-sium excretion) early in the course of the disease.

1. Drug-related nephropathy
   a. Analgesic nephropathy is the prototypical drug-related chronic interstitial nephritis.
      (1) Analgesic nephropathy occurs more commonly in women than in men. Patients usual-ly are over 45 years of age and from low socioeconomic classes and have frequent headaches or coincident psychiatric disease.
      (2) Intravenous urography reveals abnormality in more than 90% of cases, and papillary necrosis is seen in more than 50%. Half of patients are hypertensive, and anemia is common and often out of proportion to the degree of clinically apparent renal disease.
      (3) Several agents have been implicated (e.g., acetaminophen, phenacetin, and aspirin), but none has been specifically proven culpable. The risk for analgesic nephropathy ap-pears to be increased in patients who use more than 3 g/day of such agents.
      (4) Treatment of progressive analgesic nephropathy is supportive. Removal of the inciting agent rarely arrests the deterioration of renal function.
   b. Gold nephropathy is a frequent and important complication of parenteral gold therapy for rheumatoid arthritis. Gold accumulation leads to immune-complex membranous glomer-ulonephritis and nephrotic syndrome. Cessation of gold therapy at the first sign of pro-teinuria is recommended and often results in regression of signs of renal disease. It is not yet known if oral gold preparations are equally nephrotoxic.
   c. Lithium nephrotoxicity. Lithium carbonate, used in the treatment of bipolar disorder, is fil-tered freely and undergoes significant (i.e., 60%–70%) reabsorption in the proximal tu-bules. Lithium toxicity results in antidiuretic hormone (ADH)-unresponsive nephrogenic diabetes insipidus, incomplete distal renal tubular acidosis, and, rarely, azotemia.

2. Toxin-related nephropathy
   a. Cadmium nephropathy. Cadmium is a highly toxic by-product of zinc production, which has numerous industrial applications. During long-term exposure, cadmium accumulates in the kidney while blood and urine cadmium concentrations remain normal. Cadmium probably leads to end-stage renal disease, although the true incidence is not known.
   b. Lead nephropathy and **saturnine gout** are well-recognized sequelae of chronic lead intox-ication.
      (1) The earliest cases of lead intoxication involved miners, paint manufacturers, and distillers of "moonshine" liquor. Lead poisoning also has been reported in children who have ingested lead-based paint. Individuals who recover from acute lead poison-ing occasionally are found later to be victims of chronic lead-related renal disease.
      (2) Clinical manifestations of lead nephropathy include reduced GFR, reduced renal

plasma flow (RPF), minimal or no proteinuria, normal urinary sediment, hyperuricemia and low urate clearance, and, occasionally, hypertension, hyperkalemia, and acidemia.

(3) Treatment includes removal of lead exposure and chelation therapy with sodium or calcium **ethylenediaminetetraacetic acid (EDTA)** or penicillamine (in appropriate cases).

c. Copper nephrotoxicity is rare but occasionally is seen in Wilson's disease. Clinically, copper nephropathy may resemble cadmium nephropathy (proximal tubular disease) or acute tubular necrosis. D-Penicillamine is the treatment of choice.

d. Mercury nephropathy. Mercury is associated with several renal lesions, including membranous and proliferative glomerular disease with nephrotic syndrome, proximal tubular atrophy and Fanconi's syndrome with the development of chronic renal failure, and oliguric acute tubullar necrosis. Chelation therapy with British antilewisite (**BAL or dimercaprol**) and hemodialysis may reduce mortality if initiated promptly (i.e., within 48 hours following exposure).

3. Crystalline nephropathy

a. Uric acid produces renal injury in three ways.

(1) Uric acid stones may develop in concentrated acid urine.

(2) Acute uric acid nephropathy (acute crystalline obstruction of renal tubules) may accompany sudden or extreme elevations in serum uric acid (i.e., serum levels exceeding 25 mg/dl), as occurs in **tumor lysis syndrome**.

(3) Gouty nephropathy is a syndrome of interstitial fibrosis and decreased renal function and perhaps is related to cortical microtophi and a nephrotoxic influence of hyperuricemia in some gouty patients. Lead nephropathy (saturnine gout) may account for a significant percentage of patients with renal insufficiency and gout.

b. Oxalic acid also produces tubulointerstitial disease. Elevated urine levels of oxalic acid may lead to the formation of calcium oxalate stones or may mimic the syndrome of acute uric acid nephropathy (acute crystalline obstruction). **Primary hyperoxaluria** is an inherited disease of oxalate overproduction, which terminates in renal failure with extensive deposition of oxalate crystals throughout the body (a condition termed **oxalosis**). **Ethylene glycol poisoning** may lead to renal failure in part by the hyperoxaluria that results from the metabolism of ethylene glycol to oxalate. The use of **methoxyflurane** in anesthesia has been linked to an increased oxalate production with resultant nephrotoxicity. Increased oxalate absorption often is seen following ileojejunal bypass surgery for obesity and may lead to **nephrocalcinosis**. Mild hyperoxaluria may result from pyridoxine or thiamine deficiency.

4. Miscellanous nephropathies

a. Amyloidosis

(1) Definition and classification. Amyloidosis is a disorder of unknown etiology, which involves the deposition of eosinophilic, amorphous material. The major classifications of amyloidosis are **primary amyloidosis** (occurring without pre- or coexisting illness), **secondary amyloidosis** (occurring in the presence of chronic inflammatory disease), and **heredofamilial amyloidosis**.

(2) Clinical features. Amyloid deposition may be focal and restricted to the kidneys or systemic and generalized. Proteinuria is universal, with nephrotic syndrome developing in 76% of patients. Hypertension occurs in 50% of patients. Kidney size occasionally is increased but decreases with advanced disease.

(3) Clinical course. Progressive deterioration of renal function is the rule.

(4) Diagnosis is unequivocally established by biopsy demonstrating amyloid protein by green birefringence with Congo red stain.

(5) Therapy. There is no effective treatment for primary amyloidosis, although alkylating agents and colchicine have been advocated. Treatment of secondary amyloidosis is limited to the treatment of the underlying inflammatory disease. Amyloidosis recurs in the transplanted kidney.

b. Sarcoidosis (see also Chapter 2, section XIV A)

(1) Definition. Sarcoidosis is a granulomatous disease of unknown etiology. Renal involvement may be secondary to noncaseating granulomatous replacement of the renal interstitium.

(2) Clinical features. Renal size usually is normal, and mild nonselective proteinuria is common. Hypercalcemia, hypercalciuria, or both frequently complicate sarcoidosis due to increased synthesis of 1,25-dihydroxycholecalciferol [$1,25\text{-}(OH)_2D_3$].

(3) Clinical course. The hypercalcemia may induce acute renal failue, and the hypercalciuria may lead to nephrocalcinosis or calcium nephrolithiasis. Hyperglobulinemia, when present, may be associated with distal renal tubular acidosis. Although glomerulonephritis has been noted among patients with sarcoidosis, the existence of a true sarcoid glomerulopathy is not fully established.

(4) **Therapy.** Steroids are indicated for the management of hypercalcemia.

C. Renal papillary necrosis

1. **Definition.** Renal papillary necrosis results from ischemic necrosis of the renal medulla or renal papillae. There are two forms. The **papillary form** involves the entire papilla, whereas the **medullary form** begins with focal areas of infarction in the inner medullary zone.

2. **Etiologic factors.** Conditions associated with renal papillary necrosis include diabetes mellitus, urinary tract obstruction, severe pyelonephritis, analgesic abuse, sickle cell hemoglobinopathy, extreme hypoxia and intravascular volume depletion in infants, and renal allograft rejection.

3. **Clinical features.** The clinical presentation of renal papillary necrosis varies with the stage and extent of disease. Patients with sickle cell trait may have completely asymptomatic renal papillary necrosis, which is discovered incidentally during urography for unrelated complaints. Infection frequently complicates renal papillary necrosis and leads to clinical pyelonephritis. The necrotic papillae may be sloughed and produce typical ureteral colic or ureteral obstruction. Azotemia is an uncommon presenting sign.

4. **Clinical course.** The course of renal papillary necrosis is a function of the underlying disease. End-stage renal disease may develop, particularly among diabetics.

5. **Diagnosis.** Intravenous urography can establish the diagnosis of both forms of renal papillary necrosis. Radiographically, the affected calyces appear irregular and fuzzy early in the disease process. As the lesion progresses, sequestration of the necrotic tissue leads to sinus formation and the appearance of a sinus tract or **arc shadow** on the urogram. In advanced renal papillary necrosis, the sequestrum may be sloughed and surrounded by contrast material—the so-called **ring sign**. Calcification, calicectasis, and medullary cavities may be present in this stage.

6. **Therapy** includes relief of obstruction, prevention and prompt eradication of infection, and control of pain (colic). Surgery occasionally is necessary to control hemorrhage or to relieve obstruction.

XIV. RENAL TRANSPORT DEFECTS

A. Meliturias.
Excessive quantities of **sugars** may gain access to the urine due to an increased filtered load (as in the hyperglycemia of diabetes mellitus) or to failure of appropriate reabsorption in the nephron.

1. **Primary renal glycosuria** is an autosomal recessive disorder recognized by constant glycosuria from birth in the absence of abnormal carbohydrate metabolism (i.e., hyperglycemia, ketosis, and other meliturias). Two variants are described. **Type A** patients have massive glycosuria at low plasma glucose concentrations, whereas **type B** patients have some glycosuria at low plasma glucose levels but normal reabsorption at higher levels. A glucose tolerance test distinguishes these syndromes from diabetes. No therapy is indicated for this harmless disorder.

2. **Other meliturias are recognized.**
   a. **Essential pentosuria (L-xylulosuria)** is an autosomal recessive defect in the metabolism of glucuronic acid, which is found primarily among Jews. L-Xylulosuria occurs secondary to a deficiency of nicotinamide-adenine dinucleotide phosphate (NADP)-linked xylitol dehydrogenase.
   b. **Essential fructosuria** also is an autosomal recessive error of metabolism, which is a result of defective phosphofructokinase activity.

B. Aminoacidurias

1. **Cystinuria** is an autosomal recessive defect in the transport of cystine, lysine, ornithine, and arginine. The low solubility of cystine accounts for the symptoms and complications of cystinuria in that it predisposes to the formation of renal cystine stones, which may lead to renal failure. Therapy consists of a life-long alkaline diuresis to prevent stone formation or D-penicillamine in refractory cases.

2. **Hypercystinuria** is a selective defect in cystine transport. It is autosomal recessive and clinically similar to cystinuria.

3. **Dibasic aminoaciduria** is a selective defect in lysine, ornithine, and arginine (but not cystine)

transport. Autosomal recessive and dominant forms are recognized. Symptoms include amino acid–induced diarrhea, malnutrition, hyperammonemia, and growth and mental retardation. Therapy consists of a low-protein diet.

4. **Iminoglycinuria** is a benign, autosomal recessive disorder of proline, hydroxyproline, and glycine transport.

5. **Hartnup disease** is an autosomal recessive defect in the transport of neutral α-amino acids. Hartnup disease patients have a reduced ability to convert tryptophan to niacin, resulting in **pellagra**—a syndrome characterized by photosensitive erythema, cerebellar ataxia, neuropsychiatric symptoms, and delerium. Therapy is oral nicotinamide.

C. Fanconi's syndrome

1. **Definition.** Fanconi's syndrome refers to a collection of proximal tubular defects, which may exist in varying number and severity and which may be inherited or acquired.

2. **Etiology**
   a. **Inherited causes** of Fanconi's syndrome include cystinosis, Lowe's syndrome, Wilson's disease, tyrosinemia, galactosemia, glycogenosis, and fructose intolerance.
   b. **Acquired causes** of Fanconi's syndrome include transplant dysfunction, myeloma, Sjögren's syndrome, hyperparathyroidism, potassium depletion, amyloidosis, nephrotic syndrome, interstitial nephritis, heavy metal toxicity, and outdated tetracycline.
   c. An **idiopathic** form of Fanconi's syndrome also exists.

3. **Clinical features and course**
   a. Symptoms and signs of Fanconi's syndrome include glycosuria, aminoaciduria, phosphaturia, bicarbonaturia, vasopressin-resistant polyuria, rickets or osteoporosis, short stature, and uremia.
   b. The natural history of Fanconi's syndrome depends heavily on the course and prognosis of the underlying disease or diseases.

4. **Therapy** is designed to replace lost urinary solutes and to correct the underlying disease or diseases. Phosphate, vitamin D, and bicarbonate should be given when indicated by laboratory and clinical data.

XV. RENAL VASCULAR DISEASE

A. Renal arterial occlusion: thrombosis and embolism.
Occlusive disease of the renal arterial system encompasses a broad spectrum of clinical syndromes and pathophysiology. Arterial blood flow may be interrupted by in situ thrombosis or by embolism from distant endovascular sites. Occlusion may be sudden and complete or gradual, with resultant functional renal artery stenosis.

1. **Etiology**
   a. **Renal arterial thrombosis** may develop spontaneously in the context of atherosclerosis, aneurysm, arteritis, hypercoagulable states, sickle cell disease, and thrombotic microangiopathy. Thrombosis also may develop as a complication of external trauma, instrumentation with angiography catheters, arterial surgery, and renal allograft transplantation.
   b. **Renal arterial embolism** may be caused by a clot, tumor fragment, or infectious coagulum. Cardiac conditions that may lead to renal arterial embolism include a dilated left atrium, artificial heart valves, myocardial infarction, infective endocarditis, marantic endocarditis, and myxoma. Noncardiac conditions that may cause renal arterial embolism include atheromatous plaques and paradoxical, fat, or tumor embolism.

2. **Clinical features and diagnosis**
   a. **Acute, complete renal arterial occlusion** usually presents as flank pain, hematuria, fever, nausea, tissue necrosis [as evidenced by elevated lactate dehydrogenase (LDH) and serum glutamic-oxaloacetic transaminase (SGOT)], and acute renal failure. The diagnosis is confirmed using radionuclide scanning or angiography. Bilateral occlusion and occlusion of a solitary functioning kidney produce severe anuric acute renal failure.
   b. **Chronic or segmental occlusion** produces symptoms and signs commensurate with the degree of ischemic damage.

3. **Therapy**
   a. Therapy for renal arterial thrombosis is surgical removal of the clot to restore renal blood flow. Best results are obtained when the operation is conducted within 48–72 hours following the onset of disease.
   b. Therapy for renal arterial embolism, which usually is diffuse and involves large numbers of smaller arterial branches, is anticoagulation with heparin and resolution of the underlying focus of emboli.

B. Renal vein thrombosis. Obstruction of renal venous drainage by a clot may be due to extension of clots in the vena cava, invasion of the renal vein by tumor, severe dehydration in infants, renal amyloidosis, and certain glomerular diseases associated with nephrotic syndrome, particularly membranous glomerulonephritis.

1. Clinical features and diagnosis. The clinical presentation varies depending on whether the condition is acute or chronic. Slowly evolving renal vein thrombosis may be completely asymptomatic, whereas acute renal vein thrombosis may produce pain, hematuria, costovertebral angle tenderness, and, ultimately, signs of worsening renal function. The affected kidney appears to be enlarged when visualized with the aid of intravenous urography. Selective venography is diagnostic.

2. Clinical course. Renal vein thrombosis generally is not a cause of glomerular disease. Renal vein thrombosis may develop during nephrosis due to loss of anticoagulant proteins and procoagulant deactivators in the urine protein.

3. Therapy is controversial, as is the belief that renal vein thrombosis predisposes to pulmonary embolism. Current therapy is long-term (3–6 months) anticoagulation with warfarin sodium. Longer treatment is recommended if embolic phenomena occur.

C. Renal artery stenosis. In experimental animals, it has been clearly shown that partial reduction in the luminal size of one or both renal arteries produces **renovascular hypertension**, which is mediated in most cases by increased renin production with resultant activation of angiotensin and aldosterone. In humans, renal artery stenosis is a recognized cause of renovascular hypertension. However, the coincidence of radiographically demonstrated renal artery stenosis and clinically demonstrated renovascular hypertension does not establish a causal relationship.

1. Incidence and etiology. Among prepubertal children, the primary lesion responsible for renal artery stenosis is medial **fibromuscular dysplasia**. Adults over 50 years of age suffer **renal artery atherosclerosis**, which is twice as common in men as in women. Rare causes include Takayasu's arteritis, arterial wall disease (e.g., hematoma, dissecting aneurysm, and tumor), and external arterial compression due to tumor, fibrosis, or cyst.

2. Clinical features include a nearly continuous abdominal or flank bruit, hypokalemia, mild metabolic alkalosis, and asymmetric kidney size. None of these is a constant finding, and often there is no feature to distinguish renal artery stenosis from essential renovascular hypertension.

3. Diagnosis. Diagnostic strategies vary as a function of clinical suspicion.
   a. Rapid sequence intravenous urography shows disparity in renal length and a delayed and persistent nephrogram on the affected side.
   b. If surgical repair is contemplated or a definitive diagnosis is required, renal angiography (either standard or digital subtraction) is appropriate. Stenotic segments are reliably identified by this study.
   c. Proof that angiographically demonstrated renal artery stenosis is etiologically important in the hypertensive diathesis requires that the renal vein renin from the affected side be identified as 1.5 times greater than that from the unaffected side. Although volume depletion and furosemide administration increase this test's sensitivity, up to 30% of renal vein renin studies may be misleading or nondiagnostic. The ultimate diagnosis relies on demonstration of normal blood pressure with correction of the renal artery stenosis.

4. Therapy. Therapeutic options are antihypertensive drugs, percutaneous transluminal angioplasty, and surgical repair of the affected vessel.

D. Microangiopathy: hemolytic-uremic syndrome and thrombotic thrombocytopenic purpura (TTP). As members of the disease group termed **microangiopathic hemolytic anemia**, hemolytic-uremic syndrome and TTP are similar clinical syndromes, which share features with DIC, malignant hypertension, postpartum renal failure, sepsis, and systemic sclerosis.

1. Clinical features
   a. TTP characteristically presents as fever, microangiopathic hemolytic anemia, thrombocytopenia, fluctuating neurologic signs, purpura, and renal failure. Gastrointestinal involvement (e.g., mucosal bleeding and jaundice) is common. The course usually is fulminant; more than 50% of patients die within 6 weeks of the onset of TTP.
   b. Hemolytic-uremic syndrome is primarily a pediatric disorder characterized by microangiopathic hemolytic anemia, thrombocytopenia, and acute renal failure. The disorder may occur in epidemics and has been reported to follow shigellosis. Hemolytic-uremic syndrome usually has a sudden and dramatic onset, with renal failure the dominant clinical

feature. As in TTP, other organ systems may be involved. Renal function returns in most patients who recover from systemic disease. Relapses have been reported.

2. Diagnosis
   a. Laboratory findings are similar in both disorders. Anemia is a constant finding, occurring in association with a variety of structurally damaged red cells in the peripheral circulation. The reticulocyte count and fibrin split products are elevated, a leukocytosis is common, and the serum LDH and indirect bilirubin levels are elevated. Thrombocytopenia is severe (i.e., < 20,000 platelets/mm^3). The bone marrow shows erythroid hyperplasia with adequate or increased megakaryocytes. Azotemia is common, and the degree of renal failure is characteristically severe. Urinalysis shows hematuria, pyuria, hemoglobinuria, and granular casts.
   b. Renal biopsy findings also are similar. Arterioles and small arteries are occluded by eosinophilic, hyaline thrombi containing fibrin and platelet aggregates, which cause impressive vascular dilatation. Microinfarcts commonly occur but without inflammatory infiltrates or signs of vasculitis. Renal lesions are focal and almost completely confined to the arterial side.

3. Therapy. Controlled trials comparing individual treatment programs have not been performed. Therapeutic methods currently in use include antiplatelet drugs (e.g., aspirin, sulfinpyrazone, and dipyridamole), glucocorticoids, exchange transfusion, plasmapheresis, and, rarely, splenectomy.

4. Prognosis has improved with modern therapy. Untreated TTP is almost universally fatal within 1 year. However, 1-year survival rates for treated patients range from 40% to 80%. Less than 5% of patients with hemolytic-uremic syndrome die within 1 month.

E. Systemic sclerosis (scleroderma) is a generalized disturbance of connective and vascular tissue, which leads to fibrosis of the affected tissue. Systemic sclerosis may be a very localized disease (called **morphea**) or a lethal, systemic disease. Renal involvement is a common cause of morbidity and death. The incidence of renal involvement in systemic sclerosis is not solidly established but, based on autopsy series, is estimated to range from 42% to 80%. Clinical evidence of renal involvement (i.e., azotemia, hypertension, and active urinary sediment) is seen in about 45% of systemic sclerosis patients. In one study, subtle vascular and hemodynamic abnormalities were seen in 80% of patients.

1. Clinical features and course
   a. Acute renal disease occurs in the context of rapidly accelerated generalized disease activity, with prominent malignant hypertension. Renal failure can ensue precipitously if the blood pressure is uncontrolled. Pathologically, acute renal disease is quite similar to other microangiopathic diseases. The interlobular arteries show marked intimal thickening and mucoid proliferation, which may lead to cortical necrosis. Glomerular changes usually are mild and nonspecific, often consisting of only mesangial prominence. Interstitial edema with some mononuclear infiltrate is common. Unlike isolated malignant hypertension, systemic sclerosis does not primarily affect arterioles but does produce adventitial fibrosis.
   b. Chronic renal disease may be present in systemic sclerosis patients with little or no clinical signs of renal involvement. Kidney size usually is normal, and the earliest sign of disease is proteinuria, which is noted in 30% of patients. Nephrotic syndrome is rare, and hematuria, urinary casts, and pyuria usually are absent. Hypertension complicates chronic renal disease frequently (i.e., in 25%–50% of patients) and is a harbinger of impending deterioration of renal function. Renal failure occasionally develops in systemic sclerosis patients who have neither proteinuria nor hypertension.

2. Therapy
   a. Treatment of acute renal disease is, to a large degree, the control of accelerated hypertension. Captopril, enalapril, minoxidil, and nitroprusside may be required. Propranolol and furosemide are frequently used adjunctive agents.
   b. Treatment of chronic renal disease is less clear-cut. It is not known whether some vasoactive therapy during early, nonazotemic, nonhypertensive stages of the disease is protective. Similarly, the role of treatment for patients with abnormal renal biopsies but no clinical renal disease is unclear.

F. Sickle cell nephropathy

1. Pathology
   a. Sickle cell trait and sickle cell disease are associated with a variety of renal complications. The renal medulla is relatively anoxic and hyperosmolar—factors that favor erythrocyte sickling. Most damage occurs in the renal papillae.

b. Medullary infarction resulting from occluded (sickled) vessels produces a spectrum of tubular disorders, including impaired urine concentration. Due to the location of injury, these patients behave as though they have been papillectomized. Papillary necrosis also is seen. Patients with sickle cell trait are affected less severely than those with sickle cell disease.

2. Clinical features
- **a. Impaired secretion of potassium and hydrogen ion** occurs, and a frequent biochemical finding is hyperkalemia with a hyperchloremic (normal anion gap) metabolic acidosis (see Part II: section IV D 2).
- **b. Hematuria** represents the most dramatic of the renal abnormalities in sickle cell disease. Although usually self-limited, life-threatening exsanguination occurs in rare cases.
- **c. Glomerular disease** including nephrotic syndrome has been documented in sickle cell disease. Membranoproliferative-like lesions have been reported, as has typical membranous glomerulonephritis.

3. Clinical course. Although GFR frequently is supranormal early in the course of sickle cell nephropathy, gradual deterioration of renal function is common. Progression to end-stage renal disease occurs in some cases.

4. Therapy. Careful fluid management to maintain adequate intravascular volume, both during crises and at other times, clearly is important. Volume depletion is injurious to renal function and is more likely to occur due to the urine concentrating defect. Patients who are prone to hyperkalemia or acidosis should be advised to reduce their dietary intake of potassium and protein. Hemodialysis is a useful renal replacement therapy, which does not increase the number or severity of crises nor the transfusion requirement in most patients. Sickle cell damage does afflict a kidney allograft.

G. Radiation nephritis. High doses of ionizing radiation are destructive to the kidney and urinary tract. Delivery of at least 2000 rads over a period of several weeks can induce disease. Radiation-induced nephritis most commonly results from inadvertent exposure during radiotherapy for abdominal or retroperitoneal tumor.

1. Immediate radiation nephrotoxicity results in decreased renal blood flow, with tubular function and blood pressure remaining normal.

2. Acute radiation nephritis develops within 6–12 months after exposure. Clinical signs are edema, hypertension, headache, exertional dyspnea, anemia, cylindruria, proteinuria, and microscopic hematuria. Death occurs in nearly 50% of patients and is due to severe azotemia and hypertension. Patients who recover from the acute phase may have some persistent proteinuria.

3. Chronic radiation nephritis may follow acute radiation nephritis or develop de novo up to 10 years following exposure. Clinical signs are fairly nonspecific and include fatigue, nocturia, hypertension, hyperuricemia with clinical gout, uremia, anemia, proteinuria, cylindruria, and hyposthenuria.

XVI. TUMORS OF THE URINARY TRACT

A. Renal tumors

1. Benign renal tumors
- **a. Renal adenomas**, the most common benign renal tumors, are small (approximately 3 mm) and usually are detected incidentally. Debate exists as to whether these lesions represent early stages of renal cell carcinoma.
- **b. Hamartomas (angiomyolipomas)** occur in the kidney; 50% of cases are associated with **tuberous sclerosis**. This benign tumor usually is bilateral and multiple. Hematuria is the major manifestation among tuberous sclerosis patients, and treatment is selected on the basis of the severity of bleeding; that is, partial renal infarction or nephrectomy.
- **c. Hemangiomas** are benign submucosal medullary lesions, which usually are unilateral and should be considered in the differential diagnosis of hematuria. These lesions usually are too small for angiographic detection. Treatment, as with hamartomas, is chosen to address the severity of hemorrhage.

2. Malignant renal tumors
- **a. Renal cell carcinoma (hypernephroma, adenocarcinoma of the kidney)**
  - **(1) Epidemiology.** This neoplasm is three times more common in men than in women and usually occurs in the sixth or seventh decade of life. A toxin or an environmental factor is thought to be associated with its development but has not been identified. The only

circumstance in which hypernephroma is familial is in association with **von Hippel-Lindau syndrome**.

(2) **Clinical features.** Most patients present with painless gross hematuria. Anemia and various gastrointestinal complaints occur in 25% of patients. Fever, hypertension, and an abdominal mass are inconsistent findings, appearing in less than 15% of patients. Because renal cell carcinomas can produce several hormones and hormone-like substances, these tumors are associated with many hormone-mediated syndromes (e.g., hypercalcemia, erythrocytosis, and Cushing's syndrome). Metastases can involve almost any extrarenal site. The long bones and lungs are most commonly involved, with the initial presentation occasionally being a pathologic fracture or an abnormal chest x-ray without abnormal urinary findings. Primary tumors can be microscopic even in the presence of extensive metastatic disease.

(3) **Diagnosis.** In 95% of cases the diagnosis is confirmed by arteriography, which may reveal neovascularization, puddling of contrast material in necrotic areas, tortuous vessels, aneurysms, arteriovenous shunting, premature venous opacification, and poorly demarcated tumor margins. Urine cytology rarely is helpful.

(4) **Therapy.** Surgical removal of the affected kidney is the only effective therapy. Extremely large or vascular neoplasms may require preoperative infarction. In some cases, enucleation of tumor from a solitary kidney (unilateral disease) and enucleation or nephrectomy plus enucleation of tumor in the contralateral kidney (bilateral disease) have been successful. A solitary metastasis may be cured by surgical removal.

(5) **Prognosis.** The prognosis for patients with renal cell carcinoma varies with the degree of tumor involvement. The 10-year survival rate following radical nephrectomy is 60% for patients with local disease and 7% for those with distant metastases. Few patients with disseminated disease survive longer than 8–10 years.

b. **Nephroblastoma (Wilms' tumor)** is an embryonal renal tumor, which is recognized before the age of 8 years in 80% of cases and is rare in neonates. The tumor usually is unilateral. Hepatic or pulmonary metastases are found at presentation in one-third of patients.

(1) **Pathology.** Both glandular and sarcomatous elements are present. Many Wilms' tumors secrete renin.

(2) **Clinical features and diagnosis.** Most patients present with hematuria, hypertension, and a palpable abdominal mass. Urography demonstrates the mass lesion and distortion of the collecting system.

(3) **Therapy and prognosis.** Treatment consists of surgical removal of the primary tumor and all metastatic lesions. Adjuvant chemotherapy (with actinomycin D, vinblastine, doxorubicin, and cisplatin) and radiotherapy have greatly improved 5-year survival rates, which now approach 60%.

B. Urothelial tumors

1. **Incidence.** Although transitional cell carcinoma of the renal pelvis occurs, more than 90% of urothelial malignancies are bladder cancers. Every year, 30,000 new cases of bladder neoplasia arise in the United States.

2. **Risk factors** include urban domicile, male sex, advanced age, cigarette smoking, and, possibly, ingestion of cyclamate and saccharin. In addition, exposure to certain industrial carcinogens has been implicated in or strongly associated with the development of bladder cancer.

   a. Substances that have been implicated in the development of bladder cancer include those used in the manufacture of chemicals, dyes, pigments, paint, rubber, and cable and those used in the printing and petroleum industries.

   b. Substances that have been associated with the development of bladder cancer include those used by rodent controllers, fuel workers, coal miners, tar and pitch workers, and metal engineers.

3. **Clinical features.** Painless hematuria is the most common presentation. Large tumors within the bladder can give rise to voiding symptoms. Tumors spread hematogenously, by lymphatics, or by local extension.

4. **Diagnosis.** The diagnosis is based on urine cytology and early cystoscopy with biopsy. CT scanning is well-suited to examine the retroperitoneum and pelvis for metastatic disease. There are no specific biochemical or serologic markers for this disease.

XVII. KIDNEY INVOLVEMENT IN LYMPHOMA AND LEUKEMIA

A. Acute or chronic renal failure may develop during the course of hematologic malignancy in direct, structural ways, such as:

1. Ureteral obstruction from retroperitoneal nodes

2. Compression or invasion of ureters by tumor or retroperitoneal fibrosis

3. Renal lymphomatous or leukemic infiltration

4. Renal artery or vein obstruction

5. Rupture of renal pelvis or ureter

B. **Renal failure may result from humoral, metabolic, or immune disturbances**, such as:

1. Hypercalcemia and hyperphosphatemia

2. Amyloidosis

3. Cryoglobulinemia

4. Glomerulonephritis (e.g., medullary cystic disease in Hodgkin's disease; other glomerulopathies in non-Hodgkin's lymphoma)

C. **Renal failure may be a consequence of therapy.** Examples include:

1. Radiation nephritis

2. Chemotherapy nephrotoxicity

3. Tumor lysis syndrome (i.e., hyperuricemia and hyperphosphatemia)

4. Uric acid nephropathy and uric acid stones

XVIII. THE KIDNEY IN PREGNANCY

A. **General physiologic effects**

1. Under the hormonal influence of pregnancy, renal size increases by 1 cm or more (radiographically); the renal pelvis, calyces, and ureters dilate, as in hydronephrosis; GFR and RPF increase 25%–40%; a primary respiratory alkalosis develops; and the osmostat resets downward. Uric acid clearance nearly doubles and renal excretion of glucose increases, while blood glucose levels remain normal.

2. Clinically, the enlargement of the collecting system should not be mistaken for obstruction. The serum creatinine and BUN values decrease below 0.8 mg/dl and 13 mg/dl, respectively. Serum bicarbonate concentration is 4–5 mEq/L lower than in the pregravid state, and serum osmolality is 10 mOsm/kg lower with a corresponding drop of 5 mEq/L in serum sodium concentration. The serum uric acid is reduced to 3–4 mg/dl, and 24-hour urine glucose may exceed 20 g at term in the absence of diabetes.

B. **Urinary tract infections** that occur in pregnant women frequently are due to the rich nutrient content of the urine and to the urinary stasis resulting from ureteral dilatation.

1. **Clinical conditions. Symptomatic bacteriuria** represents the most common renal problem seen by obstetricians. Although asymptomatic bacteriuria occurs with equal frequency in pregnant and nonpregnant women (i.e., in 4%–7% of all women), clinical infection (i.e., cystitis or pyelonephritis) develops in 40% of pregnant women. (There is some concern that asymptomatic bacteruria increases the rate of prematurity, particularly if there is kidney involvement.) **Acute bacterial interstitial nephritis** occurs in 1%–2% of pregnant women, with signs and symptoms that are comparable to those seen in nonpregnant women. Lower tract infection also presents with typical symptoms.

2. **Laboratory findings and diagnosis** are the same in both pregnant and nonpregnant women.

3. **Therapy.** Although an overwhelming majority of pregnant women respond well to antibiotic therapy without fetal morbidity, antibiotic therapy must be chosen with respect to possible toxic effects on the fetus. Sulfonamides displace albumin-bound bilirubin and may cause kernicterus; tetracycline has obvious dental and osseous toxicity. Ampicillin is the drug of choice when no allergy exists. Cephalosporins also are safe. Asymptomatic bacteriuria should be treated for 10–14 days. Clinical pyelonephritis should be treated for 6 weeks, owing to the very high rate of relapse.

C. **Acute renal failure** complicates 1 in 2000–5000 pregnancies and has a bimodal pattern of occurrence. The first peak occurs in the first trimester and is related to septic abortion. The second peak occurs between 34 and 40 weeks gestation and is related to preeclampsia, hemorrhage, and intravascular volume depletion.

1. Clinical conditions

 a. Cortical necrosis is a special case of acute renal failure complicating pregnancy. Acute cortical necrosis accounts for 5% of cases of acute renal failure in the general population but 10%–30% of cases among pregnant women. Cortical necrosis may complicate any phase of pregnancy, particularly with abruptio placentae. The necrosis can be patchy or extensive. Some women recover variable amounts of renal function; however, most cases ultimately progress to end-stage renal disease.

 b. Idiopathic postpartum renal failure is a rare cause of renal failure peculiar to pregnancy. These patients present several weeks after an uncomplicated delivery with renal failure and severe hypertension. The exact etiology is unknown; however, the pathologic lesion strikingly resembles the hemolyic-uremic syndrome/TTP complex. It is unknown whether a virus, retained placental tissue, or drugs induce this condition by deranging coagulation or endothelial cell function. Dilatation and curettage to remove any placental fragments is worth consideration. Some patients improve with anticoagulation.

2. Prognosis. Pregnancy-related acute renal failure has a better outlook for recovery than renal failure that is induced by medical or surgical complications. Nonetheless, maternal mortality is significant, ranging between 10% and 25%.

D. Hypertension. Blood pressure declines early in pregnancy, reaching diastolic levels that are 15 mm lower than prepregnancy levels by 22 weeks gestation. Blood pressure then rises gradually to prepregnancy values by term. This blood pressure drop is accompanied by a constant cardiac output, which suggests decreased peripheral resistance as a mechanism.

1. Clinical conditions. Hypertensive disorders of pregnancy are classified for clinical purposes as follows:

 a. Preeclampsia-eclampsia

 b. Chronic hypertension, which, in most women, is essential hypertension recognized before pregnancy. A secondary cause rarely is present and may, as in the case of pheochromocytoma, result in disastrously high maternal mortality. A standard evaluation for hypertension should be conducted in women with high blood pressure who contemplate pregnancy.

 c. Chronic hypertension with superimposed preeclampsia

 d. Late or transient hypertension, which, in most cases, occurs in the third trimester and resolves within 10 days of delivery but tends to recur in subsequent pregnancies. Many of these women may ultimately develop essential hypertension.

2. Therapy. The treatment of hypertension during pregnancy is very difficult. Overly enthusiastic lowering of maternal blood pressure may diminish uteroplacental blood flow, leading to fetal compromise. For many reasons, some of which remain controversial, diuretics should not be used routinely. The special case of preeclampsia-eclampsia is discussed below. Diastolic blood pressures above 100 mm Hg in noneclamptic women are best treated with hydralazine or methyldopa.

E. Preeclampsia-eclampsia (toxemia of pregnancy)

1. Definition. Preeclampsia is a syndrome of **hypertension** (frequently malignant), **proteinuria**, **edema**, and, in its extreme, a **microangiopathic hemolytic anemia** with vascular endothelial destruction. This is primarily, but not exclusively, a disease of young primiparas. The hallmark of this disease is the **labile vasospasm** reflecting a vascular sensitivity to the pressor effects of endogenous peptides and catecholamines. Blood pressure may fluctuate widely, but sustained 4- to 6-hour periods of hypertension are reliable signs of disease. Preeclampsia that is associated with maternal convulsions and coma is referred to as **eclampsia**.

2. Pathology. The renal histopathology is glomerular capillary endotheliosis, with swelling of capillary endothelial cells in the absence of hypercellularity. Vacuolization is common.

3. Clinical features and diagnosis. The initial clinical presentation may be mild or severe; however, sustained hypertension newly appearing in the third trimester of a first pregnancy is a suitable criterion for a presumptive diagnosis of preeclampsia. Untreated, fulminant preeclampsia progresses rapidly to maternal convulsions, anuric renal failure, and death.

4. Therapy includes hospitalization and bed rest, prompt delivery if the fetus is mature, parenteral magnesium sulfate for impending convulsions, and careful titration of blood pressure to a diastolic range of 95–105 mm Hg. Ganglionic blockers induce meconium ileus in the fetus and are to be avoided. Diuretics are not recommended.

Part II: Fluid and Electrolyte Disorders

I. WATER METABOLISM

A. Normal physiology

1. **Regulation of water intake.** Increased thirst is the normal response to water loss. The neural center that controls the release of **antidiuretic hormone (ADH)** is anatomically close to the thirst center and responds to increased body fluid tonicity.
   a. **Tonicity** refers to the shift of water through biomembranes produced by osmotically active particles such as glucose and sodium. Urea exerts virtually no tonicity since it easily crosses all membranes and produces no osmotic shift of water.
   b. **Osmolality** is a function of the number of molecules in solution independent of effects on water movement.

2. **Regulation of water output**
   a. **Proximal tubular reabsorption.** Of the 200 L/day of water that are filtered at the glomerulus, 125 L are reabsorbed in the proximal tubule.
   b. **Osmotic gradient formation in the medulla.** Glomerular filtrate not reabsorbed in the proximal tubule enters the loop of Henle, where active sodium reabsorption without water reabsorption causes dilution of the urine and increases the concentration of solutes in the medullary interstitium.
   c. **Collecting tubular transport.** Water that reaches the collecting tubule either is excreted (if ADH is absent, causing the tubule to be impermeable to water) or is reabsorbed (if ADH is present, causing the tubule to be permeable to water). Thus, ADH affects the osmolality of urine, which may range from 1200 mOsm/kg to 50 mOsm/kg.

B. Hyponatremia

1. **Definition.** Hyponatremia refers to serum sodium concentration of less than 135 mEq/L.
   a. **Pseudohyponatremia** (isotonic hyponatremia) results from the shift of water from the intracellular fluid to the extracellular fluid, which is caused by the presence of osmotically active particles (e.g., glucose) in the extracellular fluid space. Serum sodium concentration is reduced, but the osmolality of the extracellular fluid is normal or even above normal.
   b. **True hyponatremia** (hypotonic hyponatremia) is clinically significant when serum sodium concentration is less than 125 mEq/L and the serum osmolality is less than 250 mOsm/kg.

2. **Etiology**
   a. **Decreased renal water excretion**
      (1) **Decreased GFR.** A decrease in the filtered load of water to less than 10% of normal results in a clinically significant decrease in the ability of the kidney to excrete water.
      (2) **Increased proximal tubular reabsorption.** An increase in proximal tubular reabsorption of filtered fluid from the normal 65% to more than 90% may impair the capacity of the kidney to excrete water. Increased proximal tubular reabsorption occurs when the kidney is hypoperfused (e.g., in states of excessive fluid loss from diarrhea or vomiting). Decreased effective renal perfusion in diseases such as congestive heart failure, cirrhosis, or nephrotic syndrome also stimulates proximal tubular reabsorption. This group of disorders is characterized by a low urine sodium concentration, indicating increased renal reabsorption of sodium, high BUN, and the physical finding of either true volume depletion or of one of the edematous conditions.
      (3) **Increased collecting tubular reabsorption** of water is induced by nonosmotically stimulated ADH secretion. This condition is characterized by relatively normal urine sodium excretion (if intake is normal), a high urine osmolality, and signs of body water expansion resulting from retention of excessively ingested water.
   b. **Increased fluid intake.** Fluid intake in excess of 1 L/hr exceeds normal excretory capacity and leads to hyponatremia. This is seen in patients who are given excessive hyponatremic intravenous fluids and in psychiatric patients who drink excessively.
   c. **Syndrome of inappropriate ADH secretion (SIADH)** results from nonosmotically stimulated ADH release associated with the following disorders.
      (1) **Tumor.** Several tumors have been reported to produce an ADH-like peptide, most notably the oat cell carcinoma of the lung.
      (2) **CNS disease.** Excessive ADH release has been documented in postseizure patients as well as in those with cerebral trauma, brain tumors, and psychiatric disturbances.
      (3) **Pulmonary disease.** SIADH has been described with pulmonary tumors, infections, and bronchospastic disease. The mechanism is believed to be stimulation of the so-called **J receptors** in the pulmonary circulation, which lead to pituitary ADH release.
      (4) **Hypopituitarism.** Individuals with glucocorticoid deficiency may have excessive ADH

release, resulting from the loss of glucocorticoid tonic inhibition of ADH release. Primary adrenal insufficiency involving both glucocorticoid and mineralocorticoid production may be associated with a syndrome of renal sodium wasting, which exacerbates the hyponatremia.

(5) Drug-induced SIADH. Drugs that may produce SIADH include chlorpropamide and clofibrate, both of which may increase ADH release as well as sensitize the renal tubule to the effects of ADH. Thiazide diuretics, which may directly lead to ADH release, also may cause hyponatremia through excessive renal sodium excretion or through potassium depletion. CNS-active drugs such as phenytoin also produce SIADH.

(6) Idiopathic SIADH. Elderly patients may have no apparent reason for SIADH and yet maintain sustained hyponatremia. This condition may be related to the increase in ADH release that occurs with advancing age.

(7) Reset osmostat. In chronically ill and malnourished patients, serum sodium concentration is adjusted to maintain an abnormally low serum osmolality. Increased water intake leads to dilution of the urine and excretion of the water load, whereas water restriction leads to an increased urine osmolality and ADH release yet persistent hyponatremia.

3. Clinical features. CNS dysfunction may develop as the tonicity of the extracellular fluid falls and water diffuses down an osmotic gradient into the brain cells, leading to cellular edema. Sustained hyponatremia at a serum sodium concentration below 125 mEq/L may lead to permanent CNS dysfunction. Acute hyponatremia with a decrease in serum sodium concentration to below 125 mEq/L over a period of hours almost always is associated with acute CNS disturbances such as obtundation, coma, seizures, and death if untreated.

4. Diagnosis
  a. Physical examination may reveal:
    (1) Volume depletion (e.g., in cases related to drugs such as diuretics)
    (2) Volume expansion (e.g., in cases related to cirrhosis or congestive heart failure)
  b. Laboratory data
    (1) Urine osmolality is greater than 50–100 mOsm/kg in the presence of plasma hypotonicity.
    (2) Urine sodium concentration is high when plasma volume is expanded in SIADH but is low when effective arterial blood volume is reduced, as in edematous conditions. A urine sodium concentration less than 20 mEq/L strongly argues against SIADH.
  c. Water loading test. When an intravascularly volume expanded individual is given 20 ml water/kg orally or intravenously over a period of 20–40 minutes, the normal response is excretion of 80% of this water load within 4 hours and reduction of urine osmolality below 100 mOsm/kg. Failure to achieve these effects suggests an impairment in the kidney's ability to excrete water.

5. Therapy
  a. Fluid restriction. All patients who are severely hyponatremic should reduce free water intake to approximately 700 ml/day.
  b. Inhibition of water reabsorption
    (1) Demeclocycline has been shown to alter ADH-induced water flow in the collecting tubule. This drug must be given in doses of 600–1200 mg/day and requires 4–5 days to achieve its peak action. Demeclocycline cannot be administered to patients with liver disease, heart failure, or kidney disease since it may accumulate to toxic levels in these conditions.
    (2) Furosemide. Acute administration of furosemide combined with large amounts of saline may lead to increased water excretion. This effect is relatively transient and can be achieved only with acute infusions of furosemide.
  c. Hypertonic infusions. The infusion of 3% or 5% sodium chloride rapidly raises the tonicity of the extracellular fluid. (Serum sodium concentration should not increase faster than 2 mEq/L/hr.) Because extracellular fluid expansion may lead to pulmonary edema, hypertonic saline usually is given in combination with bumetanide or furosemide and should be used only in the treatment of symptomatic patients. Elevation of serum sodium concentration to 125 mEq/L usually alleviates the dangers of brain edema. The amount of hypertonic saline (in mEq) needed to raise the serum sodium concentration ($[Na^+]$) is calculated using the following equation:

$$(\text{normal serum } [Na^+] - \text{current serum } [Na^+]) \times \text{total body water.}$$

6. Complications
  a. Acute hyponatremia. Acute reduction of serum osmolality can produce intracranial hy-

pertension and brain damage, particularly if the serum sodium concentration falls below 125 mEq/L over a period of hours.

    b. Chronic hyponatremia. It has been postulated that chronic hyponatremia (serum sodium concentration of < 125 mEq/L) may lead to alterations in cognitive function, but this remains controversial.

C. Hypernatremia

    1. Definition. Hypernatremia refers to serum sodium concentration that is above normal. Clinically significant effects are produced at serum sodium levels greater than 155 mEq/L. Hypernatremia always implies hypertonicity of all body fluids since the rise in the extracellular fluid osmolality obligates movement of water from the intracellular space, producing increased intracellular osmotic activity and cell dehydration.

    2. Etiology

      a. Extrarenal causes

        (1) Decreased fluid intake. Adequate water intake is required to maintain the tonicity of body fluids in the face of continuous water losses through the skin as well as losses through the urine and gastrointestinal tract. In cool environments, this intake equals approximately 700 ml/day. If intake is less than external losses, body fluid osmolality rises.

        (2) Increased skin losses. Profuse sweating may lead to excess water losses through the skin. In addition, burns and other widespread inflammatory lesions of the skin may cause marked fluid losses.

        (3) Increased gastrointestinal losses. Diarrhea and protracted vomiting also may result in water deficits.

      b. Renal causes

        (1) Osmotic diuresis. The presence of osmotically active, nonreabsorbable solute in the glomerular filtrate prevents water and sodium reabsorption and leads to increased renal water losses. Hyperglycemia with glycosuria is a common cause of osmotic diuresis. Since water losses are relatively greater than sodium losses, the serum sodium concentration rises progressively during osmotic diuresis.

        (2) Decreased ADH effect

          (a) Central diabetes insipidus (i.e., failure of ADH synthesis or release) may occur in the following settings.

            (i) Tumor. ADH deficiency may occur either through direct invasion of the neurohypophysis or through increased intracranial pressure compressing the brain stem.

            (ii) Histiocytosis, particularly Hand-Schüller-Christian disease, has a predilection for neurohypophyseal involvement, producing ADH deficiency.

            (iii) Sarcoidosis also may involve the neurohypophysis, producing diabetes insipidus.

            (iv) Trauma. Classically after resection of the pituitary stalk, there is a phase of acute ADH release followed by a prolonged period of central diabetes insipidus.

          (b) Nephrogenic diabetes insipidus (i.e., failure of renal water conservation despite high levels of plasma ADH) may occur in the following settings.

            (i) Renal disease. Structural renal disease impairs the integrity of the renal medulla and, thereby, the urine concentrating ability.

            (ii) Hypercalcemia. Elevation of serum calcium concentration to above 12 ml/dl may impair urine concentrating ability, most likely as a result of increased medullary blood flow and dissipation of medullary hypertonicity.

            (iii) Hypokalemia. Reduction of serum potassium concentration below 3.5 mEq/L leads to a direct stimulation of thirst and a mild impairment of urine concentrating ability.

            (iv) Lithium ingestion blocks ADH-stimulated osmotic water flow in the collecting tubule.

            (v) Demeclocycline therapy. This tetracycline antibiotic alters ADH-induced water flow through a direct effect on the cell membrane.

            (vi) Sickle cell anemia. Reduced medullary blood flow produced by sickling erythrocytes within the vasa recta also may impair urine concentrating ability.

            (vii) Amyloidosis. Deposition of amyloid fibrils in the collecting tubule cells reduces transepithelial water flow.

            (viii) Urinary tract obstruction and the postobstructive state are associated with nephrogenic diabetes insipidus.

3. Clinical features

a. **CNS disorders.** Generalized CNS depression including obtundation, coma, and seizures develops in young children and elderly patients. Intracerebral hemorrhage may occur due to tearing of bridging veins.

b. **Extracellular volume depletion.** Although two-thirds of water deficits are derived from the intracellular fluid, there also is mild contraction of extracellular fluid volume.

c. **Abnormal urine output.** If the kidneys cause water losses, polyuria (i.e., urine output that is inappropriately high given the level of plasma osmolality or extracellular fluid volume) may be present. If the kidneys are normal and water losses are extrarenal, urine volume typically is reduced.

4. Diagnosis

a. **Dehydration test.** Urine concentrating ability may be tested after overnight dehydration to determine whether a patient has renal water wasting.

  (1) Water deprivation begins at 8:00 P.M. and lasts 14 hours, after which the urine osmolality should exceed 800 mOsm/kg. The patient then is given a subcutaneous dose of ADH as 5 units aqueous vasopressin. The urine osmolality should not be further increased by this maneuver.

  (2) However, if the urine osmolality is less than 800 mOsm/kg after water deprivation or if it increases by greater than 15% after ADH administration, some degree of ADH deficiency is present.

  (3) If the urine osmolality does not exceed 300 mOsm/kg after water deprivation and there is no further increase after ADH administration, some form of nephrogenic diabetes insipidus is present.

b. **Plasma ADH assay.** In nephrogenic diabetes insipidus, the urine osmolality may not be a true reflection of ADH release, and, thus, plasma ADH levels should be measured.

c. **Assay of urine osmolality and composition.** It is useful to measure the solute composition of the urine in the evaluation of polyuria. Urine osmolality of less than 150 mOsm/L suggests a primary defect in water conservation. Urine osmolality of greater than 150 mOsm/L during polyuria suggests an osmotic diuresis. After measuring urine osmolality, the urine should be analyzed for sodium, glucose, and urea to determine the etiology of the diuresis.

d. **Physical examination** generally is not useful in determining the etiology and pathogenesis of polyuria.

5. Therapy

a. **Free water** may be administered orally, which is the preferred route, or intravenously as a 5% dextrose solution. Infusion of a fluid with a tonicity of less than 150 mOsm/L is dangerous and may lead to acute hemolysis.

b. **Vasopressin** may be administered in several different forms. Currently, the agent of choice for the treatment of ADH deficiency is **1-deamino-8-D-arginine vasopressin (dDAVP or desmopressin)**, which may be administered as a nasal spray in a dose of 10–20 μg every 12 hours.

c. **Thiazide diuretics** stimulate proximal tubular reabsorption of sodium and water as a result of volume depletion. This action reduces the delivery of fluid to the distal nephron and, thereby, reduces the degree of polyuria.

d. **Other drugs** such as clofibrate, carbamazepine, and chlorpropamide enhance the renal tubular effects of ADH and, possibly, contribute to the stimulation of ADH release in certain settings.

6. Complications.
Diseases of water conservation are dangerous only if patients are not allowed access to water. In such settings, severe volume depletion and cellular dehydration may occur.

II. SODIUM METABOLISM

A. **Normal physiology.** Sodium is the primary osmotic component of the extracellular fluid, which contains approximately 3000 mEq of sodium. The sodium content of the extracellular fluid determines the volume of that space and the "fullness," or effective volume, of the systemic circulation. A less than 1% change in renal sodium excretion can produce major changes in extracellular fluid volume.

1. **Renal handling.** Approximately 30,000 mEq/day of sodium are filtered at the glomerulus. If sodium intake is approximately 200–300 mEq/day, the entire glomerular filtrate of sodium must be reabsorbed, less 1% (typical amount of ingested sodium), in order to maintain sodium homeostasis. Although only 10%–15% of the glomerular filtrate is reabsorbed in the distal tubule and collecting duct, this is the major regulatory site for determining final urine sodium composition.

2. Hormonal regulation. Aldosterone stimulates sodium reabsorption in the proximal cortical collecting duct. Other hormones may alter renal tubular handling of sodium, but none is as well studied as aldosterone. Aldosterone release from the adrenal gland is governed by the secretion of **renin**.

   a. Renin is an enzyme that catalyzes the conversion of **angiotensinogen** to the decapeptide **angiotensin I** (in plasma). Angiotensin I is converted to the octapeptide **angiotensin II** (in the lung and kidney) by angiotensin-converting enzyme. Angiotensin II is a potent vasoconstrictive agent as well as a potent stimulus for increased aldosterone release from the adrenal gland.

   b. Renin secretion by the kidney is stimulated by renal hypoperfusion, adrenergic stimulation, and circulating catecholamines. Renin is released from the **juxtaglomerular apparatus**, which is located between the afferent and the efferent arterioles of the glomeruli.

B. Edema

1. Definition

   a. Edema generally is defined as an increase in the interstitial compartment of the extracellular fluid.

   (1) Normally, the extracellular fluid volume equals approximately 14 L and accounts for one-third of the total body water. About 25% of the extracellular fluid is represented by plasma volume and is contained within the circulation. The other 75% or 11 L is represented by the interstitial fluid between cells.

   (2) If the interstitial fluid volume increases by approximately 2 L, clinically evident edema may result; edema may be **observable** (as **swelling**) or **palpable** (as **pitting**).

   b. Although edema generally is a function of increased extracellular fluid volume, in some instances increased transcapillary hydrostatic pressure (e.g., as occurs in the portal circulation in cirrhosis) also may contribute to edema.

2. Pathophysiology.
Edema, or the pathologic increase in the extracellular fluid volume, primarily is a function of excessive renal tubular reabsorption of sodium. Decreased renal perfusion (e.g., as occurs in congestive heart failure with reduced cardiac output, in cirrhosis with reduced effective arterial blood volume, and in the nephrotic syndrome) is the proximate cause of the increased renal sodium reabsorption, which represents the body's attempt to maintain adequate effective arterial blood volume.

3. Etiology

   a. Congestive heart failure. When cardiac output is reduced, effective arterial blood volume also is decreased, which triggers the release of renin and aldosterone. These effects combined with alterations in renal hemodynamics stimulate an increase in the proximal tubular reabsorption of sodium.

   b. Cirrhosis. The primary cause of sodium retention in liver disease may be ascites formation, which occurs due to high pressure in the portal circulation. This leads to extracellular fluid volume depletion and secondary renal sodium retention. When hypoalbuminemia occurs, effective arterial blood volume is reduced, stimulating renal sodium retention.

   c. Nephrotic syndrome. Hypoalbuminemia leads to reduced effective arterial blood volume as a result of renal protein losses, which stimulate renal tubular reabsorption of sodium.

   d. Chronic renal failure. When the GFR falls to less than 10 ml/min, the kidney is unable to filter and, therefore, excrete a normally ingested sodium load, which leads to edema.

   e. Excessive mineralocorticoid activity. Tumors of the adrenal gland and tumors that secrete large amounts of adrenocorticotropic hormone (ACTH) may be associated with marked sodium retention.

4. Clinical features

   a. Peripheral edema. Sodium retention may manifest as swelling in the dependent regions of the body.

   b. Pulmonary edema. If pulmonary venous pressure acutely rises above 18 mm Hg, pulmonary edema may develop.

5. Diagnosis

   a. Physical examination. Peripheral edema may be identified by the persistence of an indentation following palpation of the soft tissues in the dependent areas. Pulmonary edema is identified by the physical findings of rales or wheezes or by chest x-ray.

   b. Urine sodium assay reveals a urine sodium level that is less than sodium intake and that usually is significantly less than 20 mEq/L.

6. Therapy

   a. Dietary sodium restriction is essential for the management of edema. A sodium intake of 1 g (23 mEq)/day is the lowest practical intake level that can be achieved.

b. Diuretics. Several diuretic agents are useful for increasing sodium excretion.

   (1) Loop diuretics, such as furosemide and bumetanide, are particularly effective. Side effects of these drugs include intravascular volume depletion, hypokalemia, metabolic alkalosis, and hypercalcemia (with thiazide congeners only). Hypomagnesemia also may occur due to the use of loop-active and distal nephron–active diuretics.

   (2) Potassium-sparing diuretics, such as amiloride and triamterene, act primarily to block sodium reabsorption and secondarily to block potassium secretion in the distal tubule. Use of these agents may lead to potassium retention and increased sodium excretion.

   (3) Aldosterone antagonists. Spironolactone is a competitive aldosterone antagonist, the use of which also leads to potassium retention and increased sodium excretion.

III. POTASSIUM METABOLISM

A. Normal physiology. Potassium is a primary cationic component of the intracellular fluid, which contains approximately 3000 mEq of potassium. In comparison, the extracellular fluid contains very little potassium—about 65 mEq. The ratio of extracellular to intracellular potassium concentration is an important determinant of electrical activity in excitable membranes (e.g., the cardiac conduction system and somatic nerve endings). The normal dietary potassium intake of 40–60 mEq/day must be excreted by the kidney to preserve potassium homeostasis. Also, dietary potassium intake must be taken up rapidly by cells in preparation for renal excretion; otherwise, the serum potassium rapidly rises to life-threatening levels.

1. Extrarenal handling. Cellular uptake of potassium is influenced by the following extrarenal factors.

   a. Insulin. High insulin levels stimulate cellular uptake of potassium.

   b. Epinephrine. This β_2-active catecholamine directly stimulates cellular uptake of potassium. This may be particularly important during severe exertion, when serum potassium levels rise due to muscle ischemia.

   c. Dopamine also stimulates cellular uptake of potassium and may be important in handling acute potassium loads.

   d. Total body potassium. Individuals with a high total body potassium content may have a reduced capacity for cellular uptake of potassium.

2. Renal handling. Most urine potassium is the result of distal tubular secretion. Several factors are known to alter potassium secretion.

   a. Aldosterone secretion. Aldosterone directly stimulates potassium secretion and sodium reabsorption in the collecting tubule of the kidney.

   b. Sodium reabsorption. The delivery of fluid and sodium to the collecting tubule also stimulates potassium secretion. This mechanism accounts for the increased potassium secretion caused by diuretics, which act at more proximal sites in the nephron to block sodium reabsorption.

   c. Acid-base imbalance. Cell potassium content is an important determinant of potassium secretion.

      (1) In **metabolic alkalosis**, potassium ions enter cells in exchange for hydrogen ions, thereby stimulating potassium secretion.

      (2) In **metabolic acidosis**, the reverse is true; that is, potassium secretion is depressed.

B. Hypokalemia

1. Definition. Hypokalemia is defined as serum potassium concentration of less than 3.5 mEq/L. Since most of the potassium content of the body is within cells and cell potassium concentration is about 155 mEq/L, cell potassium can be severely depleted without causing large changes in serum potassium.

2. Etiology. Hypokalemia can result from extrarenal or renal causes.

   a. Extrarenal causes

      (1) Dietary deficiency and gastrointestinal losses

         (a) Inadequate dietary intake. Because potassium conservation in the kidney is limited, a severe reduction of intake to less than 10 mEq/day can lead to a large negative potassium balance and hypokalemia.

         (b) Diarrhea can lead to severe potassium depletion as the potassium content of diarrheal fluid may be as high as 100 mEq/L.

         (c) Vomiting. Although the potassium content of vomitus is relatively small, the secondary effects of intravascular volume depletion, which produce secondary hyperaldosteronism and the associated metabolic alkalosis, stimulate renal potassium excretion.

(2) Potassium redistribution

(a) Insulin administration. A therapeutic or replacement dose of insulin can drive potassium into cells, producing acute hypokalemia.

(b) Epinephrine infusions also can produce acute hypokalemia by an independent action involving β_2-receptors.

(c) Folic acid and vitamin B$_{12}$ therapy for patients with megaloblastic anemia stimulates cell proliferation and produces acute hypokalemia as potassium is used in cell synthesis. This effect also may be seen in patients with rapidly growing tumors.

(d) Acute alkalemia. Infusion of large amounts of bicarbonate stimulates potassium entry into cells in exchange for hydrogen ion.

(e) Hypokalemic periodic paralysis. In this rare syndrome, potassium levels fall acutely—without a loss of potassium from the body—prior to episodes of paralysis. This syndrome commonly is associated with thyroid disease in Orientals and probably represents a defect in catecholamine sensitivity.

b. Renal causes. Any hyperactivity of the normal components of renal potassium excretion can produce negative potassium balance via increased renal losses.

(1) Drug-induced renal losses

(a) Diuretics that act proximal to the site of potassium secretion stimulate urinary excretion of potassium by increasing the delivery of sodium and fluid to the distal tubules.

(b) Antibiotics. Carbenicillin and ticarcillin are antibiotics that act as nonreabsorbable anions in the distal tubule and, thereby, stimulate potassium secretion. Significant hypokalemia is commonly seen.

(c) Gentamicin. Tubular defects with magnesium wasting and secondary potassium wasting occasionally may be seen in patients treated with large doses of gentamicin.

(d) Amphotericin B. This antifungal agent causes damage to the apical membrane of the renal tubular cell, thus increasing potassium loss from the cell. Hypokalemia is a sign of amphotericin toxicity in the kidney.

(2) Hormone-induced renal losses

(a) Primary hyperaldosteronism

(i) Primary adrenal adenomas are associated with hypokalemia, hypertension, and metabolic alkalosis. Occasionally, patients may have hypertension with normal serum potassium levels.

(ii) Diffuse bilateral adrenal hyperplasia may be associated with a milder hypokalemia than is seen with primary adrenal adenoma.

(iii) Ectopic ACTH syndrome. Massive mineralocorticoid increase and renal potassium wasting may occur in patients with oat cell lung carcinoma—a tumor that produces and secretes ACTH.

(iv) Exogenous mineralocorticoid

Licorice ingestion. Licorice produced in Europe (anise) contains a mineralocorticoid-like component, **glycyrrhizic acid**, the ingestion of which may lead to the development of hypokalemia with hypertension and metabolic alkalosis.

Tobacco chewing. Certain tobacco compounds also contain a mineralocorticoid-like constituent, and the use of such tobacco may cause the development of hypokalemia and metabolic alkalosis.

(b) Secondary hyperaldosteronism

(i) Renin-secreting tumor. This rare entity, diagnosed by arteriography, is characterized by intrarenal tumors of the juxtaglomerular apparatus. Severe hypertension and hypokalemia may occur.

(ii) Renal artery stenosis in rare cases may be associated with hypokalemia and hypertension due to severe secondary hyperaldosteronism produced by hyperreninemia. The initial finding of hypokalemia suggests a favorable hypotensive result from correction of the vascular lesion.

(iii) Malignant hypertension. Severe underperfusion of the kidney may occur in malignant hypertension and may lead to hyperreninemia, secondary hyperaldosteronism, and hypokalemia.

(iv) Disorders with reduced effective arterial blood volume produce only mild hypokalemia despite hyperreninemia and hyperaldosteronism. Reduced tubular flow rate reduces potassium secretion.

In **congestive heart failure**, secondary hyperaldosteronism may develop, causing mild hypokalemia even in the absence of diuretic use.

In **cirrhosis**, severe hypokalemia is common due to poor diet (low intake) and secondary hyperaldosteronism.

(3) Potassium loss due to primary renal tubular disorders

  (a) Renal tubular acidosis is characterized by potassium wasting, which may be secondary to sodium depletion and metabolic acidosis or directly attributable to tubular defects in potassium conservation. Potassium wasting is a feature of distal (type I) as well as proximal (type II) renal tubular acidosis of any etiology.

  (b) Bartter's syndrome occurs in children as well as adults and is characterized by renal potassium wasting, metabolic alkalosis, and polyuria. Blood pressure usually is normal or reduced, but renin and aldosterone levels are extremely high. The pathogenesis is not well understood, but a primary defect in renal conservation of sodium chloride is considered a likely cause.

  (c) Chronic magnesium depletion produces a syndrome of renal tubular potassium wasting without other associated defects in ion transport. The potassium wasting can be severe and is unresponsive to potassium repletion until magnesium deficits have been corrected.

(4) Potassium loss due to surreptitious diuretic use is associated with a clinical presentation identical to that of Bartter's syndrome, including hypokalemia, magnesium wasting, metabolic alkalosis, hyperreninemia, and hyperaldosteronism. Laxative abuse is associated with similar presentations.

3. Clinical features

  a. Neuromuscular disorders. Potassium depletion may cause weakness, paralysis, and coma.

  b. Cardiac disorders. Arrhythmia, particularly in the presence of digitalis intoxication, is a hallmark of severe hypokalemia.

  c. Endocrine disorders. Hypokalemia is associated with abnormalities in pancreatic insulin release. Glucose intolerance has been shown to worsen as a result of diuretic-induced hypokalemia.

  d. Polyuria. The polyuria of hypokalemia primarily is a function of polydipsia.

4. Diagnosis

  a. Physical examination. The presence or absence of hypertension is a useful differentiating feature in the approach to the patient with hypokalemia.

  (1) If the patient is hypertensive, the hypokalemia may be caused by excessive mineralocorticoid activity. Since many hypertensive patients are treated with diuretics, any hypokalemia could be a side effect of such therapy.

  (2) If the patient is normotensive, the hypokalemia represents either a gastrointestinal or a primary renal loss of potassium.

  b. Serum electrolyte assay rarely is useful for evaluating the specific cause of hypokalemia. An exception is the finding of combined acidosis and hypokalemia, which suggests renal tubular acidosis.

  c. Urine potassium assay. Urine potassium levels below 20 mEq/L suggest extrarenal potassium losses, whereas levels exceeding 30 mEq/L suggest renal losses. However, urine potassium levels may fall to low values even with primary renal losses during severe potassium depletion (i.e., serum potassium concentration of < 2.0 mEq/L).

  d. Renin-aldosterone axis assay

  (1) Noninvasive tests

  (a) Renin stimulation test. This test is used to determine whether excessive mineralocorticoid activity is due to excessive renin production or to a primary adrenal disorder. To evaluate renin production, 40 mg of furosemide are administered followed by measurement of plasma renin in both the supine and upright positions.

  (i) In normal individuals, renin levels are increased several-fold following furosemide administration, and the levels increase further when the individual assumes the upright position.

  (ii) In individuals with renin suppression due to extracellular fluid volume expansion secondary to excessive mineralocorticoid activity, renin levels are suppressed following furosemide administration and are not stimulated when the individual assumes the upright position.

  (b) Aldosterone suppression test. To document that aldosterone production is independent of normal inhibitory stimuli, 1–2 L of saline are infused followed by measurement of plasma aldosterone in both the supine and upright positions. Individuals in whom aldosterone levels are not suppressed to below normal values may have primary aldosterone overproduction.

  (2) Invasive tests include measurement of bilateral renal venous renin as well as adrenal venous aldosterone and cortisol concentrations. This information is necessary to establish a definitive diagnosis of primary aldosteronism and to define the presence of unilateral or bilateral adrenal disease. The hypertension associated with bilateral adrenal hyperplasia does not respond to adrenalectomy, whereas hypertension of aldosteron-oma is responsive to tumor removal.

e. Urine chloride assay. In cases of mineralocorticoid excess, Bartter's syndrome, and diuretic abuse, urine chloride levels tend to be elevated in the presence of metabolic alkalosis and hypokalemia. The absence of elevated urine chloride levels is highly suggestive of gastrointestinal potassium losses. Severe potassium depletion (i.e., serum potassium concentration of < 2.0 mEq/L) may impair renal reabsorption of chloride and lead to increased chloride excretion.

f. Diuretic assay. If Bartter's syndrome is suspected, the urine must be analyzed for chloride and diuretics, including loop-active agents and thiazides, before a diagnosis of a primary tubular disorder can be established. Such diuretic assays are commercially available.

5. Therapy. In many cases, hypokalemia can be corrected by administration of potassium salts.

a. Forms of potassium salts. Potassium may be administered with a variety of anions. Potassium chloride is the preferred form of therapy since many patients have concurrent chloride deficits. In cases of hypokalemia with coincident renal tubular acidosis, potassium citrate, potassium lactate, or potassium gluconate may be given.

b. Routes of administration. Potassium may be given intravenously or orally.

   (1) Intravenous potassium solutions should not exceed a concentration of 100 mEq/L, and the rate of administration should not exceed 60 mEq/hr. Normally, potassium deficits are on the order of 300–1000 mEq/L. These deficits should be replaced slowly, over days, except when digitalis intoxication or life-threatening arrhythmias are present.

   (2) Oral potassium is absorbed effectively and should be substituted for intravenous potassium whenever possible. Several potassium salts may be given in wax matrix capsules, which avoid the problem of gastrointestinal ulceration caused by earlier enteric-coated potassium preparations. A variety of potassium salts also are available as liquid suspensions.

c. Chronic potassium therapy. The need for potassium supplementation in patients receiving diuretics with mild hypokalemia is debated. However, serum potassium levels probably should be maintained above 3.5 mEq/L. This may be accomplished with oral potassium supplementation. Although some foods are high in potassium, it is difficult to administer adequate potassium salts as food constituents to overcome these deficits.

C. Hyperkalemia

1. Definition. Hyperkalemia is defined as serum potassium concentration of greater than 5.5 mEq/L.

2. Etiology. Pseudohyperkalemia may be caused by release of potassium from coagulated cells and platelets after blood is withdrawn for analysis. Measurement of plasma potassium is required to eliminate this artifact. **True hyperkalemia** may result from extrarenal or renal causes.

a. Extrarenal causes

   (1) Insulin deficiency. Hyperkalemia may occur in diabetic patients due to a lack of insulin and to the presence of associated renal abnormalities [see Part II: section III C 2 b (2)].

   (2) Cell lysis syndromes. Acute cell necrosis following either chemotherapy or a massive crushing injury produces hyperkalemia by rapid cellular release of potassium.

   (3) Succinylcholine therapy. The muscle relaxant succinylcholine may produce hyperkalemia in susceptible individuals with generalized muscle or neurologic disease.

   (4) Hyperkalemic periodic paralysis is a rare and poorly understood syndrome that may be associated with an acute shift of extracellular potassium. [The hypokalemic form of this syndrome, which is more common, is discussed in Part II: section III B 2 a (2) (e).]

   (5) Hyperosmolality. Acute increases in extracellular fluid osmotic activity may produce a transcellular shift of potassium and hyperkalemia. Diabetic patients given intravenous glucose on the suspicion of hypoglycemia may develop this entity if hyperglycemia occurs.

   (6) Acidosis. Mineral acidosis may be associated with an acute shift of potassium from the intracellular to the extracellular fluid as hydrogen ions and chloride ions enter cells.

b. Renal causes. The renal capacity to excrete potassium is approximately 500–1000 mEq/day, which is 10–20 times the normal intake. Any impairment of the normal components of renal potassium excretion may reduce this excretory capacity so that normal intake may produce hyperkalemia.

   (1) Severe renal failure. When the GFR falls to below 10 ml/min, hyperkalemia may occur, even with normal intake. At a GFR above this, hyperkalemia is not a result of glomerular insufficiency per se but is a result of a specific disorder in tubular potassium transport or an extrarenal potassium disturbance.

    (2) Aldosterone insufficiency. Aldosterone is the major hormonal determinant of renal potassium secretion.

       (a) Acquired aldosterone deficiency may occur as a result of renal disease that is associated with reduced renin production. (Recall that renin is an enzyme that cleaves precursor molecules to produce the aldosterone secretagogue, angiotensin II.) Primary adrenal disease also may be associated with reduced aldosterone production. Aldosterone deficiency may be produced by:

         (i) Interstitial renal disease

         (ii) Lead nephropathy

         (iii) Diabetic nephropathy*

         (iv) Obstructive uropathy

         (v) Angiotensin antagonist therapy

         (vi) Addison's disease

       (b) Inherited aldosterone deficiency. Several adrenal enzyme defects associated with deficiency of the 17- or 21-hydroxylase enzymes may be associated with aldosterone deficiency.

       (c) Drug-induced aldosterone deficiency. Nonsteroidal anti-inflammatory drugs act to reduce renin secretion and may produce hyperkalemia through aldosterone deficiency.

    (3) Aldosterone resistance. The following conditions are characterized by tubular defects associated with elevated aldosterone levels but impaired potassium secretion.

       (a) Sickle cell nephropathy

       (b) SLE

       (c) Amyloidosis

       (d) Interstitial renal disease

       (e) Obstructive nephropathy

       (f) Hereditary aldosterone resistance

       (g) Use of triamterene, amiloride, or spironolactone

3. Clinical features

  a. Neuromuscular disorders. By altering transmembrane electrical potential, severe hyperkalemia may alter muscle function or neuromuscular transmission, leading to severe weakness or paralysis.

  b. Cardiac disorders. Cardiac arrhythmias may occur at any level above normal but generally are noted only when serum potassium concentration exceeds 6 mEq/L. As serum potassium level rises, a series of electrocardiographic changes may be seen, including:

    (1) Prolongation of the P-R interval

    (2) T-wave peaking

    (3) Prolongation of the QRS interval

    (4) Ventricular tachycardias, ventricular fibrillation, and asystole

4. Diagnosis

  a. Ruling out pseudohyperkalemia. In vitro lysis of erythrocytes, leukocytes, or platelets can produce hyperkalemia as a result of intracellular potassium release (pseudohyperkalemia). All hyperkalemic patients should be checked for pseudohyperkalemia by measuring both plasma and serum potassium concentrations and by inspecting the serum for discoloration suggesting hemolysis.

  b. Urine potassium assay. Although there is only a rough correlation between urine and serum potassium levels, hyperkalemia induced by increased intake or increased cell lysis should be associated with urine potassium levels exceeding 50 mEq/L. Values less than 30 mEq/L in the setting of hyperkalemia suggest impaired renal secretion of potassium.

  c. Renin-aldosterone axis assay. In certain patients, evaluation of aldosterone and renin levels may help to define the etiology of hyperkalemia.

5. Therapy for hyperkalemia is divided into acute and chronic phases.

  a. Acute antagonism and redistribution

    (1) Calcium. The intravenous administration of 1–2 ampules of calcium chloride acutely antagonizes the cardiac effects of hyperkalemia. Electrocardiographic changes may transiently improve, but serum potassium level remains elevated.

    (2) Glucose and insulin. The intravenous infusion of 25 g (1 ampule) of dextrose plus 15 units of insulin lowers serum potassium within 10–15 minutes.

    (3) Sodium bicarbonate. The intravenous infusion of 44 mEq (1 ampule) of sodium bicarbonate acutely stimulates cellular uptake of potassium.

---

*Insulin deficiency in this condition may potentiate the hyperkalemia.

b. Acute removal
   (1) Diuretics. Furosemide, bumetanide, and, especially, acetazolamide increase potassium excretion in individuals with adequate renal function.
   (2) Aldosterone. The administration of aldosterone as either desoxycorticosterone acetate (15–20 mg/day, intramuscularly) or fludrocortisone acetate (0.2–0.6 mg/day, orally) may increase potassium excretion. Acute administration of desoxycorticosterone acetate in individuals who are aldosterone deficient may also act, in hours, to increase potassium excretion.
   (3) Dialysis. A 4-hour hemodialysis treatment effectively removes potassium and lowers the serum potassium level by approximately 40%–50%. Peritoneal dialysis is less effective, but the acute administration of glucose that accompanies infusion of the dialysate stimulates cellular uptake of potassium.
   (4) Cation-exchange resins. The administration of sodium polystyrene sulfonate binds potassium in the gastrointestinal tract. Two mEq of sodium are exchanged for every one mEq of potassium removed, so that a substantial sodium load may result. Sorbitol is administered orally to prevent severe constipation. Cation-exchange resins can remove 50–100 mEq of potassium over a 6-hour period and may be given orally or rectally.
c. Chronic removal. After the acute removal of potassium, potassium homeostasis may be maintained with any of the following agents.
   (1) Aldosterone may be administered in the forms and dosages described above in section III C 5 b (2).
   (2) Diuretics. Furosemide or acetazolamide may be used in combination with fludrocortisone acetate to increase potassium excretion.
   (3) Cation-exchange resins may be given on a chronic basis to increase gastrointestinal excretion of potassium.

IV. ACID-BASE METABOLISM

A. Normal physiology. Acid-base balance refers to the maintenance of the hydrogen ion concentration of body fluids by three control systems: body buffers (e.g., bicarbonate), the lungs, and the kidneys. Because hydrogen ions (protons) are highly reactive species, even slight changes in hydrogen ion concentration can cause marked alterations in physiologic processes.

1. Hydrogen ion concentration and pH. The hydrogen ion concentration of body fluids is low compared with the concentrations of other ions. It is more convenient, therefore, to express the concentration as **pH**, or the **negative logarithm of hydrogen ion concentration**. The pH of the extracellular fluid is maintained at about 7.4. Although it cannot be measured directly, the pH of the intracellular fluid most likely is between 6.8 and 7.0.

2. Generation and elimination of hydrogen ion. Normal metabolic processes generate large amounts of carbonic as well as noncarbonic (nonvolatile) acids, which enter the body fluids and must be buffered and eliminated.
   a. Carbonic acid. Hydrogen ions are produced through complete oxidation of glucose and fatty acids to carbonic acid. Upon dehydration, carbonic acid forms a volatile end product (carbon dioxide), which can be eliminated by the lungs.
   b. Nonvolatile acid is produced through incomplete metabolism of glucose and fatty acids to organic acids (e.g., acetoacetic and β-hydroxybutyric acids) as well as metabolism of proteins such as methionine and phosphoprotein to sulfuric and phosphoric acids, respectively. Approximately 1 mEq of nonvolatile acid per kg of body weight is produced daily and is excreted primarily by the kidneys.

3. Henderson-Hasselbalch equation. The bicarbonate–carbonic acid (HCO_3^-/CO_2) system is the major buffer component of the extracellular fluid. Acid-base disturbances often are characterized in terms of changes in either the bicarbonate (base) or dissolved carbon dioxide (acid) component of this buffer pair. The classic expression of acid-base state is based on the Henderson-Hasselbalch equation, which relates three variables—pH, carbon dioxide tension (PCO_2), and plasma bicarbonate concentration ($[HCO_3^-]$)—and two constants—pK and S as:

$$pH = pK + \log \frac{[HCO_3^-]}{S \times PCO_2},$$

where: pK = the negative logarithm of the dissociation constant for carbonic acid (6.1), and S = the solubility constant for carbon dioxide in plasma (0.03 mmol/L/mm Hg). Normally, the plasma $[HCO_3^-]$ is 24 mmol/L and the arterial PCO_2 is 40 mm Hg. Thus:

$$pH = 6.1 + \log \frac{24}{1.2} = 7.4.$$

4. Respiratory regulation of arterial PCO$_2$. By regulating the rate of alveolar ventilation, the lungs may retain or excrete carbon dioxide and in this way regulate the "acid" component of the bicarbonate buffer system.

5. Renal regulation of plasma bicarbonate content. The kidneys regulate the plasma bicarbonate content by generating new bicarbonate in the process of hydrogen ion secretion. This process replenishes the bicarbonate used to buffer acid produced by incomplete metabolism of neutral foodstuffs and by metabolism of acid precursors in the diet. There are two important aspects of hydrogen ion metabolism in the kidney: the reabsorption of bicarbonate ion and the secretion of hydrogen ion.

    a. Reabsorption of bicarbonate ion. Approximately 4300 mEq of bicarbonate are filtered daily at the glomerulus, virtually all of which is reabsorbed into the proximal tubules. The remaining minute portion of the filtered bicarbonate is reabsorbed into the distal and collecting tubules. Proximal tubular reabsorption of bicarbonate occurs indirectly by the following process.*

      (1) Filtered bicarbonate ion together with secreted hydrogen ion form carbonic acid within the tubular lumen. Sodium ion reabsorption is linked to this secretion of hydrogen ion to maintain electroneutrality.

      (2) Carbonic anhydrase in the brush border of the proximal tubule catalyzes the dehydration of carbonic acid to carbon dioxide and water. Being readily diffusible, carbon dioxide diffuses into the proximal tubular cell, where intracellular carbonic anhydrase catalyzes its rehydration to carbonic acid.

      (3) The bicarbonate ion formed by the dissociation of carbonic acid is passively reabsorbed into the peritubular blood along with equimolar amounts of sodium ion, which is actively transported into the peritubular blood. The hydrogen ion formed by the dissociation of carbonic acid within the cell serves as a source of another hydrogen ion to be secreted.

      (4) The entry of sodium ion into the tubular cell is balanced electrochemically by two mechanisms: the passive inward diffusion of chloride ion from the tubular lumen into the cell and the exchange of hydrogen ion for sodium ion. The net result of either chloride ion diffusion into the cell or sodium-hydrogen exchange is a reabsorption of sodium chloride or sodium bicarbonate, respectively, into the peritubular capillaries.

    b. Addition of "new" bicarbonate. In addition to conserving bicarbonate, the kidneys add newly synthesized bicarbonate to the plasma **via secretion of hydrogen ion.**

      (1) The addition of new bicarbonate does not involve the bicarbonate reabsorbed into the proximal tubule but, rather, the bicarbonate generated within the distal tubular cell via the hydration of carbon dioxide and the dissociation of carbonic acid. This process is similar to that for the reabsorption of the filtered bicarbonate; since the secreted hydrogen ion does not result in bicarbonate reabsorption in the distal tubule, the formed bicarbonate in the cell is "new."

      (2) The renal contribution of new bicarbonate is accompanied by the excretion of an equivalent amount of acid in the urine in the form of titratable acid, ammonium ion, or both.

        (a) Titratable acid formation and secretion. The exchange of hydrogen ion for sodium ion converts dibasic sodium phosphate or sulfate in the glomerular filtrate into monobasic sodium phosphate or sulfate, which is excreted in the urine as titratable acid. The hydrogen ion secreted into the distal tubules, therefore, can react with filtered phosphate rather than filtered bicarbonate.

        (b) Ammonia formation and secretion. Unlike phosphate, ammonia enters the tubular lumen not by filtration but by tubular synthesis and secretion, which normally are confined to the distal and collecting tubules. Virtually all of the nonpolar ammonia that enters the tubular lumen immediately combines with hydrogen ion to form ammonium ion, which is nondiffusible because it is lipid insoluble. The renal excretion of ammonium ion results in the addition of bicarbonate to the plasma.

6. Concept of compensation. Compensation can be defined as the physiologic response to an alteration in either the **respiratory** or **metabolic** (renal) component of acid-base balance in order to restore the body pH value toward normal. Physiologic compensation generally is not complete. In the Henderson-Hasselbalch equation, changes in the "numerator" (metabolic component) are associated with secondary changes in the "denominator" (respiratory component), which restore the log ratio toward 24:1.2 (i.e., 20:1), and, therefore, return pH toward normal. Conversely, changes in the respiratory component are associated with compensatory changes in the metabolic component in order to restore pH toward normal.

---

*The material contained in sections IV A 5 a and b has been adapted from Bullock J: Acid-base physiology. In *Physiology.* Media, PA, Harwal Publishing, 1984, pp 238–241.

B. Respiratory acidosis

1. **Definition.** Respiratory acidosis is characterized by an increased blood PCO_2 (i.e., to a value greater than 40 mm Hg) and a decreased blood pH (i.e., acidemia).

2. **Etiology.** Respiratory acidosis is associated with a reduced capacity to excrete carbon dioxide via the lungs. Causes include all disorders that reduce pulmonary function and carbon dioxide clearance.

   a. **Primary pulmonary disease** that is associated with alveolar-arterial mismatch may lead to carbon dioxide retention, usually as a late manifestation.

   b. **Neuromuscular disease.** Any weakness of the pulmonary musculature that leads to reduced ventilation (e.g., myasthenia gravis) may produce carbon dioxide retention.

   c. **Primary CNS dysfunction.** Any severe injury to the brain stem may be associated with reduced ventilatory drive and carbon dioxide retention.

   d. **Drug-induced hypoventilation.** Any agent that causes severe depression of CNS or neuromuscular function may be associated with respiratory acidosis.

3. **Clinical features**

   a. **CNS disorders.** Since blood flow to the brain is regulated by blood PCO_2, respiratory acidosis is associated with increased blood flow to the brain and increased cerebrospinal fluid (CSF) pressure. These effects may lead to a variety of symptoms of generalized CNS depression.

   b. **Cardiac disorders.** The acidemia in respiratory acidosis is associated with reduced cardiac output and pulmonary hypertension—effects that may lead to critically reduced blood flow to vital organs.

4. **Diagnosis**

   a. **Acute respiratory acidosis.** Acute carbon dioxide retention leads to an increase in blood PCO_2 with minimal change in plasma bicarbonate content. For each 10 mm Hg rise in PCO_2, the plasma bicarbonate level increases by approximately 1 mEq/L and the blood pH decreases by approximately 0.08. Serum electrolyte levels are close to normal in individuals with acute respiratory acidosis.

   b. **Chronic respiratory acidosis.** After 2–5 days, renal compensation (i.e., increased hydrogen ion secretion and bicarbonate production in the distal nephron) occurs such that the plasma bicarbonate level steadily increases. Arterial blood gas analysis shows that for each 10 mm Hg rise in PCO_2, the plasma bicarbonate level increases by 3–4 mEq/L and the blood pH decreases by 0.03.

5. **Therapy**

   a. **Correction of the underlying disorder.** Attempts should be made to correct muscular dysfunction or to correct reversible pulmonary disease, if either of these is the cause of the respiratory acidosis. In the case of drug-induced hypoventilation, vigorous attempts should be made to clear the offending agent from the body.

   b. **Respiratory therapy.** A blood PCO_2 of more than 60 mm Hg may be an indication for assisted ventilation if CNS or pulmonary muscular depression is severe.

C. Respiratory alkalosis

1. **Definition.** Respiratory alkalosis is characterized by a decreased blood PCO_2 and an increased blood pH (alkalemia).

2. **Etiology.** Respiratory alkalosis is associated with excessive elimination of carbon dioxide via the lungs. Causes include any disorder that is associated with inappropriately increased ventilatory rate and carbon dioxide clearance.

   a. **Anxiety** (hysterical hyperventilation) is the most common cause of respiratory alkalosis.

   b. **Salicylate intoxication** initially causes overstimulation of the respiratory center, resulting in respiratory alkalosis. This may be the only acid-base abnormality noted in adults with salicylate intoxication, although metabolic acidosis may develop due to the salicylate load, which enhances the hyperventilation.

   c. **Hypoxia.** Any disorder associated with a decreased oxygen tension (PO_2) of blood may lead to an increased inspiratory rate and, thus, respiratory alkalosis.

   d. **Intrathoracic disorders.** Any inflammatory or space-occupying lesion in the lung may be associated with primary stimulation of ventilatory rate, leading to a low PCO_2. Such conditions include:

      (1) Pulmonary embolism

      (2) Pneumonia

      (3) Asthma

      (4) Pulmonary fibrosis

      e. Primary CNS dysfunction. CNS disorders that may be associated with inappropriate stimulation of ventilation include:

        (1) Cerebrovascular accident (CVA)

        (2) Tumor

        (3) Infection

        (4) Trauma

      f. Gram-negative septicemia. An early manifestation of gram-negative septicemia or bacteremia is a primary stimulation of ventilation with respiratory alkalosis. The mechanism is unknown.

      g. Liver insufficiency. The most common acid-base disorder in liver disease is primary respiratory alkalosis through a direct CNS effect.

      h. Pregnancy. Primary stimulation of ventilation is typically seen throughout pregnancy.

  3. Clinical features. Acute alkalemia may be associated with several organ system disorders.

      a. CNS disorders. A generalized feeling of anxiety may be present and may progress to more severe obtundation and even precoma.

      b. Neuromuscular disorders. Acute alkalemia may produce a tetany-like syndrome, which may be indistinguishable from that of acute hypocalcemia.

      c. Cardiac disorders. A stimulation of cardiac output may occur with mild alkalemia; depression of cardiac function may occur when blood pH exceeds 7.7.

  4. Diagnosis

      a. Acute respiratory alkalosis. Increased respiratory rate leads to a loss of carbon dioxide via the lungs, which in turn increases the blood pH. For each 10 mm Hg decrease in blood PCO_2 acutely, the plasma bicarbonate level decreases by 2 mEq/L and the blood pH increases by 0.08. Serum chloride level also is increased.

      b. Chronic respiratory alkalosis. Within hours after an acute decrease in arterial PCO_2, hydrogen ion secretion in the distal nephron decreases, leading to a decrease in plasma bicarbonate. For each 10 mm Hg decrease in blood PCO_2 chronically, the plasma bicarbonate level decreases by 5–6 mEq/L and the blood pH increases by only about 0.02. Serum chloride level also is elevated.

  5. Therapy. The primary goal of therapy is to correct the underlying disorder. Use of carbon dioxide–enriched breathing mixtures or controlled ventilation may be required in cases of severe respiratory alkalosis (pH > 7.6).

D. Metabolic acidosis

  1. Definition. Metabolic acidosis is characterized by a decreased blood pH and a decreased plasma bicarbonate concentration. This condition may be caused by one of two basic mechanisms: the loss of bicarbonate or the accumulation of an acid other than carbonic acid (e.g., lactic acid).

  2. Etiology. The causes of metabolic acidosis may be divided into those associated with a normal anion gap and those associated with an increased anion gap. **The anion gap reflects the concentrations of those anions that actually are present in serum but are routinely undetermined**, including negatively charged plasma proteins (mainly albumin), phosphates, sulfate, and organic acids (e.g., lactic acid). An increase in the anion gap represents an increase in one of these moieties, usually organic acids. No change in the anion gap, with decreases in both plasma bicarbonate concentration and serum pH, suggests a primary loss of bicarbonate or the addition of mineral acid.

      a. Metabolic acidosis with an increased anion gap

        (1) Ketoacidosis refers to a condition of increased **ketone body** (ketoacid) formation, which leads to titration of bicarbonate and consequent metabolic acidosis. Ketoacidosis occurs as a complication of diabetes mellitus, prolonged starvation, and prolonged alcohol abuse.

        (2) Lactic acidosis. Decreased oxygen delivery to tissues results in increased lactate production, with accompanying severe metabolic acidosis. Lactic acidosis is a characteristic feature of many conditions associated with low tissue perfusion (e.g., shock and sepsis).

        (3) Renal failure. The accumulation of various organic and inorganic anions associated with reduced GFR accounts for the increased anion gap in severe renal failure.

        (4) Intoxication. The ingestion of a variety of chemical agents may result in the accumulation of organic acids (e.g., lactic acid). Such intoxicants include:

          (a) Salicylate

          (b) Methanol

          (c) Ethylene glycol

b. Metabolic acidosis with a normal anion gap (hyperchloremic metabolic acidosis)

(1) **Renal loss of bicarbonate** may occur due to the following conditions.

(a) **Proximal tubular acidosis** is characterized by decreased proximal tubular reabsorption of bicarbonate leading to excessive urinary excretion of bicarbonate. Causes include cystinosis, SLE, multiple myeloma, heavy metal poisoning, Wilson's disease, and nephrotic syndrome.

(b) **Distal tubular acidosis** is characterized by a decreased distal tubular capacity for hydrogen ion secretion and, therefore, the inability to generate new bicarbonate. Causes include heavy metal poisoning, amphotericin B toxicity, SLE, obstructive uropathy, Sjögren's syndrome, and other hyperglobulinemic conditions.

(c) **Hyperkalemic renal tubular acidosis.** Hyperkalemia, particularly that associated with hyporeninemic hypoaldosteronism, is characterized by reduced ammonia excretion, reduced bicarbonate production, and, thus, the inability to buffer nonvolatile acids derived from the diet. Acidosis (i.e., reduced plasma bicarbonate) is due to reduced ammonia production and, therefore, reduced capacity to excrete hydrogen ion and to generate "new" bicarbonate [see Part II: section IV A 5 a (3) (b) and b (2)].

(d) **Loss of organic anions.** In diabetic ketoacidosis, loss of ketoacids in the urine produces a loss of metabolic precursors of bicarbonate as these ketoacids are metabolized in the liver using hydrogen ions in various oxidation-reduction reactions in the Krebs cycle.

(e) **Carbonic anhydrase inhibition.** Drugs such as acetazolamide (a diuretic) and mafenide (a topical treatment for burns) inhibit the action of carbonic anhydrase and thereby reduce proximal tubular reabsorption of bicarbonate.

(2) **Gastrointestinal loss of bicarbonate** also produces this syndrome and may occur due to:

(a) Diarrhea

(b) Pancreatic fistulas

(c) Ureterosigmoidostomy

(3) **Mineral acid administration.** Hyperchloremic metabolic acidosis also is produced by administration of hydrochloric acid or any of its metabolic precursors, including:

(a) Ammonium chloride

(b) Arginine hydrochloride

(c) Calcium chloride (oral only)

3. Clinical features of metabolic acidosis usually are related to the underlying disorder. A blood pH of less than 7.2 may lead to reduced cardiac output. Acidosis also may be associated with resistance to the vasoconstrictive action of catecholamines, resulting in hypotension. Kussmaul's respiration may be prominent as the ventilatory rate increases in response to the fall in serum pH.

4. Diagnosis

a. Serum electrolyte assay shows a decreased bicarbonate and a variable chloride content, depending on whether the acidosis is associated with a normal or an increased anion gap.

b. Arterial blood gas analysis also demonstrates a decreased bicarbonate level, with a compensatory decrease in blood PCO_2. Winter's formula predicts that, in pure metabolic acidosis, the PCO_2 should be 1.5 times the bicarbonate concentration plus 8 ($\pm$ 2) mm Hg. Variance from this predicted response to pure metabolic acidosis suggests a complicating respiratory dysfunction. (A PCO_2 that is lower than predicted suggests primary respiratory alkalosis; a PCO_2 that is higher than predicted suggests a CNS disorder of pulmonary function, leading to inappropriate carbon dioxide retention.)

5. Therapy. Metabolic acidosis may be treated with alkali when the blood pH is less than 7.2, with therapy aimed at elevating the pH above this point. Sodium bicarbonate is the preferred alkali.

a. The required amount of bicarbonate can be calculated on the basis that bicarbonate occupies a space that accounts for approximately 50% of body weight. Thus, the amount of sodium bicarbonate needed to raise the plasma bicarbonate from 6 mEq/L to 13 mEq/L is calculated as: 7 mEq/L $\times$ 0.5 $\times$ kg of body weight. This is a rough approximation, and repeated measurements of plasma bicarbonate and blood pH must be made in patients so treated.

b. Underestimation of bicarbonate requirements can occur if bicarbonate losses persist during administration (proximal tubular acidosis) or if ongoing organic acid production is sufficiently rapid to consume administered bicarbonate in a buffering reaction (lactic acidosis). In the presence of proximal tubular acidosis, the chronic bicarbonate requirement is 2–4 mg/kg/day.

E. **Metabolic alkalosis**

1. **Definition.** Metabolic alkalosis is characterized by an increased blood pH and an increased plasma bicarbonate concentration.

2. **Etiology.** Increased plasma bicarbonate levels result from either **increased endogenous production of bicarbonate** (in the stomach or kidney), with reduced renal excretion, or **exogenous administration of bicarbonate or other alkali**. Since the renal capacity for bicarbonate excretion is several thousand mEq/day, it is clear that some impairment in renal bicarbonate excretion is mandatory for the maintenance of metabolic alkalosis and a sustained rise in plasma bicarbonate. Metabolic alkalosis is dependent on the factors that initiate alkalemia (generation phase) and on the factors that maintain alkalemia (maintenance phase).

   a. **Vomiting.** Loss of gastric hydrochloric acid by any means causes an increase in plasma bicarbonate since the source of hydrogen ion for gastric secretion is the dehydration of carbonic acid within the parietal cells. The concomitant decrease in extracellular fluid volume produced by vomiting, plus the chloride deficits, reduces the GFR and increases the rate of proximal tubular reabsorption of sodium and bicarbonate to maintain the metabolic alkalosis. Potassium deficits also develop because of renal potassium wasting, and this may potentiate increased proximal tubular reabsorption of bicarbonate.

   b. **Diuretics.** Inhibition of sodium chloride reabsorption above the distal tubule leads to increased flow rate and, therefore, hydrogen ion secretion in the distal convoluted tubule and collecting tubule. Increased hydrogen ion secretion causes increased generation of bicarbonate. The volume depletion produced by the sodium deficits following diuretic use reduces the GFR, stimulates proximal tubular reabsorption of bicarbonate, and maintains metabolic alkalosis.

   c. **Excessive mineralocorticoid action** on the distal convoluted tubule and collecting tubule stimulates hydrogen ion secretion, thereby raising the plasma bicarbonate level. Potassium depletion also produced by this mechanism results in stimulation of proximal tubular secretion of hydrogen ion. This combination of events leads to a sustained increase in plasma bicarbonate.

   d. **Administration of alkali** either as sodium bicarbonate (e.g., during cardiac resuscitation) or as organic ions (e.g., lactate, citrate, and acetate, which are metabolically converted to bicarbonate by hepatic action) results in an increased plasma bicarbonate level. However, unless renal reabsorption of bicarbonate is stimulated, plasma bicarbonate is not sustained at an elevated level.

   e. **Rapid correction of hypercapnia.** Following sustained respiratory acidosis, renal bicarbonate production is elevated as a compensatory event by a stimulation of hydrogen ion secretion. If arterial PCO_2 then is acutely reduced by mechanical ventilation, a transient state of hyperbicarbonatemia and elevated blood pH ensues (a condition termed **posthypercapnic metabolic alkalosis**).

3. **Clinical features** of metabolic alkalosis generally are dominated by the underlying disease state. However, symptoms of tetany may be the most pronounced clinical features.

4. **Diagnosis**

   a. Serum electrolyte assay shows an increased bicarbonate level and a decreased chloride level. Hypokalemia is a frequent finding.

   b. Arterial blood gas analysis reveals an elevated bicarbonate level and a variable PCO_2 value. Since a decrease in ventilation is required to elevate the PCO_2, hypoxia also may result. Thus, carbon dioxide retention does not typically occur as compensation for the elevated plasma bicarbonate level.

   c. Urinary indices are useful in the diagnosis of metabolic alkalosis. If extracellular fluid volume contraction is not present (e.g., due to excessive mineralocorticoid activity) or if renal reabsorption of sodium chloride is inhibited (e.g., due to diuretic use), urine chloride levels are elevated. If extracellular fluid volume depletion also is present (e.g., due to vomiting), urine chloride level typically is unmeasurably low. Rarely, severe potassium depletion (i.e., serum potassium concentration of < 2 mEq/L) is associated with urinary chloride wasting in the presence of extracellular fluid volume depletion.

5. **Therapy** involves correction of the underlying disease state as well as reduction of renal avidity for bicarbonate. The latter effect is accomplished by extracellular volume expansion with sodium chloride–containing solutions.

   a. The metabolic alkalosis caused by excessive mineralocorticoid activity is highly dependent on potassium depletion. Administration of potassium chloride corrects this disorder.

   b. In individuals who have posthypercapnic metabolic alkalosis, judicious administration of acetazolamide or other inhibitors of proximal tubular bicarbonate reabsorption is an adjunct to therapy.

V. CALCIUM METABOLISM

A. Normal physiology

1. Calcium exists in serum in three forms. About 40% of serum calcium is bound to protein, about 5%–15% is complexed with anions such as citrate and phosphate, and the remaining portion is nonbound, ionized calcium. The ionized component of serum calcium is the most important clinically. For example, hypoalbuminemia lowers serum calcium by reducing the protein-bound component; the ionized calcium concentration, however, is unaffected in hypoalbuminemia, and the patient is asymptomatic.

2. Ionized calcium homeostasis is maintained by a balance of calcium input into the blood from the gastrointestinal tract and bone and calcium output from the blood into the urine and lower gastrointestinal tract. Calcium transport across the gastrointestinal tract is influenced strongly by **1,25-dihydroxycholecalciferol** [1,25-$(OH)_2D_3$, or **calcitriol**], which is the active metabolite of vitamin D, and by **parathyroid hormone (PTH)**. PTH raises serum calcium by increasing calcium release from bone, by reducing renal excretion of calcium, and by stimulating renal activation of vitamin D to calcitriol. This is the second of two steps in the metabolic activation of dietary vitamin D. The first step takes place in the liver, and the product is **25-hydroxycholecalciferol** [25-$(OH)D_3$, or **calcifediol**]. Serum calcium level is the principal regulator of PTH release.

B. Hypocalcemia is defined as serum calcium concentration of less than 8.5 mg/dl. **Hypoalbuminemia** lowers the total serum calcium by reducing the protein-bound component. Generally, the total serum calcium level is decreased 0.8 mg/dl for each 1 g/L decrement in serum albumin. However, **PTH deficiency** is the primary determinant of hypocalcemia. For a complete discussion of hypocalcemia, see Chapter 9, section III B.

C. Hypercalcemia results from disorders that cause either increased gastrointestinal absorption or increased bone resorption of calcium. Normal serum calcium level may reach 10.5 mg/dl in men and 10.2 mg/dl in women. Values exceeding these may indicate true hypercalcemia, but serum protein level also must be monitored to confirm that an increased level of protein does not explain the increased total serum calcium. **Hyperparathyroidism** is the result of oversecretion of PTH, which in turn causes hypercalcemia. A full discussion of hypercalcemia can be found in Chapter 9, section III A.

VI. PHOSPHATE METABOLISM

A. Normal physiology

1. **Phosphate function.** Phosphate may be the single most important dynamic constituent required for cellular activity. Virtually all bodily functions are powered by the high-energy phosphate bonds of ATP. In addition, phosphate is the major anion and chief buffer of the intracellular fluid. Its primary role in the renal excretion of hydrogen ion makes phosphate a major constituent of acid-base metabolism as well.

2. **Phosphate distribution.** About 85% of the total body store of phosphate is in bone. Phosphate also is found in the intracellular and extracellular fluid compartments. Plasma phosphate exists primarily in the form of inorganic phosphate, the majority of which is free (not bound to protein). The inorganic phosphate content of the extracellular fluid is a prime determinant of intracellular inorganic phosphate, which is the source of phosphate for ATP. Intracellular phosphate deficits may result in reduced cell energy production and, therefore, generalized cell dysfunction.

3. **Phosphate homeostasis** involves the balance of phosphate intake and phosphate output ("external" balance) as well as the maintenance of normal phosphate distribution within the body ("internal" balance).
   a. **External phosphate balance.** Normal dietary intake of phosphate is 1200 mg/day, which is provided primarily by dairy products, and normal phosphate excretion is 1200 mg/day (800 mg in the urine and 400 mg in the stool). The gastrointestinal tract is a passive component of external phosphate balance, whereas renal phosphate handling is closely regulated.
      (1) Normally, 90% of filtered phosphate is reabsorbed in the proximal tubule, with only a minute portion reabsorbed distally. The main regulator of renal phosphate handling is PTH. A high PTH level inhibits phosphate reabsorption, and a low PTH level stimulates it.
      (2) PTH-independent control of renal phosphate reabsorption also is exerted by dietary phosphate content and other hormones such as calcitonin, thyroid hormone, and GH.

b. Internal phosphate balance also is regulated since intracellular phosphate levels are 200–300 mg/dl and extracellular levels are 3–4 mg/dl. Increased insulin levels, hydrogen ion shifts, and intracellular metabolic disturbances all alter the phosphate distribution in the body.

B. Hypophosphatemia

1. **Etiology.** Hypophosphatemia can result from extrarenal or renal loss of phosphate.
   a. **Extrarenal causes**
      (1) **Dietary deficiency and gastrointestinal losses**
         (a) **Inadequate dietary intake.** Most food contains some phosphate. Inadequate dietary intake of phosphate is unusual and only occurs under specific iatrogenic circumstances.
         (b) **Antacid abuse.** Large amounts of aluminum- or magnesium-containing antacids bind phosphate in the gastrointestinal tract, increase gastrointestinal phosphate losses, and may produce hypophosphatemia.
         (c) **Starvation.** During prolonged starvation, cell breakdown liberates phosphate into the extracellular fluid. The amount of phosphate in remaining, intact cells, however, is preserved at normal levels. As urinary plus stool loss of liberated, extracellular phosphate exceeds dietary intake, negative phosphate balance occurs. Although hypophosphatemia does not follow immediately, severe phosphate deficits may develop upon refeeding as cellular uptake of phosphate is stimulated by new cell growth and macromolecule synthesis.
      (2) **Redistribution of body phosphate**
         (a) **Increased glycolysis.** Any condition associated with increased glycolysis within cells causes organic phosphate compounds to accumulate as the phosphorylated carbon residues in the Embden-Meyerhof pathway, with depletion of intracellular organic phosphate. Serum phosphate level falls as phosphate diffuses into cells, causing hypophosphatemia. Reduction of intracellular inorganic phosphate through this mechanism may be drastic and lead to ATP depletion and, thus, reduced cellular energy. In uncomplicated cases, phosphorylated compounds are metabolized through the Krebs cycle, causing ATP repletion. With more severe phosphate depletion, ATP deficits may lead to cell dysfunction.
         (b) **Respiratory alkalosis.** Hyperventilation is associated with reduced serum phosphate due to increased cellular uptake of phosphate. Glycolysis within cells is stimulated by acute elevation of cellular pH.
         (c) **Sepsis.** Hypophosphatemia is a known concomitant of gram-negative sepsis and may coexist (although independently) with hypophosphatemia due to respiratory alkalosis.
         (d) **Epinephrine** also stimulates cellular uptake of phosphate. This effect is independent of cellular phosphate uptake due to insulin-mediated glycolysis or to other alterations of glucose metabolism.
   b. **Renal causes**
      (1) **Excess PTH.** Any condition associated with normal renal function but elevated PTH levels can produce renal phosphate wasting. This may occur with primary hyperparathyroidism as well as the various states of secondary hyperparathyroidism.
      (2) **Primary renal tubular defects.** Conditions such as cystinosis, heavy metal poisoning, multiple myeloma, SLE, and Wilson's disease may be associated with generalized proximal tubular defects and renal phosphate wasting.
      (3) **Specific transport defects for phosphate** have been designated as **hypophosphatemic vitamin D–resistant rickets**, which may be familial or sporadic and exists in both child-onset and adult-onset forms. In each of these conditions, decreased phosphate transport in the proximal tubule produces excessive renal phosphate wasting.
      (4) **Glycosuria.** Phosphate and glucose compete for transport in the proximal tubule. All glycosuric conditions are associated with excessive renal losses of phosphate.

2. **Clinical features**
   a. **CNS disorders.** Cellular ATP deficiency may produce obtundation, coma, and seizures. Peripheral neuropathy and Guillain-Barré syndrome also have been described.
   b. **Hematologic disorders.** Hemolytic anemia due to cellular ATP depletion and abnormal membrane integrity has been described but is rare. Thrombocytopenia, reduced platelet function, and reduced white cell phagocytic activity have been described but are of uncertain clinical significance.
   c. **Muscular disorders.** Dysfunction of skeletal muscle has been described and attributed to ATP deficits. Acute rhabdomyolysis may be particularly prevalent in alcoholic patients who are acutely hypophosphatemic. Paralysis of respiratory muscles with respiratory failure also may be seen.

d. Bone disorders. Increased bone resorption with abnormal mineralization occurs in chronic hypophosphatemia.

e. Cardiac disorders. Reduced cardiac function has been described in patients with severe hypophosphatemia and in experimental animals. However, the clinical importance of this finding has not been established.

3. Diagnosis. Hypophosphatemia causes complete elimination of phosphate from the urine. A urine phosphate level of more than 100 mg/L strongly suggests renal phosphate wasting. A low urine phosphate level suggests antacid-induced phosphate depletion or increased cellular uptake of phosphate. Glucose infusion is the cause of hypophosphatemia in most hospitalized patients.

4. Therapy. All hypophosphatemic patients should be treated. In general, this involves correction of the underlying condition, such as discontinuation of glucose infusions. In individuals with severe hypophosphatemia and preexisting phosphate depletion (e.g., alcoholic patients), symptomatic hypophosphatemia should be treated with phosphate supplementation. Oral phosphate is preferred, and 1500–2000 mg/day may be given in divided doses. If the patient is comatose or is unable to take oral phosphate, intravenous phosphate may be administered twice daily in 250-mg doses, provided that serum phosphate measurements are taken at 12-hour intervals. Infusion of phosphate must be discontinued if the serum phosphate level rises to 1.5 mg/dl.

5. Complications. The greatest danger of hypophosphatemia lies in the injudicious administration of intravenous phosphate. Acute hypocalcemia due to the formation of calcium phosphate may lead to shock, acute renal failure, and death. For this reason, intravenous phosphate should be administered only when there is clear evidence of specific clinical disturbances attributable to hypophosphatemia.

C. Hyperphosphatemia

1. Etiology

a. Renal failure. Since the kidney is the main regulator of the serum phosphate level, renal failure commonly is associated with hyperphosphatemia. This disorder is not seen until the GFR has decreased to 25% of normal. Serum phosphate level generally does not exceed 10 mg/dl in renal failure. Values exceeding this suggest an additional etiologic factor.

b. Cell lysis syndromes

(1) Rhabdomyolysis. Acute muscle breakdown of any etiology is associated with the release of cellular phosphate and, therefore, hyperphosphatemia. Severe hyperphosphatemia (i.e., a serum phosphate concentration of > 25 mg/dl) may be seen in cases associated with acute renal failure.

(2) Tumor lysis syndrome. Malignant disorders associated with a high sensitivity to chemotherapy or radiotherapy result in rapid cell death with such treatments. This may lead to massive release of phosphate and other intracellular substances into the extracellular fluid. Severe hypocalcemia, cardiovascular collapse, and renal failure due to calcium, urate, and phosphate deposition in the kidney have been described in this condition.

c. Exogenous phosphate administration by any route (i.e., intravenous, oral, or via phosphate enemas) may result in severe and unpredictable hyperphosphatemia.

d. Hypoparathyroidism. Since the level of PTH determines the rate of renal phosphate handling, any condition associated with parathyroid insufficiency or a lack of organ response to PTH may be characterized by hyperphosphatemia.

e. Tumoral calcinosis is a rare disorder characterized by hyperphosphatemia, soft tissue calcified masses, and normocalcemia. Rather than a disorder of calcium metabolism, this condition is due to a specific increase in the renal reabsorption of phosphate. Tumoral calcinosis may represent a heritable condition.

f. Miscellaneous causes. GH excess, hyperthyroidism, and sickle cell anemia are associated with hyperphosphatemia due to excessive renal reabsorption of phosphate. However, this finding is of no clinical significance in these disorders.

2. Clinical features. Hypocalcemia, hypotension, and renal failure may be seen in severe hyperphosphatemia. Milder cases, typically seen in chronic renal failure, are associated with secondary hyperparathyroidism. The treatment of hypercalcemia with phosphate may result in cardiac and renal calcification.

3. Diagnosis. Hyperphosphatemia in the absence of renal insufficiency is due to either cell lysis or tumoral calcinosis. The etiologic diagnosis of hyperphosphatemia is made on the basis of the patient history, physical examination, and laboratory data.

4. Therapy. Acute hyperphosphatemia may be a medical emergency that requires immediate therapy. In cases of tumor lysis syndrome, acute hemodialysis may be required and is an effective treatment. Administration of large amounts of phosphate-binding gels may be useful in the long-term treatment of hyperphosphatemic conditions.

VII. MAGNESIUM METABOLISM

A. Normal physiology. Magnesium is the second most abundant intracellular cation. (Potassium is the most abundant.)

1. Magnesium distribution. More than 50% of the total body store of magnesium is in bone, with most of the remaining portion found in soft tissues, mainly muscle. Less than 1% of body magnesium is in the extracellular fluid, 20%–30% of which is bound to protein and the rest of which exists as free cation.

2. Magnesium homeostasis. Magnesium is absorbed into the small intestine, but this is primarily an unregulated process. During dietary deprivation of magnesium, stool magnesium losses result in hypomagnesemia. The kidney efficiently conserves magnesium during dietary deprivation and excretes any excess magnesium due to excessive intake.

B. Hypomagnesemia

1. Definition. Clinically important hypomagnesemia occurs when serum magnesium concentration falls below 1.0 mEq/L, although it has been proposed that even mild degrees of hypomagnesemia may be associated with a variety of clinical disorders.

2. Etiology
  a. Extrarenal causes
   (1) Dietary deficiency and gastrointestinal losses
     (a) Inadequate dietary intake. Nutritional hypomagnesemia may develop after prolonged starvation as well as postoperatively.
     (b) Malabsorption. Generalized malabsorption syndrome, chronic diarrhea, diffuse bowel injury, and chronic laxative abuse all are associated with reduced gastrointestinal absorption of magnesium. Since gut losses of magnesium can occur even in an individual with a normal gastrointestinal tract, any disorder associated with reduced magnesium intake can result in hypomagnesemia.
   (2) Redistribution of body magnesium. Acute cellular uptake of magnesium has been described in individuals who are in alcohol withdrawal, in patients who are given insulin, and in respiratory alkalosis patients. Also, following parathyroidectomy for severe osteitis fibrosa cystica, acute bone formation may cause rapid accumulation of magnesium and calcium in bone and consequent hypomagnesemia.
  b. Renal causes
   (1) Primary tubular disorders. A number of tubular disorders, including Bartter's syndrome, renal tubular acidosis, and postoperative diuresis, are characterized by a defect in renal magnesium conservation and hypomagnesemia. Hypomagnesemia also may develop in patients following renal transplantation.
   (2) Drug-induced tubular losses. Diuretics such as thiazides, furosemide, and ethacrynic acid typically produce varied degrees of hypomagnesemia. Cisplatin produces marked renal magnesium wasting and clinically severe hypomagnesemia even with small doses of this chemotherapeutic agent. Gentamicin also may produce a toxic injury to the renal tubule, with magnesium and potassium wasting occurring in the absence of reduced GFR.
   (3) Hormone-induced tubular losses. Hyperaldosteronism is associated with magnesium wasting, although the renal tubular mechanism responsible is unknown. Since PTH is an important determinant of renal tubular magnesium handling, hypoparathyroidism is associated with renal magnesium wasting and hypomagnesemia.
   (4) Ion- or nutrient-induced tubular losses. Because calcium and magnesium compete for transport in the ascending limb of the loop of Henle, hypercalcemia is associated with reduced renal magnesium transport. Phosphate depletion and alcohol consumption each are associated with decreased renal reabsorption of magnesium by unknown mechanisms.

3. Clinical features. Muscle twitching, tremor, and muscle weakness are commonly seen. These physical signs are due to the direct effect of magnesium on neuromuscular function as well as the hypocalcemic effect of hypomagnesemia. Severe chronic hypomagnesemia leads to decreased glandular secretion of PTH as well as impaired bone response to PTH, and both of these effects lead to hypocalcemia. Also, hypomagnesemia produces a defect in renal potassium reabsorption, which eventually produces potassium depletion. Thus, all of the clinical signs of hypocalcemia and hypokalemia may be seen in hypomagnesemic patients. The clinical presentation of hypokalemia includes cardiac arrhythmias, particularly in the patient given digitalis.

4. **Therapy.** In most patients, magnesium deficits can be repleted by a normal diet. If ongoing losses occur, magnesium supplementation is necessary. Even in severe magnesium deficiency, however, 50% of an administered dose of magnesium is excreted in the urine. Symptomatic deficits usually amount to 1–2 mEq/kg of body weight. If oral magnesium therapy is required, magnesium oxide, given four times daily in doses of 250–500 mg, generally is tolerated and has 25%–50% absorption. If parenteral therapy is necessary, 12 ml (49 mEq) of 50% magnesium sulfate in 1 L of 5% dextrose in water (D5W) is given over 3 hours and 80 mEq in 2 L of D5W are given over the remainder of the 24-hour period. An additional 49 mEq of magnesium sulfate in 1 L of D5W are given daily for a subsequent 3 days.

C. Hypermagnesemia

1. **Etiology.** Since the kidneys can excrete several hundred mEq of magnesium each day, hypermagnesemia usually is iatrogenic and only occurs, in a sustained fashion, in patients with impaired renal function who ingest magnesium as either laxatives or antacids. Acute magnesium intoxication may occur in women who are treated for toxemia of pregnancy with intravenous magnesium salts that are administered at an excessive rate. Muscular paralysis can develop at serum magnesium levels of 10 mEq/L.

2. **Therapy.** Calcium ion is a direct antagonist to magnesium and should be given to seriously ill patients with magnesium intoxication. Hemodialysis may be required following cessation of magnesium therapy.

STUDY QUESTIONS

Directions: Each question below contains five suggested answers. Choose the **one best** response to each question.

1. A 54-year-old man who has been maintained on chronic peritoneal dialysis for the past year is seen in the emergency room. He has been very careful regarding technique, but over the last 24 hours has noticed a mild, cramping abdominal pain. No other pertinent history is elicited. He does not note any cloudiness of the dialysis fluid. On physical examination he has a temperature of 101° F, but all other vital signs are normal. Abdominal examination reveals the presence of a catheter in place with no erythema but mild peri-umbilical tenderness. Peritoneal fluid analysis reveals a white blood cell count of 300/mm³ (80% neutrophils). The most appropriate diagnosis is

(A) uremic peritonitis
(B) bacterial peritonitis
(C) cholecystitis
(D) perforated gastric ulcer
(E) acute pancreatitis

2. A 19-year-old woman enters the emergency room complaining of dysuria and frequency over the last 24 hours. She denies any past problems of this nature and specifically denies any vaginal discharge or other history of gynecologic symptoms. She has recently been married, and prior to this time was not sexually active. Physical examination reveals a body temperature of 101° F but, otherwise, normal vital signs. Palpation of the costovertebral angles reveals no tenderness, and gynecologic examination reveals no evidence of vaginitis or cervicitis. The hemogram is normal, except for a white blood cell count of 11,000/mm³. Electrolytes as well as blood urea nitrogen (BUN) and creatinine levels are normal. Urinalysis reveals 8–10 white blood cells per high-power field with many gram-negative rods. The proper course of action is to treat with

(A) ampicillin and continue therapy for 10 days, at which time the patient need return only if symptomatic
(B) ampicillin but schedule intravenous urography
(C) ampicillin but schedule cystoscopy
(D) ampicillin and schedule a repeat culture 4 days after discontinuation of therapy
(E) a single dose of intramuscular gentamicin

3. A 78-year-old man enters the hospital because of abnormalities of urination. Today the patient is passing large amounts of urine; however, there are days on which he passes no urine at all. On physical examination now, the patient has a blood pressure of 180/90 mm Hg but the rest of the physical examination is normal. Laboratory studies reveal a blood urea nitrogen (BUN) level of 120 mg/dl and a serum creatinine level of 4.2 mg/dl. Urinalysis reveals a specific gravity of 1.010, urine that is negative for protein, glucose, ketone bodies, and blood, and an occasional white blood cell per high-power field on microscopic examination. The most likely etiology of this patient's renal insufficiency is

(A) obstructive uropathy
(B) acute glomerulonephritis
(C) acute interstitial nephritis
(D) acute tubular necrosis
(E) chronic renal failure of unspecified nature

4. A 71-year-old man is seen in the surgical intensive care unit for acute renal failure. The patient had an operation for removal of gallstones, after which there was a persistent drainage from his biliary catheter associated with spiking fevers to 102° F. The patient has been taking gentamicin (70 mg every 8 hours) and cephalothin (2 g four times a day) for the past 10 days. Over the last 4 days the serum creatinine level has increased at a rate of 1 mg/dl/day, but there has been no diminution in urine output of 1.5 L/day. There has been no history of hypotension at any time during this hospitalization. Physical examination shows normal blood pressure and vital signs. Results of laboratory studies show a creatinine level of 7.1 mg/dl, and renal ultrasonography reveals no evidence of obstruction. The most likely cause of this patient's acute renal failure is

(A) sepsis
(B) trauma to the ureter during surgery
(C) gentamicin nephrotoxicity
(D) acute glomerulonephritis
(E) cephalothin-induced acute renal failure

5. A 32-year-old man has acute renal failure following a mismatched blood transfusion, during which acute intravascular hemolysis occurred, leading to hemoglobinuric acute tubular necrosis. When the man's family asks what his chance for recovery is, they should be told that he

(A) is unlikely to recover renal function but has an excellent chance of long-term survival on dialysis

(B) has a poor prognosis, both for recovery of renal function and for long-term survival on dialysis

(C) has a 90% chance of recovering renal function and being otherwise normal

(D) has a 20% chance of recovering renal function and being otherwise normal

(E) should be prepared for renal transplantation as the only effective means of therapy

6. Which of the following statements best describes polycystic kidney disease in adults?

(A) Ninety percent of patients with polycystic kidney disease die of renal failure

(B) The most common clinical manifestation of polycystic kidney disease is pain

(C) Polycystic kidney disease is transmitted as a sex-linked autosomal recessive trait

(D) Bilateral renal cystic disease may be equated with polycystic kidney disease

(E) Fifteen percent of patients with polycystic kidney disease have associated berry aneurysms

7. Which of the following physiologic changes occurs during a normal pregnancy?

(A) Hyperuricemia

(B) Proteinuria

(C) Hypertension

(D) A 40% increase in the glomerular filtration rate (GFR)

(E) Metabolic alkalosis

Directions: Each question below contains four suggested answers of which **one or more** is correct. Choose the answer

A   if **1, 2, and 3** are correct
B   if **1 and 3** are correct
C   if **2 and 4** are correct
D   if **4** is correct
E   if **1, 2, 3, and 4** are correct

8. Factors that commonly contribute to the hyperkalemia seen in patients with mild-to-moderate renal failure (i.e., a serum creatinine of 2–4 mg/dl) include

(1) intrinsic impairment in renal potassium secretion

(2) elevated potassium intake

(3) 25% reduction of glomerular filtration rate (GFR)

(4) aldosterone deficiency

9. A patient who received a kidney transplant less than 1 month ago is experiencing a failure of kidney function. This may be due to

(1) acute rejection of the transplanted kidney

(2) stenosis of the renal artery in the transplanted kidney

(3) rejection of the transplanted ureter, leading to obstruction

(4) drug-induced renal dysfunction

Directions: The groups of questions below consist of lettered choices followed by several numbered items. For each numbered item select the **one** lettered choice with which it is **most** closely associated. Each lettered choice may be used once, more than once, or not at all.

Questions 10–16

Match each clinical condition with the simple acid-base disturbance associated with it.

(A) Respiratory alkalosis
(B) Respiratory acidosis
(C) Metabolic alkalosis
(D) Metabolic acidosis

10. Myasthenia gravis

11. Cardiogenic shock

12. Early gram-negative septicemia

13. Heroin overdose

14. Normal pregnancy

15. Diuretic abuse

16. Diabetic coma

Questions 17–20

For each renal disorder listed below, select the clinical feature with which it is most closely associated.

(A) Nodular glomerulosclerosis
(B) Positive fluorescent antinuclear antibody
(C) Glomerular capillary endotheliosis
(D) Necrotizing granulomatous vasculitis
(E) Positive Congo red staining with amyloid

17. Lupus nephritis

18. Diabetic nephropathy

19. Toxemia of pregnancy

20. Wegener's granulomatosis

ANSWERS AND EXPLANATIONS

1. The answer is B. *(Part I: IV C 4)* The most common cause for this clinical picture is acute bacterial peritonitis. This complication occurs in 10%–20% of renal patients maintained on chronic ambulatory peritoneal dialysis (CAPD). The typical organism is a staphylococcal agent derived from the skin. Peritonitis may become a recurrent problem in patients on CAPD and may be due to contamination of the peritoneal catheter or the presence of an intra-abdominal abscess. Initial treatment should be aimed at eradicating staphylococcal organisms. Although uremic peritonitis does occur in dialysis patients as do a variety of intra-abdominal disorders (e.g., ulcers, cholecystitis, and pancreatitis), in this clinical setting the physician must consider primarily bacterial peritonitis and ignore these less likely entities.

2. The answer is D. *(Part I: X B, C, D, E)* The patient should be treated with ampicillin for 10 days, and then urine should be cultured 4 days after the drug is withdrawn. Urinary tract infection is common in young women when they become sexually active. It is likely due to urethral trauma during intercourse, leading to bacterial contamination of the bladder. Generally, a single course of ampicillin is sufficient, and no specific culture need be obtained at the time of initiation of therapy as long as the patient has a good response to treatment. A culture should be obtained following withdrawal of the drug, however, to be certain that reinfection has not occurred and that a longer course of ampicillin is not required. There is no indication for more active diagnostic studies at this point since their yield is extremely low. Gentamicin would not be an appropriate choice of therapy because these initial infections nearly always are due to *Escherichia coli*, which are sensitive to ampicillin in the majority of cases.

3. The answer is A. *(Part I: IX A, C)* The incidence of prostatism in elderly men is so great that it must be considered the primary cause of renal insufficiency until proven otherwise. This patient's history is classic in that he had 1 or 2 days on which he seemed to pass no urine followed by days of high urine flow, a pattern that is caused by the gradual accumulation of large amounts of urine in the collecting system under pressure, which eventually may overcome some degree of obstruction. The high pressure is transmitted back to the kidney and results in renal insufficiency. Acute glomerulonephritis and acute interstitial nephritis are ruled out by the normal results of urinalysis. The possibility of acute tubular necrosis should be considered, but there is no information in the history that suggests recent surgery or nephrotoxic drug intake that would have produced acute tubular necrosis. The best way to screen for obstructive uropathy is renal ultrasonography, which would demonstrate dilatated upper tract calyces.

4. The answer is C. *[Part I: II A 3 a (3)]* Approximately 5%–10% of patients treated with gentamicin develop a nonoliguric form of acute renal failure. Although the patient has received normal doses of gentamicin, its accumulation in the kidney has produced a late form of acute renal failure; the serum creatinine level then rises while an inappropriately high dosage is maintained. This exacerbates the renal insufficiency and prolongs the course of acute renal failure. The nonoliguric nature of this patient's clinical condition also is a typical finding in gentamicin nephrotoxicity. Although the patient could have obstructive uropathy, the negative results of ultrasonography strongly indicate otherwise. Cephalothin can produce an acute interstitial nephritis, but the patient's clinical course is much more compatible with the more common drug-induced disease of gentamicin nephrotoxicity. Acute glomerulonephritis usually is associated with hypertension and an active urinary sediment containing casts, protein, and red blood cells.

5. The answer is C. *(Part I: II D 3)* The prognosis for acute renal failure is completely a function of the underlying disease producing this condition. In post-surgical patients who are at great risk for sepsis and bleeding, the rate of recovery may be as low as 10%–15%, particularly among elderly individuals. While the mortality rate among patients with acute renal failure due to medical illness (e.g., following a mismatched blood transfusion) is approximately 30%, complete recovery of kidney function is likely as long as no other illness supervenes. The kidney function in patients who have had an episode of acute renal failure is clinically normal in over 90% of those who survive the acute episode. A small number of patients may develop end-stage renal failure, but these individuals typically have had a modest degree of renal insufficiency prior to the occurrence of acute renal failure.

6. The answer is E. *(Part I: XII A)* About 15% of patients with polycystic kidney disease have associated berry aneurysms. While other organs (e.g., the liver, lung and pancreas) may have cystic changes, the possibility of subarachnoid hemorrhage due to intracranial aneurysm represents the most serious complication with the exception of kidney disease in these patients. Approximately 50% of patients with polycystic kidney disease never have clinical findings of renal failure; the most common clinical manifestation is hypertension, although pain and hematuria also are common occurrences.

7. The answer is D. *(Part I: XVIII A 1, 2)* The glomerular filtration rate (GFR) increases by approximately 40% in pregnancy. In fact, a fall in serum uric acid level typically occurs, as does a rise in uric acid clearance. Proteinuria normally is not seen in pregnancy, and the finding of increased urinary protein excretion suggests the presence of underlying renal disease or preeclampsia. The blood pressure typically falls in pregnancy; therefore, any degree of elevation represents important hypertension. Finally, respiratory alkalosis, not metabolic alkalosis, typically occurs, and this leads to a fall in serum bicarbonate level.

8. The answer is C (2, 4)). *(Part I: I B 1; Part II: III C 2 b)* In mild renal failure, the intrinsic capacity of the kidney to secrete potassium is still adequate. Unless there is a specific impairment in this system, specifically a reduced amount of aldosterone or massive potassium intake, individuals can easily maintain potassium balance and demonstrate a minimal (if any) elevation in serum potassium level. A reduced glomerular filtration rate (GFR) only becomes a factor when it falls below 10–20 ml/min, which is 10%–20% of the normal GFR.

9. The answer is E. *(Part I: IV D)* The most common cause of reduced kidney function in patients following renal transplantation is acute tubular necrosis (ATN) due to kidney damage during the transplantation procedure. The next most common cause is acute rejection, in which both cellular and humoral immunity are brought to bear in attacking the transplanted kidney. Stenosis of the transplanted renal artery occurs in 15% of cases, leading to hypertension and renal insufficiency. Since the ureter also is foreign tissue, rejection of this portion of the renal structure may occur, leading to obstruction or leak of urine into the abdominal cavity. Drug-induced renal dysfunction is an important problem because of the nephrotoxicity of cyclosporine, a drug commonly used to prevent rejection episodes.

10–16. The answers are: 10-B, 11-D, 12-A, 13-B, 14-A, 15-C, 16-D. *[Part II: IV B 2 b, c, C 2 f, h, D 2 a (1), (2), E 2 b]* Diseases (e.g., myasthenia gravis and other myopathies) that lead to thoracic wall dysfunction and hypoventilation lead to carbon dioxide retention and respiratory acidosis.

Conditions of tissue hypoperfusion, including severe decreases in cardiac output, lead to anaerobic glycolysis, increased lactate production, and decreased hepatic lactate metabolism. The result is lactic acidosis, a metabolic acidosis that is characterized by an increased anion gap.

Tachypnea and hyperpnea are early clinical signs of endotoxemia. The resulting decrease in PCO_2 leads to a pure respiratory alkalosis. As septicemia proceeds to septic shock, lactic acidosis may supervene.

Drugs that depress the central ventilatory center (e.g., heroin) will induce hypoventilation, carbon dioxide retention, and respiratory acidosis.

During normal pregnancy, progesterone stimulates the ventilatory center, producing a mild respiratory alkalosis.

The chloruresis and volume depletion induced by diuretic use leads to augmented proximal reabsorption of sodium bicarbonate, causing metabolic alkalosis.

Diabetic ketoacidosis is a metabolic acidosis associated with a wide anion gap. It occurs secondary to ketone body formation in the insulin-deficient state.

17–20. The answers are: 17-B, 18-A, 19-C, 20-D. *[Part I: XI L 3, M 1 a (2), N 3; XIII B 4 a; XVIII E 1, 2]* The glomerular abnormalities of systemic lupus erythematosus (SLE) form a disease spectrum, and there are four associated major lesions. These include the focal proliferative, diffuse proliferative, membranous, and mesangial forms of lupus nephritis. Serologic studies of the four lesions determine differing levels of anti-DNA antibodies and complement components, but common to all four are immunofluorescent findings positive for antinuclear antibody.

All lesions in the kidney of individuals with diabetes mellitus are grouped under the term, diabetic nephropathy. The foremost clinical feature of diabetic glomerular disease is an overt proteinuria, which develops after a prolonged course of diabetes mellitus. Although diffuse glomerulosclerosis is the most common lesion (found in 90% of all diabetic individuals) and is responsible for the proteinuria, the nephrosis, and the renal failure, it is neither specific for nor diagnostic of diabetes. In contrast, the other major renal lesion associated with diabetes, nodular glomerulosclerosis (Kimmelstiel-Wilson syndrome), is both specific for and diagnostic of diabetes; however, it is not responsible for the nephrosis or the renal failure.

Preeclampsia is the toxemia of pregnancy, and it comprises a syndrome that incudes hypertension, edema, and proteinuria. Eclampsia includes the preeclamptic spectrum of symptoms with associated maternal convulsions and coma. The primary pathologic renal feature is glomerular capillary endotheliosis.

Necrotizing granulomatous vasculitis (Wegener's granulomatosis) is characterized by upper or lower respiratory tract symptoms of necrotizing vasculitis and granulomatous inflammation. The kidneys are involved in approximately 50% of patients. Individually, the vasculitis and granulomatous inflammation are not specific for Wegener's granulomatosis; both must be histologically evident for diagnosis. The most recognizable presentation of the condition is the occurrence of necrotizing lesions.

A diagnosis of amyloidosis (i.e., systemic or focal accumulation of amyloid in tissue) is made by biopsy and positive Congo red staining of amyloid protein.

7
Allergic and Immunologic Diseases

Donald P. Goldsmith
Thomas E. Klein
Stephen J. McGeady

I. IMMUNODEFICIENCY DISORDERS. In this chapter, discussion of hereditary and acquired immunodeficiency disorders is limited to disorders of adaptive immunity (both humoral and cellular), defects of the complement system, and abnormalities of phagocytes. It is important to recognize that, although not ordinarily considered immunodeficiencies, other lesions (e.g., loss of skin through burns) also can seriously compromise host defenses.

A. Introduction

1. **Definition of immunity.** The human immune system includes a variety of components that function to defend the body against foreign and potentially harmful agents—living or nonliving.
   a. **Natural immunity** results from, among other things, the presence of **physical barriers** (e.g., skin and mucous membranes), **protein elements with antimicrobial activity** (e.g., **complement** and lysozymes), and **phagocytes** (e.g., granulocytes and monocytes/macrophages). Natural immunity is not specific; it resists all foreign agents (antigens) equally.
      (1) The **complement system** is a complex group of serum proteins that are significant in host defense. They cause lysis of microorganisms, produce chemotactic factors, and promote phagocytosis (**opsonization**). There are nine complement components and several regulatory proteins, which keep the complement system in check. Deficiencies of both the complement components and the regulatory proteins are known.
      (2) **Phagocytes** are ultimately responsible for removing pathogenic organisms and unwanted material from the body. Other components of the immune system enhance their efficiency by producing chemotactic factors and by recognizing foreign material and coating it with antibody and complement (which promote opsonization by the phagocytes). When phagocytes are deficient, either in number or in function, the host is in serious danger of many types of infection.
   b. **Adaptive immunity** is provided by antibodies (**humoral immunity**) and by small lymphocytes (**cellular immunity**) and is directed at specific antigens. Adaptive immunity demonstrates **immunologic memory**, which means that the defenses are deployed more quickly and generally are more potent when an individual is re-exposed to an antigen than after initial exposure.
      (1) **Antibody (humoral) immunity.** Antibodies are protein molecules of a type called **immunoglobulins**. When the amino acids of the immunoglobulin are arranged so that the protein binds to an antigen, an **antibody** is formed.
         (a) Five classes, or **isotypes**, of immunoglobulins are known to exist and are designated IgG, IgA, IgM, IgD, and IgE. **IgM** is found mostly intravascularly, whereas **IgG** exists equally in intravascular and extravascular fluids. IgA seems to be a secretory immunoglobulin and, in a modified form called **secretory IgA**, is found in all body secretions.
         (b) Immunoglobulins are synthesized by plasma cells, which differentiate from **B lymphocytes**, or **B cells**, with immunoglobulin on their cell surface. Ordinarily, almost all B cells have IgM on their surface. When they are stimulated to produce antibody, however, some B cells switch to other immunoglobulin isotypes. B cells exist in lymphoid tissue and in the circulation.
         (c) Clinical disease has been associated with deficiencies of IgG, IgA, and IgM; the consequences of IgD and IgE deficiencies, however, are unclear. Syndromes in which all immunoglobulins are deficient as well as isolated deficiencies of IgG, IgA, and IgM have been described.
      (2) **Cellular immunity** involves the action of thymus-dependent (**T**) **lymphocytes**, or **T cells**.
         (a) Antigen-specific T cells are responsible for delayed hypersensitivity and for resis-

tance to certain microbial pathogens. T cells modulate the activities of macrophages, B cells, and other T cells.

  (b) Cellular immunodeficiencies occur when antigens are unable to activate T cells to release the many soluble factors that lead to a cellular immune response. In some of these syndromes the T cells are absent altogether, whereas in others they are present but malfunctioning. Cellular immunodeficiencies may exist alone or in combination with antibody deficiency syndromes.

2. Incidence of immunodeficiency disorders. Insofar as these disorders represent a diverse group of conditions, it is impossible to cite an overall incidence. The **selective deficiency of IgA** is the most common primary immunodeficiency, occurring in 0.2% of the general population, or in 1 in 500 individuals. In general, antibody deficiency syndromes are most common, followed by cellular immunodeficiencies. Phagocyte and complement deficiencies are quite rare, together constituting only about 10% of all primary immunodeficiencies. The incidence of **acquired immune deficiency syndrome (AIDS)** is increasing rapidly. In 1985, there were over 12,000 AIDS patients in the United States alone.

B. Antibody deficiency syndromes are characterized by an inability to produce antigen-specific antibody molecules.

1. General considerations. The following is a general discussion of the clinical features common to most antibody deficiency syndromes as well as the standard diagnostic and therapeutic approach to these disorders. A more detailed discussion of each of the antibody deficiency syndromes follows (see section I B 2–9).

  a. Clinical features
  (1) In most cases, patients present with **recurrent sinopulmonary infections** due to high-grade extracellular encapsulated bacteria. Most commonly seen are infections of the lungs, sinuses, and middle ear caused by *Hemophilus influenzae, Streptococcus pneumoniae,* and *Streptococcus pyogenes.* These patients also are prone to fatal infections (e.g., sepsis and meningitis) caused by these same organisms. In hereditary antibody deficiencies, the onset of infection usually is at the end of the first year of life since maternal antibody protects for a time.
  (2) Patients with antibody deficiencies are relatively resistant to viral illnesses, although they have been reported to be more vulnerable to **hepatitis viruses. Paralytic polio** also has developed in some hypogammaglobulinemic patients who have received the live, attenuated poliovirus vaccine.
  (3) Also common in antibody-deficient patients is **intestinal infestation** with *Giardia lamblia,* which leads to diarrhea and malabsorption.
  (4) **Pneumonia** due to *Pneumocystis carinii* has been seen in hypogammaglobulinemic patients, especially in association with neutropenia. Despite the recurrent infections, these individuals may appear robust, grow normally, and live many years.

  b. Diagnosis and classification. The diagnosis of antibody deficiency syndromes is based on quantitative measurement of the immunoglobulin isotypes present in the serum and demonstration of specific antibody activity. The syndromes are classified on the basis of the presence or absence of B cells, the mode of inheritance, and specific clinical features.
  (1) **Immunoglobulin isotypes are measured** by radial immunodiffusion on agar gel, radioimmunoassay, enzyme-linked immunosorbent assay (ELISA), and laser nephelometry.
  (2) **Specific antibody formation is assessed** by measuring antibody against antigens to which the population is commonly exposed or antigens commonly used for immunization. Naturally occurring antibodies to the blood group substances A and B, called **isohemagglutinins,** and antibodies to diphtheria and tetanus antigens often are measured.
  (3) **B cells are identified** on the basis of surface immunoglobulin by immunofluorescent labeling with anti-immunoglobulin or with monoclonal antibodies against specific B-cell markers.

  c. Therapy
  (1) The treatment of choice for most antibody deficiency syndromes is replacement therapy with immune human serum globulin. The gamma globulin may be administered as intramuscular injections of immune globulin human [USP], which is 95% IgG, or by intravenous infusion of specially treated immune human serum globulin preparations. (Immune globulin human [USP] is unsuitable for intravenous administration because it contains IgG aggregates that fix complement and, as a result, may produce anaphylactoid reactions.)
    (a) The usual dose of the intramuscular preparation is 0.6 ml (100 mg)/kg of body weight, with a serum IgG level of 200 mg/dl as the goal of therapy. (Serum IgG levels higher than 200 mg/dl have not been proven to be clearly beneficial to the

patient.) Disadvantages of intramuscular injection therapy include the pain associated with the large injections, the variable serum IgG levels achieved, and the possibility of local nerve or muscle damage.

(b) Three specially prepared immune human serum globulin products currently are available for intravenous administration. These are Gamimune N (manufactured through exposure to low pH), Sandoglobulin (manufactured through exposure to low pH and trace pepsin), and Gammagard (manufactured through an ion-exchange adsorption process). All of these chemical manipulations reduce the tendency of the IgG to aggregate and, thus, the risk of anaphylactoid reactions. With the availability of products suitable for intravenous infusion, higher serum IgG levels should be achievable without undue discomfort to the patient. The intravenous preparations are considerably more expensive than the intramuscular ones but are preferred due to the decreased discomfort of administration and the more reliable serum levels achievable.

(2) Despite the administration of immune human serum globulin, most patients with hypo- or agammaglobulinemia have significant numbers of infections. This is especially true if they have developed chronic sinopulmonary disease prior to the institution of gamma globulin therapy. These infections are best treated with the appropriate antibiotic based on culture results. In some cases, the chronic administration of antibiotics is justifiable.

2. X-Linked agammaglobulinemia is characterized by very low levels or complete absence of all immunoglobulins in serum and secretions. (In a variant form of this syndrome, growth hormone also is deficient.) Affected boys are unable to produce antibody in response to antigen stimulation. Cellular immunity, however, is intact in these individuals.

a. Etiology. The gene responsible for this inherited condition is located on the X chromosome. Evidence suggests that the basic defect in X-linked agammaglobulinemia is an inability of the immunoglobulin genes, which are not on the X chromosome, to rearrange properly to perform protein synthesis. This immunoglobulin dysfunction is secondary to the absence of an enzyme that is coded by genes on the X chromosome.

b. Clinical features (see section I B 1 a)

c. Diagnosis of X-linked agammaglobulinemia is based on demonstration of extremely low levels or absence of immunoglobulin in serum and secretions, absence of antibody production, and absence of circulating B cells in an individual with a family history that indicates an X-linked recessive inheritance pattern.

d. Therapy (see section I B 1 c)

e. Complications

(1) X-Linked agammaglobulinemia may be complicated by a progressive and fatal autoimmune disorder that has many of the features of **dermatomyositis.**

(2) Patients may develop an echoviral meningoencephalitis. This condition usually is fatal, although some reports indicate that a very large or intrathecal infusion of gamma globulin may be curative.

(3) The incidence of malignancies (primarily lymphomas and leukemias) in this condition is reported to be 6%.

(4) Chronic lung disease with bronchiectasis is a common sequela of recurrent pulmonary infections.

(5) If the severe complications of X-linked agammaglobulinemia do not occur, patients may live for many years.

3. Autosomal recessive agammaglobulinemia also is characterized by deficiency of all immunoglobulin isotypes and an inability to produce antibody. Some B cells may be present in the circulation of affected patients.

a. Etiology. The defect in this inherited disorder is not understood as well as that in X-linked agammaglobulinemia.

b. Clinical features (see section I B 1 a)

c. Diagnosis of autosomal recessive agammaglobulinemia is made in the same way as for the X-linked condition, but with a family history confirming an autosomal recessive mode of transmission.

d. Therapy (see section I B 1 c)

e. Complications are similar to those in X-linked agammaglobulinemia.

4. Immunoglobulin deficiency with increased IgM is characterized by very low serum levels of IgG and IgA but normal or very high serum levels of IgM and, generally, very little capacity to produce antibody. Affected patients reveal normal numbers of circulating B cells.

a. Etiology. This also is an inherited condition, the inheritance of which has been described as being X-linked, autosomal recessive, or autosomal dominant. Although the precise cause of the syndrome is not known, it is thought that an enzyme necessary for switching from IgM to other immunoglobulin isotypes is missing.

b. Clinical features (see section I B 1 a)

c. Diagnosis is based on demonstration of deficiency or absence of IgG and IgA in serum but normal or markedly increased serum levels of IgM and, occasionally, IgD. There may be specific antibody formation by IgM alone. IgM-bearing B cells exist in normal numbers in the circulation, and all parameters of cellular immunity are normal.

d. Therapy (see section I B 1 c)

e. Complications. Patients with immunoglobulin deficiency with increased IgM generally have a better prognosis than those with either X-linked or autosomal recessive agammaglobulinemia. Complications that sometimes occur include neutropenia, thrombocytopenia, and hemolytic anemia, which may resolve when immune human serum globulin is given. These patients also are prone to chronic lung disease.

5. Selective IgA deficiency is characterized by the presence of little or no serum and secretory IgA in an otherwise immunologically intact individual who has normal numbers of IgA-bearing B cells.

a. Etiology. The defect in IgA deficiency is believed to be abnormal terminal differentiation of IgA-bearing B cells. The cause is unknown, although some inherited cases have been described.

b. Clinical features. Although the tendency toward sinopulmonary infections also exists in IgA deficiency, the severity of the infections is considerably less than that described for most other immunodeficiency syndromes, with severe or life-threatening infections being quite uncommon.

c. Diagnosis is based on the following findings:

(1) Serum IgA level below 5 mg/dl and absence of IgA in secretions

(2) Normal serum levels of all other immunoglobulins and normal antibody formation

(3) No defects or only minor defects of cellular immunity

(4) Normal numbers of circulating B cells

d. Therapy

(1) IgA deficiency never is treated with gamma globulin products. These products contain insignificant amounts of IgA, and infused IgA does not reach the secretions. Most importantly, however, IgA-deficient individuals often form antibodies to IgA, and, if this occurs, the administration of immune human serum globulin products or plasma containing IgA can precipitate anaphylactoid reactions. If an IgA-deficient patient requires blood or plasma, it should be taken from another IgA-deficient individual.

(2) Generally, IgA-deficient patients are treated with antibiotics as needed for bacterial infections, to which these patients seem to be particularly vulnerable.

e. Complications. Selective IgA deficiency generally is a benign disorder compatible with a normal life span. However, several conditions can coexist at greater than normal frequency.

(1) Autoimmune diseases of many types have been reported in IgA-deficient patients, particularly rheumatoid arthritis and systemic lupus erythematosus (SLE).

(2) Allergic disorders, including asthma and allergic rhinitis, occur more frequently in IgA-deficient individuals.

(3) Although there have been occasional reports of malignancies in IgA-deficient individuals, it is uncertain whether the incidence of cancer actually is increased in this common disorder.

(4) Anaphylactoid reactions to IgA delivered in plasma or plasma products may occur.

6. Antibody deficiency with normal immunoglobulin levels occasionally occurs and is characterized by normal numbers of circulating B cells but no antibody production.

a. Etiology. The cause of this condition is unknown but may reflect abnormal mobilization of the genes that code for antibody diversity—a situation that would permit synthesis of immunoglobulin but preclude production of normal antibody.

b. Clinical features (see section I B 1 a)

c. Diagnosis is based on demonstration of normal or increased immunoglobulin levels but an inability to form specific antibodies. Some patients have a deficiency of an IgG subclass but normal levels of total IgG; others lack the capacity to respond to antigens despite the presence of all immunoglobulin isotypes. In some patients, the inability to respond is selective, and antibody formation to some antigens may be normal. These patients have normal numbers of circulating B cells and normal cellular immunity.

d. Therapy (see section I B 1 c)

e. Complications. This condition may be complicated by chronic pulmonary disease.

7. Common variable immunodeficiency (also called **acquired agammaglobulinemia**) is the name given to a group of immune disorders characterized by very low levels of immunoglobulins and the inability to produce antibody despite the presence of normal numbers of circulating B cells. The defect may appear at any time in life in an individual who previously demonstrated normal antibody production.

   a. Etiology. This mixed group of disorders may be inherited or acquired. A few cases may involve abnormalities of T cells, in which inadequate **helper T-cell** activity or excessive **suppressor T-cell** activity causes the antibody deficiency.

   b. Clinical features (see section I B 1 a)

   c. Diagnosis is based on demonstration of deficiency or absence of all major immunoglobulin isotypes and absence of antibody production. Common variable immunodeficiency is characterized by the presence of normal numbers of B cells in the circulation and tissues. Cellular immunity apparently is intact, although the aberrations of T-cell function noted above may preclude B-cell development in some patients.

   d. Therapy (see section I B 1 c)

   e. Complications

   (1) Chronic pulmonary disease develops often, as in other antibody deficiency syndromes.

   (2) Gastrointestinal disorders are common and varied, including malabsorption, nodular lymphoid hyperplasia, and pernicious anemia.

   (3) The incidence of malignancy in this syndrome is approximately 8%.

8. Immunodeficiency with thymoma is characterized by very low levels of all immunoglobulins, deficient antibody formation, and very few circulating B cells in a patient with a thymoma. Some impairment of cellular immunity as well as other hematologic abnormalities may exist in this condition.

   a. Etiology. Immunodeficiency with thymoma is a syndrome of uncertain etiology. Although unproven, it is suspected that the thymoma either secretes a factor that inhibits immunoglobulin production or produces excess suppressor T cells.

   b. Clinical features (see section I B 1 a)

   c. Diagnosis is based on demonstration of marked hypogammaglobulinemia, absence of antibody formation, and absence of circulating B cells in a patient with a thymoma. Evidence of depressed cellular immunity also may be seen.

   d. Therapy (see section I B 1 c)

   e. Complications. Immunodeficiency with thymoma may be complicated by a variety of conditions, including:

   (1) Disorders related to recurrent sinopulmonary infections

   (2) Aplastic anemia, thrombocytopenia, diabetes mellitus, and a myasthenia-like condition

   (3) Malignancy, which develops in 20% of patients who are followed for many years and may involve the thymoma itself, although the tumor usually is benign

9. Transient hypogammaglobulinemia of infancy is characterized by diminished levels of immunoglobulins but the ability to produce specific antibody.

   (1) Etiology. This disorder is thought to be caused by a prolonged delay in the onset of immunoglobulin synthesis in the infant. Although some delay is normal, the lag is greatly prolonged in these infants. A lack of helper T cells has been suggested as the cause of the delay but is unproven.

   (2) Clinical features are similar to those described for selective IgA deficiency (see section I B 5 b).

   (3) Diagnosis is based on demonstration of diminished levels of IgG, IgA, and occasionally IgM in an individual with normal numbers of circulating B cells, normal antibody synthesis, and normal parameters of cellular immunity. Since selective IgA deficiency may have a similar presentation, the immunoglobulin levels must be followed serially and shown to normalize in order to make a definite diagnosis of transient hypogammaglobulinemia.

   (4) Therapy. Although these infants and young children have a significant number of pyogenic infections, it is unclear whether administration of immune human serum globulin is beneficial. Some immunologists believe that exogenous gamma globulin may further delay the onset of immunoglobulin production in these patients.

   (5) Complications. Transient hypogammaglobulinemia of infancy generally is an uncomplicated, benign condition.

C. Cellular immunodeficiencies

1. General considerations. The following is a general discussion of the clinical features common to most cellular immunodeficiencies as well as the standard diagnostic and therapeutic approach to these disorders. A more detailed discussion of each of the cellular immunodeficiencies follows (see section I C 2–7).

a. Clinical features. Patients characteristically present with recurrent infections due to opportunistic organisms and low-grade pathogens. Affected individuals are particularly susceptible to infections with intracellular pathogens including viruses, fungi, protozoa, and some bacteria. Common pathogens include *Candida albicans* and *P. carinii*, but virtually any organism may produce infection in the more severe forms of cellular immunodeficiency.

(1) The severe cellular immunodeficiencies have a clinical course characterized by recurrent infections, chronic diarrhea, and wasting. These patients seldom survive longer than 1 or 2 years.

(2) Many of the cellular immunodeficiencies are characterized by only a partial deficiency of cellular immunity and, thus, have a more benign course and a better prognosis.

b. Diagnosis and classification

(1) The diagnosis of cellular immunodeficiencies is based on a demonstrated decrease in the number or function of the T cells responsible for mediating these reactions.

  (a) Quantitative assessment of T cells is done either by counting the peripheral blood lymphocytes that bind sheep erythrocytes to form a rosette or by immunofluorescent labeling of these cells with T-cell–specific monoclonal antibodies. The latter technique also is used to subdivide the T-cell population into **helper T cells** or **suppressor T cells.**

  (b) Functional assessment of T cells most commonly involves in vitro stimulation of peripheral blood mononuclear cells with polyclonal mitogens, antigens, or the cells of an unrelated donor (**allogeneic cells**). In vivo assessment of T-cell function involves skin testing with ubiquitous antigens for delayed hypersensitivity or grafting skin from an unrelated donor to observe for rapidity of graft rejection.

(2) The cellular immunodeficiencies are classified by etiology (when known), by association with other clinical or laboratory defined abnormalities, and by clinical presentation.

c. Therapy and prognosis. Although significant progress has been made in the treatment of cellular immunodeficiencies, these disorders continue to carry a guarded prognosis.

2. **DiGeorge syndrome (thymic hypoplasia)** is characterized by T-cell deficiency that occurs with normal immunoglobulin levels and the capacity for some antibody production. (Completely normal antibody production requires T-cell help.) Hypoparathyroidism also is present in DiGeorge syndrome.

a. Etiology. DiGeorge syndrome is an inherited disorder due to failure of the third and fourth pharyngeal pouches to develop in the embryo. This causes the absence of both the thymus and the parathyroid glands. Absence of the thymus denies the T cell a critical developmental stage and results in cellular immunodeficiency. Absence of the parathyroid glands leads to hypoparathyroidism.

b. Clinical features. Affected infants present with hypocalcemia and tetany secondary to hypoparathyroidism. Typical facial abnormalities at birth include low-set ears with notched pinnae, micrognathia, ocular telorism, and a fish-shaped mouth. These patients also often have cardiovascular abnormalities, particularly of the great vessels. If they survive the early problems, patients later are afflicted by life-threatening infections, chronic diarrhea, and wasting.

c. Diagnosis of DiGeorge syndrome is based on clinical evidence of hypoparathyroidism (e.g., hypocalcemia, hyperphosphatemia, and tetany) and indications of cellular immunodeficiency. The severity of the defect in cellular immunity is quite variable due to the varying degree of thymic hypoplasia.

(1) A common finding is that of abnormally low numbers of T cells.

(2) In vitro lymphocyte stimulation produces variable results, showing sometimes normal and sometimes diminished T-cell function.

(3) B-cell numbers usually are increased, and immunoglobulin levels are normal. Patients have some capacity for antibody formation but usually have an impaired response.

(4) An important clue to the diagnosis of this syndrome is a chest x-ray showing absence of a thymic shadow and the presence of the typical cardiovascular anomalies.

d. Therapy. DiGeorge syndrome has been treated successfully by transplantation of a thymus obtained from an aborted fetus. It is critical that the fetus be less than 12 weeks gestational age, otherwise the thymus would contain cells with the capacity to react to the human leukocyte antigen (HLA) factor of the new host, causing a fatal graft-versus-host reaction. In some cases of thymic hypoplasia, the patient seems to improve spontaneously without therapy. This may reflect the presence of small foci of thymic tissue in abnormal locations, which become functional with time. This occurrence cannot be predicted.

e. Complications

(1) The absence of parathyroid glands leads to chronic hypoparathyroidism.

       (2) The abnormalities of the heart and aortic arch produce severe cardiovascular dysfunction.

       (3) The immunodeficiency leads to recurrent and sometimes fatal infection.

  3. Purine nucleoside phosphorylase (PNP) deficiency. This syndrome is characterized by PNP deficiency, cellular immunodeficiency, and reduced antibody formation.

    a. Etiology and pathogenesis. PNP is an enzyme that functions in the purine salvage pathway. Absence of PNP causes accumulation of metabolites of this pathway, particularly inosine and deoxyguanosine. These products selectively inhibit proliferation of some lymphocytes, resulting in cellular immunodeficiency but somewhat preserved antibody production.

    b. Clinical features (see section I C 1 a)

    c. Diagnosis

      (1) The diagnosis of PNP deficiency syndrome is based on demonstration of the following:

        (a) A progressive decrease in the function and number of T cells

        (b) Absence of PNP from red cells, white cells, and fibroblasts

        (c) Preservation of antibody-mediated immunity and B-cell numbers

      (2) The progressive nature of this condition suggests that there is a maternal contribution to metabolism of the purine salvage pathway in utero, which is lost at birth, leading to progressive damage to the lymphoid system.

    d. Therapy

      (1) PNP deficiency has been treated by infusion of normal red cells, which have been frozen and irradiated to destroy any lymphocytes. Since red cells are rich in PNP, they provide at least a partial replacement of the missing enzyme.

      (2) The definitive treatment is bone marrow transplantation from a suitable donor (i.e., an HLA-identical sibling). However, no successful bone marrow transplants have been reported to date.

    e. Complications. PNP deficiency is associated with all of the infectious complications common to the cellular immunodeficiencies.

  4. Severe combined immunodeficiency (SCID) is a group of disorders characterized by complete absence of both cellular and humoral immunity.

    a. Types. Several subtypes have been described, including SCID that is associated with:

      (1) Absence of granulocytes, termed **reticular dysgenesis**

      (2) Diminished numbers of both T cells and B cells

      (3) Diminished numbers of T cells but normal amounts of B cells

      (4) Diminished numbers of both T cells and B cells and absence of HLA antigens from the cells, termed **bare lymphocyte syndrome**

      (5) Deficiency of the enzyme, **adenosine deaminase (ADA)**

      (6) A normal amount of immunoglobulin but no specific antibody production, termed **Nezelof's syndrome**

    b. Etiology and pathogenesis. SCID usually is inherited; it is caused by an insult to the developing immune system. The type of insult and the level of development at which the lesion occurs determine the particular subtype of SCID.

      (1) Reticular dysgenesis reflects an insult to the hemopoietic stem cell, which precludes normal development of lymphoid cells and granulocytes.

      (2) SCID with diminished numbers of both B cells and T cells reflects a lesion of the progenitor cell of these lymphocyte lines.

      (3) SCID with decreased T-cell and normal B-cell numbers reflects an insult that occurs somewhat later in differentiation (i.e., after the lymphocyte subclasses have divided but before B-cell function has been attained).

      (4) The bare lymphocyte syndrome reflects the dependence of the immune system on HLA antigens for cellular interactions. When HLA antigens fail to be expressed on the cell surface, the cells cannot interact and a profound immunodeficiency results. It is likely that an enzymatic defect in the developing lymphocytes is responsible for failure of these antigens to be expressed.

      (5) SCID with ADA deficiency results from the accumulation of adenosine and its metabolites in the absence of ADA in the purine salvage pathway. These metabolites are selectively toxic to lymphoid cells and result in the immunodeficiency.

      (6) Nezelof's syndrome is thought to result from abnormal thymic development and a B-cell dysfunction that permits immunoglobulin production but precludes antibody formation.

    c. Clinical features. SCID, regardless of subtype, demonstrates the characteristic morbidity associated with cellular immunodeficiencies (i.e., wasting and recurrent infections). In SCID, however, the illness is more severe and begins almost at birth.

    d. Diagnosis is based on demonstration of complete absence of both cellular and humoral immunity.

        (1) Reticular dysgenesis is suggested by very low numbers of circulating lymphoid cells and granulocytes, with no demonstrable cellular immune function.

        (2) SCID with decreased numbers of T cells and B cells is suggested by the absence of immune function, with decreased numbers of peripheral lymphocytes bearing T- and B-cell markers.

        (3) SCID with decreased T-cell and normal B-cell numbers is suggested by diminished T cells but normal numbers of peripheral lymphocytes with surface immunoglobulins or B-cell markers demonstrated by monoclonal antibodies.

        (4) The bare lymphocyte syndrome is suggested by the finding of peripheral lymphocytes that are devoid of HLA antigens. B cells and T cells typically are diminished in number, although normal numbers occasionally are described.

        (5) SCID with ADA deficiency is diagnosed when the typical findings of combined immunodeficiency are accompanied by absence of ADA.

        (6) Nezelof's syndrome is suggested by the absence of cellular immune function, with normal or increased quantities of immunoglobulins but an inability to form any specific antibody.

    e. Therapy. All subtypes of SCID are best treated by bone marrow transplantation. Until recently, this procedure was available only to SCID patients fortunate to have an HLA-identical sibling. However, bone marrow transplantation now can be accomplished using specially treated marrow from a parent.

        (1) It has been shown that treatment of the parent's bone marrow with **soy bean agglutinin** (a lectin derived from soy beans) and **neuraminidase-treated sheep red cells** followed by gradient centrifugation removes the more mature cells from the marrow. The remaining, immature stem cells then can be transplanted to the child with SCID without causing a graft-versus-host reaction.

        (2) This procedure has proved successful in fully reconstituting immunity or, at least, restoring cellular immunity in more than 50 children with SCID. Earlier attempts to reconstitute immunity in SCID patients using fetal liver or thymus tissue or cultured thymic epithelium seldom were successful.

    f. Complications. SCID is complicated mainly by an exquisite susceptibility to infection, which usually leads to early death. Other complications include an often fatal graft-versus-host reaction if viable lymphocytes are transfused into the patient.

5. Cellular immunodeficiencies associated with defects in other systems. Patients with these disorders have partially impaired cellular immunity and some defect in antibody production. The defect in the other system usually is as clinically troublesome as the immunodeficiency.

    a. Wiskott-Aldrich syndrome. Patients with this disorder have a cellular immunodeficiency and diminished IgM levels and are prone to bleeding disorders because their platelets are small, few in number, and short-lived. The immune deficit is progressive.

        (1) Etiology. Wiskott-Aldrich syndrome is inherited as an X-linked condition. The precise defect is unknown, but it is clear that the diverse manifestations of this disorder cannot be traced to a single cell line aberration or differentiation abnormality. The cause of the progressive deterioration of immune function also is unclear.

        (2) Clinical features. Wiskott-Aldrich syndrome is recognized clinically as a triad of eczema, thrombocytopenia, and susceptibility to infections. Patients usually present with petechiae (due to thrombocytopenia) and eczema in the first 6 months of life, with the vulnerability to infections apparent soon afterward. Since the immunodeficiency includes both humoral and cellular components, there may be pyogenic infections in addition to infections with viral and opportunistic organisms.

        (3) Diagnosis. Wiskott-Aldrich syndrome should be suspected in a boy who presents with thrombocytopenia, eczema, and immunodeficiency.

            (a) The antibody defect is variable but often includes decreased serum IgM, increased serum IgA and IgE, and inability to produce antibody to polysaccharide antigens.

            (b) The cellular immune defect is characterized by decreased lymphocyte responsiveness to mitogens and antigens in vitro and by decreased delayed hypersensitivity in vivo. The cellular immunodeficiency becomes more pronounced with advancing age.

        (4) Therapy. Bone marrow transplantation, with preoperative immunosuppression by cytotoxic agents, has proved corrective of both the immunodeficiency and the thrombocytopenia.

        (5) Complications. Wiskott-Aldrich syndrome has severe complications, including:

            (a) Severe, life-threatening hemorrhage or intracranial bleeding secondary to thrombocytopenia

(b) Lymphoreticular malignancies, which have a predilection for the central nervous system (CNS)

b. Ataxia-telangiectasia. Patients with this disorder have a selective IgA deficiency and impaired cellular immunity and antibody production, which leaves them prone to infection. The loss of immunity is progressive.

(1) Etiology. Ataxia-telangiectasia is inherited as an autosomal recessive condition. Specific causes are unknown, but it is certain that a single differentiation defect cannot explain the characteristic abnormalities of the lymphoid system, blood vessels, and CNS.

(2) Clinical features. Ataxia-telangiectasia is a syndrome consisting of oculocutaneous telangiectasia and progressive cerebellar ataxia. Patients usually present first with recurrent sinopulmonary infections that lead to bronchiectasis; the cerebellar ataxia and oculocutaneous telangiectasia appear later, although the presentation may be quite variable.

(3) Diagnosis. Ataxia-telangiectasia should be suspected in a patient who presents with progressive cerebellar ataxia, oculocutaneous telangiectasia, and immunodeficiency.

(a) The antibody defect is variable but most often includes a selective IgA deficiency and a decreased ability to form antibody.

(b) The cellular defect often includes a decreased number of circulating T cells and an abnormally low (but not absent) responsiveness to T-cell mitogens and to antigens in vitro.

(c) Most patients with ataxia-telangiectasia have an elevated α-fetoprotein level without accompanying liver disease or malignancy.

(4) Therapy. Bone marrow transplantation has not been successful in treating this disorder; the procedure does not correct the neurologic abnormality.

(5) Complications. Ataxia-telangiectasia may be complicated by:

(a) Progressive neurologic deterioration

(b) Lymphoreticular malignancy

6. Cellular immunodeficiencies associated with selective immune defects

a. X-Linked lymphoproliferative syndrome (Duncan's disease) is an unusual disorder in which the immune system does not adequately resist Epstein-Barr virus infections.

(1) Etiology. X-Linked lymphoproliferative syndrome is inherited as an X-linked recessive condition. The exact defect is unknown but seems to reflect an abnormal cellular immune response to Epstein-Barr virus combined with the capacity of this virus to infect lymphoid cells selectively and to transform or destroy them.

(2) Clinical features. X-Linked lymphoproliferative syndrome may not be clinically evident until the affected individual is exposed to Epstein-Barr virus. Once infected, patients may succumb to an acute and possibly fatal episode or may develop aplastic anemia, hypogammaglobulinemia, or B-cell malignancies subsequent to the infection.

(3) Diagnosis. X-Linked lymphoproliferative syndrome should be suspected in a male whose kindred demonstrate abnormally severe Epstein-Barr virus infections or untoward sequelae. Infection with this agent may result in clinical and laboratory findings consistent with lymphoma, hypogammaglobulinemia, or aplastic anemia. The specific immune defect is not demonstrable by immunologic testing but appears to reflect an impaired response to Epstein-Barr virus.

(4) Therapy. X-Linked lymphoproliferative syndrome is treated symptomatically. Patients who survive the Epstein-Barr virus infection are treated appropriately for hypogammaglobulinemia, aplastic anemia, or neoplasm. Increased understanding of the hereditary aspects of this disorder may make therapy with Epstein-Barr virus–specific gammaglobulin, interferon, or antiviral agents feasible.

(5) Complications of X-linked lymphoproliferative syndrome represent sequelae of Epstein-Barr virus infection and include hypogammaglobulinemia, B-cell neoplasia, aplastic anemia, and death.

b. Hyperimmunoglobulinemia E (Buckley's syndrome, Job's syndrome) is associated with high serum IgE levels and susceptibility to staphylococcal abcesses and, occasionally, infection by opportunistic organisms.

(1) Etiology. Hyperimmunoglobulinemia E often is familial and is inherited as an autosomal recessive condition. The precise defect is unknown, although abnormalities in cellular immunity are clearly present. Inadequate suppressor T-cell activity toward IgE has been shown, but it is not clear how this defect would predispose to the infections observed.

(2) Clinical features. Hyperimmunoglobulinemia E presents as dermatitis, cold staphylococcal abscesses of the skin, and pulmonary infections. The infections begin early in infancy and are recurrent.

(3) Diagnosis. Hyperimmunoglobulinemia E should be suspected in a patient who demonstrates a susceptibility to staphylococcal infections in association with extremely high IgE levels. There is an abnormality of cellular immunity, which may be illustrated by abnormal lymphocyte responses to allogeneic cells in vitro; other aspects of T-cell function are intact. Antibody formation is diminished but present.

(4) **Therapy.** Hyperimmunoglobulinemia E is treated with chronic β-lactamase–resistant penicillin for staphylococcal infections and appropriate antimicrobials for other infections. Skin abscesses may require local drainage. Long-term survival can be expected with vigorous treatment.

(5) **Complications** seen in hyperimmunoglobulinemia E include structural lung disease with pneumatocele formation secondary to chronic staphylococcal infection.

c. **Chronic mucocutaneous candidiasis (CMCC)** involves susceptibility to *Candida albicans* and, occasionally, to other organisms. Endocrinopathies occasionally coexist.

(1) **Etiology.** CMCC is of uncertain etiology. The cellular immunodeficiency is largely limited to *C. albicans* infections and is of variable severity.

(2) **Clinical features.** Individuals with CMCC have chronic candidiasis of the mucous membranes, skin, and nails. The syndrome has several subtypes, which vary widely in severity and associated organ failure.

(a) **Early-onset CMCC.** This form of CMCC presents in infancy or within the first 2 decades as candidiasis of the oral mucosa followed by nail and then skin involvement. Infection may be severe and disfiguring due to granuloma formation. About 50% of patients with early-onset CMCC have endocrine disease.

(b) **Late-onset CMCC**, which may be seen in elderly individuals, is the mildest form of CMCC. Infection may be limited to a single nail or to the buccal mucosa. Endocrinopathy is rare.

(c) **Familial CMCC** is inherited as an autosomal recessive condition and is characterized by mild-to-moderate candidiasis. Endocrinopathy is seldom encountered.

(d) **Juvenile familial polyendocrinopathy with CMCC** is characterized by mild-to-moderate candidiasis. Endocrinopathy is invariably present and consists of hypoparathyroidism, Addison's disease, or both.

(3) **Diagnosis.** CMCC is diagnosed on the basis of clinical and laboratory findings.

(a) Immunologically, CMCC is a poorly characterized group of syndromes. A complete or partial defect in resistance to *C. albicans* often can be demonstrated by anergy on skin testing or by failure of T-cell response to stimulation with *Candida* antigen in vitro. Other aspects of immune function appear to be intact. Immunologic findings are similar in all four subtypes of CMCC.

(b) In the CMCC subtypes that involve endocrine disorders, there are decreased serum levels of the hormone or hormones produced by the affected endocrine organ or organs. Autoantibodies to the affected gland may be found.

(4) **Therapy.** CMCC can be treated in several ways, depending on the severity of the condition.

(a) The milder forms of CMCC do well with symptomatic treatment and hormone replacement therapy, if endocrinopathy is present.

(b) The more severe forms are treated with intensive antifungal therapy, any of several immunologic enhancement maneuvers (e.g., transfer factor injections, thymus extracts, and fetal thymus or bone marrow transplantation), and hormone replacement, when appropriate. None of the immunologic enhancement procedures has had lasting success in a significant number of patients, although some therapeutic success has been claimed for each. Patients with severe CMCC seldom survive past the third decade due to severe pulmonary disease.

(5) **Complications** of CMCC include severe psychological disturbances, which are seen in more severely afflicted patients and may be due to the chronic and sometimes disfiguring nature of the disease.

7. **Acquired immune deficiency syndrome (AIDS)** is a newly described immune disorder, which apparently did not exist in developed nations until the late 1970s. Currently, AIDS is defined by clinical criteria, as no specific serologic or immunologic markers have been identified. For a complete discussion of AIDS, see Chapter 8, section VI D 4.

D. **Phagocyte disorders.** This section considers primarily disorders of **polymorphonuclear leukocytes (neutrophils)**, as these are the most common. Since mononuclear phagocytes are the cells that initiate immune reactions, disorders of these cells might cause disruption of cellular as well as humoral immunity. However, disorders of mononuclear phagocytes are seldom seen.

1. **General considerations.** The following is a general discussion of the features that are common to most neutrophil disorders. More specific information concerning individual disorders follows (see section I D 2–4).

a. Clinical features. Neutrophil disorders cause patients to be vulnerable to infection by a variety of organisms; however, the following emerge as the most commonly isolated pathogens in these syndromes: *Staphylococcus aureus, Escherichia coli, Streptococcus pneumoniae, Pseudomonas aeruginosa,* and *C. albicans.* The infections vary in location and severity.

b. Diagnosis of neutrophil disorders is based on studies that evaluate the number or function of circulating neutrophils or their precursors in bone marrow.

   (1) In **neutropenias**, a circulating neutrophil count below 2000/mm³ is indicative of a deficiency.

   (2) Chemotactic defects are diagnosed by evaluating the ability of neutrophils to migrate toward a chemotactic stimulus.

   (3) Microbicidal disorders are diagnosed by evaluating the ability of neutrophils to kill microorganisms or to reduce dye through chemical changes that reflect the generation of bactericidal products.

c. Therapy. In general, neutrophil disorders are treated symptomatically, with antimicrobial therapy for the infections that accompany them.

   (1) Continuous antimicrobial therapy, usually with trimethoprim-sulfamethoxazole, may be helpful in some situations, such as chronic granulomatous disease.

   (2) Leukocyte or neutrophil transfusions from normal donors have been used successfully in life-threatening infections.

   (3) Bone marrow transplantation is a reasonable consideration in the most severe phagocyte disorders. Since these patients have otherwise normal immune function, bone marrow transplantation must be preceded by immunosuppressive therapy. For this reason, transplantation is attempted only when other therapy is not feasible.

2. Neutropenia (see also Chapter 3 section III B 3 b) is an absolute decrease in the number of circulating neutrophils. In rare cases, this disorder is inherited. Most often, neutropenia occurs secondary to exposure to agents that are directly toxic to neutrophils or that decrease neutrophil production by the bone marrow. The danger of infection increases with the severity and duration of the neutropenia. When the number of circulating neutrophils is less than 500/mm³, the patient is in great danger of severe infection.

a. Hereditary neutropenia occurs in several forms, which vary widely in severity. The following are examples.

   (1) Infantile genetic agranulocytosis

      (a) Etiology. This rare, life-threatening disorder is believed to be inherited as an autosomal recessive trait. Although the precise defect is not known, the disorder involves maturation arrest of myeloid cells in the bone marrow.

      (b) Clinical features. Infantile genetic agranulocytosis is characterized by severe neutropenia and recurring infections in very young patients. Fulminating infection may ensue.

      (c) Diagnosis. The diagnosis is established in an infant who demonstrates neutropenia in the absence of antineutrophil antibodies. Bone marrow examination reveals decreased neutrophil precursors beyond the myelocyte stage.

      (d) Therapy (see section I D 1 c)

   (2) Cyclic neutropenia

      (a) Etiology. This rare, autosomal recessive disorder is characterized by episodes of neutropenia recurring every 15–35 days, between which neutrophil levels return to normal. Although the exact cause is uncertain, the periodic nature of the neutropenia suggests a recurring insult to, or inhibition of, the bone marrow.

      (b) Clinical features. Cyclic neutropenia is accompanied by a compensatory increase in circulating monocytes. The infections in this condition are less severe than those occurring in infantile genetic agranulocytosis, with manifestations limited to fever, malaise, and aphthous stomatitis.

      (c) Diagnosis. The diagnosis is made on the basis of the characteristic clinical presentation. The patients occasionally demonstrate antineutrophil antibodies. The bone marrow shows normal numbers of neutrophil precursors.

      (d) Therapy (see section I D 1 c)

b. Secondary neutropenia

   (1) Etiology. Secondary neutropenia usually has an apparent etiology and often can be predicted. For example, immunosuppressive agents (e.g., cyclophosphamide) are known to be toxic to the bone marrow. Also, autoimmune phenomena related to collagen vascular diseases may result in reduced numbers of circulating neutrophils (e.g., Felty's syndrome in rheumatoid arthritis).

   (2) Clinical features. Secondary neutropenia may be severe and in rare cases is fatal due to the development of fulminating infection.

(3) Diagnosis. This disorder should be suspected in patients using high-risk drugs and in those with coexisting conditions known to be associated with neutropenia.

(4) Therapy (see section I D 1 c)

3. Chemotactic defects and adherence disorders include lazy leukocyte syndrome, neutrophil actin dysfunction, and deficiency of the cell membrane glycoproteins, LFA-1 and Mac-1.

a. Lazy leukocyte syndrome

(1) Etiology and pathogenesis. This disorder is believed to be due to neutrophils having abnormal receptors for chemotactic factors, resulting in the inability of neutrophils to respond to chemotactic stimuli. Thus, mature neutrophils collect in the marrow, unresponsive to signals summoning them to the periphery.

(2) Clinical features. Lazy leukocyte syndrome is associated with recurrent pyogenic infections of the respiratory tract and gingivitis.

(3) Diagnosis is based on finding neutropenia and defective leukotaxis in a patient who demonstrates mature neutrophils in the bone marrow.

(4) Therapy (see section I D 1 c)

b. Neutrophil actin dysfunction

(1) Etiology and pathogenesis. This structural (polymerization) abnormality of the protein, actin, is inherited as an autosomal recessive condition. Because neutrophils require actin for movement and phagocytosis, these activities are abnormal.

(2) Clinical features. Neutrophil actin dysfunction has led to fatal pulmonary infection.

(3) Diagnosis is based on demonstration of defective neutrophil phagocytosis and locomotion accompanied by a paucity of microtubules and microfilaments on electron microscopy of the neutrophils.

(4) Therapy (see section I D 1 c)

c. LFA-1 and Mac-1 deficiency

(1) Etiology and pathogenesis. Without the cell membrane glycoproteins, LFA-1 and Mac-1, the neutrophil is unable to move and adhere properly. This impairs neutrophil function and leads to a susceptibility to infection. This is an inherited defect with variable inheritance patterns.

(2) Clinical features are the same as for lazy leukocyte syndrome [see section I D 3 a (2)].

(3) Diagnosis is based on the demonstration of defective neutrophil adherence in the absence of the cell membrane glycoproteins, LFA-1 and Mac-1. The commercially available monoclonal antibody, OKM1, detects this antigen.

(4) Therapy (see section I D 1 c)

4. Microbicidal disorders result in susceptibility to infection by the organisms described above (see section I D 1 a) as well as others. Affected individuals show very poor resistance, and once established, infections often progress despite appropriate antibiotic therapy. Two well-characterized microbicidal disorders of neutrophils are chronic granulomatous disease and Chédiak-Higashi syndrome.

a. Chronic granulomatous disease is a group of disorders characterized by an inability of neutrophils and macrophages to kill organisms after ingesting them.

(1) Etiology and pathogenesis. Chronic granulomatous disease is the result of an inherited deficiency of one of the cellular enzymes involved in phagocyte oxidative metabolism. Deficiencies of glucose-6-phosphate dehydrogenase, glutathione peroxidase, and NADPH oxidase have been described. These result in deficient production of oxidation products, including hydrogen peroxide, hydroxyl radicals, and superoxide anions, which the cell needs to kill ingested organisms. Both X-linked and autosomal inheritance patterns have been described.

(2) Clinical features include lymphadenopathy, hepatosplenomegaly, pneumonia, and multiple abscess formation.

(3) Diagnosis. The diagnosis of chronic granulomatous disease is easily made using the **nitroblue tetrazolium dye (NBT) test**. Failure of neutrophils and monocytes to change the dye color from its usual yellow to blue is diagnostic of chronic granulomatous disease. The dye conversion reflects the generation of respiratory burst products, including hydrogen peroxide and others, which fail to be generated in this disorder.

(4) Therapy (see section I D 1 c)

b. Chédiak-Higashi syndrome is a disorder characterized by neutrophils with abnormally large granules.

(1) Etiology and pathogenesis. Chédiak-Higashi syndrome is inherited as an autosomal recessive condition. The genetic defect is thought to involve an abnormal function of cellular microtubules, which precludes normal fusion of cytoplasmic lysosomes to the vacuole containing the ingested microorganism.

(2) Clinical features include lymphadenopathy, hepatosplenomegaly, pneumonia, and recurrent infections. In addition, there are characteristic physical abnormalities such as partial oculocutaneous albinism and rotatory nystagmus.

(3) **Diagnosis** of Chédiak-Higashi syndrome is based on finding the above-mentioned physical anomalies in a patient with extremely large, characteristic granules in the peripheral blood neutrophils. Bacterial killing is abnormal, and, because of their large granules, neutrophils have impaired movement.

(4) **Therapy** (see section I D 1 c)

E. Complement system defects

1. **Complement component deficiencies** have been described for each of the nine complement components. The clinical manifestations of these deficiencies vary depending on which component is lacking.

   a. **Etiology.** All complement component deficiencies are inherited as autosomal recessive traits. The nature of the genetic defect is not known.

   b. **Clinical features.** Complement component deficiencies show two general patterns.
      (1) Deficiencies of the activation proteins of the classical pathway—that is, C1 (q, r, and s), C4, and C2—most often are associated with autoimmune phenomena. A lupus-like syndrome is common.
      (2) In contrast, deficiencies of the proteins of the membrane attack unit—that is, C5, C6, C7, and C9—seem to predispose to systemic infections, especially by *Neisseria* species. Gonococci and meningococci both cause recurrent disseminated disease.

   c. **Diagnosis.** Several techniques may be used for the diagnosis of complement component deficiencies.
      (1) Immunochemical assays such as radial immunodiffusion and immunoelectrophoresis are available for complement components.
      (2) Functional assays, measuring hemolysis, also may be used, in which all but the complement component being measured are added to a red cell/anti-red cell antibody system. The serum to be tested then is added. The ability of serum to complete the reaction and produce hemolysis is a reflection of the presence and functional integrity of the complement component being measured.

   d. **Therapy.** Complement component deficiencies are treated symptomatically. Infections are treated with appropriate antimicrobial agents, and autoimmune phenomena are treated as indicated.

   e. **Complications.** Complement component deficiencies generally are not complicated by other than their basic presenting clinical abnormality.

2. **Deficiencies of regulatory proteins** of the complement system have been described in two instances—C1 esterase inhibitor deficiency and C3b inactivator deficiency—both of which are inherited.

   a. **C1 esterase inhibitor deficiency** (see also sections IV D 7 a and IV E 7 a)
      (1) **Etiology.** This disorder is inherited as an autosomal dominant trait. The nature of the genetic defect is unknown.
      (2) **Clinical features.** Deficiency of C1 esterase inhibitor produces recurrent attacks of hereditary angioedema of the skin and upper respiratory tract.
      (3) **Diagnosis.** Both quantitative and functional assays are available for the diagnosis of C1 esterase inhibitor deficiency.
      (4) **Therapy.** C1 esterase inhibitor deficiency is treated with attenuated androgens. The most widely used agents are danazol and stanozolol, which generally restore the inhibitory protein to normal levels in almost all patients. Infusion of normal plasma probably does more harm than good in these patients by supplying C1 substrate and, thus, fuel for the reaction.
      (5) **Complications.** The angioedema may result in life-threatening obstruction of the upper airways.

   b. **C3b inactivator deficiency**
      (1) **Etiology.** This disorder is inherited as an autosomal recessive trait. The nature of the genetic defect is unknown.
      (2) **Clinical features.** Deficiency of C3b inactivator predisposes to recurrent staphylococcal infections by depletion of C3 through unchecked consumption.
      (3) **Diagnosis.** The absence of C3b inhibitor usually is demonstrated by radial immunodiffusion, although a functional (hemagglutination) assay also is available.
      (4) **Therapy** is symptomatic treatment of accompanying infections.

II. MECHANISMS OF IMMUNE REACTIONS.
Gell and Coombs classified immune reactions (also called **hypersensitivity reactions**) into four distinct types: immediate hypersensitivity (type I) reactions, cytotoxic (type II) reactions, immune complex–mediated (type III) reactions, and delayed hypersensitivity (type IV) reactions.

A. Immediate hypersensitivity reactions

1. **Definition.** Immediate hypersensitivity reactions occur when an antigen binds to preformed, cell-bound IgE molecules, causing the release of mediators. The interaction between the antigen and IgE antibody may be explained by the **bridging hypothesis**. IgE molecules bind to IgE receptors on the membranes of mediator cells (mast cells or basophils). An antigen binds to one IgE molecule and then to a second, creating a bridge between the molecules. Cross-linking requires that an antigen be divalent or multivalent.

2. **Mechanism**
   a. **Antigen.** An antigen is a substance that stimulates an immune response when it is appropriately presented to the immune system. Not all antigens stimulate an IgE response; antigens that induce an IgE response in allergic individuals usually are innocuous to non-allergic individuals. Antigens are more **immunogenic** (i.e., effective in stimulating an immune response) if first processed by macrophages. Antigens are classified as **complete antigens** or **haptens**.
      (1) **Complete antigens** can independently induce an IgE response. These antigens are composed primarily of protein constituents with many cross-links and have molecular weights ranging from 10,000 to 70,000 daltons. Relatively larger molecules appear to be more immunogenic, but those with molecular weights greater than 70,000 daltons have difficulty penetrating mucosal surfaces of the respiratory and digestive systems.
      (2) **Haptens** elicit an immune response only when combined with tissue- or serum-derived carrier proteins. Haptens are partial antigens and, alone, are unable to stimulate macrophages, T cells, or B cells. Many drugs act as haptens and induce IgE responses in the hapten-carrier state.
   b. **IgE antibody**, or **reagin**, is known to induce immediate hypersensitivity. (In some animal species, including humans, IgG antibody also may be pivotal in the immediate hypersensitivity response.)
      (1) **Chemical properties.** IgE is a glycoprotein that contains 12% carbohydrate. Its molecular weight is 190,000, sedimentation constant is 8S, and electrophoretic mobility is measured in the gamma region. Similar to other immunoglobulins, IgE is composed of two light and two heavy chains.
      (2) **IgE production** occurs in B cells in the spleen and in lymphoid tissues of the tonsils and adenoids as well as in the bronchi, peritoneum, and respiratory and intestinal mucosa.
         (a) **Regulation** of IgE production is not well understood but involves cooperation between B cells and IgE-specific helper T cells and suppressor T cells.
         (b) **Ontogeny.** IgE antibody production begins in the fetus by 11 weeks gestation. (Unlike IgG, IgE does not cross the placenta.) IgE levels peak by age 10–15 years and then decline to the normal range.
      (3) **Function.** Although IgE antibody is integral to the immediate hypersensitivity response, it is not essential for the maintenance of health. Individuals with low IgE levels do not have more frequent infections, but higher IgE levels may be protective against helminthic infections. IgE antibody also may be important to the general inflammatory process by activating cells with subsequent mediator release when appropriate. A survival advantage of IgE is suggested by the fact that 25% of the general population has clinically significant allergic disease mediated by IgE antibodies.
      (4) **Sensitization**
         (a) **Respiratory system.** Airborne allergens may be 2–60 μm in size. Aerosolized particles up to 5 μm in size penetrate the airways beyond terminal bronchioles, but most pollens are larger and do not pass below the carina. Direct sensitization after contact with nasal mucous membranes occurs, but the effect of larger pollens on airways below the carina would appear to be indirect.
         (b) **Gastrointestinal system.** Sensitization through the gastrointestinal tract also is indirect because there is relative impermeability to macromolecules; some antigens also may be altered by digestive enzymes.
   c. **Mediator cells** have IgE receptors and release mediators when sensitized by IgE molecules.
      (1) **Mast cells**—the primary effectors of immediate hypersensitivity—are of variable size and shape, contain metachromatic granules, and are located around arterioles and venules in subcutaneous and submucosal tissues. Up to 500,000 IgE molecules may exist on the surface of one mast cell.
      (2) **Basophils** circulate in the blood and are found in some inflammatory infiltrates. Their metachromatic granules are larger than those of mast cells and also contain heparin and histamine in a protein-mucopolysaccharide matrix.
   d. **Mediators** are classified either as preformed and prepackaged in secretory granules or as newly formed constituents released after initiation of the immediate hypersensitivity reaction. The release of mediators is dependent on the influx of extracellular calcium and is initiated by the cross-bridging of two IgE molecules on the surface of the mediator cell.

(1) Preformed mediators are responsible for the early and late manifestations of immediate hypersensitivity reactions.

    (a) Histamine acts at two distinct tissue receptor sites, H_1 and H_2, causing smooth muscle contraction and increased vascular permeability. H_1 receptors are blocked by compounds such as **chlorpheniramine**. H_2 receptors mediate gastric acid secretion as well as chronotropic and inotropic effects on the heart; H_2 receptors are blocked by compounds such as **cimetidine**. Histamine also regulates microvascular circulation, which promotes tissue growth and repair.

    (b) Eosinophil chemotactic factors of anaphylaxis (ECF-A) are tetrapeptides that attract eosinophils. These substances probably function in hypersensitivity reactions as negative feedback controls by attracting eosinophils, which then metabolize other mediators.

    (c) Neutrophil chemotactic factor (NCF) preferentially attracts neutrophils; its significance is speculative, however, since neutrophils are not prominent in immediate hypersensitivity reactions.

    (d) Serotonin is stored in preformed granules in platelets and is released under the influence of **platelet activating factor (PAF)**. Serotonin may induce bronchoconstriction and is known to cause increased capillary permeability. Its role in the immediate hypersensitivity reaction, however, is uncertain. Serotonin appears to function primarily as a neurotransmitter.

    (e) Other mediators

        (i) Heparin is responsible for the metachromatic staining property of the granules of mast cells and basophils, but its biologic function in immediate hypersensitivity reactions is uncertain.

        (ii) The role of other preformed constituents, such as granuloproteins, also is unknown.

(2) Newly formed mediators are formed after initiation of the immediate hypersensitivity response but are released relatively early in the inflammatory process.

    (a) Slow-reacting substance of anaphylaxis (SRS-A) is derived from arachidonic acid and is a mixture of leukotrienes. Immediately after the onset of an antigen-antibody reaction, histamine is higher in concentration than SRS-A, but within minutes this is reversed. Like histamine, SRS-A has potent smooth muscle contracting properties. In animal models, SRS-A also stimulates release of thromboxane, which is thought to amplify the SRS-A response. Histamine and SRS-A may act synergistically on certain smooth muscles, but SRS-A is not inhibited by antihistamines. **Epinephrine** is capable of modifying smooth muscle contraction caused by SRS-A.

    (b) PAF promotes platelet aggregation and release of mediators, particularly serotonin. Although PAF causes smooth muscle contraction in animal models and stimulates human neutrophil responses in vitro, its importance in immediate hypersensitivity reactions is uncertain.

    (c) Kinins are generated by Hageman factor, kininogen, and prekallikrein. **Bradykinin**, a nonapeptide, is the principal biologically active derivative of the kinin pathway; its actions include smooth muscle contraction, increased vascular permeability, and dilation of peripheral blood vessels, which may lead to hypotension. The importance of bradykinin in the immediate hypersensitivity reaction is uncertain.

    (d) Prostaglandins, thromboxanes, and leukotrienes are derived from arachidonic acid, which is liberated by phospholipases from cell membrane phospholipids. All of the substances have many diverse pharmacologic actions, including smooth muscle contraction, increased permeability and dilation of capillaries, and increased pain threshold. Their importance in immediate hypersensitivity reactions is under investigation.

3. Clinical features of immediate hypersensitivity reactions include the signs and symptoms of allergic rhinitis (see section III D) and of urticaria and angioedema (see sections IV A and IV B). **IgE-mediated anaphylaxis** caused by antibiotics (e.g., penicillin), foreign proteins, foods, and therapeutic agents typifies an immediate hypersensitivity reaction, although anaphylaxis also may be caused by an immune complex–mediated reaction, as in the case of a blood transfusion–associated reaction. Various organ systems may be involved within seconds to minutes after introduction of the causative agent.

    a. Skin. Erythema, pruritus, urticaria, and angioedema may occur.

    b. Respiratory system. Rhinorrhea, laryngeal edema, and lower airway obstruction may occur and progress to asphyxia. Hoarseness, dysphonia, and chest tightness also may be experienced.

    c. Gastrointestinal tract. Nausea, vomiting, diarrhea, and fecal urgency or incontinence may develop.

    d. Cardiovascular system. Hypotension (causing lightheadedness or syncope) and vascular collapse (manifesting as shock) may be primary events or may be related to respiratory obstruction and asphyxia.

4. **Diagnosis** of immediate hypersensitivity reactions can be made by a complete history, physical examination, and appropriate investigations (see sections III E and IV E).

    a. The diagnosis of anaphylaxis usually is not difficult to make because of the striking clinical manifestations. Seizures, dysrhythmias, vasovagal reactions, and hereditary angioedema may have similar presentations.

    b. **Immediate skin reactions** are the most sensitive diagnostic procedures for identifying the antigens causing IgE-mediated reactions.

       (1) **Technique**

           (a) **Puncture.** A drop of antigen is placed on the skin, and the skin then is punctured through the drop with a 26–27 G needle. The epidermis is penetrated, but blood should not appear.

           (b) **Intradermal.** Enough antigen to raise a 3-mm wheal (approximately 0.02 ml) is injected intradermally, bevel up.

       (2) **Time of appearance and resolution.** This reaction begins almost immediately and completely resolves usually within 60–90 minutes.

       (3) **Physical appearance.** Arteriolar dilatation leads to an erythematous flare surrounding a centrally located, relatively soft wheal (localized hive) where the antigen has been applied. This wheal often is raised more than 1 mm above the skin surface.

       (4) **Pathogenesis.** Interaction between an allergen and mast cell–bound IgE antibodies leads to mediator release, increased capillary permeability, and accumulation of tissue fluid (visible wheal).

5. **Therapy**

    a. **Transient symptoms**, mild wheezing, and evanescent pruritus can be treated with oral or parenteral antihistamines, with or without subcutaneous epinephrine. Close monitoring is advisable.

    b. **Systemic manifestations** and more intense symptoms (e.g., airway obstruction and hypotension) require acute care.

       (1) **Delay of absorption of the allergen eliciting anaphylaxis** is important if anaphylaxis is due to an insect sting or an injection of antibiotic or allergy extract. Delay of absorption can be achieved by administration of subcutaneous epinephrine at the site of the injection and by applying a tourniquet between the heart and the site of the injection.

       (2) **Enhancement of oxygenation** can be achieved by administration of subcutaneous epinephrine in a contralateral appendage, supplemental oxygen, a nebulized β-sympathomimetic (e.g., isoproterenol), or aminophylline and by intubation, if necessary.

       (3) **Reversal of hypotension** may require the administration of isotonic saline or a colloidal solution, an α-agonist (e.g., *l*-norepinephrine acid tartrate), dopamine, and corticosteroids.

B. **Cytotoxic reactions**

1. **Definition.** Cytotoxic reactions occur when either IgG or IgM molecules bind to cell-bound antigen, which leads to complement activation, membrane attack, and subsequent cell cytolysis. Examples of cytotoxic antibody-mediated reactions include **Rh-hemolytic disease of the newborn** and **drug-induced Coombs-positive hemolytic anemia**. Penicillin-induced hemolytic anemia is an example of the latter and is used here as a model of cytotoxic reactions.

2. **Mechanism.** In penicillin-induced hemolytic anemia, the red blood cells of patients treated with penicillin become coated with penicilloyl and, possibly, penaldoyl metabolites. The metabolite–red cell complexes can stimulate formation of high-titer IgG antibodies. These antibodies may bind to the metabolite–red cell complex and result in extravascular hemolysis due to erythrophagocytosis in the reticuloendothelial system.

3. **Clinical features.** Patients who develop penicillin-induced hemolytic anemia usually have been treated with high-dose penicillin therapy (over 10 million units of penicillin per day). A rapid drop in hematocrit signals hemolysis, which is associated with reticulocytosis. (Cephalosporins and cisplatin also have been implicated in drug-induced Coombs-positive hemolytic anemias.)

4. **Diagnosis.** A strong positive direct but negative indirect Coombs antiglobulin reaction can be demonstrated in approximately 3% of patients treated with high-dose penicillin therapy, but hemolysis develops in only a few patients. The diagnosis is established by the presence of extravascular hemolysis and reticulocytosis. There is no evidence of intravascular hemolysis, as erythrophagocytosis occurs in the reticuloendothelial system.

5. **Therapy** for cytotoxic reactions includes treating the underlying cause of the reaction as well

as the ensuing symptoms of such a reaction. In the case of penicillin-induced hemolytic anemia, discontinuing the causative agent, penicillin, is the most prudent measure. Red blood cell transfusions may be indicated. The treatment of other examples of cytotoxic reactions, such as Rh-hemolytic disease of the newborn, must emphasize prevention of such reactions.

C. Immune complex–mediated reactions

1. **Definition.** Immune complex–mediated reactions occur when immune (antigen-antibody) complexes deposit in tissues or on endothelial surfaces, which leads to complement activation and further tissue injury. **Serum sickness** is the classic example of an immune complex–mediated reaction. The most common cause of serum sickness was heterologous serum but is now penicillin.

2. **Mechanism**
   a. **Antigen.** Immune complexes are formed in the presence of intravascular antigen and antibody. The concentration and duration of exposure of the antigen are important factors that determine the quantity and chronicity of complex formation. Antigens may be exogenous or autogenous.
      (1) **Exogenous antigens** include drugs (penicillin), hormones (insulin), vaccines (tetanus), and infectious agents (hepatitis B). Infectious agents can replicate and cause chronic immune complex formation.
      (2) **Autogenous antigens** include tumors as well as altered immunoglobulin (rheumatoid factor), nuclear (DNA), and cytologic (thyroglobulin) matter. Autogenous antigens are a source of chronic immune complex formation.
   b. **Antibody.** Immune complexes have a greater tendency to activate complement and cause tissue injury if a proper relationship exists between the concentration of antigen and antibody. Small complexes do not activate complement, and large complexes are cleared rapidly from the intravascular space. The quantity of the antibody response is an important determinant of the size of the complex formed. The type of antibody produced also is important, as antibodies differ in their ability to activate complement and to bind to antigen.
   c. **Complement activation.** The complement system is activated by intravascular complexes containing a single IgM or two adjacent IgG molecules. The complement system modifies the immune response by causing increased local vascular permeability, attraction of neutrophils, accumulation of monocytes, release of leukocytes, and phagocytosis. In addition, **membrane attack complexes** are formed, which result in irreversible membrane damage and osmotic lysis.

3. **Clinical features.** Filtering membranes are affected by immune complex–mediated reactions. Necrotic and fibrinoid lesions in arteries and cellular destruction of postcapillary venules are seen. Signs of immune complex–mediated reactions and serum sickness include palpable purpura, arthritis, urticaria, serositis, vasculitis, urinary abnormalities, lymphadenopathy, and peripheral neuropathy (see section V D 1 b)
   a. Renal glomeruli are most commonly affected. Findings include decreased glomerular filtration, proteinuria, and increased urinary sediment.
   b. Turbulent blood flow through areas of arterial bifurcations predispose to necrotizing arteritis.
   c. The choroid plexus is a filter for the cerebrospinal fluid (CSF) and, therefore, is a common location of immune complex deposition.
   d. Membranes of peripheral blood cells may be affected by immune complex reactions. Thrombocytopenia, anemia, and leukopenia may develop.
   e. Immune complex formation occurs in selective IgA deficiency and malignancies without the expected findings of tissue destruction.

4. **Diagnosis** of immune complex–mediated reactions ideally can be made by identifying the causal antigen and antibody. However, this usually is difficult, and other methods must be employed.
   a. **Serologic assays**
      (1) Cryoprecipitates, which are antigen-antibody complexes that become insoluble and precipitate after incubation at 4° C, may be detected in type III reactions.
      (2) Complement assays may demonstrate decreased levels of C3, C4, or **total hemolytic complement** (CH_{50}). Decreases in other complement components also may be seen.
      (3) Circulating immune complexes also can be demonstrated by other specialized techniques involving cell receptors and antiglobulins.
   b. **Biopsy** of affected tissues can be studied by routine histologic, electron-microscopic, or immunohistochemical methods.
   c. **The Arthus reaction** is an immune complex–mediated reaction due to excessive antibody production and can be elicited by a skin test.

    (1) **Technique.** An appropriate amount of the antigen (usually 0.1 ml) is injected intradermally, bevel up.

    (2) **Time of appearance and resolution.** This reaction develops within 2–4 hours after challenge, maximally intensifies by 6–12 hours, and then gradually subsides over the next few hours.

    (3) **Physical appearance.** Nonpruritic, diffuse swelling develops at the challenge site. The lesion is erythematous and sometimes petechial. If particularly severe, skin necrosis may evolve with subsequent fibrosis.

    (4) **Relevance.** If diphtheria toxoid is administered intradermally, an Arthus reaction will develop when circulating levels of antitoxin antibodies are high. Skin tests with suspected antigens in hypersensitivity pneumonitis also will result in an Arthus reaction when specific circulating antibodies are present.

5. Therapy

  a. Elimination of the causal antigen is the most effective method of treatment. This is possible for immune complex–mediated reactions that occur with pneumococcal pneumonia and infective endocarditis but is not feasible in hepatitis B virus–induced chronic hepatitis.

  b. Pharmacologic management is aimed at minimizing vascular localization as well as the formation and consequences of immune complexes.

    (1) **Antihistamines** reduce vascular permeability and may be clinically effective. The combined use of H_1- and H_2-receptor blocking agents may have a greater potential for reducing vascular permeability.

    (2) **Anti-inflammatory agents**, both steroidal and nonsteroidal, effectively treat common symptoms of immune complex disease. Neutrophil migration is inhibited by glucocorticoids.

    (3) **Cytotoxic drugs**, such as azathioprine and cyclosporine, have been effective in life-threatening immune complex disease.

    (4) **Plasmapheresis** removes circulating immune complexes and also has been effective.

D. Delayed hypersensitivity reactions

1. Definition. Delayed hypersensitivity reactions are T-cell dependent reactions manifesting as inflammation at the site of antigen exposure. Reactions usually peak 24–48 hours after exposure to the eliciting antigen.

2. Mechanism. T cells are triggered by specific antigens to produce soluble products called **lymphokines**.

  a. Lymphokines stimulate the proliferation of lymphocytes and the aggregation and activation of macrophages, and they inhibit the migration of macrophages and neutrophils.

  b. The action of lymphokines results in an infiltration of recruited cells, which primarily are activated and stimulated **monocytes**. Other cells found in delayed hypersensitivity reactions include **neutrophils** and **basophils**, the latter of which may accumulate due to the production of specific lymphokines.

3. Clinical features. Delayed hypersensitivity reactions can occur in response to antigen exposure on skin (e.g., contact dermatitis). Delayed hypersensitivity reactions also occur in response to tumors as well as viral, bacterial, fungal, and parasitic infections. Rashes, tissue necrosis, and microbial phagocytosis may ensue. The prototypical delayed hypersensitivity reaction is the tuberculin skin test reaction.

4. Diagnosis is aided considerably by the **delayed skin reactivity test**.

  a. Technique. An appropriate amount of antigen (0.1 ml) is injected intradermally, bevel up.

  b. Time of appearance and resolution. This reaction appears 24–36 hours after application of the antigen, reaches maximal reactivity 24 hours later, and recedes over the next 24–48 hours.

  c. Physical appearance. There is nonpitting, localized, relatively hard and nonpruritic induration. Induration more than 4 mm in diameter is considered positive. If this reaction is excessive, localized ulcerations may occur with possible scar formation.

  d. Relevance. Since delayed reactivity is the expected response to many diverse antigens (i.e., many viruses, all fungi, and some bacteria), lack of reactivity to these antigens suggests an immunodeficient state. When some low molecular weight chemicals interact with skin proteins, haptens may be formed, which then provoke delayed hypersensitivity skin reactions in certain sensitive individuals.

5. Therapy

  a. Corticosteroids decrease the inflammatory response by redistributing lymphocytes to the bone marrow or intravascular space. Corticosteroids also affect macrophage migration and decrease the density of epidermal Langerhans cells, which are important in processing topically applied antigens.

    b. Cytotoxic drugs augment delayed hypersensitivity responses by limiting the activity of suppressor T cells.

    c. Anticoagulant drugs, such as heparin, can suppress delayed hypersensitivity reactions in animals by a mechanism that is unclear. The clinical potential of this relationship has not been defined.

III. ALLERGIC RHINITIS

A. Definition. This symptom complex is characterized by nasal blockage, rhinorrhea, sneezing, and pruritus and is caused by the release of mast cell mediator secondary to repeated antigen exposure. There are two major classifications of allergic rhinitis.

    1. Seasonal allergic rhinitis has periodic symptoms that occur only during the pollinating season of the antigen to which the patient is sensitive.

    2. Perennial allergic rhinitis has continuous or intermittent symptoms that occur year-round.

B. Incidence. Although accurate estimates are difficult to obtain, it is believed that 15%–20% of adults have allergic rhinitis. In one survey of college students in Rhode Island, 26% had symptoms of allergic rhinitis. There is no apparent male or female predilection for allergic rhinitis, and no ethnic or racial patterns have been identified. Symptoms may begin at any age but develop in most patients before age 20. A history of allergic disorders in the immediate family is very common.

C. Etiology. Various aeroallergens (e.g., spores, pollens, and organic dusts) are responsible for symptoms of allergic rhinitis.

    1. Common characteristics of aeroallergens
        a. Aeroallergens usually are less than 50 μ in size.
        b. The allergens are lightweight and, therefore, are easily windborne. (Heavier, insect-borne pollens do not cause allergic rhinitis.)
        c. The allergens are released into the environment in very large numbers.
        d. The allergenic constituents usually are proteins with molecular weights of 10,000–40,000 daltons.
        e. Seasonal patterns for each pollen are consistent from year to year, but quantities of pollen vary depending on environmental conditions.

    2. Specific seasonal allergens
        a. Ragweed pollen is the most significant cause of allergic rhinitis in the midwestern and eastern United States. Its season usually runs from late summer to early fall (mid-August to early October).
        b. Tree pollens elicit symptoms in early spring; **grass pollens** are the major offenders in late spring and early summer. Since roses are fully blooming in late spring, sensitivity to grass pollen often is mistaken as "rose fever." In the southeast and southwest regions of the United States, however, grass pollinates from early spring to late fall and may lead to nearly perennial symptoms.
        c. Mold spores initially appear in the air in early spring, reach peak levels in July and August, and subside after the first frost. In the United States, the clinically most important spores are *Alternaria* and *Cladosporium*. The highest mold-spore counts are registered when a windy period follows a few days of rainy and damp weather.

    3. Specific perennial allergens
        a. House dust has many diverse constituents, but the common house mite is considered one of the primary antigenic components.
        b. Epidermal antigens are produced primarily by pets such as cats, dogs, and rabbits.
        c. Indoor molds (i.e., spores found in homes) are most commonly *Aspergillus* and *Penicillium*.
        d. Nonspecific irritants, which probably are not true allergens, include cigarette smoke, air pollution, perfumes, cooking odors, and chemical fumes.
        e. Occupational allergens include materials such as platinum salts, wood dust, and laundry detergent enzymes, which are known to produce both allergic rhinitis and asthma in association with IgE antibodies.

D. Clinical features

    1. Characteristic symptoms
        a. Sneezing is characteristic, often with paroxysms of 15–20 sneezes in quick succession, which are likely to occur in the early morning hours.

    b. Pruritus of the nose, palate, and pharynx is common and may lead to the "allergic salute" (i.e., repeated pushing up on the end of the nose, usually by a child).

    c. A thin, watery nasal discharge usually is present and is associated with varying amounts of nasal obstruction and postnasal drainage.

    d. Excess lacrimation and ocular pruritus and soreness commonly occur.

    e. Loss of olfaction and taste may result from chronic severe nasal congestion.

    f. Headache or earache may ensue if eustachian tube and paranasal sinus drainage is significantly impaired. This condition can lead to the development of otitis media or sinusitis.

  2. Characteristic physical findings usually are seen during the height of the offending pollen season or at the time of maximal exposure to other antigens.

    a. The nasal cavity characteristically contains thin nasal secretions, and the mucosal surface is edematous, boggy, and usually pale or bluish in color. Mouth breathing is common.

    b. Nasal polyps can be seen but are not common, and their presence should suggest cystic fibrosis in children and aspirin intolerance in adults.

    c. Conjunctival findings include injection and swelling, excess lacrimation, granularity, and occasionally chemosis. Infraorbital shiners (infraorbital congestion) may develop.

    d. Continual rubbing of the nose frequently produces a transverse crease across the lower third of the nose.

    e. Severe chronic nasal congestion in children sometimes leads to a broadened nose and narrowed palatal arch.

E. Diagnosis

  1. Laboratory findings

    a. Accurately applied **skin tests** with potent and appropriate antigens are the best diagnostic procedures to identify the antigens causing IgE-mediated allergic rhinitis.

    b. The **radioallergosorbent test (RAST)** is reserved for patients with extensive eczematoid dermatitis, significant dermatographism, or a complicated history without corroborative skin tests.

    c. An increased IgE level supports the diagnosis, but total IgE levels are increased in only 30%–40% of patients with allergic rhinitis. Therefore, the clinician must consider the multiple other causes of elevated IgE levels.

    d. Peripheral eosinophilia may be seen but is a very inconsistent finding in patients with allergic rhinitis.

    e. A stained smear of nasal secretions at the time of clinically active disease often shows a higher number of eosinophils, but this finding also may be seen in eosinophilic nonallergic rhinitis, hyperplastic sinusitis, and in normal infants less than 6 months of age.

    f. In selected patients with negative skin tests and RAST studies, conjunctival and nasal mucosal challenges may be helpful.

  2. Differential diagnosis

    a. Nasal congestion with mild rhinorrhea sometimes is seen in **pregnancy** and in patients with **hypothyroidism**.

    b. Decongestant nasal spray abuse, birth control pills, and such medications as propranolol, clonidine, and reserpine commonly are associated with nasal blockage.

    c. Vasomotor rhinitis is a syndrome characterized by nasal blockage and rhinorrhea without evidence of immunologic nasal disease. Exacerbations are caused by changes in body or environmental temperatures, relatively high humidity, emotional stress, chemical fumes, tobacco smoke, and alteration of body position. Response to medical therapy often is poor.

    d. Symptoms of **eosinophilic nonallergic rhinitis** are similar to those of vasomotor rhinitis; however, in the former condition, nasal eosinophilia is present, nasal polyps are common, and symptoms usually respond to medical management.

    e. Infectious rhinitis occurs more often in patients with underlying allergic rhinitis and usually is associated with reddened nasal mucosa, thick nasal secretions, sore throat, cervical adenopathy, and low-grade fever.

    f. A symptom complex known as the **aspirin triad** consists of nasal polyps, chronic sinus disease, and asthma, with exacerbation of symptoms after administration of aspirin or other nonsteroidal anti-inflammatory agents.

    g. Anatomic abnormalities may cause nasal obstructive symptoms and should be recognized on nasal examination. The most common of such abnormalities is a partially deviated septum.

F. Therapy. Management is stepwise and involves avoidance of any offending allergens and provocative substances, administration of selective pharmacologic agents, and, in some instances, initiation of immunotherapy.

1. **Avoidance.** This aspect of management is most successful when a single antigen (e.g., an antigen in animal dander) is responsible for symptoms. In patients with multiple sensitivities, however, sensible, environmental precautions are recommended and appear to limit severe exacerbations.

2. **Pharmacologic agents**
   a. **Antihistamines** are useful in controlling rhinorrhea and pruritus. Many different agents are available, and because of marked individual variation in efficacy and production of side effects, the clinician should be familiar with one or two preparations from the three major classes of antihistamines. If a drug from one class is ineffective, it is unlikely that another one from that same class will be better; therefore, it is best to choose a preparation from another class.
      (1) **Ethanolamines** (e.g., diphenhydramine) are effective but often produce significant sedation and atropine-like side effects.
      (2) **Ethylenediamines** (e.g., pyrilamine) also are effective; these antihistamines produce less sedation than ethanolamines and minimal gastrointestinal side effects.
      (3) **Alkylamines** (e.g., chlorpheniramine) are effective and produce minimal sedation.
   b. **Sympathomimetic medications**
      (1) **Oral** administration of α-adrenergic agents (e.g., phenylpropanolamine and pseudoephedrine) is effective in reducing nasal congestion but not rhinorrhea. CNS stimulation may occur, but this effect often is negated when adrenergic agents are used in combination with an antihistamine.
      (2) **Topical** application of short-acting phenylephrine or long-acting oxymetazoline decreases nasal congestion, but regular administration for more than 3–4 days results in severe rebound nasal congestion (medicamentous rhinitis).
   c. **Cromolyn sodium.** A 4% solution of cromolyn sodium now is available in the United States for topical nasal use. This medication requires frequent administration but has been shown to benefit both seasonal and perennial allergic rhinitis. The use of cromolyn sodium is now preferred to corticosteroid treatment.
   d. **Corticosteroids**
      (1) **Systemic** corticosteroids significantly improve symptoms during the height of a specific pollen season. This treatment is rarely indicated, however, and use of long-term oral corticosteroid therapy for perennial allergic rhinitis is contraindicated.
      (2) **Topical.** New, highly effective and rapidly metabolized topical steroid preparations (e.g., beclomethasone dipropionate and flunisolide acetate) are quite beneficial in seasonal and perennial allergic rhinitis. These agents also are useful during withdrawal of topical sympathomimetic drugs in patients with severe medicamentous rhinitis. These newer preparations have fewer corticosteroid-induced side effects than systemic agents, and localized atrophy of the nasal mucosa has not been identified with their long-term use. Continued use of the topical steroids, however, is not recommended; these medicines should not be administered continuously for more than 3 weeks.

3. **Immunotherapy.** Clinically significant symptoms may persist after environmental avoidance measures have been instituted and appropriate medications have been taken. In such patients, a trial of immunotherapy with those antigens to which the patient cannot regularly avoid is indicated. Recently performed double-blind studies have clearly demonstrated the efficacy of this management technique, with patients experiencing significant improvement after 1 year of therapy. The treatment program, however, is time-consuming and in most patients does not provide complete relief.

IV. URTICARIA AND ANGIOEDEMA may occur simultaneously or separately as manifestations of immediate hypersensitivity reactions. The two conditions have similar etiologies, pathophysiologic processes, and clinical characteristics and, for this reason, are considered together in this chapter. Because **urticaria** is seen more commonly (with or without angioedema), it is the term used here to refer to either or both conditions. Distinctions have been made where it is important to do so.

A. **Definition and description.** Episodes of urticaria that persist less than 6 weeks are termed **acute**; those lasting longer than 6 weeks are considered **chronic**.

1. **Urticaria** (also called **hives**) is a well-circumscribed, migratory, and often pruritic cutaneous eruption, which may occur on any area of the body. Individual lesions (called **wheals**) seldom last longer than 24–48 hours.
   a. **Gross examination.** The lesions usually are multiple and occasionally coalesce, and they

vary in size from a few millimeters to several centimeters. Typically, the wheals have serpiginous borders and centers that blanch with pressure.

   b. **Microscopic examination** reveals engorgement and dilation of small venules, capillaries, and lymphatics in the superficial dermis; widening of the dermal papillae; flattening of the rete pegs; swelling of collagen fibers; and the presence of a minimal perivascular infiltrate consisting predominantly of mononuclear cells occasionally accompanied by eosinophils.

   c. **Papular urticaria** describes urticaria-like lesions most often seen on the extremities and exposed areas of children as a result of bites from insects such as bedbugs, fleas, and mites. These lesions are more persistent than ordinary hives.

2. **Angioedema.** Similar pathophysiologic changes are seen with angioedema but are confined to the deeper dermis and subcutaneous tissue, where there are fewer sensory nerve endings. Angioedema, therefore, usually is not pruritic. It presents as colorless areas of well-demarcated, nonpitting edema.

B. **Epidemiology**

1. **Acute urticaria** is relatively common and experienced at least once by 10%–20% of the population, appearing more often in atopic individuals.

2. **Chronic urticaria** has no predilection for atopic individuals and occurs more often in females. The peak incidence is between the third and fourth decades; however, chronic urticaria has been reported in children as young as 1 month of age. Children are more likely than adults to have chronic urticaria without angioedema, and the median duration of lesions is shorter in children than in adults.

C. **Pathogenesis.** Urticaria and angioedema result from a number of mechanisms, with the final common pathway involving the mediators of immediate hypersensitivity. The physiologic changes seen in urticaria mimic the **triple response of Lewis**, with:

1. **Erythema** due to capillary dilatation

2. **Flare**, or secondary erythema, due to arteriolar dilatation mediated by axon reflexes

3. **Wheal**, or edema, caused by extravasation of fluid with increased vascular permeability

D. **Clinical syndromes according to etiology.** Several environmental factors, iatrogenic agents, and diseases are associated with urticaria.

1. **Drug sensitivity** is very common, with lesions induced by mechanisms such as IgE antibody activity, direct release of histamine, or inhibition of prostaglandin synthesis. Further details of drug allergy are discussed in section V.

   a. **Histamine release.** A variety of agents cause direct cell degranulation, including:

      (1) Radiographic contrast media

      (2) Narcotic analgesics (meperidine and the chemically dissimilar opiates, codeine and morphine)

      (3) Antimicrobial agents (chlortetracycline, polymyxin, quinine, and stilbamidine)

      (4) Muscle relaxants (curare)

      (5) Vasoactive drugs (atropine, amphetamine, and hydralazine)

      (6) Miscellaneous agents (bile salts, thiamine, dextran, and deferoxamine)

   b. **Inhibition of prostaglandin synthesis.** Acetylsalicylic acid (aspirin) and other nonsteroidal anti-inflammatory agents inhibit cyclo-oxygenase in vitro and may cause urticaria. From 20%–50% of adults with chronic urticaria are aspirin intolerant; children with chronic urticaria are less likely to be sensitive to aspirin. Symptoms occur from minutes to hours after aspirin ingestion and may persist for weeks. Aspirin may aggravate urticaria that is due to other causes.

2. **Food sensitivity.** Acute urticaria is more common in atopic than in nonatopic individuals.

   a. **Food antigens**—particularly those derived from eggs, milk, nuts, fish, and shellfish—more frequently affect younger individuals. Certain food antigens cause direct histamine release.

   b. **Food dyes**—especially the azo dye **tartrazine** (yellow dye number 5)—induce lesions through an unspecified mechanism. Approximately 15% of aspirin-sensitive individuals also are sensitive to tartrazine.

   c. **Food additives** such as benzoates and sulfites also cause urticaria through an unspecified mechanism. Antibiotics added in the food chain can induce lesions through an immediate hypersensitivity response.

   d. **Natural salicylates** are found in trace amounts in blueberries, bananas, green peas, and licorice but do not appear to cause urticaria even in aspirin-sensitive individuals.

   e. **Mold-containing foods** such as brewer's yeast, baker's yeast, cheeses, alcoholic beverages, and mold-contaminated (spoiled) foods do not seem to cause urticaria even in individuals who are sensitive to inhaled mold spores.

3. **Seasonal or perennial inhalant allergens** occasionally cause hives, which invariably are also associated with respiratory tract symptoms.

4. **Infections** caused by bacterial, fungal, helminthic, and, particularly, viral agents also are implicated as causes of urticaria. Urticaria, which is presumably due to complement activation by immune complexes, may precede infection-related symptoms, particularly in infectious mononucleosis and viral hepatitis. Focal bacterial infection such as dental abscess, sinusitis, and urinary tract infections often are considered when patients with chronic urticaria are evaluated.

5. **Insect sensitivity.** Stings by the Hymenoptera species may result in acute urticaria, which sometimes is associated with anaphylaxis. Caterpillar-induced direct histamine release (**contact sensitization**) may cause acute urticaria, and exposure to fleas and mites may cause papular urticaria.

6. **Physical agents** (i.e., environmental, mechanical, thermal, and solar factors) reproducibly induce urticaria in susceptible individuals. Physical urticaria sometimes may be transferred via a **Prausnitz-Küstner reaction**, although specific sensitizing IgE-mediated antigens have not been identified. Elevated plasma histamine levels have been documented in patients with physical urticaria.
   a. **Dermatographism** is a wheal and flare reaction induced by firm stroking of the skin. Up to 5% of the population has this condition, which may present immediately or 6–8 hours after the skin is stroked. Dermatographism may exacerbate chronic urticaria that is due to other causes.
   b. **Heat urticaria** may be localized or generalized.
      (1) **Localized heat urticaria** is extremely rare and occurs when a warm stimulus contacts the skin.
      (2) **Generalized heat urticaria**, or **cholinergic urticaria**, is associated with factors that involve cholinergic nerve fibers, such as emotional stress, sweating, exercise, and a hot shower. Characteristic lesions are 2- to 3-mm wheals surrounded by a prominent erythematous flare.
   c. **Cold urticaria** is induced by exposure to a cold stimulus and may be generalized or limited to only exposed areas. Symptoms often are maximal upon warming. Acquired, inherited, and cholinergic forms exist.
      (1) **Acquired cold urticaria** may occur transiently in association with drugs (e.g., griseofulvin) or infections (e.g., infectious mononucleosis). Acquired cold urticaria also is associated with cryoglobulinemia, cryofibrinogenemia, and cold hemagglutinin disease.
      (2) **Familial cold urticaria** is a rare autosomal dominant condition characterized by burning papular lesions accompanied by chills, arthralgia, myalgia, and headache, which occur approximately 30 minutes after exposure to a cold stimulus.
      (3) **Cold-induced cholinergic urticaria** is a very rare syndrome characterized by small punctate wheals, which result from exposure to a cold environment. These lesions are indistinguishable from generalized heat urticaria.
   d. **Aquagenic urticaria** is a rare disorder characterized by small perifollicular wheals, which develop after contact with water of any temperature.
   e. **Solar urticaria** occurs within minutes after brief exposure to sunlight and lasts for a few hours. Systemic symptoms may occur with prolonged exposure. Six types have been identified, based primarily on the different wavelengths that induce the lesions. Patients with **erythropoietic protoporphyria** develop urticaria at wavelengths of 4000 Å because of a genetic deficiency of the mitochondrial enzyme, **ferrochelatase** (heme synthetase), which inserts the iron into protoporphyrin IX to form heme.
   f. **Exercise-induced urticaria** may occur in a heterogeneous group of patients, which may include those with other forms of physical urticaria. Typically, exercise precipitates characteristic cutaneous lesions, sometimes with the development of bronchospasm and hypotension (**exercise-induced anaphylaxis**).
   g. **Pressure urticaria** typically presents within minutes to several hours after pressure is applied to the skin. The lesions of pressure urticaria may be painful.
   h. **Vibratory angioedema** is a rare disorder characterized by occasionally severe pruritus and angioedema that occur within minutes after exposure to a vibratory stimulus. An autosomal dominant inheritance pattern has been identified.

7. **Hereditary diseases.** All hereditary forms of urticaria and angioedema are rare. In addition to the three hereditary disorders described in section IV D 6 c, e, h, there are three important hereditary diseases associated with urticaria or angioedema.

   a. Hereditary angioedema is the most common hereditary disease in this category.
      (1) Etiology and pathogenesis. Hereditary angioedema is an autosomal dominant disorder characterized by a deficiency of the C1 esterase inhibitor, which leads to measurable levels of C1. Consequently, C4—a substrate of C1—is excessively consumed, causing diminished serum levels of C4 even when the patient is free of symptoms. C4 levels are undetectable during an attack. C2—another substrate of C1—usually is not diminished when the patient is asymptomatic but is decreased during an attack.
      (2) Clinical features. Hereditary angioedema is characterized by recurrent attacks of cutaneous and mucosal edema without urticaria or pruritus. Cutaneous swelling occurs most often on the face and extremities. Mucosal edema may involve the larynx and result in airway obstruction, which is the most common cause of death in this disease. Gastrointestinal tract involvement may result in intense abdominal pain simulating a surgical abdomen. Traumatic (triggering) episodes only sometimes are evident prior to the onset of symptoms.
   b. Heredofamilial urticaria (Muckle-Wells syndrome) is a progressive disorder, which is inherited as an autosomal dominant trait and is characterized by amyloidosis, nerve deafness, limb pain, fever, nephrosis, and hyperglycinuria.
   c. C3b inactivator deficiency is a very rare, autosomal recessive disorder characterized by spontaneous activation of the alternative complement pathway, histaminuria, and nonpruritic urticaria (see section I E 2 b).

8. **Neoplasms**
   a. Urticaria occasionally occurs in patients with neoplasms, although the association may be coincidental. Malignancies of the colon, rectum, and lung as well as leukemia and lymphoma have been seen most often.
   b. Malignancies and angioedema have been reported with an acquired deficiency of C1 esterase inhibitor.

9. **Hormone disorders.** Urticaria has been associated with hyperthyroidism, parathyroid lesions, and hypercalcemia. Chronic urticaria may be worse during menstruation, and cyclic urticaria may occur coincidentally with menstruation. There is little evidence to support autosensitization to endogenous hormones.

10. **Connective tissue diseases.** Urticaria has been associated with various connective tissue diseases, including SLE, Sjögren's syndrome, polymyositis, and leukocytoclastic vasculitis. Urticaria also is seen in serum sickness. In these diseases, lesions may be secondary to activation of complement by immune complexes.

11. **Psychogenic causes.** Emotional stress may exacerbate urticaria that is associated with other specific causes. In addition, psychological factors are thought to play a role in certain patients when other causes have not been identified.

12. **Miscellaneous causes.** Urticaria has been associated with some unusual causes, such as direct contact with an electric current and the presence of implanted materials (e.g., tantalum staples). Urticaria also is seen in **urticaria pigmentosa** and **systemic mastocytosis**.
   a. Urticaria pigmentosa is caused by the proliferation of mast cells in the skin. This cutaneous disorder typically occurs in childhood and is characterized by hyperpigmented (tan) lesions that urticate after the skin is stroked (**Darier sign**).
   b. Systemic mastocytosis is considered to be a generalized form of urticaria pigmentosa. Mast cell infiltrates are present in various organ systems and release histamine, resulting in flushing, headache, and, occasionally, hypotension.

13. **Idiopathic urticaria.** A specific etiology is identified in only 15%–20% of patients with chronic urticaria. In the remaining majority of patients, atopy is not characteristic and IgE levels are normal. Mild dermatographism may be present, and mast cell liability is thought to be a feature due to the elevated total skin levels of histamine in these patients.

E. **Diagnosis.** A careful history and physical examination may eliminate the need for extensive laboratory evaluations and may reveal an obvious cause of acute urticaria. Establishing the etiology of chronic lesions usually is more difficult and may require a complete blood count and erythrocyte sedimentation rate assessment as well as urinalysis. The following are recommended evaluations for specific types of urticaria and angioedema.

1. **Drug sensitivity.** Resolution of urticaria after elimination of suspected medication is helpful but may be only coincidental and not diagnostic. Reliable skin tests are not available for most drugs; however, skin tests and challenges for some drugs are described in section V E.

2. **Food sensitivity.** As with drugs, resolution of lesions with elimination of suspected foods may be coincidental and not diagnostic. Percutaneous food skin tests and double-blind food or food additive challenges may be diagnostic.

3. **Inhalant allergens.** Evaluation for inhalant sensitivity is discussed in section III D 1.

4. **Infections.** Evaluations include cultures and radiography guided by clinical circumstances.

5. **Insect sensitivity.** Skin tests for specific insect venoms are reliable and preferred over specific in vitro tests (e.g., RAST).

6. **Physical agents**
   a. **Dermatographism** is present if the skin urticates after firm stroking.
   b. **Heat urticaria**
      (1) Localized heat urticaria is suspected if the skin urticates after coming in contact with a warm stimulus.
      (2) Patients with generalized heat urticaria develop localized urticaria within 20 minutes after an intradermal injection of 0.05 ml of 0.02% methacholine chloride. This skin test may not be positive during the refractory period immediately after an episode of generalized heat urticaria. A controlled exercise challenge also may precipitate generalized heat urticaria.
   c. **Cold urticaria**
      (1) Cold urticaria is diagnosed by placing an ice cube on the patient's forearm for 4 minutes and observing that, within the next 10 minutes, pruritus and a hive in the shape of the ice cube develop. Positive cold hemagglutinins and elevated levels of cryoglobulins and cryofibrinogens also may be present.
      (2) Patients with cold-induced cholinergic urticaria do not respond to the ice cube test but develop generalized hives after exercise in a cold environment.
   d. **Aquagenic urticaria** is diagnosed by the development of urticaria in response to local application of tap water at various temperatures.
   e. **Solar urticaria** can be diagnosed by controlled challenge with different wavelengths of light. Erythropoietic protoporphyria is characterized by normal excretion of urinary porphyrin as well as elevated red cell protoporphyrin and fecal protoporphyrin and coproporphyrin levels.
   f. **Exercise-induced urticaria** is diagnosed by exercise challenge. Caution must be taken, however, because bronchospasm or hypotension may develop.
   g. **Pressure urticaria** is assessed by application of pressure followed by observation for up to 24 hours.
   h. **Vibratory angioedema** is diagnosed by gently vibrating a patient's forearm with a laboratory vortex for 4 minutes.

7. **Hereditary diseases**
   a. Hereditary angioedema is diagnosed most easily by decreased levels of C4 and correspondingly low levels of CH_{50}, an absence of C1 esterase inhibitor, and diminished levels of C2 during attacks. Normal levels of C1 esterase inhibitor are present in patients with deficient function of this protein. A functional assay is available to identify these patients.
   b. C3b inactivator deficiency is diagnosed by low levels of inactive C3 by-products.

8. **Neoplasms** associated with acquired C1 esterase inhibitor deficiency show low levels of C1 esterase inhibitor, C4, and—unlike hereditary angioedema—decreased C1q levels.

9. **Hormone disorders** that cause urticaria are assessed by clinically appropriate assays, such as serum thyroxine or parathyroid hormone (PTH) levels.

10. **Connective tissue diseases** are identified by skin biopsy with immunofluorescence and by assessment of:
    a. Rheumatoid factor
    b. Erythrocyte sedimentation rate
    c. Immunoglobulin levels
    d. Complement (CH_{50}, C3, and C4)
    e. Autoantibody status

11. **Psychogenic causes** of urticaria are not easily identified. No characteristic personality profile exists for these patients.

12. **Miscellaneous causes.** Urticaria pigmentosa and systemic mastocytosis are diagnosed by characteristic collections of mast cells on tissue biopsy.

13. **Idiopathic urticaria** is diagnosed in the absence of known causes.

F. **Therapy**

   1. **Elimination of etiologic factor.** All precautions must be taken to eliminate any possible underlying cause of the urticaria, such as a drug or food, an inhalant, or a physical agent. In

addition, any underlying illnesses, such as an infection, a neoplasm, or a hormone or connective tissue disease, should be treated appropriately.

2. Antihistamines. Initial therapy for urticaria and angioedema includes an H_1-receptor blocker, particularly hydroxyzine. If more than a single agent is necessary, improvement may occur with addition of a second H_1-receptor blocker of a different class, an adrenergic agent, or an H_2-receptor blocker such as cimetidine or ranitidine.

3. Corticosteroids. If oral corticosteroids are needed (only for severe and recalcitrant urticaria), an every-other-day regimen is suggested with tapering as rapidly as possible. Topical corticosteroids are not useful.

4. Recommendations for specific types of urticaria and angioedema
   a. Cold urticaria generally responds to an H_1-receptor blocker, but cyproheptadine may be more useful and usually renders the ice cube test negative.
   b. Solar urticaria is treated with avoidance of sunlight, protective garments, and topical preparations that absorb or reflect light. Preparations containing zinc oxide and titanium oxide screen out the visible spectrum.
   c. Pressure urticaria usually is unresponsive to most antihistamines, and low doses of corticosteroids may be needed.
   d. Vibratory angioedema often responds to diphenhydramine.
   e. Hereditary angioedema attacks may be prevented by the use of attenuated androgens, such as danazol, stanozolol, or oxymetholone. Acute attacks are treated with subcutaneous epinephrine and analgesics. Acquired C1 esterase inhibitor deficiency may also be treated with attenuated androgens.

V. DRUG ALLERGY

A. Definition. Drug allergy is a hypersensitivity response that occurs in a susceptible individual due to the production of specific antibodies or sensitized lymphocytes directed against the drug or its metabolites. Reactions usually occur after a latency period of several days. It is important to differentiate drug allergy from other adverse reactions, which may or may not be drug related.

1. Drug-related reactions
   a. Drug overdose may cause adverse reactions as a result of excessive drug concentrations (e.g., seizures due to supratherapeutic serum levels of theophylline).
   b. Drug side effects are undesirable but unavoidable reactions not associated with excessive drug concentrations (e.g., tremulousness induced by metaproterenol).
   c. Teratogenic drug effects are developmental defects in a fetus caused by drugs taken by the mother during pregnancy (e.g., facial deformities associated with hydantoin).
   d. Secondary drug effects are consequences of a drug's primary pharmacologic activity (e.g., the release of microbial antigens, endotoxins, or both during treatment of syphilis with penicillin).
   e. Drug interaction occurs when one drug changes the action of another drug by altering its metabolism, absorption, or binding (e.g., sedation induced by the simultaneous ingestion of tranquilizers and alcohol).
   f. Drug intolerance occurs when a small dose of a drug causes a characteristic but heightened pharmacologic effect (e.g., intoxication due to ingestion of a minimal amount of alcohol).
   g. Drug idiosyncracy is a qualitatively abnormal response to a drug, which is distinctly different from its pharmacologic action (e.g., hemolysis due to primaquine administration in a patient with glucose-6-phosphate dehydrogenase deficiency).

2. Reactions unrelated to drugs
   a. Psychogenic reactions are caused by vasovagal responses or anxiety (e.g., extreme diaphoresis with injections).
   b. Other symptoms are caused by the underlying disease and not by the administered drug (e.g., a coincidental viral skin eruption may occur in a patient treated with antibiotics).

B. Incidence. Less than 10% of all drug reactions are believed to be allergic in nature. The incidence of drug allergy depends primarily on the administered drug. Some commonly used drugs are associated with reaction rates exceeding 2%, including ampicillin and other semisynthetic penicillins, trimethoprim-sulfamethoxazole, corticotropin, and erythromycin. However, the overall incidence of drug allergy is less than 1% per drug course. Among hospitalized patients, the risk of death due to an allergic reaction to penicillin is 1 in 50,000.

C. Etiology and pathogenesis. Most drugs have molecular weights of less than 1000 and, therefore, are incomplete antigens. However, a native drug or any of its metabolites may covalently bind to a high molecular weight carrier (usually a protein) to produce an allergic reaction. The moiety bound to the carrier—called a **hapten**—usually is a drug metabolite. This hapten-carrier complex can elicit an allergic reaction by any of four immune mechanisms of tissue injury described in section II. In some instances, more than one of these mechanisms may be involved.

D. Clinical features. Allergic drug reactions may be multisystemic or organ specific.

1. Multisystemic drug reactions

  a. Systemic anaphylaxis may occur immediately after oral or parenteral administration of a drug and is characterized by palpitations, urticaria, angioedema, respiratory distress, and seizures. Hypotension, coma, and death occur less commonly. Agents that cause anaphylactic or anaphylactoid reactions include antimicrobials, radiocontrast media, allergenic extracts, vaccines, chymopapain, and insulin.

  b. Serum sickness may occur from a few hours to 3 weeks after drug administration and is characterized by urticaria, angioedema, arthralgia, and low-grade fever. Lymphadenopathy, peripheral neuropathy, and glomerulonephritis are seen less commonly. Recovery is virtually complete after discontinuation of the drug, but some clinical manifestations may linger for days or weeks. Fever rarely persists beyond 48 hours.

  c. Drug-induced SLE resembles spontaneous SLE and is thought to be mediated by an immune complex (type III) mechanism. Malaise, fever, serositis, and pleuritic pain are frequent occurrences; renal, hepatic, and cutaneous findings are less common. The incidence of drug-induced SLE is dose related and commonly is seen with procainamide and hydralazine. Symptoms usually subside within 1 week after discontinuation of the causative drug, although serum antinuclear antibody level may remain elevated for months.

  d. Vasculitis of the skin and other organs may occur as a manifestation of drug allergy. **Leukocytoclastic vasculitis** refers to a characteristic histologic picture of leukocyte nuclei destruction, particularly in small vessels such as postcapillary venules. Systemic symptoms include fever, malaise, edema, arthritis, headache, and glomerulonephritis. Characteristic palpable purpuric lesions often are seen on the lower extremities. Urticaria and erythema multiforme also may be present. Vasculitis occasionally continues after the offending drug has been discontinued.

  e. Fever may be the only manifestation of drug allergy. Drugs also may produce fever through nonallergic mechanisms (e.g., as occurs with amphetamine intoxication) or through adverse drug reactions that lead to hemolysis and hepatitis. Fever may begin 7–10 days after starting a medication if there was no prior drug sensitization. Ancillary findings of drug-induced fever usually are milder than would be expected from the observed temperature. Drug-induced fever remits rapidly upon discontinuation of the causative drug.

2. Organ-specific drug reactions may involve the skin, blood elements, lungs, liver, or kidneys.

  a. Skin eruptions are the most common manifestations of drug allergy.

   (1) A **maculopapular or morbilliform rash** is seen most commonly, with or without pruritus.

   (2) Contact dermatitis occurs after topical therapy with a sensitizing agent and appears erythematous, indurated, and vesicular. Symptoms usually improve within 48 hours after the offending agent has been discontinued.

   (3) Photosensitivity reactions may be phototoxic or photoallergic.

    (a) Phototoxic reactions resemble sunburn and are not immunologically mediated. They occur on first contact with the causative agent after exposure to sunlight. The causative drug absorbs and concentrates energy in the skin, leading to this erythematous response.

    (b) Photoallergic reactions resemble eczematoid dermatitis, require prior exposure, and are immunologically mediated. A possible mechanism is that ultraviolet energy stimulates hapten-carrier conjugation, which results in tissue injury.

   (4) Fixed eruptions are edematous, well-circumscribed, pigmented lesions that reappear at the same location whenever the implicated drug is readministered. Pruritus is unusual, and there are no systemic symptoms. Lesions may be single or multiple and several centimeters in diameter, and they may remain pigmented long after the drug has been discontinued.

   (5) Exfoliative dermatitis is a potentially fatal reaction characterized by a diffuse, erythematous, scaly eruption that may lead to massive desquamation. Exfoliative dermatitis may be associated with systemic symptoms and may lead to secondary infections. The pathogenesis is unclear.

   (6) Urticaria and angioedema may occur alone or as part of a serum sickness reaction. Drug-induced angioedema often involves the face and periorbital region. Lesions may appear within hours or days after initiation of almost any drug therapy and usually sub-side within days after cessation of such therapy.

(7) **Toxic epidermal necrolysis** (also called **Lyell's disease**) appears as generalized erythema that progresses to bullae and desquamation. Fluid loss, secondary infection, severe morbidity, and death may occur. The most frequently implicated drugs include sulfonamides, penicillins, antiepileptic drugs, allopurinol, phenylbutazone, and phe-nolphthalein.

(8) **Erythema multiforme** is characterized by macular, papular, urticarial, or purpuric lesions that may progress to vesicles and bullae involving the skin and mucous membranes (a condition called **Stevens-Johnson syndrome**). Fever and malaise are common. In rare cases, pulmonary infiltrates and renal involvement may lead to death. Sulfonamides, penicillins, and phenytoin are commonly implicated in erythema multiforme.

(9) **Erythema nodosum** usually appears on the lower extremities as bilateral, subcutaneous, erythematous nodules that are warm and tender. Mild systemic symptoms also are noted. The lesions resolve completely after discontinuation of the causative drug. Implicated drugs include oral contraceptives, penicillins, sulfonamides, bromides, and iodides.

b. **Hematologic reactions** may involve all cell lines.

(1) **Eosinophilia** is a frequent finding during therapy with drugs such as cephalosporins, erythromycin, penicillins, sulfonamides, tetracyclines, digitalis, and phenothiazines and occasionally is the only manifestation of drug allergy. Eosinophilia may be a harbinger of more significant allergic reactions.

(2) **Anemia.** Most cases of drug-induced anemia are unexplained. One theory is that antigen-antibody complexes are absorbed into the red cell membrane, with subsequent activation of complement leading to hemolysis. Alternatively, a drug or its metabolite may be incorporated into the red cell membrane and function as a hapten; subsequent antibody formation then may result in hemolysis. All patients treated with penicillin demonstrate red blood cells coated with covalently bound penicillin metabolites, but few demonstrate a positive Coombs test and develop hemolysis. Drug-induced autoimmune hemolytic anemia is rare.

(3) **Granulocytopenia** may be induced by either immune or toxic reactions.

(a) **Immunologically mediated agranulocytosis** usually has an explosive onset associated with chills, fever, malaise, and a skin rash. Symptoms start after a latency period during treatment, but after recovery there may be an abrupt recurrence following administration of only a minute dose. Aminopyrine has been implicated in this process, with the identification of **leukoagglutinins**.

(b) **Toxic depression of granulopoiesis** usually is not associated with systemic hypersensitivity and has a less abrupt onset with a slower recurrence. No leukoagglutinins have been identified.

(4) **Thrombocytopenia** usually is caused by IgG antibody–drug complexes that affix to platelets and lead to complement activation. Acute hemorrhagic episodes are possible in sensitized individuals and may be preceded by fever and chills. Prompt improvement is expected after discontinuation of the drug.

(5) **Bone marrow aplasia** is due to either a pharmacologic effect (in the case of alkylating agents or antimetabolites) or an idiosyncratic reaction (in the case of chloramphenicol). Immune mechanisms have not been implicated in the development of bone marrow aplasia.

c. **Pulmonary reactions** that may be attributed to drugs include bronchial asthma and pulmonary infiltration.

(1) **Asthma**, as a manifestation of an IgE-mediated reaction to a drug, usually is accompanied by other signs or symptoms of anaphylaxis. Inhaled drugs such as pituitary snuff, acetylcysteine and cromolyn sodium may produce bronchospasm without other systemic effects. Aspirin may induce bronchospasm in susceptible individuals, most likely by inhibiting prostaglandin synthesis.

(2) **Pulmonary infiltrates** are characterized by acute or chronic symptoms of fever, cough, dyspnea, pleural effusion, hilar adenopathy, and, occasionally, bronchospasm. Physical findings usually are limited to coarse bilateral basilar rales. Peripheral eosinophilia also may be noted. Chest x-ray demonstrates either diffuse alveolar or focal migratory infiltrates. Implicated drugs include nitrofurantoin and cromolyn sodium, the latter of which has been shown to stimulate production of **migration inhibition factor** from lymphocytes in vitro.

d. **Hepatic reactions** include cholestasis and hepatocellular changes. There is little immunologic evidence to support hypersensitivity as the cause, but these reactions often are associated with other signs of allergy.

(1) Cholestasis, often preceded by eosinophilia, may be seen after administration of erythromycin estolate, phenothiazines, and troleandomycin. Resolution of cholestasis is expected after the provocative agent has been discontinued.

(2) Hepatocellular changes often are accompanied by fever, skin rashes, and eosinophilia. Halothane may produce potentially fatal hepatitis in sensitized individuals. Chronic active hepatitis and severe hepatic necrosis may occur with various drugs, but most patients with hepatocellular damage completely recover after the causative agent has been eliminated.

  e. Renal complications of drug allergy may be related to systemic vasculitis, but interstitial nephritis is the most typical allergic reaction. Fever, skin rashes, and eosinophilia occur; a type II reaction also is seen, with antitubular basement membrane antibody, IgG, and complement deposition in a linear pattern along the renal tubular basement membrane. Phenytoin, sulfonamides, and, more commonly, methicillin have been implicated in this reaction, which usually resolves after termination of therapy. Interstitial nephritis occasionally is fatal.

E. Diagnosis. Drug allergy may be substantiated by clinical criteria, skin tests, in vitro tests, or provocative challenges.

  1. Clinical criteria. A representative drug reaction occurs after a 7- to 10-day latency period, presenting as symptoms that do not resemble the pharmacologic action of the drug. Allergic reactions occur more frequently with intermittent and repetitive high-dose parenteral drug administration but also may be elicited by minute doses. If allergic symptoms subside after the suspected drug has been discontinued, drug allergy is suggested.

  2. Skin tests

    a. Immediate skin tests are useful for the diagnosis of IgE-mediated reactions, but false-positive wheal-flare reactions may be seen with drugs that cause the direct release of histamine from mast cells, such as atropine and the opiates (see section IV D 1 a). Simultaneous testing of controls also may be required because false-positive results may be seen with concentrated compounds. Drugs that show positive immediate skin tests at reasonable concentrations include penicillin, insulin, cephalosporins, chymopapain, succinylcholine chloride, and cisplatin.

    b. Delayed skin tests (patch technique) are valuable for the diagnosis of contact sensitivity to topical medications but not for suspected parenterally or orally administered medications.

  3. In vitro tests are limited because most drugs are not immunogenic and produce reactions only after forming a hapten-carrier complex. However, antibody formation and cellular immunity can be assessed.

    a. Antibody formation is assessed by measuring total serum antibody levels or specific IgE levels, which may rise during a drug reaction. Antibodies also can be detected against specific hematopoietic cells. Hemagglutinating IgE and IgM drug-specific antibodies can be measured in drug-induced serum sickness, and antitubular basement membrane antibodies can be detected in drug-induced interstitial nephritis.

    b. Cellular immunity can be demonstrated by measuring drug-dependent lymphocyte proliferation and lymphokine production (usually done only in a research laboratory).

  4. Provocative challenges—employing small initial oral, parenteral, or inhalational doses followed by an incremental increase—have been designed for penicillin, aspirin, nonsteroidal anti-inflammatory drugs, tartrazine, sulfites, and local anesthetics. Provocative challenges may cause severe anaphylaxis and must be performed under controlled conditions with extreme caution. Provocative challenges also may induce desensitization.

F. Therapy

  1. Avoidance measures involve preventing drug administration either prior to or after sensitization has occurred. If a drug reaction occurs during the administration of multiple medications, all suspicious drugs should be discontinued if possible. If a systemic reaction occurs after subcutaneous or intramuscular administration, absorption may be inhibited by application of a tourniquet proximal to the injection site and by subcutaneous administration of epinephrine at the injection site.

  2. Pharmacologic management

    a. Symptomatic management of drug reactions may range from the treatment of pruritus with antihistamines to the treatment of hypotension with α-adrenergic agonists. Oxygen, aminophylline, corticosteroids, fluid management, intubation, and mechanical ventilation may be required for severe anaphylactic reactions.

  b. Prophylactic management of drug reactions using combinations of H_1 and H_2 blockers, ephedrine, and corticosteroids has been described. The risk of another anaphylactoid reaction to repeat administration of radiocontrast media is reduced by pretreatment with 50 mg of prednisone 13 hours, 7 hours, and 1 hour before the procedure and with 50 mg of diphenhydramine and 25 mg of ephedrine 1 hour prior to the procedure.

3. Desensitization is indicated if no alternative therapy is available. Treatment is started at very low doses, and allergic symptoms are treated as necessary. Successful desensitization regimens have been described for penicillin and insulin, but extreme caution is required as fatalities have been reported.

  a. Penicillin desensitization may be performed by the intravenous or oral route.

  b. Insulin desensitization may be necessary, even after switching to a less reactive or more purified insulin. The causative agents in insulin-induced reactions may be noninsulin proteins or nonproteins such as protamine or zinc. Allergy to human insulin also has been reported. Skin tests show that pork insulin usually is less immunogenic than beef insulin. If a patient is evaluated within 48 hours after a systemic reaction, desensitization without skin tests may be started with the original agent. If insulin therapy has been interrupted for longer than 48 hours, skin tests are helpful followed by a more cautious desensitization program using the least reactive agent.

STUDY QUESTIONS

Directions: Each question below contains five suggested answers. Choose the **one best** response to each question.

1. Cyproheptadine is specifically effective treatment for which of the following types of urticaria?

(A) Generalized heat (cholinergic) urticaria
(B) Cold urticaria
(C) Solar urticaria
(D) Exercise-induced urticaria
(E) None of the above

2. Antibody deficiency syndromes are diagnosed by

(A) in vitro lymphocyte stimulation of immunoglobulin synthesis
(B) delayed skin reactivity tests
(C) skin allograft rejection time
(D) clinical criteria alone
(E) quantitative immunoglobulin assay and in vivo stimulation

3. What is the treatment of choice for the antibody deficiency syndromes?

(A) Bone marrow transplantation
(B) Injection of commercial gamma globulin preparations
(C) Transplantation of a fetal thymus gland
(D) Continuous prophylactic antibiotics
(E) Reverse isolation of the patient

4. Complement component deficiencies involving the components C1, C4, and C2 are most often characterized by

(A) a tendency to develop graft-versus-host disease if viable leukocytes are infused
(B) gram-negative bacterial infections
(C) lupus-like syndromes
(D) recurrent acute viral infections
(E) recurrent gram-positive bacterial infections

5. Deficiencies of the complement components C5–C9 are most often characterized by

(A) severe allergic manifestations
(B) recurrent infections by *Neisseria* species
(C) autoimmune diseases
(D) a high incidence of malignancies
(E) an association with antibody deficiency syndromes

6. Which of the following conditions is treated effectively with danazol?

(A) Solar urticaria
(B) Cold urticaria
(C) Hereditary angioedema
(D) Generalized heat (cholinergic) urticaria
(E) None of the above

Directions: Each question below contains four suggested answers of which **one or more** is correct. Choose the answer

A if **1, 2, and 3** are correct
B if **1 and 3** are correct
C if **2 and 4** are correct
D if **4** is correct
E if **1, 2, 3, and 4** are correct

7. Frequent complications of the antibody deficiency syndromes include

(1) lymphomas and leukemias
(2) chronic diarrhea and wasting
(3) hereditary angioedema
(4) structural lung disease

8. The treatment of cellular immunodeficiency syndromes often involves

(1) replacement of lymphokines
(2) continuous antibiotic coverage to prevent infections
(3) replacement of supraphysiologic amounts of immunoglobulins to offset the cellular defect
(4) bone marrow transplantation, but this varies with the specific syndrome

9. Phagocyte disorders are treated by

(1) infusion of fresh whole plasma
(2) prophylactic antibiotics
(3) chemical immunopotentiators
(4) bone marrow transplantation

Directions: The groups of questions below consist of lettered choices followed by several numbered items. For each numbered item select the **one** lettered choice with which it is **most** closely associated. Each lettered choice may be used once, more than once, or not at all.

Questions 10–15

For each disease, select the immune mechanism with which it is associated.

(A) Immediate hypersensitivity (type I) reaction
(B) Cytotoxic (type II) reaction
(C) Immune complex–mediated (type III) reaction
(D) Delayed hypersensitivity (type IV) reaction

10. Rh-hemolytic anemia of the newborn

11. Penicillin-induced anaphylaxis

12. Penicillin-induced hemolytic anemia

13. Contact dermatitis

14. Serum sickness

15. Drug-induced systemic lupus erythematosus

Questions 16–20

Match each description of an immunodeficiency disorder with the disorder it best describes.

(A) X-Linked agammaglobulinemia
(B) Severe combined immunodeficiency
(C) Common variable immunodeficiency
(D) Immunoglobulin deficiency with increased IgM
(E) Selective IgA deficiency

16. An antibody deficiency syndrome occasionally associated with cyclic neutropenia, thrombocytopenia, or hemolytic anemia

17. A hypogammaglobulinemia associated with normal numbers of circulating B cells

18. A syndrome characterized by agammaglobulinemia and a profound cellular immunodeficiency

19. A relatively mild antibody deficiency syndrome associated in some cases with infections, allergic disorders, and autoimmunity

20. A syndrome that may be caused by a defect in the rearrangement of the immunoglobulin genes resulting in an inability to assemble the immunoglobulin molecule

ANSWERS AND EXPLANATIONS

1. The answer is B. *(IV F 4 a)* Cyproheptadine hydrochloride is a piperidine antihistamine. Although cyproheptadine does not alter histamine release following cold exposure, it does render the ice cube test negative. Drowsiness is the most common side effect.

2. The answer is E. *(I B 1 b)* In antibody deficiency syndromes, there is quantitative or qualitative deficiency in antibody production or both. Quantitative deficiency is detected by measurement of the absolute level of each immunoglobulin isotype in the serum. Antibody deficiencies are defined further by evaluating the patient's capacity to produce specific antibody after in vivo stimulation; the amount of specific antibody produced is then noted.

3. The answer is B. *(I B 1 c)* In antibody deficiency states, the vulnerability of the host to infection is related directly to the absence of antibody to specific pathogenic organisms. This deficiency can be offset quite adequately by parenteral administration of commercial gamma globulin, which contains the pooled IgG from 2000 donors. Although successful bone marrow transplantation would provide a definitive resolution to the deficiency, the risks of that procedure are too great to justify its routine use.

4. The answer is C. *[I E 1 b (1)]* Deficiencies of all nine complement components have been described. Deficiencies of the early components of the classical pathway (i.e., C1, C4, and C2) have been associated with autoimmune diseases, and the symptom complex described most often has been similar to systemic lupus erythematosus.

5. The answer is B. *[I E 1 b (2)]* The complement system is thought to be important in host defense against certain microorganisms. Deficiencies of the components of the membrane attack unit (i.e., C5–C9) have been associated with recurrent infections by *Neisseria gonorrhoeae* and *Neisseria meningitidis*.

6. The answer is C. *(IV F 4 e)* Danazol is an attenuated androgen, which is effective in preventing attacks in patients with hereditary angioedema. Long-term treatment with low doses of danazol does not induce significant damage to the liver. Undesirable side effects of danazol, such as cholestasis and liver damage, have been observed in patients receiving relatively high doses for other diseases.

7. The answer is D (4). *(I B 1 a)* The antibody deficiency syndromes predispose to sinopulmonary infections with highly pathogenic organisms. The frequency and virulence of these infections often result in structural pulmonary disease, particularly bronchiectasis, which may then become progressive. The long-term prognosis for patients with antibody deficiency syndromes often is related to the pulmonary disease. Although lymphomas and leukemias have been reported in cases of X-linked agammaglobulinemia, these malignancies are rare. Chronic diarrhea and wasting are complications of severe cellular immunodeficiency.

8. The answer is D (4). *[I C 3 d (2), 4 e, 5 a (4), 6 b (4) (b)]* Without specific treatment, patients with cellular immunodeficiencies succumb to repeated infections. Although treatment of these disorders has had inconsistent success using lymphokines, patients have remained disease free for as long as 18 years after bone marrow transplantation. Some patients with cellular immunodeficiencies exhibit only a partial deficiency; the severity of the infections of these patients must be evaluated to gauge the need for bone marrow transplantation.

9. The answer is C (2, 4). *(I D 1 c)* Phagocyte defects represent a group of immunodeficiency disorders that vary in terms of severity and that may be cyclic, temporary, or permanent. Treatment depends upon the specific type of defect and may involve prophylactic antibiotic therapy. In severe disorders, attempts are made to provide a source of phagocyte precursors through bone marrow transplantation. In general, the severity of the problem and the long-term prognosis determine the therapeutic approach.

10–15. The answers are: 10-B, 11-A, 12-B, 13-D, 14-C, 15-C. *[II A 2 a (2), 3, B 1, C 1, D 3; V D 1 a, c, 2 a (2)]* An Rh-negative mother is sensitized for Rh-positive fetal blood by a fetomaternal transfusion at delivery. Immunoglobulin G (IgG) antibodies then develop, which can cross the placenta in a subsequent pregnancy to cause fetal red cell hemolysis (erythroblastosis fetalis) in the Rh-positive fetus. The cell-bound antigen in this example of a cytotoxic (type II) reaction usually is the D antigen, although other Rh blood group antigens (i.e., C or E) also can be the sensitizing antigen in an Rh-positive mother.

Systemic anaphylaxis occurs in about 15 in 100,000 patients treated with penicillin, resulting in an estimated 300 deaths per year in the United States. Anaphylaxis occurs within minutes after penicillin administration and is mediated by cell-bound IgE molecules.

Penicillin-induced hemolytic anemia is due to a hapten-cell interaction. Penicillin reacts with red cells to form stable penicilloyl–red cell complexes, which stimulate the formation of high-titer IgG antibodies. The cytotoxic IgG antibody is hapten specific, and the red cell destruction is primarily extravascular. The mechanism of most other drug-induced hemolytic reactions is different and is due to an immune complex–mediated reaction. In such a case, the red cell is an "innocent bystander" in complement-activated destruction of immune complexes; hemolysis may be intravascular, extravascular, or both.

There are four types of contact dermatitis: irritant, phototoxic, allergic, and photoallergic. Irritant contact dermatitis is not immune mediated and results from contact with a substance that chemically damages the skin. Phototoxic contact dermatitis also is not immune mediated and occurs when a substance damages the skin after contact and subsequent exposure to sunlight. Allergic contact dermatitis often is used synonymously with contact dermatitis and is an acquired delayed hypersensitivity reaction to an immunologically reactive substance. Photoallergic contact dermatitis is similar to allergic contact dermatitis but requires allergen and ultraviolet light exposure to produce skin damage.

Serum sickness is an immune complex–mediated disease that may be caused by heterologous sera (e.g., antitetanus antibody), homologous sera (e.g., human gamma globulin), antimicrobial agents (e.g., penicillins and sulfonamides), and other drugs (e.g., thiouracils, hydantoins, and hydralazine). IgG and IgM antibodies mediate this process.

Drug-induced systemic lupus erythematosus is associated with procainamide, hydralazine, chlorpromazine, isoniazid, D-penicillamine, phenytoin, and sulfasalazine and is primarily an immune complex–mediated reaction. Laboratory findings include an elevated erythrocyte sedimentation rate, leukopenia, mild anemia, and positive serum antinuclear antibody.

16–20. The answers are: 16-D, 17-C, 18-B, 19-E, 20-A. (*I B 2 a, 4 e, 5 b, e, 7, C 4 d*) Sometimes, an antibody deficiency syndrome is accompanied by another immune abnormality or hematologic derangement. This occurs most commonly in the syndrome of immunoglobulin deficiency with increased IgM, which usually is associated with cyclic neutropenia, thrombocytopenia, or hemolytic anemia. The coexistence of neutropenia with antibody deficiency may predispose an individual to different types of infections, especially pneumonia caused by *Pneumocystis carinii*.

The antibody deficiency syndromes represent a spectrum of defects in the development and function of the B-cell line from pre-B cell through plasma cell. In common variable immunodeficiency, there are normal numbers of B cells in the peripheral blood, and the defect presumably is one of terminal differentiation of the B cells. The presence of normal numbers of B cells distinguishes this syndrome from the congenital agammaglobulinemias.

The occurrence of severe hypogammaglobulinemia may be a manifestation of a more global immunodeficiency syndrome. When there is an association of hypogammaglobulinemia with cellular immunodeficiency, the condition is referred to as severe combined immunodeficiency. Treatment of the antibody deficiency state in this condition usually is only partially effective because of the cellular immune defect.

When the antibody defense of the mucous membranes is impaired, there is increased vulnerability to local infections and access of allergens and food macromolecules to the body. These events are thought to occur in selective IgA deficiency, accounting for the constellation of clinical symptoms.

Attempts have been made to explain antibody deficiency syndromes in terms of molecular biology. In the case of X-linked agammaglobulinemia, an abnormality in the rearrangement of genes coding for synthesis of immunoglobulin molecules has been identified.

8

Infectious Diseases

Thomas Fekete

I. GENERAL PRINCIPLES OF HUMAN-MICROBE INTERACTION. The normal human body harbors a complex microbial ecosystem. Generally, these **commensal** organisms (referred to as the **indigenous flora**) are considered to be nonpathogenic. Infection and disease may result, however, when the body is challenged by a known pathogen or when the body's defense system is disturbed, allowing uncontrolled growth or invasion by the indigenous flora.

A. Normal human-microbe ecology. Microorganisms can interact with humans in the following ways.

1. **Most indigenous organisms seldom cause disease.** Many of the organisms normally found on the skin and mucous membranes (e.g., *Staphylococcus epidermidis*, *Corynebacterium* species, and *Hemophilus* species other than *Hemophilus influenzae*) are ubiquitous but may cause disease in unusual settings (e.g., when host defenses are significantly impaired or when artificial material, such as a catheter or a prosthetic joint, is present).

2. **Some indigenous organisms may cause disease in other body sites.** Many bacteria that normally exist in one body site may cause morbidity elsewhere. For example, α-hemolytic (viridans) streptococci often exist as commensals in the oropharynx but can cause endocarditis if they are inoculated into the blood and settle on a previously damaged heart valve. Also, enteric aerobes and anaerobes, which normally exist in high density in the colon, can cause peritonitis and abscess formation if the colon is perforated and these bacteria spill into the abdominal cavity.

3. **Transient organisms may cause disease.** The body's normal flora may allow the temporary growth of certain microbes, which disappear spontaneously but may cause disease while present. For example, patients with invasive meningococcal disease first have pharyngeal carriage of *Neisseria meningitidis*, but only a tiny fraction of individuals with meningococci in the pharynx ever develop systemic disease.

4. **Pathogenic organisms usually cause disease.** Most viruses as well as *Chlamydia* and *Rickettsia* rarely are isolated from humans except during or following an acute illness. Some pathogenic bacteria include *Brucella* and *Salmonella* species, *Neisseria gonorrhoeae*, and *Mycobacterium tuberculosis*.

B. Host defense mechanisms. Although many of the microorganisms to which man is exposed have little intrinsic ability to cause illness, the human body has several important ways of protecting itself.

1. **Anatomic barriers** are integral in preventing infection. These include physical barriers, such as intact skin and mucous membranes, and functional barriers, such as the muscular protection of the glottis and bladder neck.
   a. **Herpetic whitlow** occurs when broken skin comes into contact with herpes simplex virus.
   b. Similarly, nonsterile intravenous injection of drugs may allow skin flora to enter the bloodstream and lead to the development of **endocarditis**.
   c. Mechanical devices such as indwelling bladder catheters and endotracheal tubes allow bacterial colonization of normally sterile sites, and this colonization may lead to infection.

2. **Cellular immunity.** The cellular arm of the immune system has several components (Table 8-1).
   a. **Neutrophils** (polymorphonuclear leukocytes) are phagocytic cells that are important for ingesting and killing microorganisms that breach normal body defenses.
   (1) When neutrophils are reduced substantially in number (a condition termed

Table 8-1. The Human Immune System

Component	Source	Function	Causes of Diminished Function	Opportunistic Organisms
Cellular immunity				
Neutrophil	Bone marrow	Phagocytosis; acute inflammation	Genetic disorders Chronic granulomatous disease Myeloperoxidase deficiency Acquired causes Cytotoxic therapy Leukemia Aplastic anemia Drug reaction	Endogenous flora; enteric bacilli; *Pseudomonas aeruginosa; Candida* species; *Aspergillus* species
Eosinophil	Bone marrow	Modulate hypersensitivity reactions to multicellular parasites	Idiopathic; corticosteroid therapy	None known
Monocyte/ macrophage	Bone marrow	Release lymphokines; interact with lymphocytes; phagocytosis	Cytotoxic therapy; lympho-reticular malignancy	. . .
T lymphocyte	Thymus; bone marrow	Modulate activity of B lymphocytes, macrophages, and T lymphocytes	Genetic disorders; autoimmune disease; lymphoreticular malignancy; AIDS*, organ transplantation; corticosteroid therapy	*Mycobacterium* species; fungi; *Listeria* species; *Nocardia* species
Humoral immunity				
Antibody	Plasma cells	Facilitate phagocytosis; inactivate toxins	Genetic disorders; multiple myeloma; splenectomy	Viruses; pyogenic bacteria
Complement	Liver	Enhance phagocytosis; direct cell destruction	Genetic disorders; severe liver disease	*Neisseria* species (in association with deficiency of complement components C5–C9)

*AIDS = acquired immune deficiency syndrome.

neutropenia), fungi and pyogenic bacteria that are commensals of the skin or gut, such as *Candida albicans* and *Escherichia coli*, can cause serious infections.

(2) Functional abnormalities of neutrophils may result in syndromes of varying type and severity.

    (a) For example, patients with **chronic granulomatous disease**, which is due to a deficiency of NADPH oxidase, are prone to infections by catalase-producing organisms such as *Staphylococcus aureus*, many gram-negative bacilli, and fungi. These infections start early in life and tend to be severe and recurrent.

    (b) Conversely, patients with **lazy leukocyte syndrome** tend to have mild, easily treatable infections associated with the upper respiratory tract.

b. **Monocytes** and their tissue forms, **macrophages**, also are important for the ingestion of pathogenic microbes as well as for the production of lymphokines and other modulators of the immune system. Some microorganisms are especially resistant to macrophages and may find refuge from antimicrobials in these cells, especially when drugs with poor cellular penetration are used. Examples of these bacteria are *Salmonella*, *Legionella*, and *Mycobacterium* species.

c. **Lymphocytes** are the third component of the cellular immune system. **T lymphocytes**, or **T cells**, have many roles in modulating the activities of other T cells, monocytes, and **B lymphocytes**, or **B cells**.

(1) Antigen–specific T cells are responsible for delayed hypersensitivity and for controlling infections caused by a variety of agents, including species of *Mycobacterium*, *Pneumocystis*, and *Cryptococcus*.

(2) T cells are broadly divided into **helper T cells** and **suppressor T cells** based on their effect on the immune system in terms of augmenting or diminishing the immune response. For example, helper T cells increase the ability to fight infection, and suppressor T cells increase the ability to reject foreign material.

(3) T cells also seem to have a pivotal role in the manifestations of autoimmune diseases.

3. **Humoral immunity** (see Table 8-1)

a. **Antibody-mediated immunity** involves the production of antibody by activated B cells, which are stimulated by exposure to the proper antigen and to helper T cells to differentiate into **plasma cells**. Plasma cells essentially are factories for the production of **immunoglobulins**, which they excrete into their environment. Immunoglobulins facilitate phagocytosis and activate complement and, thus, lead to a more rapid clearance of the antigen. The absence or profound deficiency of immunoglobulins leads to recurrent infections due to virulent encapsulated bacteria (e.g., *H. influenzae* and *Streptococcus pneumoniae*) and to a lesser degree by viruses (e.g., enteroviruses).

b. Another host defense is provided by the **complement system**—a cascading series of glycoproteins that either tag foreign material to promote phagocytosis or directly damage or destroy infective organisms. Severe complement deficiencies can predispose to infections. For example, the reduced production of one or more of the late complement components (i.e., C5–C9) permits overwhelming neisserial infections.

C. **Microbial virulence factors** also are important in determining the likelihood of infection. In order to infect a host, microorganisms or their products must adhere to host tissue.

1. **Some microbes invade host cells or breach barriers** to reach the susceptible body sites and, along the way, are able to avoid or overcome host defenses. In some situations (e.g., chicken pox or measles), microbes can easily infect an otherwise healthy individual who has normal host defenses but no prior exposure to the microbe.

2. **Some microbes cause disease at the contact site with the host.** An example is *Giardia lamblia*, which is confined to the lumen of the small bowel and causes abdominal cramping and diarrhea.

3. **Some microbes have a special ability to produce a toxin or virulence factor** to cause disease. For example, a toxin elaborated by some strains of *Staphylococcus aureus* (enterotoxin F or, more recently, toxic shock syndrome toxin 1 [TSST-1]) is responsible for **toxic shock syndrome** (see section VI D 2), and the virulence (Vi) antigen enables the enteric pathogen, *Salmonella typhi*, to cause **typhoid fever**.

4. **In some situations, microbes work in groups to cause disease** when an individual organism lacks an essential virulence or survival quality to act alone. An example is **delta hepatitis**, which can occur only in the presence of ongoing hepatitis B infection.

5. Since the development and use of antimicrobial agents for the prevention or treatment of infections, **microorganisms that are resistant to antibiotics may have a propensity for causing infections**. This is especially true in settings such as hospitals, where antibiotic use is widespread.

D. Epidemiologic considerations. In addition to host and microbial characteristics, environmental circumstances also help determine the nature and severity of an infection.

1. Contagious diseases are infections that can occur only after direct physical contact with or aerosol exposure to an infected human. Examples are syphilis, tuberculosis, and measles. Smallpox was successfully eradicated because it was possible to identify every case and, therefore, to direct preventive efforts to those individuals who were at risk for being exposed.

2. Vectors and fomites
   a. When an animal is a host or carrier of a disease without becoming ill itself, that animal is a **vector** of infection. Most vectors are lower animals such as insects and ticks. In general, infections that are related to animals or their products (e.g., meat, milk, or eggs) are called **zoonoses**.
   b. When an object is passively responsible for transmitting infection, it is called a **fomite**. In general, the impact of fomites on human infection is small outside the special setting of the hospital, where enhanced patient susceptibility and a high concentration of virulent organisms coexist.

3. Geography. For reasons of ecology, some diseases occur exclusively or at substantially greater frequency in certain areas. For example, malaria no longer is transmitted by mosquito bites in the United States. When considering such a disease in a diagnosis, a history of travel to or a residence in an appropriate area is very important. Duration of exposure can also be important, as in filariasis, which leads to elephantiasis only after repeated exposure to the mosquito vector over a period of months to years.

4. Season. Many infections occur more commonly during a particular time of the year. This may be due to certain activities that might expose an individual to risk and that are seasonal in nature (e.g., hunting and fishing) or to environmental factors that favor the growth of the microbe or its insect vector.
   a. It is well known that influenza infections occur most commonly in the winter.
   b. Because of their association with aerosols produced by air-conditioning cooling towers, most *Legionella* infections occur in the summer.

II. USE OF ANTI-INFECTIVE THERAPY

A. General principles. Because the use of antibiotics can be life-saving, it is important to recognize when to initiate treatment. However, any type of medical intervention presents potential hazards, and the indiscriminate use of antibiotics is no exception. In general, there are three settings that prompt antimicrobial therapy.

1. Organism-based treatment
   a. When cultures or stains from a patient demonstrate a credible microorganism, appropriate antibiotic treatment is initiated.
      (1) For example, a urethral exudate with gram-negative, intracellular diplococci is presumptive evidence for gonorrheal urethritis, and chemotherapy is warranted on the basis of this test alone. The selection of penicillin, tetracycline, spectinomycin, or a cephalosporin depends on the likelihood of drug resistance and on whether oral or injectable therapy is preferred.
      (2) Also, blood cultures positive for *Streptococcus sanguis* in a patient with a history of mitral valve disease and a fever call for prompt therapy with high doses of intravenous penicillin for bacterial endocarditis.
   b. New techniques for recognizing specific antigens of microorganisms also may be used to help initiate therapy. An example is the finding of cryptococcal antigens in the cerebrospinal fluid (CSF) in a patient with chronic meningitis. This would call for amphotericin B and flucytosine.
   c. Isolation of an organism allows in vitro testing of antibiotic susceptibility, but for many microbes, resistance patterns are predictable enough to permit treatment without these further tests.

2. Syndrome-based treatment
   a. Syndrome-based treatment is initiated when:
      (1) The clinical picture strongly suggests specific organ disease
      (2) The tests needed to make a microbiologic diagnosis are not available or practical
      (3) The most likely causative organisms all respond to the same treatment
         (a) For example, if gram-negative diplococci are not found on the Gram stain of a urethral exudate, tetracycline therapy for nongonococcal urethritis may be initiated.
         (b) It is known that *Chlamydia trachomatis* and *Ureaplasma urealyticum* may cause

nongonococcal urethritis; however, it seldom is practical to distinguish them as both organisms respond to tetracycline.

b. **Empiric therapy** is given when the diagnosis is uncertain but clinical experience suggests that the patient outcome in a particular setting is improved with antimicrobial therapy.
   (1) Generally, empiric therapy is initiated while awaiting the results of diagnostic tests to identify a specific causative organism.
   (2) In patients with severe neutropenia from cancer chemotherapy, a fever may trigger the use of antibiotics while culture results are being awaited since these patients may succumb to a treatable infection between the onset of fever and the report of positive cultures, and a substantial number of these patients improve on antibiotics without a pathogen ever being found.
   (3) **Prophylaxis** is used when a specific infection or complication is to be avoided. Generally, this form of empiric therapy is restricted to a fixed and brief period during which there is a risk of infection. Examples include the use of penicillin prior to dental procedures in patients with heart valve disease and the use of perioperative antibiotics in surgery of the large bowel.

B. **Dosage and route.** When considering the use of antibiotics, the appropriate dosage and route of administration must be established.

1. **Dosage**
   a. Dosing usually is based on pharmacologic and clinical data related to the size and age of the patient, the desired level of the drug in the target tissue, the drug's rate of elimination (often estimated by examining kidney and liver function), and the expected penetration of the drug into the infected tissue.
   b. Guidelines for proper dosing usually are provided with the drug itself and are widely available in publications. Occasionally, blood or tissue levels of the drug must be measured to assure safe and effective concentrations.

2. **Route.** In general, parenterally administered (i.e., intravenous or intramuscular) drugs are more reliably absorbed than orally administered drugs and are used:
   a. In patients who cannot tolerate orally administered drugs
   b. In patients in whom institution of therapy is urgent
   c. When no oral form of the drug exists

C. **Cost** of antibiotic treatment has become more important with the proliferation and availability of similar drugs and with the increased attention to financial matters in both inpatient and outpatient therapy. When all other factors are equal, the cost of administration may influence which drug is prescribed in a particular setting. With intravenously given drugs, there is a cost of diluents and of labor involved in preparing and infusing the drugs. The cost of administration is lower with intramuscularly given drugs and is lowest with oral agents.

D. **Specific antibiotic spectrum.** The range, or **spectrum**, of microorganisms inhibited or killed by an antibiotic is a very important consideration in deciding which drug to use. The results of in vitro testing are very helpful in selecting an antibiotic that is most likely to be effective against an infective organism. Even when the particular organism has not been tested, it may be assumed—on the basis of either local patterns of antibiotic susceptibility or general experience in treating certain syndromes—that a given drug is likely to be effective in that setting.

E. **Toxicity and side effects.** Although life-threatening toxicity rarely occurs with antibiotic treatment, the specific risks of each drug administered should be familiar to the physician so that side effects can be anticipated and minimized.

1. **Allergic reactions**—sometimes fatal—can occur with almost any pharmaceutical but are more common with the β-lactam antibiotics than with other antimicrobials.

2. Chloramphenicol is associated with **bone marrow suppression**, including irreversible aplastic anemia.

3. Many drugs can cause **renal dysfunction**, the most prominent being the aminoglycosides. This toxicity is reversible and usually of minor clinical significance, but recovery may take weeks or months. In very rare instances, dialysis may be needed temporarily.

4. **Abnormalities in blood coagulation** (e.g., changes in the levels of clotting factors or in the number or function of platelets) have been associated with several β-lactam antibiotics and sometimes result in clinically significant bleeding.

5. **Ototoxicity** is an infrequent but potentially debilitating side effect of aminoglycosides and vancomycin. Either auditory or vestibular impairment can occur, and often it is irreversible.

F. Adult immunization

  1. It is important for adults to have immunity to all of the childhood diseases except pertussis. (Although pertussis may occur in adults, it usually is mild, and the available vaccines are not well tolerated when administered to adults.)

   a. If there has been no previous vaccination, a series of tetanus and diphtheria vaccines should be administered.

   b. Killed poliovirus vaccine should be given to adults who are not already immune—especially those with children who are about to receive live poliovirus vaccine.

   c. Because rubella in a pregnant woman can result in a devastating infection of the fetus, all women of child-bearing age should be immune to rubella. Serum tests for antibody to rubella are widely available to help identify adults who need vaccination.

   d. If there is no history of mumps or measles illness or vaccination, the appropriate live virus vaccines for these illnesses should be given.

  2. Special vaccination issues pertain to the elderly and to chronically ill patients—especially those with cardiac or pulmonary disease. All such patients should receive pneumococcal vaccination once and, in the appropriate season, should have annual influenza vaccination.

  3. Travelers to countries where yellow fever is endemic (most of tropical Africa and South America) should receive this vaccine. Depending on the length of exposure, cholera and typhoid immunizations may be recommended for certain travelers. Gamma globulin is recommended for prevention of hepatitis A for travelers who expect to encounter poor sanitary facilities—especially those resulting in human fecal contamination of food or water.

  4. Homosexual men, intravenous drug users, hemophiliacs, and any health care workers who might be exposed to blood or secretions from people with **hepatitis B** should consider immunization to protect against this agent.

  5. Asplenic individuals should have pneumococcal and meningococcal vaccinations, even though protection from these infections is incomplete. In the case of elective splenectomy, the immunizations should be performed before surgery.

III. EFFECTIVE USE OF THE MICROBIOLOGY LABORATORY. In order to maximize the usefulness of any microbiology laboratory, it is necessary to be familiar with its specific capabilities and procedures. The following are some general guidelines.

A. Obtaining and handling specimens

  1. Fresh specimens are superior to old ones. This is especially true when quantitative results are important (e.g., colony counts of urine cultures) or when the target organism is fragile (e.g., protozoal trophozoites in stools). If immediate delivery of a specimen is not possible, it is best to make certain how to maintain the specimen until it can be processed.

   a. Some bacteria (e.g., gonococci) are very sensitive to cold and should not be refrigerated.

   b. Specimens to be cultured for anaerobes should be maintained in a prereduced, oxygen-free environment. Even so, it is best to place these specimens in a medium that supports anaerobic life and to transport them to the laboratory for immediate plating.

  2. Large specimens are better than small ones. In most cases it is preferable to have adequate material to culture than to have only a swab—the laboratory technologist should have the final choice as to which portion to use. Infections that are associated with a low density of microorganisms (e.g., fungal meningitis) may require that a larger volume or multiple specimens be submitted to permit isolation of the pathogen.

  3. Biological hazards should be labeled and handled properly. Such hazards include serum from patients with hepatitis B or acquired immune deficiency syndrome (AIDS). When highly infective organisms are isolated in the laboratory, the pure cultures may pose a hazard to the technologist. Specimens that may contain *Brucella*, *Francisella*, or *Salmonella* species should be clearly marked so that appropriate precautions can be taken.

B. Interpreting negative and positive cultures. When a diagnosis rests on identifying an organism obtained from a clinical specimen, it is crucial to recognize what is real and what represents simple contamination by other body flora or inanimate sources. Laboratory results are more credible when a specimen has been stained and shown to contain the appropriate cell type (e.g., neutrophil or alveolar macrophage in sputum) and lacks evidence of contamination (e.g., squamous epithelial cells in sputum or urine). When exceptional care and attention have been lavished on getting a good specimen, almost any positive results are significant.

  1. If antibiotics have been administered, the potential for positive cultures is reduced, and the predictive value of negative cultures also is diminished.

2. When cultures are truly negative, the use of special media and growth conditions should be discussed. Supplementary nutrients or suppression of other organisms may be necessary to permit growth and identification.

3. Cultures that are repeatedly positive for a given organism may be more convincing than a single positive specimen. This is especially true for blood cultures. Specimens taken from normally sterile sites such as cerebrospinal, joint, and pleural fluids usually are reliable when obtained aseptically. However, if they are culture-positive for commensals, repeat cultures are extremely helpful.

4. Corroborative tests such as antigen detection and seroconversion (i.e., the development of antibodies to a pathogen) can establish the significance of a single culture-positive specimen or establish a diagnosis when cultures have not been obtained or are negative.

C. Interpreting antimicrobial susceptibility tests. The laboratory can provide useful information about the specific microbe causing an infection by in vitro testing of its antimicrobial susceptibility pattern. For many bacteria, these tests can be done rapidly, with results sometimes available in hours. However, **the conditions used in susceptibility testing do not necessarily simulate conditions in the patient**.

1. The results of susceptibility testing may show the microorganism to be susceptible, intermediately susceptible, or resistant to the drug being tested. This information presupposes that the drug concentration at the site of infection will be similar to what usually is found in serum. It also assumes that the organism will be inhibited or killed at the infection site if it is exposed to such a drug concentration.

2. Another way to express the susceptibility is to determine the actual concentration of antibiotic needed to inhibit the microorganism. This usually is done by exposing the microbe to varying concentrations of the drug and observing which is the lowest one to inhibit growth (called the **minimum inhibitory concentration**, or **MIC**). The lower the MIC, the more susceptible the organism. In some instances, however, clinical experience shows that a drug is ineffective despite in vitro data that suggest it would work. For example, cephalosporins are not useful in treating infections caused by methicillin-resistant *S. aureus*, although blood and tissue levels in excess of the MIC are easily achievable.

3. Direct measurement of serum or tissue levels of the drug being used may be desirable so that the dosage can be adjusted to avoid toxicity and to maximize therapeutic benefit. This is especially true for patients who may have less predictable blood or tissue levels of antibiotic due to altered drug metabolism or excretion secondary to renal or hepatic dysfunction.

IV. RISK FACTORS FOR INFECTION. Sometimes it is possible to identify patient characteristics that modify the likelihood or severity of an infection. Although some of these risk assignments have been accepted without adequate validation, there is sound evidence that a substantially increased risk of infection exists among certain groups of individuals. In general, the intensity of exposure and the degree of the metabolic derangement correlate with the potential hazard of infection.

A. Diabetes. In general, diabetics are not known to have infections more frequently than individuals without glucose intolerance. However, there are a few significant differences.

1. Diabetics tend to have more **foot and lower leg ulcers**, which may become infected. When such soft tissue infections occur, they are more likely to involve gram-negative rods, and they are more difficult to cure than those occurring in normal individuals.

2. Diabetics have more **genital infections** with *Candida* species—especially vulvovaginal candidiasis. Urinary tract infections may be more severe in diabetics, and the increased morbidity probably is related to bladder dysfunction in those patients with diabetic neuropathy. It is often recommended that urinary infections be more vigorously treated in diabetics.

3. Some **rare diseases** occur almost exclusively in diabetics.
a. Malignant otitis externa is a painful, rapidly progressive, and locally destructive disease of the external auditory canal, which may extend to the temporal bone and the brain. *Pseudomonas aeruginosa* is the causative agent. (For additional information see section V C 1 a.)
b. Rhinocerebral mucormycosis is a fungal infection that starts in the nose or paranasal sinuses and is locally destructive. It is found in patients with severe metabolic acidosis, such as diabetics with ketoacidosis.
c. Synergistic gangrene is a soft tissue infection, which often is due to streptococci and obligate anaerobes. It may involve the skin or the underlying fascial structures and tends to progress relentlessly unless treated with extensive surgical debridement.

B. **Alcoholism.** The incidence of infection in alcoholics is related to the degree of liver dysfunction in these individuals.

1. It is generally believed that alcoholics have a greater incidence of pneumococcal, aspiration, and gram-negative bacillary **pneumonias** than the general population. Tuberculosis, anaerobic lung abscess, and empyema also are more common.

2. When ascites is present, alcoholics may develop **spontaneous bacterial peritonitis**, which is a bacterial infection of ascitic fluid that occurs in the absence of bowel perforation. This infection, usually caused by gram-negative aerobic bacilli or streptococci, also occurs in non-alcoholic patients with ascites.

C. **Intravenous drug use.** Several infections clearly are more common in intravenous drug users than in comparable individuals who do not use such substances.

1. **Infections related to unsterile techniques.** Intravenous drug users are prone to a variety of suppurative complications because, in most cases, the preparation of the drug is not aseptic, the equipment is unsterile, and the skin cleansing is inadequate.
   a. The most serious is **bacterial endocarditis**, which often occurs on the tricuspid valve (a valve rarely infected in other populations). Usually, the bacterium responsible is *S. aureus*.
   b. **Superficial skin infections** also are frequent, and **infectious arthritis**—usually caused by *P. aeruginosa*—is seen commonly.
   c. **Tetanus** also occurs more frequently, as a consequence of improperly cleaned wounds and low levels of immunity.
   d. **Fever** in an intravenous drug user must be evaluated carefully since these pyogenic bacterial infections can progress rapidly if treatment is delayed.

2. **Infections related to sharing needles.** Some contagious diseases can be efficiently transmitted via the small amount of blood in used needles and syringes. For example, the incidence of hepatitis B and AIDS clearly is increased in intravenous drug user populations. Non-A, non-B hepatitis and delta hepatitis also seem to be more common.

D. **Homosexuality**

1. **Homosexual men.** The increased risk of infections in sexually active homosexual men was first recognized in the mid-1970s. Because the symptoms often involve the alimentary tract, this problem was loosely labeled the **gay bowel syndrome**. The etiologic agents include *Shigella* species, *N. gonorrhoeae*, *G. lamblia*, *C. trachomatis*, *Entamoeba histolytica*, *Treponema pallidum*, hepatitis A virus, and papillomavirus. Hepatitis B virus and non-A, non-B hepatitis virus have been recognized as being hyperendemic among American homosexual men living in urban communities. Recently, the outbreak of AIDS has been focused in this same population.

2. **Homosexual women.** The incidence of infectious diseases is not known to be increased among homosexual women.

E. **Occupation** may predispose to certain infections by permitting exposure to various infective agents.

1. In some cases, the risk of occupation-related infection is unpredictable, as in the outbreaks of **Pontiac fever**, which were related to the aerosolization of *Legionella pneumophila*–contaminated water via air-conditioning ducts throughout an office building.

2. In other cases, the risk of infection is influenced by factors outside the immediate work environment. For example, the risk of brucellosis among slaughterhouse workers is determined largely by the number of livestock infected and to a lesser extent by the degree of the worker's exposure to the blood of infected livestock.

3. When an increased risk is predictable, certain preventive measures can be instituted, such as the immunization of veterinarians against rabies.

F. **Internal prostheses.** The advances in modern surgery have made it possible to replace malfunctioning body parts, most notably joints and heart valves. When a prosthesis (or any foreign material) is inserted into the body, there is a possibility that an infection will develop at the site of insertion. Because of the way the human body reacts to foreign material, a prosthetic organ is susceptible to infection by a greater number and variety of organisms than is the native, damaged organ. In addition, the clinical presentation of these infections may be atypical, and the time interval between surgery and any manifestation of sepsis may be quite long. *S. epidermidis* is involved in many of these infections. In most cases, it is believed that the bacteria are inoculated at the time of surgery, although secondary hematogenous or percutaneous spread is possible.

1. **Diagnosis** of these infections is dependent on recognition of the characteristic clinical presentation. Infected joints almost always cause local pain and may be accompanied by erythema, tenderness, and fever. Infected heart valves are almost always associated with fever and may be associated with valve dysfunction. These infections resemble native valve endocarditis.

2. **Therapy** is most successful when it includes the removal or replacement of the prosthetic device as well as systemic antibiotic treatment.

G. Indwelling catheters

1. Like internal prostheses, catheters such as intravenous or intra-arterial lines, bladder catheters, and endotracheal tubes offer a site of diminished host responsiveness. Further, they provide a communication between the external environment and the ordinarily sterile internal environment of the body.

2. In addition to intrinsic host factors, two important elements determine the likelihood of catheter-related infection: the duration of catheterization and the degree of asepsis maintained during catheterization. The duration of catheterization is the more important factor in regard to tracheal and urethral catheters; both factors are important for vascular catheters.

   a. With long-term intravenous access with a surgically implanted catheter (e.g., for hyperalimentation or for chemotherapy and administration of blood products in certain cancer patients), the risk of infection can be reduced, although not eliminated, by meticulous attention to sterile technique during insertion, by avoiding sites that are diseased or prone to bacterial contamination.

   b. For the patient who needs intravenous access for a short or intermediate period of time and has catheters placed in the extremities, the sites should be changed every 48–72 hours. When a catheter is placed in a central vein for temporary intravenous access, the maximal duration of catheterization at a given site is not absolute; however, there is a substantial risk of infection after a few days, and catheters should be removed as soon as possible or at the first signs of sepsis.

   c. In addition, vascular catheters generally are maintained with a high degree of care to avoid infection (e.g., aseptic dressing changes and the application of antibiotic-containing ointments to the insertion site); however, the importance of these measures in preventing infection is unknown.

   d. Despite the high risk of infection with the use of catheters, there is no indication for systemic antibiotic prophylaxis before or during catheterization.

H. Granulocytopenia.
A specific risk that has been identified and carefully studied is related to the absence of adequate numbers of circulating neutrophils or **granulocytopenia**. When the absolute number of neutrophils in the blood drops below 1000/mm³, the incidence of infection increases. (This relationship becomes even more apparent at lower neutrophil counts.)

1. In the majority of granulocytopenic patients, the underlying disease is a lymphoma or leukemia, although reduced neutrophil levels can be seen in association with aplastic anemia, drug-induced agranulocytosis, and cytotoxic chemotherapy. These patients most often become infected with indigenous flora, usually pyogenic bacteria and fungi.

2. The indigenous flora of granulocytopenic patients also may be altered during hospitalization. When infection is manifested by fever, clinical deterioration can be rapid.

I. Corticosteroids
are used to treat a wide variety of medical problems. Although steroids typically cause an increase in the number of circulating white blood cells, they have an immunosuppressive effect that is strongly dose-related.

1. The expression of this immunodeficiency is seen mostly in the increased incidence of infection usually controlled by cellular immunity (e.g., mycobacterial, fungal, nocardial, and cytomegaloviral infections). Steroids also alter some diagnostic tests, most notably the expression of delayed hypersensitivity.

2. Steroids also are used widely in transplantation procedures involving the kidney, heart, liver, and bone marrow. In part, the infections experienced by these patients are related to corticosteroids and the other drugs (i.e., cyclosporine and azathioprine) used to prevent organ rejection.

J. Neurologic deficits.
Neurologic dysfunction may predispose to infection if such deficits cause body defenses to be more easily breached. The following are examples.

1. Elimination of the gag reflex, whether by stroke or coma, may predispose to aspiration of oral or gastric contents.

2. A hypoesthetic limb may become secondarily infected, as in the case of leprosy that results in nerve destruction.

3. When neuromuscular control of the bladder is lost, long-term catheterization (with its attendant complications) may be necessary.

K. Age. The likelihood of acquiring certain infections varies considerably with age. In general, the maturation of the immune system is responsible for the changing pattern of infections in early childhood, and the presence of other medical illnesses accounts for most of the changes in late adulthood. The diminished immune response in the elderly and the tendency to develop atherosclerosis also may affect the likelihood of acquiring infection (e.g., the infection of arterial plaques by bacteremic salmonellosis). Age also may bear on the severity of a given infection once an individual has been exposed.

V. SPECIFIC INFECTIONS ACCORDING TO BODY SITE

A. General considerations: fever. One of the most recognized features of infectious diseases, regardless of body site, is the elevation of body temperature.

1. Normal regulation of body temperature. The normal core body temperature is about 37° (± 1°) C. Monocytes are capable of making a polypeptide called **interleukin 1**, which stimulates the hypothalamus to raise the body's temperature **set point**. The rise in set point causes alterations in circulation and perspiration, which ultimately lead to a rise in body temperature. Body temperature usually is measured by placing a thermometer in the mouth or the rectum. (Mouth breathing or the recent ingestion of very hot or cold beverages may reduce the accuracy of orally measured temperature readings, which tend to be 0.5°–1.0° C lower than rectal temperatures.) Temperature readings above 38.3° C are considered abnormal.

2. Conditions associated with fever. Almost any infectious process may be accompanied by fever, although the absence of fever at any given moment should not exclude the consideration of an infection. Fever may also occur with myocardial infarction, pulmonary embolism, drug reactions, autoimmune disease (e.g., systemic lupus erythematosus, rheumatoid arthritis, and temporal arteritis), or tumor (e.g., lymphoma and renal cell carcinoma). The actual pattern of fever rarely helps to narrow the range of etiologies for the fever.

3. Fever management. Antipyretic drugs (e.g., aspirin, acetaminophen, and nonsteroidal antiinflammatory agents) can modify a fever, but seldom completely suppress a fever caused by infection. When fever is extreme (i.e., > 42° C) or when the tachycardia and circulatory changes accompanying fever are poorly tolerated, it is wise to try to reduce body temperature. In most settings, fever merely is uncomfortable, and the attempt to eliminate it may be comparatively more unpleasant because of the shaking and sweating sometimes associated with fever lysis.

4. Beneficial effects of fever. Fever does play a role in host defense since many infective microbes prefer lower temperatures; however, the clinical significance of this protection is unknown. In addition, some elements of the immune system are more efficient at higher temperatures whereas others are less efficient. The net effect of this on recovery from infection is not known.

B. Central nervous system (CNS) infections are classified according to their location. They include meningitis, encephalitis, and intracranial abscess.

1. Meningitis
  a. Acute meningitis is an inflammatory disease involving the arachnoid layer of the meninges and the fluid that circulates in the subarachnoid space—the **cerebrospinal fluid (CSF)**.
    (1) Classification. There are two major classifications of meningitis—**bacterial** and **aseptic**. In both forms there is fever, headache, and stiff neck. However, in bacterial meningitis the CSF has a pyogenic nature, with an elevated white cell count, an increased fraction of neutrophils, an elevated protein level, and a normal or lowered glucose level. In aseptic meningitis the CSF is characterized by a mildly elevated white cell count, a normal or mildly elevated protein level, and a normal glucose level (i.e., greater than two-thirds the serum level).
    (2) Etiology. The etiologic agents of meningitis can be divided into those causing bacterial meningitis and those causing aseptic meningitis.
      (a) The causes of **bacterial meningitis** vary with the age of the patient, with *E. coli* and *Streptococcus agalactiae* occurring most frequently in infants, *H. influenzae* predominating in young children 2 months to 6 years of age, *N. meningitidis* being most common in adolescents and young adults, and *S. pneumoniae* being most

common in adults over 25 years of age. *Listeria monocytogenes* is found most commonly in cancer patients and in immunosuppressed individuals.

   (b) Aseptic meningitis usually is a viral disease or may reflect an inflammatory process adjacent to the meninges (e.g., cerebritis, brain abscess, sinusitis, or otitis). The CSF in partially treated bacterial meningitis usually has a pyogenic nature, although antibiotics may modify the disease in such a way as to create an aseptic pattern. Drug sensitivity also may cause an aseptic meningitis, as may occur with ibuprofen therapy.

(3) Clinical features. When bacteria cause meningitis, this manifestation usually is part of a systemic, bacteremic infection. An exception occurs when bacteria gain access to the meninges after trauma or surgery or via a bony defect (usually in the temporal area or the cribriform plate).

   (a) With disease due to *H. influenzae* or *S. pneumoniae*, focal infection such as pneumonia or otitis also may be apparent.

   (b) With disease due to *N. meningitidis*, there may be a characteristic systemic infection consisting of a petechial or purpuric skin rash and hypotension, which can develop very rapidly.

(4) Therapy

   (a) Antibiotics have a significant impact on the outcome of bacterial meningitis. Without treatment, death is almost certain; with treatment, however, the mortality rate is reduced to about 20% of those patients who are not moribund at the time of diagnosis. Bactericidal antibiotics should be given in dosages that permit the drug to achieve killing levels in the CSF. Because there is a barrier to virtually all drugs, reducing drug penetration from the blood into the CSF, maximum tolerated systemic dosages should be given even at the end of the course (usually a total of 2 weeks).

   (i) In adults, penicillin or ampicillin is effective against almost all of the common agents of bacterial meningitis.

   (ii) If resistant organisms are found, one of the most broad-spectrum cephalosporins (e.g., cefotaxime or ceftriaxone) should be used.

   (iii) Patients who are allergic to penicillin usually respond to chloramphenicol.

   (b) There is no specific chemotherapy for aseptic meningitis. Any underlying disease should be treated appropriately.

b. Chronic meningitis

(1) Etiology. The most common causes of chronic meningitis are tuberculosis, cryptococcal disease, malignancy, and sarcoidosis.

(2) Clinical features. Chronic meningitis may have an indolent presentation, with symptoms similar to acute meningitis or with altered mentation with or without fever. CSF abnormalities may progress with time if the underlying disease is untreated. In many of these diseases, the CSF glucose level is low. Chronic meningitis should be considered when a low CSF glucose level is noted in a patient who is found not to have acute bacterial meningitis.

(3) Therapy is directed at the underlying disease.

   (a) In cases of suspected or confirmed tuberculosis, combinations of isoniazid and rifampin are suitable since both drugs have adequate CSF penetration.

   (b) Cryptococcal meningitis responds to amphotericin B alone or in combination with flucytosine, but there is a high rate of failure or relapse.

   (c) Malignancy involving the meninges is difficult to treat and may require neural radiotherapy or intrathecal chemotherapy.

   (d) Sarcoidosis usually is treated with corticosteroids.

2. Encephalitis is an inflammatory process involving the brain.

a. Etiology. The majority of encephalitides are caused by viruses.

b. Clinical features. Encephalitis usually presents with altered mentation, seizures, or both. The CSF may be normal or have an aseptic pattern.

c. Diagnosis is made by measuring rising titers of antibody to one of the encephalitis viruses in a patient with a compatible clinical syndrome. Because herpes simplex encephalitis is treatable with antiviral agents (e.g., acyclovir or vidarabine) when the diagnosis is made before severe neurologic deterioration, an aggressive approach using brain biopsy and culture has been suggested when this etiology is suspected.

d. Differential diagnosis

(1) *Toxoplasma gondii* can cause encephalitis in a patient with diminished T-cell function (e.g., due to AIDS or organ transplant).

(2) Some intoxications and immune diseases (e.g., systemic lupus erythematosus) may have a presentation indistinguishable from encephalitis.

(3) Endocarditis also should be considered.

e. **Therapy.** With the exception of herpes simplex encephalitis, the treatment of viral encephalitis is supportive. Toxoplasmosis is treated with a long course of pyrimethamine and sulfadiazine.

3. Intracranial abscess. Suppurative infections can involve the contents of the calvarium, usually by direct spread from an infected sinus or ear.

a. **Etiology.** The bacteriology of intracranial infections reflects the types of organisms that
cause disease in more superficial contiguous structures, such as streptococci and anaerobic bacteria. Abscesses can be localized to the extradural (also called epidural) or subdural spaces or in the brain parenchyma. Rarely, hematogenous spread of bacteria can
give rise to intracranial abscesses. Less common agents are *Toxoplasma*, *Nocardia*, and
Cryptococcus species, which usually are seen in immunocompromised patients.

b. **Diagnosis. Computed tomography (CT)** of the brain is very helpful in making the diagnosis. Although early signs of disease may be subtle, within several days there usually are
characteristic lucencies with constrast-enhanced margins.

c. **Therapy.** Bacterial abscesses are treated with appropriate antibiotics, which might include
penicillin, chloramphenicol, and metronidazole. Good penetration into the brain is desirable. The usual treatment is given for infection by *Toxoplasma* (i.e., pyrimethamine and
sulfadiazine), *Cryptococcus* (i.e., amphotericin B and flucytosine), or *Nocardia* (i.e., sulfa-
methoxazole with or without trimethoprim).

C. Head and neck infections

1. Otitis. Infections of the ear can involve any of the ear's three major anatomic areas—the
outer, middle, or inner ear.

a. **Outer ear infections** tend to be minor irritations of the external auditory canal. An exception is **malignant otitis externa**—a destructive process most commonly found in diabetics
(see also section IV A 3 a). Topical antibiotic treatment is used for external otitis. Malignant
otitis externa requires antibiotics that are effective against *Pseudomonas* infection plus
surgical debridement and drainage.

b. **Middle ear infection**, or **otitis media**, typically is a disease of children, which presents as
ear pain and reduced auditory acuity. Otoscopy shows a dull tympanic membrane with or
without pus behind it. The most common causes are pneumococci, *Streptococcus
pyogenes*, and *H. influenzae*. In chronic cases, especially if multiple courses of antibiotics
have been given, enteric gram-negative rods and anaerobes may be involved. Therapy for
acute otitis media is amoxicillin, trimethoprim-sulfamethoxazole, or an oral cephalosporin. Cultures and appropriate therapy are suggested for chronic otitis media.

c. **Inner ear infections** rarely are caused by bacteria. However, several viruses may be associated with a syndrome of **vertigo** with or without **tinnitus**. No treatment is helpful.

2. Sinusitis. The paranasal sinuses have continuous exposure to the external environment via
the ostia in the nose. Under normal conditions, there are host defenses that maintain the
sterile environment of the sinuses. However, when mucociliary clearance is interrupted because of structural or functional abnormalities, infection can supervene.

a. **Etiology.** As in middle ear infections, virulent bacteria such as pneumococci and
Hemophilus species are most likely to cause acute disease, and enteric organisms are associated with more chronic infections. Bacterial sinusitis may follow and mimic viral upper
respiratory infections; however, only the bacterial infections go on to develop suppurative
complications of the CNS.

b. **Diagnosis.** Sinus radiography shows mucosal thickening or opacification or air fluid levels
in sinusitis. Tenderness and edema help to localize disease to the sinuses but are not present in all patients.

c. **Therapy.** In mild cases, antibiotics (e.g., penicillin, erythromycin, or sulfa drugs) alone or
in combination with decongestants are adequate. More advanced disease may require surgical drainage.

3. Odontogenic infections, the most common infections occurring in the oral cavity, usually are
local and respond to simple measures such as draining abscesses, restoring carious teeth, and
maintaining good oral hygiene. Sometimes, however, soft tissue infections in the mouth can
dissect through tissue planes and involve deeper structures of the face or neck. Examples are
Ludwig's angina, which is an infection extending to the floor of the mouth, and **retropharyn-
geal abscess**, which can track down to the mediastinum. The bacteriology is one of streptococci and indigenous oral anaerobes.

4. Eye infections. Normally, the eyes also are resistant to infections.

a. **Conjunctivitis.** Superficial infections of the conjunctiva usually are bacterial or viral and
resolve spontaneously. An exception is **gonorrheal conjunctivitis**—a rare disease in adults,

which must be treated vigorously with penicillin or alternative drugs effective against the gonococcus.

   b. Keratitis is an infection of the cornea. Because the transparency of the cornea is crucial for vision, diagnostic tests such as bacterial and viral smears and cultures are warranted. Initial therapy is guided by the clinical picture, since a variety of organisms can cause keratitis, including *S. aureus, P. aeruginosa,* streptococci, numerous fungi, and herpes simplex virus. It is important to recognize keratitis that is due to herpes simplex virus so that appropriate antiviral therapy can be instituted to prevent blindness.

   c. Endophthalmitis is an infection of the internal structures of the eye. It is most commonly caused by bacteria and may follow eye surgery or distant infection. Systemic and topical antibiotics are selected on the basis of the clinical findings and the Gram stain of ocular material and are administered to prevent irreversible destruction of the eye. However, the prognosis for normal visual acuity after endophthalmitis is poor.

D. Respiratory tract infections

1. **Upper respiratory infections.** Infections involving the nose, throat, larynx, airways, and adjacent structures are the most common causes of morbidity in the United States.

   a. Etiology. Upper respiratory infections almost invariably are viral; very rarely is a specific etiology sought or found.

   b. Clinical features. These infections are familiar to everyone as a cold or "flu" involving rhinorrhea, coryza, cough, a slight fever, and, sometimes, sore throat. During seasons when influenza is epidemic in a community, headache, cough, myalgia, and a more marked temperature elevation may suggest this diagnosis.

   c. Therapy for colds is symptomatic, although influenza virus infections may resolve more quickly when amantidine is administered.

   d. Prevention of most upper respiratory disease is very difficult due to the ubiquity and extreme infectivity of most epidemic viruses. Influenza is preventable in many cases by timely administration of vaccine developed against the epidemic strains that exist during a particular season. Immunization should be directed at individuals who are at greatest risk for complications of upper respiratory infection, such as elderly or chronically ill individuals.

2. **Pharyngitis** also is very common.

   a. Etiology. The major etiologic agents of pharyngitis are viruses, mycoplasma, and group A streptococci.

   b. Clinical features include sore throat that occurs with or without objective findings of erythema or exudate on the oropharynx or tonsils.

   c. Therapy
   (1) Although treatment for group A streptococcal pharyngitis may accelerate healing and reduce symptoms slightly, the major purpose of treating this disorder is to prevent subsequent **rheumatic fever**, a rare sequela of streptococcal pharyngitis.
   (2) Viral pharyngitis does not improve with any known chemotherapy.

3. **Tracheobronchitis** is an infection of the airways.

   a. Etiology. Most cases of tracheobronchitis are associated with infection by mycoplasma or by viruses, such as influenza or parainfluenza virus (in adults) or respiratory syncytial virus (in young children). Bacteria may play a role, however, in patients with chronic obstructive pulmonary disease (COPD). Also, *H. influenzae, S. aureus,* and *P. aeruginosa* are believed to be pathogenic in those with cystic fibrosis.

   b. Clinical features and laboratory findings. Cough with abundant, thick sputum is characteristic of tracheobronchitis. Fever, chest pain, and wheezing also may occur. If rales or consolidation is found, pneumonia is suggested. The white blood count and chest x-ray are unchanged from baseline in uncomplicated tracheobronchitis.

   c. Therapy. Simple supportive measures usually suffice. Antibiotics usually are given to patients with COPD, although their benefit is not clearly documented. Cystic fibrosis patients undergo chest physical therapy and receive antimicrobial agents appropriate to the sputum bacteriology.

4. **Pneumonia** is an infection of the alveoli, pulmonary interstitium, or both.

   a. Etiology. The causes of pneumonia are innumerable and include bacteria, viruses, fungi, and parasites. Identification of the specific cause of pneumonia, therefore, is necessary for effective treatment.

   b. Clinical features and diagnosis
   (1) Patient history may reveal an underlying condition. For example, the incidence of bacterial pneumonia is known to be increased in association with COPD or alcoholism. Fever is usually, but not invariably, present. Evidence of extra fluid in the lungs is noted as rales or consolidation on physical examination and increased absorption infiltrate on

chest x-ray. In addition to information gained from patient history, physical examination, and chest x-ray, the appearance of the sputum can help in making the appropriate diagnosis.

(2) Because of the vast differential diagnosis, it is helpful to consider pneumonia in two ways:

    (a) Whether it developed at home (**community-acquired**) or in a hospital or an institution (**hospital-acquired** or **nosocomial**)

    (b) Whether it had a rapid onset with chills, fever, and cough (**classical**) or a more indolent onset (**atypical**)

c. Pneumonia syndromes

(1) Classical community-acquired pneumonia

    (a) This syndrome most frequently is caused by *S. pneumoniae*. However, *Hemophilus* species and enteric gram-negative bacilli also can cause this clinical picture.

    (b) **Diagnosis.** Gram staining of expectorated sputum shows large numbers of neutrophils (i.e., > 25 per low-power field) and lancet-shaped gram-positive streptococci with their tapered ends pointed toward one another.

    (c) **Therapy**

        (i) When the presentation is truly classic—with a single shaking chill, rust-colored sputum, and a moderate fever accompanied by a Gram stain suggesting pneumococci—penicillin is the drug of choice. The decision whether to give oral or parenteral therapy is influenced by the severity of the illness and the need for hospitalization.

        (ii) Erythromycin is used in penicillin-allergic patients, when symptoms blend into those seen in the atypical form, or when the Gram stain is inconclusive.

        (iii) If the Gram staining reveals gram-negative rods, therapy appropriate for *Hemophilus* or enteric gram-negative bacilli is given—usually in the hospital.

(2) Atypical community-acquired pneumonia

    (a) **Etiology.** This syndrome usually is caused by *Mycoplasma pneumoniae*, although a variety of viruses may be responsible, including adenovirus, parainfluenza virus, and respiratory syncytial virus.

    (b) **Diagnosis.** Atypical community-acquired pneumonia is less severe than the classical form, with a less diagnostic sputum. Gram staining shows some neutrophils and a variety of bacterial forms. Cultures seldom are diagnostic.

    (c) **Differential diagnosis**

        (i) Pulmonary aspiration of oral secretions can lead to an **aspiration pneumonia**, especially in a setting of diminished protection of the airways (e.g., following unconsciousness, a seizure, or vocal cord paralysis).

        (ii) Tuberculosis is another consideration in a case of a slowly evolving pulmonary infection. However, there usually is other evidence of tuberculosis (e.g., radiographic findings, an exposure history, or a positive acid-fast smear of the sputum).

        (iii) Legionnaire's disease also may present in this way.

    (d) **Therapy**

        (i) Since *M. pneumoniae* is the most likely cause of atypical community-acquired pneumonia in an otherwise healthy, ambulatory adult, erythromycin is the drug of choice.

        (ii) When aspiration is suspected, treatment with high doses of penicillin or clindamycin is suggested.

        (iii) Tuberculosis always is treated with combinations of antibiotics (see section VI C 2).

        (iv) Legionnaire's disease usually responds to erythromycin, although some patients may require hospitalization for the intravenous administration of large doses.

(3) Classical (acute) hospital-acquired pneumonia

    (a) **Etiology.** This syndrome can be caused by a variety of bacteria. The patient usually is granulocytopenic, postoperative, or intubated. Because these patients usually have pharyngeal colonization by enteric gram-negative aerobes, the pneumonia is likely to involve these organisms. All risk factors should be taken into consideration when assessing these patients.

    (b) **Diagnosis.** Gram staining and culture of sputum are very important in determining the precise bacteriology of this infection. Sometimes, more invasive tests such as bronchoscopy and lung biopsy are needed to confirm the diagnosis.

    (c) **Therapy.** When the Gram stain suggests inflammation and shows abundant gram-negative rods, recommended treatment is a β-lactam antibiotic with activity against a wide variety of enteric gram-negative organisms, an aminoglycoside, or both. Knowledge of susceptibility patterns in the hospital can help in choosing empiric therapy. When culture results are available, more specific theapy can be given. In neutropenic patients, very broad coverage (including activity against *P. aeruginosa*) is used. If *Legionella* is seriously considered, erythromycin may be added.

(4) Atypical hospital-acquired pneumonia

(a) Etiology. This syndrome develops as an atypical pneumonia that was incubating prior to or during the patient's hospitalization (as in the case of seasonal pneumonia due to influenza or respiratory syncytial virus) or as a manifestation of underlying immunodeficiency. Noninfectious causes (e.g., pulmonary embolism, allergy, and vasculitis) always should be considered in this setting.

(b) Diagnosis. Conventional techniques used to diagnose infectious diseases may be unsuccessful. Cultures for influenza virus or for *Legionella* species may need to be obtained, and lung scanning or biopsy may be needed.

(c) Therapy. A specific diagnosis is extremely helpful in directing therapy. Empiric antibiotics directed at hospital-acquired bacterial pathogens (e.g., enteric gram-negative bacilli, *S. aureus*, or *Legionella*) may be used while awaiting the results of laboratory tests.

5. Lung abscess

a. Etiology. This infection may be the result of a pyogenic pneumonia caused by pathogens such as *S. aureus* or *S. pyogenes*. More commonly, however, lung abscess occurs as a late stage in the evolution of an untreated anaerobic or mixed flora (usually containing aerobes such as streptococci and anaerobes) pneumonia.

b. Clinical features. About half of the patients are afebrile, and some present with long-standing constitutional complaints such as weight loss. A foul smelling sputum is highly suggestive of anaerobic infection.

c. Therapy. Most lung abscesses drain into the tracheobronchial tree and can be cured with appropriate antimicrobial therapy, although the duration of therapy often is quite long.

6. Thoracic empyema

a. Etiology. This infection also is related to underlying pneumonia. Any pyogenic pneumonia may give rise to a pleural effusion, which may become infected. Rarely, anaerobic empyema is the only manifestation of thoracic infection; presumably this occurs as a sequela to an anaerobic pneumonia or lung abscess, which may not be apparent at the time of the empyema.

b. Therapy

(1) Noninfected effusions with a relatively low white cell count and a pH above 7.2 usually resolve with systemic antimicrobial therapy.

(2) Infected effusions, or those with a very low pH or a high white cell count, usually require thoracostomy drainage.

E. Gastrointestinal infections

1. Food poisoning syndromes represent a diverse collection of intoxications or infections associated with ingestion of food or beverage that has been contaminated with pathogenic organisms, toxins, or chemicals. Disregarding the purely chemical entities such as heavy metal poisoning, mushroom poisoning (see Chapter 5, section IV D 5 b), and polychlorinated biphenyl (PCB) poisoning, food poisoning syndromes can be divided into those causing **gastrointestinal symptoms** and those causing **neurologic symptoms**.

a. Gastrointestinal food poisoning is the most familiar type of food poisoning (see also Chapter 5, section IV D 4 and Table 5-1). Diarrhea, nausea, vomiting, and abdominal pain are the most common manifestations.

(1) Clinical categories usually are based on the incubation period, the food vehicle, and the nature of the gastrointestinal complaint.

(a) Preformed toxins give rise to the shortest onset syndromes. For example, the enterotoxin-mediated syndromes caused by staphylococci, *Bacillus cereus*, and *Clostridium perfringens* manifest within a few hours of ingestion of the contaminated food.

(b) Diseases that depend on the growth of bacteria require a period of hours to days to manifest, and it may be difficult to relate the illness to a specific exposure. Cultures of various leftovers sometimes are helpful; in other cases, a careful recall of foods consumed by the patient is diagnostic.

(2) Therapy. Almost all forms of gastrointestinal food poisoning are self-limited and remit spontaneously within 1 or 2 days.

b. Neurologic food poisoning syndromes are rare. However, it is usually critical to establish the diagnosis so that appropriate therapy can be instituted immediately.

(1) Botulism is an intoxication caused by a preformed toxin of *Clostridium botulinum*. Although the toxin is destroyed by heating, the duration or degree of heating may be inadequate to do so. Often a gastrointestinal prodrome occurs before the classic flaccid paralysis sets in.

(2) Fish poisoning. The other major category of neurologic intoxications is related to seafood (see also Chapter 5, section IV D 5).

(a) Consumption of contaminated shellfish can result in two types of poisoning—paralytic and neurotoxic.

(i) Paralytic shellfish poisoning results from contamination by neurotoxin-producing dinoflagellates of the genus, *Gonyaulax*. This syndrome includes paresthesias followed by muscle weakness.

(ii) Neurotoxic shellfish poisoning results from shellfish contamination by dinoflagellates of the genus, *Gymnodinium*. This syndrome is characterized by paresthesias without muscle weakness. Consumption of fleshy fish can give rise to a similar neurologic syndrome called **ciguatera** [see Chapter 5, section IV D 5 a (1)].

(b) Consumption of certain contaminated fish, such as tuna and bonito, can result in an illness resembling a histamine reaction. This syndrome is called **scombroid**.

(3) Monosodium glutamate intoxication (sometimes called **Chinese restaurant syndrome**) is characterized by a burning and tightness in the upper body accompanied by systemic symptoms such as flushing, diaphoresis, cramps, and nausea.

(4) Therapy. Neurologic food poisoning syndromes usually resolve completely but require patient reassurance and supportive medical care during the intoxication. Identifying the vehicle is crucial to prevent further cases. Specific antitoxin therapy is available for botulism and should be administered as soon as possible after the diagnosis is established. Supportive measures may include tracheal intubation for patients with botulism or paralytic shellfish poisoning.

2. Infectious diarrhea

a. Introduction. Acute diarrhea often can be attributed to microorganisms including bacteria, viruses, and protozoa. The occurrence of *any* infectious diarrhea suggests a break in optimal hygienic measures. The disease is transmitted either through fecal contamination of food or water or from human to human via fomites or by sexual contact.

b. Etiology. Determining the specific etiologic agent of diarrheal disease is not easy but was virtually impossible until recently. Since enterotoxigenic *E. coli* was identified as the most common agent of acute diarrhea in adults and rotavirus the most common agent of disease in young children, there has been increasing success in identifying the specific cause of diarrhea. In distinguishing among the various entities, it is useful to determine whether the diarrhea is caused by an invasive or a noninvasive agent.

c. Pathogenesis

(1) Invasive process. Certain agents of acute diarrhea invade the terminal ileum and colon, where they destroy mucosal cells and cause inflammation. The most common invasive agents are *Shigella*, *Salmonella*, *Entamoeba*, and *Campylobacter* species.

(2) Noninvasive process. Other agents of acute diarrhea are enterotoxigenic and adhere to mucosal cells in the small intestine, where they produce diarrheal toxins. The most common noninvasive agents are enterotoxigenic *E. coli*, *Vibrio cholerae* (rarely found in the United States), *G. lamblia*, and rotavirus.

d. Clinical features vary with respect to the presence of abdominal pain, cramps, and blood or mucus in the stool and to the frequency and nature of the bowel movements.

(1) Diarrhea due to invasive agents generally is associated with rectal bleeding, fever, and systemic symptoms such as headache.

(2) Diarrhea due to noninvasive agents usually occurs without fever and is associated with fewer systemic complaints.

e. Diagnosis. It is important to distinguish among the various infectious diarrheal diseases since their therapies are quite different.

(1) Microscopic examination

(a) Fecal leukocytes. A very useful test is to examine the stool for white blood cells using preparations stained with methylene blue.

(i) Invasive agents cause pus in the stool due to their destruction of mucosal cells in the distal small intestine and colon. [The diarrhea associated with *Clostridium difficile*, sometimes called **pseudomembranous colitis** (see Chapter 5, section V G), also is associated with pus in the stool as are several of the sexually transmitted proctitides and **inflammatory bowel diseases** (i.e., ulcerative colitis and regional enteritis, or Crohn's disease).]

(ii) Noninvasive agents do not cause the appearance of leukocytes in the stool.

(b) Trophozoites or cysts in the stool suggest the presence of protozoa such as *E. histolytica* or *G. lamblia*.

(2) Stool culture

(a) The presence of fever or the identification of fecal leukocytes suggests an invasive pathogen. When the clinical severity or the epidemiologic setting of the illness makes the precise diagnosis important, the stool can be cultured for the most common of these pathogens (i.e., *Shigella*, *Salmonella*, and *Campylobacter*).

  (b) Evaluation of the stool for protozoa (i.e., the **ova and parasite test**) also is recommended.

  (c) Culture or toxin assay for *C. difficile* is indicated for patients with persistent antibiotic-associated diarrhea or colitis.

  (3) Proctosigmoidoscopy may aid in the differential diagnosis of inflammation-related diarrhea.

  (4) Biopsy. In cases of persistent diarrhea where less invasive techniques have failed to provide a diagnosis, biopsy of the large bowel (for *E. histolytica*) or the small bowel (for *G. lamblia*) may be diagnostic.

f. Therapy

  (1) Fluid and electrolyte replacement is paramount, regardless of the agent of the diarrhea, and should be adjusted according to the patient's degree of depletion.

  (2) Specific antimicrobial therapy also may be necessary.

  (a) Among the bacterial causes of acute diarrhea, only *Shigella* infections are routinely treated; however, *Campylobacter*, *Salmonella*, and enterotoxigenic *E. coli* infections require antimicrobial treatment in special circumstances.

  (b) Antimicrobial agents usually are indicated for parasitic infections (e.g., giardiasis and amebiasis)

g. Prognosis. The prospect for complete recovery from infectious diarrhea is excellent for all patients except those who are severely immunocompromised. In almost all cases, a cause is not established or even investigated. All of the bacterial causes of infectious diarrhea can be followed by asymptomatic excretion for days to weeks after clinical resolution.

F. Hepatic infections

  1. Acute viral hepatitis is a serious health problem that is common throughout the world. Pathologically, the disease is characterized by necrosis of liver cells with portal and parenchymal infiltration.

  a. Etiology. Although many viruses have some effect on the liver, four specific hepatotropic viral agents have been characterized: hepatitis A virus, hepatitis B virus, non-A, non-B hepatitis virus, and delta agent.

  (1) Hepatitis A virus is an RNA virus that is transmitted by fecal contamination of food or water. Acute infection usually resolves completely.

  (2) Hepatitis B virus is a DNA virus that is transmitted by blood or intimate sexual contact. Acute infection progresses to a chronic state in about 10% of patients, with about 10% of that group developing cirrhosis, liver failure, or hepatoma.

  (3) Non-A, non-B hepatitis virus may be one or more viruses—none of which has been well characterized; transmission seems to be by blood contact. The risk of developing chronic infection is highest with this agent (about 20%–30%).

  (4) Delta agent is a defective RNA agent that can replicate only in the presence of hepatitis B virus. It can produce a syndrome of recurrent hepatitis in a hepatitis B carrier or a more severe coinfection with hepatitis B.

  (5) Other viruses that secondarily cause hepatitis-like syndromes include the Epstein-Barr virus and cytomegalovirus.

  b. Clinical features of acute viral hepatitis are similar regardless of etiology but are somewhat nonspecific symptoms such as general malaise, nausea, mild right upper quadrant pain, anorexia, and jaundice.

  c. Diagnosis

  (1) Characteristically, the laboratory findings include elevated serum levels of the transaminases [i.e., serum glutamic-oxaloacetic transaminase (SGOT) and serum glutamic-pyruvic transaminase (SGPT)] and bilirubin but normal or only slightly elevated serum alkaline phosphatase.

  (2) Because the hepatitis viruses are not grown in vitro, diagnostic tests measure the presence of viral antigens or of antibodies to these antigens.

  (a) For hepatitis A, the presence of immunoglobulin M (IgM) antibody to hepatitis A virus suggests acute infection.

  (b) For hepatitis B, the presence of hepatitis B surface antigen (HB_sAg) suggests either acute, early convalescent, or chronic infection. Antibody to hepatitis B core antigen (anti-HB_c) develops early in the clinical phase of the infection but does not signal improvement. Antibody to HB_sAg (anti-HB_s) is the final phase in the cycle and represents resolution of infection and development of immunity to hepatitis B. In chronic carriers, anti-HB_s does not develop.

  (c) Individuals with acute or chronic hepatitis B will develop antibody to delta virus if they are coinfected with the delta virus. This antibody is not an indicator of resistance or resolution.

(d) Currently, there is no antibody or antigen test for non-A, non-B hepatitis.

d. Therapy. Supportive care currently is the only therapy for acute hepatitis. Fulminant necrosis may lead to the consideration of liver transplantation.

e. Prevention. Since no specific therapy has been documented to improve the clinical course of viral hepatitis, prevention assumes great importance. Avoiding contact with infectious materials such as food and water (in the case of hepatitis A) or blood and body fluids (in the case of hepatitis B) is recommended. Passive immunization is available after a known exposure to hepatitis A (immune serum globulin) or hepatitis B (hepatitis B immune globulin). Active immunization also is available for individuals who are at relatively high risk for exposure to hepatitis B (e.g., intravenous drug users, homosexual men, and health care workers).

f. Complications. The most serious complication of acute viral hepatitis is **fulminant hepatitis**. This condition is characterized by progressive jaundice, hepatic encephalopathy, and ascites. Fulminant hepatitis develops in only rare cases of hepatitis A and in 1%–2% of cases of hepatitis B and non-A, non-B hepatitis. It is a more common complication of delta hepatitis; approximately one-third of cases of fulminant hepatitis follow delta hepatitis (See Chapter 5, section IX A 1 f for further discussion of complications of acute viral hepatitis.)

2. Chronic active hepatitis is a persistence of HB_sAg for longer than 20 weeks, accompanied by histologic evidence of inflammation, necrosis, or fibrosis. This may progress to cirrhosis or hepatoma after many years.

3. Chronic persistent hepatitis is twice as common as chronic active hepatitis and is characterized by mildly elevated transaminases and continued HB_sAg positivity for more than 20 weeks. Liver biopsy shows no or only minimal abnormalities.

4. Hepatic abscess (see section V G 3)

G. Intra-abdominal infections

1. Peritonitis is an inflammation of the lining of the abdominal cavity, which may result from bacterial infection or chemical irritation. Bacterial peritonitis that occurs without other abdominal disease is described as **primary** (spontaneous) **peritonitis**; when it occurs after rupture or perforation of a hollow organ it is said to be **secondary peritonitis**. It is crucial to distinguish between primary and secondary peritonitis since a ruptured viscus requires surgical repair.

a. Primary peritonitis

(1) **Etiology.** Primary peritonitis occurs at all ages and almost always is preceded by **ascites**.

(a) **In children**, primary peritonitis historically has been seen most often in association with **nephrotic syndrome** and ascites. The causative organisms usually are streptococci, pneumococci, and enteric gram-negative bacteria.

(b) **In adults**, primary peritonitis usually develops in the setting of **hepatic cirrhosis** and ascites. The causative organism most often is an enteric pathogen—usually *E. coli*. Enterococci and pneumococci also are seen.

(2) **Clinical features** include abdominal pain and distention, rebound tenderness, nausea, vomiting, fever, and hypotension.

(3) **Diagnosis.** Paracentesis of peritoneal fluid, with smear and culture for appropriate bacteria, is needed for the diagnosis. In some cases, however, exploratory laparotomy is required to rule out secondary peritonitis.

(4) **Therapy.** Systemic antibiotics are necessary for the treatment of primary peritonitis. If the Gram stain does not show a characteristic organism, empiric therapy for *E. coli*, *Klebsiella pneumoniae*, and pneumococci should be started. Because patients with advanced liver disease may be fragile, the mortality rate even in appropriately treated patients may be 20%.

b. Secondary peritonitis

(1) **Etiology.** The causes of secondary peritonitis are many, but the process is the same in most cases. Usually, enteric pathogens gain access to the abdominal cavity through a tear or necrotic defect of an abdominal organ. Common examples include ruptured appendix and perforated peptic ulcer. In most cases the infection is polymicrobial, and the causative agents are endogenous organisms.

(2) **Clinical features.** The early symptoms of secondary peritonitis are similar to those of spontaneous peritonitis. Abdominal pain combined with nausea and vomiting as well as fever are common complaints. Tachycardia and shock may develop.

(3) Diagnosis
   (a) Diagnosis may be difficult in patients who do not present with the above-mentioned symptoms, such as individuals on corticosteroid therapy. A high index of suspicion is necessary in these cases.
   (b) The single most important laboratory finding in secondary peritonitis is the presence of free air in the abdomen, as determined by chest or abdominal x-ray. Careful and repeated observation and consultation with a general surgeon will help to distinguish surgically remediable disease from mimicking conditions.
(4) Therapy. In most cases, surgical repair of the damaged viscus and drainage of abdominal pus are the cornerstones of therapy. Antibiotics with activity against enteric gram-negative bacilli and anaerobes (especially *B. fragilis*) also are important. The need for coverage of enterococci is controversial.
c. Peritonitis and peritoneal dialysis. Peritonitis is a frequent complication of peritoneal dialysis, whether it is performed acutely or on a chronic basis. Ordinarily, the dialysis need not be interrupted, and systemic or peritoneally administered antibiotics can be used for treatment.

2. Postoperative intra-abdominal abscesses often are difficult to diagnose.
   a. Etiology and pathogenesis
      (1) Postoperative abscesses develop most frequently when the bowel has been breached in the operative procedure; however, they may occur when nonviable tissue or accumulations of blood, serum, urine, or bile are present in the abdominal cavity.
      (2) Traditionally, these infections occur within several days of the operative procedure, but they may be delayed by weeks or months. Also, they tend to develop near the anatomic site of the surgery, although the contour of the abdomen may allow infected fluid to move to other locations.
   b. Diagnosis. CT and ultrasonography are the most commonly used techniques for locating these abscesses. Most importantly, there must be a high index of suspicion for patients who present with prolonged fever, abdominal pain, or both after surgery.
   c. Therapy. Once intra-abdominal abscesses have been identified they should be evacuated, either by repeat surgery or via a temporary flexible drainage catheter. Antimicrobial therapy should be administered based on the results of Gram staining and cultures. Therapy directed toward anaerobes should be considered if the fluid is foul smelling or if the Gram stain suggests a polymicrobial flora.

3. Hepatic abscess
   a. Etiology and pathogenesis. Although the liver is relatively protected from infection, bacterial (pyogenic) abscesses may develop. These may be single or multiple and often are multibacterial. Hepatic abscesses may develop due to infection or obstruction of the gallbladder or biliary tree. Bacteremia via the portal or systemic circulation also may cause hepatic abscesses.
   b. Clinical features. Although they commonly present as pain and tenderness in the hepatic region accompanied by fever and chills, hepatic abscesses also can be occult and be discovered as a source of fever of unknown origin or as a source of unexplained persistent bacteremia.
   c. Diagnosis usually is made by ultrasonography or CT scanning. Nuclear medicine scanning, such as liver/spleen or gallium scanning, can be helpful. Some diagnoses are made at laparotomy.
   d. Therapy requires drainage, most often by the open surgical route, although catheter drainage of a single hepatic abscess is an alternative approach. Antibiotic therapy is a mandatory adjunct to surgical drainage.

4. Splenic abscess
   a. Etiology and pathogenesis. Like hepatic abscesses, splenic abscesses occur infrequently. When they do develop, they usually are multiple, small, and silent manifestations of disease or infection somewhere else. Solitary splenic abscesses are less common but are more apt to be clinically evident. These usually occur in the setting of systemic bacteremia, hemoglobinopathy, splenic trauma, or intravenous drug use.
   b. Clinical features. Common symptoms include fever, pain, and tenderness in the left upper abdomen as well as splenomegaly. As noted above, symptoms may be reduced or absent in patients with multiple small abscesses.
   c. Diagnosis. CT, gallium, and liver/spleen scanning as well as ultrasonography can be used diagnostically. Blood cultures should always be obtained.
   d. Therapy should begin with broad-spectrum antibiotics and, if a specific agent can be identified, should be adjusted accordingly. Surgical drainage or splenectomy often is necessary, especially when the abscess is large and accompanied by bacteremia.

5. Cholecystitis and cholangitis are inflammatory diseases of the gallbladder and biliary tree, respectively.

    a. Cholecystitis (see also Chapter 5, section VIII B and C) is a very common medical problem.

        (1) Etiology and pathogenesis. Infection need not be present nor a very prominent feature of cholecystitis. In most cases, obstruction of the gallbladder is found, and the bile—normally sterile—may be colonized by bacteria such as *E. coli, K. pneumoniae,* or enterococci.

        (2) Clinical features include right upper abdominal pain, anorexia, nausea, vomiting, and low-grade fever with chills.

        (3) Diagnosis is made on the basis of the clinical presentation described above and evidence of gallstones or gallbladder dysfunction as demonstrated by ultrasonography or cholecystography.

        (4) Therapy. Cholecystitis usually is treated adequately with conservative measures. Cholecystectomy is recommended for recurrent disease, rupture, or empyema of the gallbladder.

    b. Cholangitis (see also Chapter 5, section VIII G) is a more serious problem than cholecystitis.

        (1) Etiology and pathogenesis. Cholangitis tends to occur with obstruction of the intrahepatic or common bile duct (usually by gallstones). Bacterial colonization (most often with *E. coli*) in this setting usually leads to infection.

        (2) Clinical features are similar to but more severe than those for cholecystitis and include right upper abdominal pain, high fever with shaking chills, and jaundice (**Charcot's triad**)—often in the setting of gallbladder disease.

        (3) Diagnosis is based on the characteristic presentation of Charcot's triad and the finding of moderate-to-severe leukocytosis with elevated serum bilirubin and alkaline phosphatase. Bacteremia is also commonly found.

        (4) Therapy usually consists of antimicrobial agents active against enteric organisms combined with decompressive surgery.

6. Appendicitis

    a. Incidence, etiology, and pathogenesis. Appendicitis is a disease that may occur at any age, with a peak incidence between the second and third decades. The pathologic process most often begins with obstruction (usually by a calculus or fecalith) and progresses to inflammation with possible perforation. Infection occurs late—around the time of rupture—and usually involves both aerobic and anaerobic fecal flora.

    b. Clinical features and laboratory data. The classic presentation is that of acute, right lower quadrant pain, anorexia, and fever. Tenderness on palpation also is very common and, when the appendix is normally located, is noted at **McBurney's point**. Moderate leukocytosis is common; severe leukocytosis suggests perforation.

    c. Differential diagnosis. The diagnosis may not be clear from the clinical information; therefore, many other illnesses should be considered. A few examples include pancreatitis, perforated ulcer, acute pelvic inflammatory disease, acute gastroenteritis, kidney stones, and ruptured corpus luteum cyst.

    d. Therapy. Since surgery is mandatory for appendicitis, prompt evaluation is important. Uncomplicated cases do not require antimicrobial therapy. However, in the case of appendiceal rupture with resultant peritonitis, appropriate antibiotics are indicated as a supplement to surgery.

H. Genital infections and sexually transmitted diseases

1. Urethritis

    a. Incidence. Urethritis is a common problem that occurs almost exclusively in sexually active individuals and is more common in men than in women.

    b. Etiology. Urethritis is classified as **gonococcal** or **nongonococcal**.

        (1) Gonococcal urethritis is caused by *N. gonorrhoeae.* In almost all cases of gonococcal urethritis, Gram staining of the urethral discharge shows gram-negative intracellular diplococci.

        (2) Nongonococcal urethritis is caused by *C. trachomatis, U. urealyticum,* or some other, yet unidentified agent. (In 25% of cases of gonococcal urethritis, one of these organisms also is present and patients may have recurrent symptoms after penicillin therapy for gonorrhea.)

    c. Clinical features

        (1) Dysuria is noted in most cases of urethritis, whether gonococcal or nongonococcal.

        (2) Urethral discharge is noted more frequently by men than by women and may be purulent (usually in gonococcal disease) or cloudy and mucoid (usually in nongonococcal disease).

d. Therapy

(1) Patients with proven gonococcal urethritis are best treated with a single dose of penicillin, ampicillin, or amoxicillin (for gonococcal infection). When penicillin resistance is anticipated, spectinomycin or ceftriaxone is suggested. Some authorities recommend a 7-day course of tetracycline to replace or follow penicillin or amoxicillin for potentially concurrent chlamydial or ureaplasmal infection.

(2) Nongonococcal urethritis is best treated with a 7-day course of tetracycline. Chlamydial and ureaplasmal infections also are treated effectively with erythromycin.

2. Pelvic inflammatory disease refers to a complex of infections involving the uterus, fallopian tubes, or ligaments of the uterus.

a. Etiology.

(1) *N. gonorrhoeae, C. trachomatis,* or a mixture of pelvic anaerobes may be involved, although it is difficult to determine which of these is responsible when instituting therapy.

(2) The presence of an intrauterine device (IUD) may predispose to pelvic inflammatory disease.

b. Clinical features and laboratory findings. The symptoms may be contemporaneous with menstruation and usually consist of lower abdominal or pelvic pain and tenderness on palpation of the cervix, uterus, or adnexae; fever is not necessarily a significant feature. A cervical discharge or pelvic mass may be present, and the white cell count may be normal or elevated.

c. Diagnosis

(1) It is important to obtain cultures for *N. gonorrhoeae.* If there is fluid in the retrouterine cul-de-sac, culdocentesis can be performed and may help to sort out the possible causes.

(2) Ultrasonography of the pelvis may demonstrate an adnexal mass or abscess, which should be followed carefully.

d. Therapy. No simple therapy is effective in all cases of pelvic inflammatory disease. Hospitalization is suggested when pain is incapacitating or when parenteral therapy is given. Examples of treatment regimens include doxycycline plus cefoxitin and clindamycin plus gentamicin.

e. Complications. The most serious long-term complications of pelvic inflammatory disease are infertility, ectopic pregnancy, and the need for hysterectomy.

3. Infectious proctitis is an inflammation of the rectal mucosa.

a. Etiology. Infectious proctitis can be caused by a variety of microorganisms. When anal sex is practiced, gonorrhea, syphilis, chlamydial infection, and herpes should be considered. When there is no history of anal sex, shigellosis and amebiasis are more likely causes.

b. Clinical features and diagnosis. Proctalgia, a change in bowel habits, and a mucoid or bloody anal discharge between bowel movements suggest this problem. A sexual history should be obtained to aid in the diagnosis, and appropriate diagnostic studies (e.g., sigmoidoscopy, culture and Gram staining of discharge, and biopsy) should be performed.

c. Therapy. When specific agents of infectious proctitis can be identified, appropriate antibiotic treatment should be administered. In general, the same regimens used to treat these pathogens in other body sites are effective in proctitis. For gonorrheal proctitis, however, cure rates are lower than for gonorrheal urethritis, and post-therapy cultures should be obtained.

4. Syndromes of genital ulcers and lymphadenopathy

a. Incidence. Ulcerative lesions of the genitalia are common outpatient problems. Men are more commonly affected by these entities than women.

b. Etiology. There are many causes, which vary in different parts of the world. In the United States, **genital herpes** is the most common cause of genital ulcers, followed by **syphilis.** Other causes include **lymphogranuloma venereum (LGV), chancroid,** and **granuloma inguinale (donavanosis)**—all of which are uncommon in the United States. (Gonorrhea is one sexually transmitted disease that **does not** cause genital ulcer syndromes.)

c. Clinical features (Table 8-2)

(1) Genital herpes initially presents as itching and soreness followed by the appearance of erythema and, eventually, the development of herpetic vesicles.

(2) Syphilis, in its primary form, presents as a painless, often solitary, chancre (ulcer) with a hard, indurated base.

(3) LGV presents as nodes that are disproportionately large as compared to the ulcer. There often is a depression between the inguinal and femoral nodes (the **groove sign**).

(4) Chancroid is characterized by multiple, painful ulcers with ragged, undermined edges and suppurative inguinal nodes.

Table 8-2. Syndromes of Genital Ulcers and Lymphadenopathy

Disease	Causative Organism	Diagnostic Tests	Clinical Findings	Therapy
Genital herpes	Herpes simplex virus	Tzanck test; culture	Lesion—usually solitary; indurated; painless Nodes—rubbery; not fluctuant	None; acyclovir
Syphilis	Treponema pallidum	Darkfield microscopy; RPR* test	Lesion—multiple; vesiculopustular; painful Nodes—firm; tender	Penicillin; tetracycline
Lymphogranuloma venereum	Chlamydia trachomatis	Culture; serologic examination	Lesion—small papule or vesicle Nodes—large; suppurative; both sides of inguinal ligament affected (groove sign)	Tetracycline; erythromycin
Chancroid	Hemophilus ducreyi	Gram stain; culture (special media needed)	Lesion—ragged; soft; dirty looking Nodes—tender; suppurative	Erythromycin; ceftriaxone; trimethoprim-sulfamethoxazole
Granuloma inguinale	Calymmatobacterium granulomatis	Biopsy with Giemsa or Wright's stain	Lesion—large; slowly advancing; rolled edges; not indurated Nodes—not prominent	Tetracycline; trimethoprim-sulfamethoxazole

*RPR = rapid plasma reagin.

(5) Granuloma inguinale is a more indolent infection characterized by a painless, beefy-red lesion with ragged edges and less prominent adenopathy.

   d. Diagnosis

   (1) When a genital ulcer is noted, a **Tzanck test** and **darkfield examination** should be performed for herpes and syphilis, respectively. All patients should undergo serologic testing for syphilis regardless of the results of these smears.

   (2) LGV should be suspected on the basis of the above-mentioned clinical picture in any patient with known exposure to *C. trachomatis*. The diagnosis is confirmed by isolation of *C. trachomatis* from pus in the inguinal nodes or by finding antibodies to *C. trachomatis* in the blood.

   (3) Chancroid is diagnosed by elimination of other causes of genital ulcers and isolation of *Hemophilus ducreyi* from the ulcers or suppurative nodes. However, *H. ducreyi* can be very difficult to grow in culture even under optimal conditions.

   (4) The diagnosis of granuloma inguinale is confirmed by demonstration of Donovan bodies in edge scrapings prepared with Giemsa or Wright's stain.

   e. Therapy. Identification and treatment of sexual contacts is always desirable.

   (1) Herpes infections are self-limited but recurrent. Acyclovir may shorten the course and reduce symptoms, but it does not affect the natural history of these infections.

   (2) Syphilis is treated with varying schedules of penicillin, depending on the stage. Tetracycline is an alternative for penicillin-allergic patients.

   (3) LGV is treated with tetracycline or erythromycin.

   (4) Chancroid is treated with erythromycin, ceftriaxone, or trimethoprim-sulfamethoxazole.

   (5) Granuloma inguinale is treated with tetracycline or trimethoprim-sulfamethoxazole.

I. Urinary tract infections (see also Chapter 6, Part I: section X)

   1. Incidence. These are the most common bacterial infections encountered in clinical practice. Outside the geriatric population, urinary tract infections occur much more frequently in women than in men. It is estimated that 20% of women have at least one of these infections in their lifetime.

   2. Etiology. Most urinary tract infections are caused by gram-negative bacteria, including *E. coli* (most commonly), *Klebsiella* species, and *Proteus* species. Less common causes include gram-positive cocci such as *Staphylococcus* species (especially *Staphylococcus saprophyticus*) and enterococci.

   3. Clinical features. It is useful to distinguish whether the infection involves the kidneys or the renal pelvis (**upper tract infection**) or is confined to the bladder, urethra, and prostate gland (**lower tract infection**).

   a. In general, symptomatic urinary tract infections, whether upper or lower, are characterized by the irritative symptoms of urinary frequency, urgency, and pain. Flank pain and fever suggest upper tract involvement.

   b. The composition of the urinary sediment is the same in both types of urinary infections and is characterized by a large number of neutrophils and a variable number of red cells. White cell casts may be noted in true upper tract infections.

   c. Quantitative urine cultures do not distinguish between upper and lower tract infections.

   4. Clinical syndromes

   a. There is standard agreement that a bacterial count exceeding 10^5 organisms/ml of urine combined with irritative voiding symptoms and pyuria indicate significant disease, not simple contamination. However, there are two clinically important situations that are not covered by this definition of urinary tract infections.

   (1) The first category—termed the **urethral syndrome**—includes patients with symptoms of true urinary tract infection but with fewer than the significant number of bacteria in the urine (i.e., 10^5/ml) as well as patients with illnesses that masquerade as urinary tract infection (e.g., vaginitis and chlamydial urethritis).

   (2) The second category—termed **asymptomatic bacteriuria**—includes patients with no symptoms of urinary tract infection but a urine bacterial count exceeding 10^5/ml. This condition is not rare and occurs most often in women and in older patients.

   b. Catheter-related infections. Bacteriuria is an inevitable concomitant of prolonged bladder catheterization. This can be delayed by careful aseptic insertion and strict closed drainage, but after 1 or 2 weeks some degree of colonization is extremely common, which ultimately progresses to bacterial counts exceeding 10^5/ml of urine.

   5. Diagnosis

   a. Diagnostic tests seldom are needed to make a decision to treat a patient with symptoms of urinary infection and an abnormal urinary sediment. In patients with previous infections or other risk factors, urine culture can be helpful.

    b. Special tests are available in research settings for distinguishing upper from lower tract infections. These include the **Fairley bladder washout technique**—an invasive and complex procedure—and the **antibody-coated bacteria test**—a noninvasive but technically difficult procedure.

    c. There is controversy concerning when to examine a patient for anatomic abnormalities as an explanation for urinary tract infections. Most evidence suggests that cystoscopy and urography seldom reveal treatable causes of infection and should be reserved for patients with frequent recurrences and jeopardized kidney function.

    d. When blood cultures are positive in the context of a urinary tract infection, involvement of the kidneys or prostate gland is implied. Fever also suggests upper tract involvement.

6. Therapy usually is directed at the agent most likely to be responsible for the infection.

    a. *E. coli* has a propensity for causing infections in otherwise healthy individuals. Thus, in the absence of cultures, antibiotics effective against *E. coli* (e.g., ampicillin or a sulfonamide) should be given.

        (1) A single dose is adequate to cure most infections in the lower tract, where urine levels of drug seem to be the most important determinant of effectiveness.

        (2) Failure to cure upper tract infections rapidly does not alter the efficacy of future therapy. Established upper tract infection may require a long course of therapy—sometimes up to several months—although briefer courses (i.e., 2 weeks) often are successful.

    b. The therapeutic approach to **asymptomatic bacteriuria** is debated. However, treatment is indicated for patients with a known structural or functional abnormality of the kidneys and for pregnant patients.

    c. Catheter-related bacteriuria may be delayed by systemic or topical antibiotics, although, when they occur, these infections are more likely to be caused by antibiotic-resistant bacteria or yeast. The use of frequent bladder catheterizations (several times daily) rather than an indwelling catheter may lessen the risk of these infections. This approach has been most effective in paraplegic patients who otherwise would require prolonged bladder drainage through an indwelling catheter.

J. Skin and soft tissue infections. Bacterial, fungal, and viral infections of the skin and related structures (e.g., hair follicles and sweat glands) are very common.

    1. Bacterial skin infections usually start in areas of trauma or previous disease.

    a. Etiology. In otherwise healthy individuals, gram-positive cocci such as *S. pyogenes* and *S. aureus* cause most skin infections. Immunocompromised individuals are subject to a wider variety of pathogens, including enteric gram-negative bacilli and *P. aeruginosa*.

    b. Clinical features. There are three major forms of bacterial skin infection—**cellulitis, abscess,** and **ulcer.**

        (1) Cellulitis is characterized by redness, warmth, and tenderness of the skin. It may involve a limited area or may spread widely and rapidly. Any part of the body can be affected. Fever and leukocytosis are common.

        (2) Abscesses represent deeper, circumscribed infections, which often start in accessory structures such as hair follicles. They may be warm or of normal skin temperature and frequently contain pus. Fever is most likely to be present in cases of large, multiple, or deep abscesses.

        (3) Ulcers are not usually the result of bacterial infection alone but reflect tissue damage from ischemia or trauma. Invariably, ulcers are colonized by bacteria and may lead to deep soft tissue or bone infection. They usually occur in dependent areas (e.g., the sacrum) or in areas of poor blood flow (such as may occur in the foot of a diabetic).

    c. Therapy

        (1) Cellulitis requires antibiotic management. Agents active against streptococci and staphylococci usually are effective, including semisynthetic penicillins (e.g., nafcillin), cephalosporins, and clindamycin.

        (2) Large abscesses must be drained; small abscesses may drain spontaneously or simply resolve. Antibiotics usually are not needed but may be useful if there is accompanying cellulitis.

        (3) Skin ulcers usually are managed by debridement and empiric antibiotic therapy with agents active against enteric gram-negative rods and anaerobes. Skin grafting may be beneficial.

    2. Fungal skin infections usually are acquired by exposure of the skin to pathogenic fungi. Exceptions are cutaneous manifestations of blastomycosis or of candidal fungemia.

    a. Clinical features. Clinically, fungal infections fall into three groups, each with a different etiology.

        (1) Dermatophytosis is a superficial infection of the epidermis due to dermatophytic fungi (i.e., *Trichophyton*, *Microsporum*, and *Epidermophyton* species). Athlete's foot and ringworm are examples. The skin usually is flaky and may be slightly discolored but is not frankly painful.

(2) **Candidiasis** is a red, tender edematous rash occurring in moist body parts due to *C. albicans*. Intertrigo is an example.

(3) **Mixed bacterial flora and fungi** (usually *Candida* species) can be involved in superficial infection. This may be evident during or after administration of antibacterial therapy.

b. Diagnosis of all fungal infections rests on potassium hydroxide preparations and fungal cultures.

c. Therapy

(1) Dermatophytoses are treated either topically, with antifungal agents such as clotrimazole, or with systemic griseofulvin or ketoconazole for infection that is widespread, refractory to topical agents, or disfiguring.

(2) Candidiasis also is treated topically, but special attention also should be given to keeping the affected area clean and dry. Oral ketoconazole is used in severe cases.

(3) Mixed bacterial/fungal infections usually do not require specific antifungal therapy.

3. **Viral skin infections** may be cutaneously inoculated, as in the case of herpes simplex, but more commonly are a manifestation of systemic viral infection or an immune response to infection. An example of this is **varicella (chicken pox)**, in which the virus is acquired via the respiratory tract and spreads to the skin following a viremia.

4. **Deep soft tissue infections**

   a. Gangrene is an infection of the skin and soft tissues caused by *Clostridium perfringens* and related species. It is characterized by cellulitis and gas in the soft tissues. Therapy is surgical debridement and an antibiotic (e.g., penicillin).

   b. Fasciitis is a rare infection of subdermal tissue planes. It usually occurs postoperatively or after rupture of an abdominal viscus and has a propensity for diabetic patients. The bacteriology is one of mixed anaerobes, streptococci, and, occasionally, gram-negative bacilli.

K. Joint infections

1. **Bacterial (pyogenic) arthritis** is an acute process that occurs in a joint following infection by any one of several microorganisms. Patients receiving intra-articular corticosteroids and patients with existing joint disease (e.g., rheumatoid arthritis) appear to be predisposed to bacterial arthritis.

   a. Etiology. The most common bacterial causes of infectious arthritis are *N. gonorrhoeae*, *S. aureus*, and streptococci. In addition, gram-negative bacilli are common agents of infectious arthritis in hospitalized or debilitated patients, and *Pseudomonas aeruginosa* is the most likely cause in intravenous drug users.

   b. Clinical features

   (1) Bacterial arthritis usually presents as an acute, single-joint (monoarticular) arthritis—most often involving the knee or another large joint. Patients commonly complain of fever and joint symptoms including pain, swelling, redness, and decreased movement.

   (2) The combined findings of tenosynovitis and a characteristic sparse vesicopustular skin rash suggest **disseminated gonococcal infection**.

   c. Differential diagnosis. Although the clinical setting of an acute monoarticular arthritis usually suggests bacterial arthritis, another entity that must be considered is **crystal-induced disease**, such as **gout** or **pseudogout** (see Chapter 10, section II A and II B).

   d. Diagnosis

   (1) The diagnosis of bacterial arthritis is based on aspiration of joint (synovial) fluid and examination for microorganisms on Gram stain and for crystals with a polarizing microscope. Samples for culture should be sent even when the Gram stain is negative.

   (2) In many cases of gonococcal arthritis, cultures from skin lesions or joint fluid are negative; however, gonococci can be cultured from other body sites (e.g., the cervix).

   e. Therapy for all bacterial arthritis involves removal of the inflammatory material—either by repeated aspiration or by surgical drainage—and administration of systemic antibiotics effective against the causative organism. The course of drug therapy should be prolonged (at least 4–6 weeks) for staphylococcal and gram-negative infections. Streptococcal septic arthritis requires only 2 weeks of therapy. In the special case of gonococcal arthritis, the response to appropriate therapy (i.e., penicillin) is rapid and therapy need only be carried out for 7–10 days; there seldom is any long-term impairment.

2. **Prosthetic joint infections** occur in less than 5% of all replaced joints and may be difficult to recognize because they can occur months to years after surgery. The bacteriology is dominated by skin flora such as *S. epidermidis*, *S. aureus*, and diphtheroids. The major clinical finding is joint pain, perhaps with some loosening of the prosthesis.

L. Osteomyelitis. Bone infections can be classified according to their pathogenesis. In general, infections of bone develop in three ways: by extension from a contiguous infection; by direct inoculation during surgery or as a result of trauma; and by hematogenous spread.

1. Osteomyelitis due to contiguous infection or inoculation. Bone infection should be suspected in a patient with a history of **trauma** or **surgery** or with obvious **soft tissue infection** overlying bone, although the bone involvement may be difficult to prove.

a. Etiology. Almost any bacterium can be responsible, including *S. aureus, P. aeruginosa*, or anaerobes.

b. Clinical features may simply be those of the adjacent infection. Pain is common, and fever is variable.

c. Diagnosis may be difficult. Radiographic evidence of osteomyelitis lags behind the symptoms and pathologic changes by about 7 to 10 days. Also, although bone scanning is very sensitive for osteomyelitis, it cannot distinguish bone infection from more superficial soft tissue infection. The definitive diagnosis rests on bone biopsy and bacterial culture.

d. Clinical course and therapy. The clinical course guides the length of treatment, but generally long courses of antibiotics are needed. Devitalized bone, poor blood supply, and adjacent infection may explain why months of treatment are required.

2. Hematogenous osteomyelitis should be suspected in a febrile patient who experiences pain and swelling over a bone but has no obvious source of infection.

a. Etiology. The bacteriology of this disease is largely *S. aureus*. However, *Salmonella* species seem to be more important in patients with sickle cell disease. Vertebral osteomyelitis also is somewhat different in that gram-negative bacilli may be introduced from the urinary tract via venous channels.

b. Diagnosis. Radiography and bone scanning are helpful. The erythrocyte sedimentation rate usually is elevated. Bone aspiration and culture are recommended for microbiologic diagnosis. Blood cultures also should be obtained.

c. Therapy. The treatment is a prolonged course of antibiotics. Nonviable bone may need to be removed surgically as it provides a site for potential relapse.

M. Intravascular infections and endocarditis. Intravascular infections manifest as **viremia, bacteremia, fungemia,** or **parasitemia,** depending on the type of infective organism demonstrated in the blood. Such infections may reflect **invasion or failure of containment at a localized site** (e.g., the bowel or lung) or a **primary infection of the blood vessels or the heart** (e.g., endocarditis).

1. Local infections lead to positive blood cultures with a frequency dependent on the site and severity of the infection and on the organism or organisms responsible for the infection.

a. For example, among hospitalized patients with pneumococcal pneumonia, 10%–25% have bacteremia. The prognosis for these patients is worse than for those without bacteremia, as the bacteremic patients tend to have more diffuse lung involvement and more virulent organisms.

b. Even when blood cultures are not positive, there may be evidence of blood-borne dissemination in the distribution of metastatic infection. Cryptococcal meningitis is believed to have a fungemic phase based on the observation that the yeast enters the body through the lungs and there is no other communication between the lungs and the meninges.

2. Septic shock is a commonly recognized clinical entity defined as a systemic infection accompanied by hypotension that is not explained by hypovolemia or intrinsic cardiac disease. In most cases, blood cultures are positive during these episodes.

a. Septic shock sometimes is called **gram-negative sepsis** based on the observation that the bacteria most frequently responsible are gram-negative enteric bacilli. It has been postulated that **endotoxin** (the lipopolysaccharide coat of gram-negative organisms) is the cause. However, an indistinguishable clinical disease can be caused by gram-positive bacteria, viruses, and yeast.

b. Antibiotic therapy is critical for patient recovery. High-dose corticosteroid therapy to supplement usual supportive measures is controversial and currently is not thought to improve survival.

3. Catheter-related infections are serious problems associated with hospitalization. Infection seldom is caused by the infusion of contaminated fluid. Rather, these infections most commonly occur at the site of cannulation.

a. Diagnosis is made by demonstrating either local skin infection at the cannulation site or positive blood cultures and the presence of the same bacteria in significant numbers on a semiquantitative culture of the catheter.

b. Therapy requires removing the catheter when local infection is present. When vascular access is crucial and the catheter has been aseptically inserted into the vena cava (e.g., a

Hickman catheter—a wide-bore catheter used for hyperalimentation, chemotherapy, or for drawing blood), conservative therapy with antibiotics alone may cure the infection. Fungal infections cannot be cured without removal of the catheter.

4. **Vascular graft infection** is one of the most serious consequences of vascular surgery. Although native blood vessels may become infected in atherosclerotic processes or in pyogenic processes involving the arterial wall itself (**mycotic aneurysm**), these events are very rare. When arteries are bypassed because of arterial insufficiency or for hemodialysis vascular access, the surgical site can become infected.

    a. **Diagnosis** rests on finding consistently positive blood cultures in a patient with such a graft. In chronic infections, immunologic disease may manifest as an elevated erythrocyte sedimentation rate, abnormal urinary sediment, and positive blood tests for circulating immune complexes.

    b. **Therapy.** The best chance of cure is with removal of the entire prosthetic device. When this is not possible, revascularization—circumventing the site of infection—can be tried. Antibiotic therapy alone cannot assure a positive outcome and must be carried out for at least 6 weeks.

5. **Endocarditis** usually results from infection of the cusp of a heart valve, although any part of the endocardium or any prosthetic material inserted into the heart may be involved.

    a. **Etiology.** A variety of organisms may cause endocarditis, although bacteria account for almost all cases. The specific agent of endocarditis depends on which cardiac structures are affected.

        (1) **Infection of normal valves** is rare and usually associated with intravenous drug use. *S. aureus* is the most common pathogen.

        (2) **Infection of previously damaged valves** usually is due to viridans streptococci. The other agents of endocarditis in this setting are enterococci, *S. aureus*, and various small gram-negative rods comprising part of the normal oral flora.

        (3) **Infection of prosthetic valves.** Staphylococci (both coagulase-positive and coagulase-negative) are the most common agents of early-onset disease (occurring < 2 months postoperatively), and streptococci are the most common agents of late-onset disease (occurring > 2 months postoperatively).

    b. **Clinical features** vary widely.

        (1) Common findings include **fever**, which is almost universal, and a **heart murmur**.

        (2) Less commonly there is evidence of **embolic disease**, such as stroke or splenic artery embolism and infarction. Most emboli are very small and may give rise to uncommon but diagnostically helpful physical findings including **Roth's spots**, **Osler's nodes**, **Janeway lesions**, and **conjunctival hemorrhage**.

    c. **Diagnosis**

        (1) Blood cultures are critical and are positive in more than 90% of cases of endocarditis. (Previous use of antibiotics may lower this figure.) Because of the continuous bacteremia of endocarditis, virtually all cultures are positive and so it is rarely necessary to obtain more than three or four cultures.

        (2) In the few patients with culture-negative endocarditis, obtaining many cultures is of little value. The microbiology laboratory should be alerted to the possibility of endocarditis in these patients so special culture techniques can be instituted.

    d. **Therapy** for endocarditis has been carefully studied. When untreated, this infection is almost uniformly fatal.

        (1) Antibiotic therapy alone provides an excellent chance of cure for streptococcal disease on a native valve and for staphylococcal disease on the tricuspid valve. The key is to provide an adequate dosage for a long enough period of time—usually 2 to 6 weeks, depending on the organism.

        (2) In medical failures, valve replacement may be a necessary adjunct to antibiotic therapy. Other indications for valve surgery include:

            (a) Fungal endocarditis (an absolute indication)

            (b) Congestive heart failure

            (c) Recurrent major emboli

            (d) Inability to provide a full course of antibiotic therapy

            (e) Inability to sterilize the blood after 10–14 days

        (3) In general, prosthetic valve disease is more difficult to treat medically or surgically.

VI. OTHER INFECTIOUS DISEASES AND SYNDROMES

  A. **Infections associated with adenopathy and splenomegaly.** Syndromes of adenopathy (both local and general), splenomegaly, and fever are common medical problems. The differential diagnosis should include tumors, rheumatic diseases, and vasculitis as well as specific infectious processes.

1. Generalized lymphadenopathy and fatigue are the classic signs of **infectious mononucleosis**.
   a. Mononucleosis most commonly is caused by the **Epstein-Barr virus** and is associated with splenomegaly, pharyngitis, and an atypical lymphocytosis.
   b. Cytomegalovirus causes a mononucleosis syndrome that is virtually indistinguishable from Epstein-Barr virus–induced mononucleosis.
      (1) Both infections tend to occur in adolescents and young adults and may be subclinical.
      (2) They are distinguished by serologic tests such as the **Monospot test**, which usually demonstrates the presence of heterophile antibody in Epstein-Barr virus infection and the absence of heterophile antibody in cytomegalovirus infection.
      (3) Specific antibodies for the two viruses also are available and can confirm the diagnosis in equivocal cases.
   c. Some cases of mononucleosis are caused by *Toxoplasma gondii*, but this infection usually is subclinical or presents as a mild "viral type syndrome" in healthy adults.
   d. Syphilis also should be considered in patients with a short duration of adenopathy and a possible exposure.

2. Splenomegaly out of proportion to adenopathy
   a. This clinical presentation is characteristic of only a few **infections**, such as malaria, schistosomiasis, and kala-azar (visceral leishmaniasis).
   b. This syndrome also should suggest a **malignancy**, such as lymphoma or Hodgkin's disease; an **infiltrative disease**, such as Gaucher's disease; a **congestive disease**, such as hepatic cirrhosis; or a **connective tissue disease**, such as lupus.
   c. Of course, **local infections**, such as splenic abscess and subphrenic abscess on the left, may manifest as a palpable spleen.

3. Localized adenopathy helps to pinpoint a potential **infection** or **tumor**.
   a. Mild lymphadenopathy in the inguinal and cervical areas is common and nonspecific and need not be pursued in the healthy individual.
   b. Lymphadenopathy in other areas is unusual without an obvious infection in the region drained by those nodes.
   c. Lymphadenopathy—which may be local or generalized and may occur with or without weight loss, malaise, and diarrhea—has been noted in individuals who are at risk for AIDS (see section VI D 4).

B. Infections associated with eosinophilia. Eosinophils are granulocytes that have limited ability to phagocytose bacteria but are prominent in hypersensitivity reactions and in infections by multicellular parasites that have an invasive phase.

1. The finding of eosinophilia (i.e., an increase in the number of circulating eosinophils above 500/mm³) should stimulate the search for an infection.
   a. Eosinophilia is seen most often with infection by helminths that are not limited to the lumen of the bowel, such as the **schistosome** (blood fluke), which belongs to the group called **trematodes**. **Pinworm** (from the helminth group called **nematodes**) does not tend to stimulate eosinophilia since it has no tissue phase.
   b. Protozoa seldom elicit eosinophilia.

2. Many noninfectious diseases may stimulate eosinophil production, release, or both. The most frequently encountered are **atopic or allergic diseases**.

3. When a drug such as an antibiotic is the allergen or hapten, eosinophilia acts as a marker for an allergic reaction to the drug. The eosinophilia tends to resolve quickly after the offending drug has been withdrawn.

C. Tuberculosis remains a major medical problem in certain immigrant and underprivileged groups in the United States as well as a widespread disease throughout the world. The diagnosis is based on identification of acid-fast bacilli—specifically, *M. tuberculosis*—on special stain or culture. The diagnosis may be difficult to establish, however, because many patients have too few bacteria to be seen on direct stain, and it takes several weeks for properly collected specimens to grow on conventional media.

1. Clinical syndromes
   a. Pulmonary tuberculosis is the most common form and, in most adults, is characterized by an increased cough (possibly with altered sputum), weight loss, hemoptysis, and fatigue. The chest x-ray usually is abnormal and shows signs of a prior exposure to *M. tuberculosis* (e.g., calcified or enlarged lymph nodes and infiltrates in the posterior segment of the upper

lobes). Most cases of pulmonary tuberculosis are believed to be a reactivation of *Mycobacteria* that was acquired months to years earlier rather than reinfection or initial infection by this bacterium.

    b. Extrapulmonary tuberculosis can develop in any organ, but the most seriously affected are the kidneys, bones, and meninges. Again, the diagnosis rests on finding *M. tuberculosis* in body fluid or tissue. Only about 40% of patients with extrapulmonary tuberculosis have clinical or radiographic evidence of lung involvement.

2. Therapy is aimed at curing the patient who has a definite diagnosis of tuberculosis. To be effective, the treatment must include at least two antimicrobial agents; single-agent treatment has a high risk of failure due to the selection of drug-resistant strains of the infecting tubercle bacillus.

    a. Because of their potency and reliability, **isoniazid** and **rifampin** are the drugs of choice for tuberculosis. Other "first-line" drugs include ethambutol, pyrazinamide, and streptomycin.

    b. Many other, "second-line" drugs are available, which are used mainly for patients who are intolerant of the first-line agents or who have drug-resistant disease. These drugs include ethionamide, kanamycin, and cycloserine.

    c. The recommended duration of therapy varies from 6 months to 2 years, depending on the regimen used.

3. Prevention

    a. Skin testing. The **tuberculin skin test** is used widely to screen certain high-risk populations, particulary those who have been exposed to an infectious individual. The test involves an intradermal injection of the **purified protein derivative (PPD)** of tuberculin. After 48–72 hours, the injection site is examined for visible and palpable induration. Because of a possible cross-reaction following exposure to other mycobacteria, a single tuberculin skin test to determine sensitization to *M. tuberculosis* is considered positive only if the area of induration measures at least 1 cm in diameter.

    b. Chemoprophylaxis. Certain individuals are at extremely high risk for the development of significant symptomatic tuberculosis. In many cases, disease can be prevented by administering isoniazid alone for 1 year, at a dosage of 300 mg/day. The high-risk groups include:

      (1) Individuals under the age of 30 who have positive skin tests for tuberculosis

      (2) Individuals of any age who previously had negative skin tests but recently had positive skin tests for tuberculosis

      (3) Individuals with positive skin tests who receive chronic corticosteroid therapy

      (4) Individuals who live in the same house or come in close contact with an infected and contagious patient

D. Newly described infections. In the past 10 years, a number of new diseases with infectious etiologies have been described. For example, several new causes of acute diarrhea have been recognized, such as *Campylobacter*, rotavirus, Norwalk agent, and *Cryptosporidium*. Some of these diarrheal agents are more common in the United States than the classic causes of infectious diarrhea, such as cholera and *Shigella* and *Salmonella* species. The following discussion highlights some of these "new" infections, all of which have been extensively studied and are important to recognize.

1. Lyme disease

    a. Etiology. Lyme disease is a multisystem infection caused by a spirochete, *Borrelia burgdorferi*, which is transmitted by tick bite.

    b. Clinical features. The first finding is a skin rash, which spreads slowly from the site of the bite and shows central clearing. This lesion, called **erythema chronicum migrans**, is the classic sign of Lyme disease. Weeks to months later, the patient may develop aseptic meningitis, carditis, or arthritis.

    c. Diagnosis is made by testing for antibody titers against *B. burgdorferi*.

    d. Therapy with penicillin or tetracycline shortens the course of the disease.

2. Toxic shock syndrome

    a. Etiology and pathogenesis

      (1) Toxic shock syndrome is caused by a toxin formed by certain strains of *S. aureus*. Individuals who do not have antibody to this toxin are uniquely susceptible to this illness.

      (2) The infection often involves vaginal colonization by toxin-producing staphylococci, and the presence of a tampon in the vagina seems to increase the risk of toxic shock syndrome. However, infections at other sites can lead to the same disease.

    b. Clinical features. Toxic shock syndrome is characterized by fever, hypotension, mucosal changes, and a characteristic desquamative rash on the hands and feet. Multisystem involvement also occurs, with gastrointestinal, renal, hepatic, hematopoietic, and muscular systems affected.

  c. **Therapy.** The treatment for the acute illness is supportive, and antistaphylococcal therapy is given to prevent recurrences.

3. Legionnaire's disease
  a. **Etiology**
    (1) Legionnaire's disease is a pneumonia caused by *L. pneumophila*, a gram-negative bacterium that dwells in warm aquatic environments.
    (2) Since *L. pneumophila* was first described, several legionnella-like organisms have been discovered, which produce a similar but distinct disease pattern.
  b. **Epidemiology**
    (1) Infection occurs when contaminated water is aerosolized and then inhaled (e.g., during nebulizer treatments). Several outbreaks of legionnaire's disease have been connected to the airborne spread of contaminated fluid from air-conditioning cooling towers.
    (2) Individuals who are particulary vulnerable to infection include cigarette smokers, people with underlying lung disease, and immunosuppressed individuals (e.g., those receiving steroid therapy).
  c. **Clinical features**
    (1) Fever occurs in almost all cases, is abrupt, and usually is associated with shaking chills. A sudden headache may precede the rapid rise in temperature.
    (2) Cough is another common symptom, which initially is nonproductive but progresses to a productive cough that may be associated with slight hemoptysis.
    (3) Other, less common symptoms include diarrhea, nausea, vomiting, and pleuritic pain.
  d. **Diagnosis.** The diagnosis is made by culturing the bacterium from infected body sites (e.g., lung tissue, pleural fluid, or sputum) or by demonstrating it by immunofluorescent techniques. When *L. pneumophila* cannot be isolated by these methods, rising titers of antibodies from the acute phase to convalescence can be diagnostic.
  e. **Therapy.** The preferred therapy for all legionella infections is erythromycin.

4. Acquired immune deficiency syndrome (AIDS)
  a. **Epidemiology.** In the United States, most cases of AIDS occur in homosexual or bisexual men. Intravenous drug users constitute the second largest group, followed by hemophiliacs. Some patients are believed to have been infected via transfusion of blood products and others via heterosexual contact. In some developing countries, such as those in central Africa, there is no clear risk factor except, perhaps, heterosexual contact.
  b. **Etiology.** AIDS is believed to be caused by a retrovirus, which has been called **human T-cell lymphotropic virus III (HTLV-III)**, **lymphadenopathy-associated virus (LAV)**, and **human immunodeficiency virus (HIV)**.
  c. **Definition and description.** AIDS causes a progressive deterioration in the cellular immune system—specifically the helper T cells. The clinical criteria currently used to define AIDS include the presence of an **opportunistic infection** or a specific, **unusual malignancy** in an individual with no other underlying disease.
    (1) **Infections associated with AIDS.** In most cases, the diagnosis of AIDS is made on the basis of finding one of the following infections.
      (a) The most frequently found infection in AIDS patients is ***Pneumocystis carinii pneumonia***, which usually presents as a mild-to-moderate nonproductive cough accompanied by dyspnea. Arterial blood gas analysis shows hypoxemia, and chest x-ray reveals bilateral infiltrates. Individuals with early or mild disease may have minimal findings. Bronchoscopy or lung biopsy usually is performed to obtain material for microscopic examination. Therapy is either high-dose trimethoprim-sulfamethoxazole or pentamidine. The prognosis for patients with this infection is about the same as for patients with other immunosuppressive diseases who are infected by *P. carinii*—about 75% survive the first episode but fewer survive subsequent attacks.
      (b) **Mycobacterial infections** also are found frequently—especially those caused by *Mycobacterium avium-intracellulare*. The typical presentation is one of fever and malaise. Specific organ involvement may be present. Because this infection cannot be contained, patients usually have disseminated disease at the time of death.
      (c) **Cytomegalovirus disease** is very common among AIDS patients and may be much more severe in these patients than it is in otherwise healthy people. The lungs and eyes are most severely and commonly involved, but almost any organ can be affected. No current treatment is effective.
      (d) **Cryptococcal meningitis** (fever, headache, stiff neck, and confusion) and **cryp-**

tosporidial diarrhea (copious, persistent watery diarrhea) tend to run a more aggressive course in AIDS patients.

(2) **Cancers typically associated with AIDS** include **Kaposi's sarcoma** and **non-Hodgkin's lymphoma.** Kaposi's sarcoma usually presents as raised purple plaques on the skin or mucous membranes. Non-Hodgkin's lymphoma presents as fever and lymphadenopathy. Although these tumors may occur in other patient populations, they are much more difficult to manage in AIDS patients. This is due, in part, to the difficulty of administering cytotoxic chemotherapy to AIDS patients without increasing their susceptibility to opportunistic infections.

(3) **Other findings** that may be present include renal failure, thrombocytopenia, or neurologic abnormalities including dementia, neuropathy, and myelopathy. These may be found before the opportunistic infection or tumor.

   d. **Diagnosis** is made by identifying one or more of these infections or tumors in an individual who reveals no other reason for immunoincompetence. Nearly all of such individuals are positive for antibody to the AIDS virus.

   e. **Therapy and prognosis**

(1) Treatment for AIDS basically is supportive and consists of attending to all treatable infections and tumors. It is important to provide emotional support as well.

(2) Experimental therapy consists of various immunomodulators and antiretroviral drugs.

(3) Even when each opportunistic infection or tumor is treated appropriately, the mortality rate among AIDS patients is very high, with only a 20% survival at 2 years.

   f. **Prevention** is possible by avoiding exposure to the causative retrovirus. For example, sexual contact with high-risk individuals and the sharing of needles are potentially hazardous activities and should be avoided. The development of a simple and reliable enzyme-linked immunosorbent assay (ELISA) screening test for antibodies to this virus as a marker for potential infectivity as well as voluntary restriction of blood donation among members of high-risk groups give hope of insuring a safe blood supply.

5. **AIDS-related complex** is one name given to a group of syndromes that are not characterized by life-threatening infections but rather by any combination of the following clinical features: thrush; weight loss; fatigue; adenopathy; and diarrhea. The adenopathy usually is prolonged (> 3 months) and involves several body sites. Node biopsy reveals follicular hyperplasia. Many individuals with this constellation of findings are antibody- or culture-positive for HTLV-III/LAV/HIV. There is no treatment for AIDS-related complex, with the exception of topical nystatin or clotrimazole or oral ketoconazole for the oral candidiasis. On short-term follow-up, some patients (~5% per year) go on to develop AIDS, but most maintain their adenopathy, fatigue, or weight loss.

6. **Asymptomatic infection with HTLV-III/LAV** seems to be more common than either AIDS or AIDS-related complex. However, the prognosis for asymptomatic patients who are antibody-positive is unknown. Since there is no effective therapy, the decision whether to look for HTLV-III/LAV/HIV is personal. Counseling about this test and its implications is very important.

STUDY QUESTIONS

Directions: Each question below contains five suggested answers. Choose the **one best** response to each question.

1. A 32-year-old sexually active man has had a soft ulcer on the shaft of his penis for the past 6 months. The ulcer measures 5 cm × 3 cm and is nontender, and there is one small 8-mm inguinal node. A scraping from the base of the ulcer is cultured and shows *Staphylococcus epidermidis*. What is the most likely cause of this man's genital ulcer syndrome?

(A) Granuloma inguinale
(B) Genital herpes
(C) Lymphogranuloma venereum (LGV)
(D) Staphylococcal skin abscess
(E) Gonorrhea

2. All of the following statements concerning fever are true EXCEPT

(A) it usually is not necessary to treat fever
(B) interleukin 1 directly stimulates an increase in metabolic activity in order to raise body temperature
(C) fever commonly is associated with myocardial infarction and pulmonary embolism
(D) orally measured temperature readings are less reliable than rectally measured readings
(E) a normal body temperature does not exclude the diagnosis of infection

3. A 35-year-old man who is dining in a seafood restaurant has a meal consisting of clams on the half shell, red snapper and bonito cooked in a Chinese sauce, fresh vegetables, and a glass of wine. About 30 minutes after eating he complains of paresthesias and a burning sensation in his upper body. This man's symptoms could be related to any of the following neurologic food poisoning syndromes EXCEPT

(A) neurotoxic shellfish poisoning
(B) monosodium glutamate intoxication
(C) ciguatera
(D) botulism
(E) scombroid

Directions: Each question below contains four suggested answers of which **one or more** is correct. Choose the answer

A   if **1, 2, and 3** are correct
B   if **1 and 3** are correct
C   if **2 and 4** are correct
D   if **4** is correct
E   if **1, 2, 3, and 4** are correct

4. The agents of tuberculosis and legionnaire's disease both enter the body via the lungs. Other characteristics that are common to both of these pulmonary diseases include

(1) symptomatic disease is more likely to occur in individuals with diminished immune function
(2) Gram staining of sputum is helpful in the diagnosis
(3) cough is a common symptom and may be associated with hemoptysis
(4) the infectious agent is transmitted from person to person via respiratory droplets

5. Chest diseases that are characterized by a purulent tracheobronchitis include

(1) cystic fibrosis
(2) *Mycoplasma pneumoniae* pneumonia
(3) chronic obstructive pulmonary disease
(4) sarcoidosis

6. Individuals with diseases that are associated with decreased helper T-cell function [e.g., renal transplant recipients and patients with acquired immune deficiency syndrome (AIDS)] are particularly prone to infection by

(1) *Staphylococcus aureus*
(2) *Mycobacterium tuberculosis*
(3) *Streptococcus pneumoniae*
(4) *Pneumocystis carinii*

7. Acute abdominal cramps and watery diarrhea develop in a 27-year-old woman who has 2 children in a day-care center. A stool smear shows numerous white blood cells. Possible agents of this woman's diarrhea include

(1) rotavirus
(2) *Shigella* species
(3) *Giardia lamblia*
(4) *Salmonella* species

8. Fever and abdominal pain are indicative of peritonitis in which of the following patients?

(1) A 65-year-old man 2 days after a bowel anastomosis
(2) A 9-year-old boy with nephrotic syndrome and ascites
(3) A 29-year-old woman on chronic peritoneal dialysis
(4) A 51-year-old man with advanced hepatic cirrhosis and ascites

9. In an individual with no symptoms of illness, which of the following organisms could be cultured from a mucosal surface?

(1) *Hemophilus parainfluenzae*
(2) *Neisseria meningitidis*
(3) Alpha-hemolytic streptococci
(4) *Rickettsia rickettsii*

Directions: The groups of questions below consist of lettered choices followed by several numbered items. For each numbered item select the **one** lettered choice with which it is **most** closely associated. Each lettered choice may be used once, more than once, or not at all.

Questions 10–14

For each condition that impairs host immune function, select the microorganisms most likely to cause disease.

(A) *Neisseria* species
(B) Catalase-producing organisms
(C) Mycobacteria and cryptococci
(D) *Streptococcus pneumoniae*
(E) *Escherichia coli* and *Klebsiella pneumoniae*

10. Chronic granulomatous disease

11. Substantial neutropenia (i.e., < 500 neutrophils/mm³ blood)

12. Deficiency in terminal complement components

13. Multiple myeloma

14. High-dose corticosteroid therapy

Questions 15–19

Several patient characteristics can increase the risk of infection. For each individual with one of these risk factors, select the infection that is most likely to develop.

(A) Brucellosis
(B) Shigellosis
(C) Rhinocerebral mucormycosis
(D) Spontaneous bacterial peritonitis
(E) Bacterial endocarditis

15. Patient with diabetes mellitus

16. Patient with alcoholic liver disease

17. Intravenous drug user

18. Slaughterhouse worker

19. Homosexual man

ANSWERS AND EXPLANATIONS

1. The answer is A. (*V H 4 b–c; Table 8-2*) Syndromes of genital ulcers and lymphadenopathy have many causes, which can be distinguished only with attention to clinical details and laboratory findings. The indolent, painless presentation of this patient's genital ulcer syndrome is classic for granuloma inguinale. However, it would be prudent to perform a serologic test for syphilis since any sexually active individual with a sexually transmitted disease may be at an increased risk for this infection as well. Genital herpes usually produces clusters of vesicular lesions, which become pustular then form crusts and heal. Even severe episodes last only a few weeks, and the lesions usually are painful. Lymphogranuloma venereum (LGV) is predominantly a disease of the inguinal nodes, which are disproportionately large as compared to the ulcer. The ulcer in LGV is slight or has healed by the time the diagnosis is made. Staphylococci seldom cause such an indolent infection over a period of time as long as 6 months, and the presence of *Staphylococcus epidermidis* on a skin surface is a normal finding. Gonorrhea does not produce genital ulcers.

2. The answer is B. (*V A 1–3*) Fever is produced indirectly by the action of interleukin 1, a polypeptide that stimulates the hypothalamus to raise the body's temperature set point. The rise in set point produces alterations in circulation and perspiration, ultimately leading to an increase in body temperature. Many body sites are used to measure body temperature, such as the mouth and the rectum; however, several factors interfere with the accuracy of orally measured temperature readings. Although fever is a common manifestation of many infections and inflammatory processes (e.g., myocardial infarction and pulmonary embolism), its absence should not exclude the consideration of an infection. An example of this is pneumonia, in which fever is a common manifestation but may not always be present—especially in elderly patients.

3. The answer is D. [*V E 1 b (1)–(3)*] All neurologic food poisoning syndromes are rare in the United States, with the exception of monosodium glutamate intoxication (also called Chinese restaurant syndrome), which is a self-limited and usually mild disorder characterized by burning and tightness in the upper body. The three seafood-related neurologic food poisoning syndromes—neurotoxic shellfish poisoning, ciguatera, and scombroid—have short incubation periods and usually manifest as paresthesias, other sensory changes, and varying degrees of weakness. Botulism rarely manifests so quickly, often is preceded by gastrointestinal symptoms, and is characterized by neuromuscular effects (typically a descending paralysis). Complete recovery usually is expected for patients with any of these neurologic food poisoning syndromes.

4. The answer is B (1, 3). [*VI C 1 a, 3 b (3), D 3 b–d*] Tuberculosis and legionnaire's disease are pulmonary diseases that are quite distinct from one another but have several common features. Infection in both cases is more likely to occur in debilitated or immunocompromised individuals and is accompanied by a specific immune response. Disease transmission, however, occurs in different ways. Tuberculosis is transmitted from person to person via respiratory droplets, whereas legionnaire's disease is spread by aerosolized contaminated water—often from air-conditioning cooling towers. Pulmonary tuberculosis is characterized by an increased cough, possibly with altered sputum and hemoptysis. In legionnaire's disease, a nonproductive cough progresses to a productive cough, which also may be associated with hemoptysis, Although Gram staining is not helpful in the diagnosis of either disease, the identification of acid-fast bacilli (specifically, *Mycobacterium tuberculosis*) on special stain or *Legionella pneumophila* on direct immunofluorescent antibody staining secures the diagnosis of tuberculosis or legionnaire's disease, respectively.

5. The answer is B (1, 3). [*V D 3 a–b, 4 b (1), c (1) (b), (2) (a)–(c)*] The microscopic manifestation of a purulent tracheobronchitis [the presence of large numbers of neutrophils (polymorphonuclear leukocytes) in the sputum (i.e., > 25 per low-power field)] is an important diagnostic feature in many pulmonary diseases. These include most bacterial pneumonias and some noninfectious diseases such as chronic obstructive pulmonary disease and cystic fibrosis. Most atypical pneumonias do not produce a strong polymorphonuclear inflammatory response, such as *Mycoplasma pneumoniae* pneumonia, which shows relatively few neutrophils on Gram staining. Sarcoidosis is a granulomatous disease of the lung parenchyma and lymph nodes and rarely involves the trachea or bronchi.

6. The answer is C (2, 4). [*I B 2 a (2), c (1), 3 a; Table 8-1*] A deficiency of the number or function of T cells can result in infection by a variety of opportunistic organisms—usually low-grade intracellular pathogens—including mycobacteria (e.g., *Mycobacterium tuberculosis*), protozoa (e.g., *Pneumocystis carinii*), and fungi (e.g., *Cryptococcus neoformans*). Functional disorders of neutrophils also cause susceptibility to a variety of organisms. An example is chronic granulomatous disease, a neutrophil dysfunction that causes vulnerability to infection by *Staphylococcus aureus*. Infections associated with highly virulent encapsulated bacteria (e.g., *Streptococcus pneumoniae*) occur more frequently in asplenic patients and in those with impaired humoral immunity.

7. The answer is C (2, 4). [*V E 2 b, c, e (1) (a)*] Children in day-care centers are prone to many infections, and they have an especially high rate of infectious diarrhea. All of the agents listed can cause diarrhea in children. Rotavirus, however, rarely causes diarrhea in adults. The presence of fecal leukocytes indicates an invasive agent of diarrhea, two of the most common of which are *Salmonella* and *Shigella* species. *Giardia lamblia*, a noninvasive agent of diarrhea, does not cause the appearance of leukocytes in the stool.

8. The answer is E (all). (*V G 1 a–c*) Peritonitis is an infection of the lining of the abdominal cavity, which can develop in many ways. Peritonitis that occurs without other abdominal disease is described as primary; that which occurs after rupture or perforation of a hollow viscus is described as secondary peritonitis. Primary infection may originate as bacteremia, which results in peritonitis only in the presence of ascites. In children, primary peritonitis usually is associated with nephrotic syndrome; in adults, this infection most commonly develops in the setting of hepatic cirrhosis. In secondary peritonitis, enteric pathogens usually enter the abdominal cavity from a perforated or necrotic abdominal organ (e.g., a ruptured appendix). Peritonitis also may develop as a complication of acute or chronic peritoneal dialysis due to the communication between the peritoneal surface and the skin. Fever, abdominal pain, and nausea are common symptoms of peritonitis, regardless of the cause.

9. The answer is A (1, 2, 3). (*I A 1–4*) Many organisms normally exist on skin and mucous membranes and generally are nonpathogenic except in unusual settings (e.g., impaired host defenses). An example of such an indigenous organism is *Hemophilus parainfluenzae*, which is part of the normal flora of the oral cavity and pharynx. Other indigenous organisms may cause disease in other body sites, such as α-hemolytic streptococci, which may exist in the normal oropharynx but can cause endocarditis if it is transported to and colonizes a previously damaged heart valve. Although strongly associated with serious meningitis in infants, *Neisseria meningitis* may exist as part of the normal pharyngeal flora in some people. On the other hand, *Rickettsia rickettsii* rarely is isolated from humans, existing exclusively in the blood and tissues of individuals with Rocky Mountain spotted fever.

10–14. The answers are: 10-B, 11-E, 12-A, 13-D, 14-C. (*I B 2 a, c, 3 a–b; Table 8-1*) The phagocytic cells (neutrophils) of patients with chronic granulomatous disease are capable of killing only organisms that produce hydrogen peroxide—not catalase. For this reason, patients with this functional disorder of neutrophils are susceptible to infection by such catalase-producing organisms as *Staphylococcus aureus*.

A quantitative decrease in neutrophils (termed neutropenia) occurs most commonly in leukemia patients and as a consequence of cytotoxic therapy. By far the most common pathogens to cause infection in this setting are aerobic gram-negative bacilli that are part of the normal bowel flora (e.g., *Escherichia coli* and *Klebsiella pneumoniae*).

In general, neisserial infections are far more common in individuals with deficiencies of the terminal complement components (i.e., C5–C9). It is important to note, however, that such complement deficiencies are very rare, and most neisserial infections occur in hosts with normal complement levels.

Multiple myeloma is, paradoxically, a tumor that causes the formation of large amounts of immunoglobulin but predisposes to infections often contained by antibodies. The reason is that antibodies specific for infecting organisms are reduced in quantity. The types of pathogens most significantly increased in patients with multiple myeloma are encapsulated bacteria such as *Streptococcus pneumoniae*.

High-dose corticosteroid therapy has many effects on immune function, the most striking of which is to predispose patients to infections normally handled by cellular immunity. These include mycobacterial and fungal (e.g., cryptococcal) infections as well as infections by herpes viruses and *Listeria* and *Nocardia* species.

15–19. The answers are: 15-C, 16-D, 17-E, 18-A, 19-B. (*IV A 3 b, B 2, C 1 a, D 1, E 2*) Certain groups of individuals are known to be at a significantly increased risk of infection. The risk factors for infection include not only illnesses but also homosexuality, intravenous drug use, occupation, and the presence of an internal prosthesis or indwelling catheter.

Diabetes is one illness that is associated with an increased incidence of certain infections. For example, foot and lower leg ulcers as well as genital infections with *Candida* species occur more frequently in diabetics than in normal individuals. One rare disease that occurs almost exclusively in diabetics is rhinocerebral mucormycosis. This infection is especially associated with metabolic acidosis (as with ketoacidosis in diabetes mellitus) and is less frequently associated with states of immunosuppression.

In alcoholics, the incidence of infection is related to the degree of liver dysfunction. Patients who have alcoholic liver disease in conjunction with ascites are prone to spontaneous bacterial peritonitis. (In rare cases, this infection also occurs in states of nephrosis leading to ascites.)

Intravenous drug use carries multiple risks for infection, most of which are related to unsterile techniques. The most serious suppurative infection associated with aseptic techniques is bacterial endocarditis. Superficial skin infections, infectious arthritis, and tetanus also are common in this setting.

Occupation may predispose to infection by exposing an individual to a variety of pathogenic organisms. A predictable case of this is the exposure of veterinarians to rabies. Slaughterhouse workers are at risk for exposure to *Brucella*, probably from mucosal contact with aerosolized animal serum if the animals they process are not disease free.

Homosexual men also are at an increased risk for infections, many of which are sexually transmitted. *Shigella* infections, which are transmitted by fecally contaminated food or by intimate sexual contact, are hyperendemic in the American male homosexual community.

I. DISORDERS OF THE PITUITARY GLAND

A. Anterior pituitary disease results from insufficient production of pituitary hormones (hypopituitarism), excessive production of pituitary hormones (acromegaly, Cushing's disease, or hyperprolactinemia), or the local effects of pituitary tumors.

1. **Pituitary tumors** make up 10% of intracranial tumors. Most are benign, but their continued slow growth in the confined sellar and suprasellar areas may cause serious neurologic damage.
   a. **Types**
      (1) Tumors arising from the pituitary itself when viewed by light microscopy are classified as **chromophobic adenomas** (85%), **eosinophilic adenomas** (10%), or **basophilic adenomas** (5%).
         (a) Eosinophilic cells produce growth hormone (GH) and prolactin.
         (b) Basophilic cells produce adrenocorticotropic hormone (ACTH), thyroid-stimulating hormone (TSH), luteinizing hormone (LH), and follicle-stimulating hormone (FSH).
         (c) The distinction of separate cell types for each hormone produced can be made by electron microscopy and immunochemical staining. Chromophobic adenomas are often shown to be hormonally active, producing ACTH, GH, or prolactin.
      (2) **Craniopharyngiomas**, the most common tumors of the hypothalamic-pituitary area in children, arise from embryonic nests of cells of Rathke's pouch. These tumors usually are located above the sella turcica, but they may produce changes within the sella itself. They may be solid or cystic, may contain cholesterol-rich fluid, and often contain areas of calcification.
      (3) **Meningiomas** and **metastatic tumors** may involve the hypothalamic-pituitary area.
   b. **Clinical features**
      (1) **Excess hormone production** by pituitary adenomas may lead to **acromegaly**, **Cushing's disease**, or **hyperprolactinemia**. In rare cases these tumors may produce excess TSH, FSH, or LH.
      (2) **Insufficient hormone production**, due to compression and destruction of pituitary and hypothalamic cells, produces the syndrome of **hypopituitarism**.
      (3) **Neurologic effects**
         (a) **Optic nerve compression**. Pituitary tumors may press upward on the inferior surface of the optic chiasm. Vision loss tends to occur first in the superior temporal quadrants, with bitemporal hemianopia in more advanced cases.
         (b) **Headache** is common.
         (c) Other neurologic manifestations such as mental status changes, cranial nerve abnormalities, vomiting, and papilledema are less common.
   c. **Diagnosis**
      (1) **Diagnostic imaging**
         (a) **Skull x-ray** may show enlargement or distortion of the sella when tumors are 10 mm or more in diameter (macroadenomas). Suprasellar calcification suggests the presence of a craniopharyngioma.
         (b) Tumors less than 10 mm in diameter (microadenomas) may be visualized with special procedures such as **computed tomography (CT)** with injection of contrast medium.
      (2) **Hormone studies.** Pituitary adenomas that secrete excess GH, ACTH, or prolactin can be commonly diagnosed by hormone measurements, even if the adenoma is too small to be visualized by diagnostic imaging.

d. Therapy
    (1) Surgery is indicated for pituitary adenomas that are causing neurologic symptoms or are producing a syndrome of hormone overproduction.
        (a) Transsphenoidal pituitary microsurgery is used for intrasellar tumors that have minimal or no suprasellar extension. Small adenomas can often be removed without damage to normal pituitary tissue.
        (b) Transfrontal resection may be necessary for large tumors that compress the optic chiasm, extend far outside of the sella turcica, or both.
    (2) Radiotherapy, used either alone or in conjunction with surgery, may decrease the size of pituitary tumors and decrease hormone production.
    (3) Medical treatment
        (a) Hormone replacement is needed if hypopituitarism is present.
        (b) Bromocriptine may decrease the size of prolactin-secreting adenomas and their hormone production.

2. Hypopituitarism
  a. Etiology
    (1) Pituitary tumors, most commonly chromophobic adenomas and craniopharyngiomas, may destroy normal hypothalamic-pituitary tissue.
    (2) Sheehan's syndrome is hypopituitarism caused by infarction of the anterior pituitary gland during childbirth. The pituitary gland doubles in size during pregnancy, largely because of hyperplasia of the lactotropes. The blood supply does not keep pace with the enlargement, however, and hypotensive episodes during a complicated delivery may lead to infarction.
    (3) Surgery for the removal of pituitary or other brain tumors may cause damage to the hypothalamus, the pituitary gland, or both.
    (4) Rarer causes of pituitary or hypothalamic destruction include **sarcoidosis, hemochromatosis, Hand-Schüller-Christian disease, tuberculosis, syphilis**, and **fungal infections**.
  b. Clinical features
    (1) GH deficiency causes growth failure in children, but it has no clinical effect in adults.
    (2) Gonadotropin (LH and FSH) deficiency causes amenorrhea and genital atrophy in women and loss of potency and libido in men. If adrenal androgens are deficient as well, because of concomitant ACTH deficiency, pubic and axillary hair may be lost, especially in women.
    (3) TSH deficiency results in the symptoms and physical changes of hypothyroidism (see section II B 2 a–b).
    (4) ACTH deficiency leads to adrenal insufficiency (see section V C). **Secondary adrenal insufficiency (caused by pituitary disease)** differs in several clinical manifestations from primary adrenal insufficiency (caused by adrenal disease).
        (a) Hyperpigmentation of the skin and mucous membranes is characteristic of primary adrenal disease. It is caused by the elevated ACTH levels that result from the negative feedback of the low plasma cortisol levels (cortisol deficiency leads to increased ACTH secretion). There is no hyperpigmentation in secondary adrenal insufficiency, since ACTH levels are low, not high.
        (b) Electrolyte changes (i.e., decreased serum sodium and increased serum potassium levels) are minimal in secondary adrenal insufficiency, since aldosterone production by the adrenal cortex (which promotes sodium retention) depends mainly on renin and angiotensin (which are undisturbed) rather than on ACTH.
    (5) Prolactin deficiency may be responsible for the postpartum failure of lactation in Sheehan's syndrome but otherwise produces no clinical manifestations.
    (6) With slow, progressive destruction of pituitary tissue, **failure of GH and gonadotropin secretion** occurs early. With continuing loss of tissue, TSH and finally ACTH and prolactin fall below normal levels.
    (7) Deficiency of individual pituitary hormones may occur. Isolated GH deficiency and isolated gonadotropin deficiency are not uncommon, especially in children. Isolated deficiencies of TSH and ACTH are very uncommon.
  c. Diagnosis
    (1) Evaluation of target-organ function is often the first step in the diagnosis of hypopituitarism; this condition is often suspected because of failure of more than one target organ (i.e., the thyroid, the adrenal glands, or the gonads). Tests of thyroid, adrenal, ovarian, and testicular function are described in sections II, V, VI, and VII, respectively.
    (2) Measurement of pituitary hormones
        (a) GH levels may be undetectable under basal conditions in normal individuals; therefore, provocative maneuvers are needed to prove inadequacy of hormone production.

   (i) Insulin-induced hypoglycemia is the most consistently effective test stimulus for GH. Regular insulin, in a dose of 0.1–0.15 U/kg, is given as an intravenous bolus, and GH is measured at 30, 60, and 90 minutes. The fall in the serum glucose level, usually maximal at 30 minutes, is followed by a rise in GH to a level greater than 8–10 ng/ml in normal individuals. The patient must be observed closely during the test; central nervous system (CNS) symptoms of hypoglycemia require immediate intravenous administration of glucose.

   (ii) Levodopa (L-dopa) is almost as consistently effective as insulin, and administration is considerably more convenient. L-Dopa is given orally in a dose of 0.5 g, and GH is measured at 30, 60, and 90 minutes.

   (iii) Arginine, glucagon with **propranolol**, and **exercise** are also used in provocative testing to stimulate GH production.

  (b) Other pituitary hormones can be measured by radioimmunoassay, but since low values cannot be distinguished reliably from normal values, the evaluation is useful only in special situations.

   (i) If thyroid function is subnormal [e.g., a low thyroxine (T_4), low triiodothyronine (T_3) uptake], the TSH level should be elevated if the disorder originates in the thyroid; a low (or low-normal) TSH value strongly suggests hypopituitarism.

   (ii) If adrenal insufficiency is present (e.g., if levels of serum cortisol are low), the ACTH level should be elevated if the disorder originates in the adrenal gland; a low (or low-normal) ACTH level strongly suggests hypopituitarism.

   (iii) In a postmenopausal woman, or in a man with inadequate testicular function (i.e., a low testosterone level), LH and FSH levels should be high; low (or low-normal) values suggest hypopituitarism.

 (3) Other provocative tests

  (a) Insulin-induced hypoglycemia stimulates cortisol production as well as GH production. Cortisol levels can be measured in the same blood samples in which GH is measured. An increase in serum cortisol of at least 10 μg/dl to a level of 20 μg/dl or higher indicates normal function of the entire hypothalamic-pituitary-adrenal axis.

  (b) The **metyrapone test** evaluates ACTH reserve function.

   (i) Metyrapone inhibits 11β-hydroxylation, the enzymatic step that produces cortisol from its precursor, 11-desoxycortisol. Oral metyrapone administration causes a fall in cortisol production, which stimulates ACTH output by the pituitary gland. The increased ACTH stimulates production of 11-desoxycortisol.

   (ii) If the serum level of 11-desoxycortisol increases as expected after metyrapone administration, it indicates that both pituitary ACTH reserve and adrenal response to ACTH are normal.

d. Therapy

 (1) The **underlying cause of** the patient's **pituitary insufficiency** (e.g., enlarging pituitary tumors or granulomatous diseases) may require treatment.

 (2) Hormone replacement

  (a) GH administration can restore normal growth to children with isolated GH deficiency or panhypopituitarism. However, the availability of GH is limited, since the only source (before government approval of synthetic GH) has been human pituitary glands obtained at autopsy.

  (b) Thyroid hormone is given in usual replacement doses (see section II B 4).

  (c) Cortisol is given in usual replacement doses (see section V B 4).

  (d) Estrogen-progesterone combinations may be given to women to restore menstrual function, and **testosterone** may be given to men to restore libido and potency. Fertility is considerably more difficult to achieve, depending on the precisely controlled administration of gonadotropins. Gonadotropin-releasing hormone (GnRH) has been successful in restoring ovulation in women and sperm production in men, but only in cases of hypothalamic insufficiency without pituitary impairment.

3. Acromegaly

 a. Etiology. Acromegaly is caused by a pituitary adenoma that produces GH. In many cases the adenoma is large enough to distort the sella turcica and can be seen on lateral skull x-ray; in other cases more sensitive tomographic methods are needed to visualize the tumor; in a few cases no tumor can be visualized. Pathologically the tumors are eosinophilic or chromophobic adenomas.

 b. Clinical features. Excess GH secretion may cause changes in bone, in soft tissues, and in metabolic processes.

  (1) Bone and soft tissue changes

   (a) In children, excess GH secretion may cause increased linear growth of long bones, resulting in **gigantism**. After closure of the epiphyses at puberty, these changes cannot occur.

Table 9-1. Skeletal and Soft Tissue Manifestations of Acromegaly

Enlargement of hands (especially fingertips) and feet
  Increased ring, glove, and shoe sizes
Coarsening of facial features
  Thick skin folds
    Brows and nasolabial creases
  Enlargement of nose
  Enlargement of mandible
    Prognathism
    Spreading of teeth
Enlargement of internal organs
  Heart, lungs, liver, spleen, and kidneys
Skin thickening and interstitial edema, with swelling and firmness of soft tissues
Osteoarthritis
Entrapment neuropathies (especially carpal tunnel syndrome)
X-ray changes
  Enlargement of sinuses
  Tufting of distal phalanges, cortical thickening

   (b) In adults, soft tissue growth and bone enlargement, especially in the acral areas of the skeleton, lead to **diverse manifestations**, many of **which affect the patient's appearance** (Table 9-1). These changes are very gradual and may not be obvious to the patient and his or her family until the present appearance is compared with that on old photographs.
   (2) Metabolic changes
      (a) Decreased glucose tolerance, a result of the anti-insulin actions of GH, is common, although overt diabetes occurs in only 10% of acromegalic patients.
      (b) A tendency to develop **hyperphosphatemia** is caused by the increased tubular re-absorption of phosphate that is induced by GH.
   c. Diagnosis. The diagnosis of acromegaly depends on the clinical manifestations plus confirmatory abnormalities in the blood levels of GH, somatomedin C, or both.
      (1) Levels of GH should be measured in the morning under basal conditions, if possible before the patient arises from bed, because exercise or stress can raise GH levels, especially in women. A level higher than 10 ng/ml favors the diagnosis of acromegaly. When GH cannot be suppressed below 5 ng/ml 1–2 hours after ingestion of 100 g of glucose, the diagnosis of acromegaly becomes more conclusive. Acromegalic patients may even show a paradoxical rise in GH after glucose administration, whereas the level falls in normal individuals. [If the basal level of GH is greatly increased (e.g., above 30–50 ng/ml), as is common in acromegaly, demonstration of nonsuppressibility of GH by glucose is not necessary].
      (2) Somatomedin C, a growth factor produced by the liver under the stimulation of GH, may be elevated in acromegalic patients whose GH level is normal or equivocal. Elevated levels of somatomedin C provide an additional index of GH activity and further evidence of the diagnosis.
   d. Therapy
      (1) Transsphenoidal pituitary adenomectomy results in prompt return to normal levels of GH in the majority of patients; permanent cure is common when the adenoma is small but uncommon when the tumor is large and extends beyond the sella turcica.
      (2) Conventional radiotherapy lowers GH levels very slowly; normal levels may not be reached until 3 to 10 years after treatment, if at all.
      (3) Bromocriptine, a dopamine agonist, reduces GH levels in many patients, but only a minority of patients achieve normal levels. This treatment is useful when surgery or radiotherapy has been only partially successful.
4. Hyperprolactinemia
   a. Etiology
      (1) Prolactin-secreting pituitary adenomas (prolactinomas) are the most common pituitary tumors. They are more common in women, usually appearing during the reproductive years and causing menstrual abnormalities and galactorrhea (the galactorrhea-amenorrhea syndrome). Men tend to have larger tumors at the time of diagnosis, which usually are suspected because of neurologic impairment and hypogonadism.
      (2) Damage to the hypothalamus or pituitary stalk by tumors, granulomas, and other processes may prevent hypothalamic dopamine from having its normal regulatory effect on lactotrope activity, resulting in hypersecretion of prolactin.

    (3) Drugs can inhibit dopamine activity and thus interfere with its regulation of prolactin secretion. These drugs include psychotropic drugs (e.g., phenothiazines, butyro-phenones, and tricyclic antidepressants), antihypertensives (e.g., methyldopa and reserpine), metoclopramide, cimetidine, and others.

b. Clinical features

    (1) Amenorrhea or menstrual irregularity is a result of the inhibition by prolactin of hypothalamic GnRH production as well as a result of direct effects of prolactin on the ovaries.

    (2) Galactorrhea is a direct result of prolactin excess.

    (3) Loss of potency and libido, with low testosterone levels, is the common endocrine manifestation in men.

c. Diagnosis

    (1) Prolactin levels are elevated. A serum level of prolactin higher than 300 ng/ml strongly suggests the presence of a prolactinoma. Functional causes of hyperprolactinemia, such as drugs, seldom raise the level higher than 100 ng/ml.

    (2) Skull x-rays and **CT scanning** with injection of contrast medium are used to visualize an adenoma.

d. Therapy. The treatment of a prolactinoma depends on the size of the tumor and the symptoms that it is causing. A small nonenlarging tumor in a woman with insignificant galactorrhea who does not desire pregancy may not require treatment. If pregnancy is desired, if the galactorrhea or amenorrhea is unacceptable, or if the tumor is enlarging or causing local symptoms, therapeutic options include surgery, administration of bromocriptine, and x-ray therapy.

    (1) Transsphenoidal surgery cures the majority of patients with small prolactinomas. Large tumors with suprasellar extension, however, are usually not cured by surgery.

    (2) Bromocriptine is remarkably effective in decreasing prolactin levels, usually to normal, which promptly relieves the galactorrhea and restores normal menses and fertility; it frequently reduces tumor size as well.

        (a) Bromocriptine is a difficult drug for many individuals to take, however, because it frequently causes nausea, headache, dizziness, and fatigue.

        (b) Initial doses of 2.5 mg once or twice daily may have to be raised to 10–20 mg daily for full effect.

        (c) Because of the poor surgical results in patients with large tumors, many physicians recommend initial treatment with bromocriptine. If the tumor shrinks, there will be a greater chance for successful surgery.

    (3) Radiotherapy may be used in conjunction with surgery and administration of bromocriptine to reduce tumor size and function further.

B. Posterior pituitary disease. Arginine vasopressin [antidiuretic hormone (ADH)] is produced by cells in the supraoptic nucleus of the hypothalamus, travels down the pituitary stalk in the axons of these cells, and is stored in the nerve endings in the posterior lobe of the pituitary gland (i.e., in the neurohypophysis). **Inadequate ADH production** may follow damage to the hypothalamus, the pituitary stalk, and, less commonly, the posterior pituitary gland, and it **results in diabetes insipidus. Excessive ADH production produces the syndrome of inappropriate secretion of ADH (SIADH).**

1. Diabetes insipidus. Diabetes insipidus that is due to ADH insufficiency is termed central diabetes insipidus; that due to renal unresponsiveness to ADH is termed nephrogenic diabetes insipidus.

a. Etiology

    (1) Approximately half of the cases of diabetes insipidus are **idiopathic**.

    (2) Injury to the hypothalamic-pituitary area may result from head trauma, brain tumors, and neurosurgical procedures.

    (3) Less common causes of diabetes insipidus include **sarcoidosis, syphilis, tuberculosis, Hand-Schüller-Christian disease**, and **encephalitis**.

b. Clinical features

    (1) Polyuria, with urine volumes of 3–15 L daily, results from the inability to reabsorb free water and to concentrate urine in the absence of adequate ADH.

    (2) Thirst results, which leads to **increased fluid intake**. A conscious patient with a normal thirst mechanism and free access to water will maintain hydration; the disease in such a patient is an inconvenience rather than a threat to life. However, rapid and life-threatening dehydration may occur in an infant or in an unconscious patient.

    (3) Laboratory abnormalities include a **dilute urine** (with osmolality less than 200 mOsm/kg and specific gravity less than 1.005) and a high-normal or slightly **elevated plasma osmolality**.

c. Diagnosis

    (1) The measurement of **plasma osmolality** in the untreated patient is helpful in distinguishing the causes of polyuria. In diabetes insipidus the loss of free water is primary and the plasma osmolality tends to be high (280–310 mOsm/kg). In psychogenic polydipsia, excessive fluid intake is primary and the plasma osmolality tends to be low (255–280 mOsm/kg).

(2) **Water deprivation.** Fluid intake is withheld until the urine osmolality reaches a plateau (i.e., an hourly increase of less than 30 mOsm/kg for 3 consecutive hours). When the urine osmolality is stable, the plasma osmolality is measured. Five units of aqueous vasopressin are then injected subcutaneously, and the urine osmolality is measured again 1 hour later. The responses typical of normal individuals and of patients with partial, complete, and nephrogenic diabetes insipidus are shown in Table 9-2. Patients with partial diabetes insipidus show an increase in urine osmolality with dehydration, but the incompleteness of their response is demonstrated by a further rise after ADH is injected.

(3) **Infusion of hypertonic saline** solution (2.5% sodium chloride administered intravenously for 45 minutes at 0.25 ml/kg/min), after a water load (20 ml/kg in 30–60 minutes), causes a sharp fall in urine flow in normal subjects because of stimulation of ADH secretion. Patients with diabetes insipidus cannot respond to this stimulus.

(4) **Differential diagnosis.** When a patient presents with polyuria and dilute urine, central diabetes insipidus must be differentiated from nephrogenic diabetes insipidus and compulsive water drinking.

  (a) **Nephrogenic diabetes insipidus** is a condition in which the renal tubules fail to respond to normal circulating levels of ADH.

   (i) The condition may be familial, starting in infancy, or it may occur later in life in association with hypokalemia, hypercalcemia, chronic renal disease, sickle cell anemia, amyloidosis, or the use of certain drugs such as lithium, demeclocycline, or methoxyflurane.

   (ii) The clinical features are the same as those caused by ADH deficiency. The difference is seen in the failure of nephrogenic diabetes insipidus to respond to administration of ADH.

  (b) **Compulsive water drinking (psychogenic polydipsia)** is a primary psychiatric abnormality that leads to polyuria and dilute urine. Differentiation from diabetes insipidus may be difficult. It is most common in young or middle-aged women who often have a history of psychiatric disorders.

d. **Therapy**

(1) **Vasopressin**

  (a) **Aqueous vasopressin** acts rapidly and is used in acute situations such as head injuries and diabetes insipidus that occurs postoperatively. Five to ten units are injected intramuscularly or subcutaneously every 4–6 hours.

  (b) **Vasopressin tannate in oil** has a prolonged action and is used for long-term management. After warming and thorough mixing of the solution, 2.5–5 units are injected intramuscularly or subcutaneously every 1–3 days.

  (c) **Desmopressin** is a synthetic analog of vasopressin that can be administered topically; 0.05–0.2 ml is applied to the upper respiratory mucous membranes twice daily by nasal cannula. This is the most convenient form of ADH treatment, but it is also the most expensive.

(2) **Chlorpropamide.** A side effect of this oral hypoglycemic agent is the potentiation of the action, secretion, or both of endogenous ADH. Patients with less than total absence of ADH often become asymptomatic when 250–500 mg of chlorpropamide are taken daily. This treatment obviates the need for vasopressin injections. Hypoglycemia must be watched for.

(3) **Thiazide diuretics** have the paradoxical effect of decreasing urine output in patients with diabetes insipidus. The volume depletion induced by the diuretic increases sodium and water reabsorption in the proximal tubule, thus blunting the effect of the defective water absorption in the distal and collecting tubules. Thiazides are only partially

Table 9-2. Response to Water Deprivation Test

Test Results	Increase in Urine Osmolality above 280 mOsm/kg with Dehydration	Further Response to ADH
Normal	+	−
Complete central diabetes insipidus	−	+
Partial central diabetes insipidus	+	+
Nephrogenic diabetes insipidus	−	−

effective, decreasing urine volume by 30%–50%. However, they are the only drugs of any value in the treatment of nephrogenic diabetes insipidus, since their action does not depend on distal tubular response to ADH.

2. Syndrome of inappropriate secretion of ADH (SIADH)

a. Etiology

(1) ADH production by **malignant tumors**, particularly oat cell carcinoma of the lung and carcinoma of the pancreas, was the originally recognized cause of SIADH.

(2) More commonly, excess ADH production is caused by other disease processes through unknown mechanisms via the hypothalamic-neurohypophyseal axis or by diseased tissue. These disease processes include **pulmonary diseases**, such as pneumonia and tuberculosis, and **CNS disorders**, such as stroke, head injury, and encephalitis.

(3) Drugs, such as chlorpropamide, carbamazepine, vincristine, and clofibrate, may stimulate hypothalamic-neurohypophyseal ADH production.

b. Pathophysiology. ADH excess causes water retention and extracellular fluid volume expansion, which is then compensated for by increased urinary sodium excretion. Clinically significant volume expansion (i.e., edema or hypertension) is not present, because of the natriuresis. However, the water retention and the sodium loss both contribute to **hyponatremia**, which **is the hallmark of SIADH**. If water intake is kept to a minimum, this sequence of events does not occur and serum sodium levels do not fall.

c. Clinical features. Hyponatremia refers to a serum sodium level below 135 mmol/L. Symptoms of lethargy, confusion, agitation, headache, nausea and vomiting, and focal neurologic abnormalities are common when the sodium level falls rapidly or when it reaches a level below about 125 mmol/L. Convulsions and coma may occur with more severe degrees of hyponatremia.

d. Diagnosis. The diagnosis of SIADH is based on the following conditions.

(1) Hyponatremia is present, with low serum osmolality.

(2) There is continued **urinary sodium excretion** (greater than 20 mmol daily) despite the low serum sodium levels. The urine osmolality is higher than the serum osmolality. (Other causes of hyponatremia, such as sodium depletion, cause renal retention of sodium, with less than 20 mmol excreted daily).

(3) Conditions that might appropriately stimulate ADH secretion because of volume depletion must be excluded. These include adrenal insufficiency, fluid loss, edematous states (e.g., heart failure, nephrosis, and cirrhosis), and renal failure.

e. Therapy

(1) The cause of SIADH should be treated when possible.

(2) Fluid restriction to 500–1000 ml daily is effective in raising the serum sodium level and is the mainstay of treatment. The limiting factor is patient compliance.

(3) If hyponatremia is severe, hypertonic saline (5%) should be administered to raise the serum sodium level above 120 mmol/L. Salt loading is only of temporary value because the additional sodium is soon excreted in the urine.

(4) If fluid restriction cannot be enforced, 300 mg of **demeclocycline** can be administered three or four times daily. Demeclocycline is an antibiotic with the useful side effect of inhibiting renal tubular response to ADH.

II. DISORDERS OF THE THYROID GLAND. The thyroid may produce too little or too much hormone; it may undergo chronic enlargement and inflammation (**chronic thyroiditis**); and it is a common site for benign and malignant tumors. Thyroid disease is suggested by symptoms of **hypothyroidism** (too little hormone secretion), **hyperthyroidism** (excess hormone secretion), or by localized or diffuse thyroid enlargement (**goiter**). Initially, thyroid disease usually is evaluated by thyroid function tests, which estimate hormone production. Information on the physical characteristics and function of separate areas of the thyroid may then be obtained, if necessary, by isotope scans and other imaging techniques.

A. Thyroid function studies

1. Serum thyroxine determination measures the total bound (99.95%) and free (0.05%) T_4 in the circulation. The serum T_4 concentration is elevated in hyperthyroidism and decreased in hypothyroidism.

a. The proteins that bind T_4, mainly **thyroxine-binding globulin**, are elevated by estrogen treatment, pregnancy, congenital thyroxine-binding globulin excess, and sometimes by liver disease.

(1) If the binding proteins are elevated, the total T_4 concentration in the blood will be high but the concentration of free T_4 (which is the active form of the hormone at the tissue level) will remain normal because it is regulated by the normally functioning T_4-TSH feedback mechanism.

(2) If the concentration of free T_4 is normal, the patient is euthyroid, and the elevated level of total T_4 is misleading.

    b. The converse is also true. Thyroxine-binding globulin levels may be lowered by androgen treatment, congenital thyroxine-binding globulin deficiency, or by the nephrotic syndrome or cirrhosis. In this case, the concentration of total T_4 is low, but the patient maintains a normal level of free T_4 and is euthyroid.

    c. Therefore, the T_4 concentration alone is not an adequate test to evaluate thyroid function. Either the T_4 concentration must be measured in conjunction with a test that evaluates protein binding (i.e., the T_3 uptake test), or free T_4 itself must be measured.

2. Serum triiodothyronine determination measures the concentration of the total bound and free T_3 in the circulation. The total T_3 measurement may give the same misleading results as the total T_4 measurement if there is an abnormality in binding proteins.

3. Triiodothyronine uptake test

    a. This test is performed by combining in a tube the patient's serum, a known amount of radiolabeled T_3, and an insoluble binder of T_3, such as a small piece of resin. The binding proteins from the patient's serum and the resin compete for the labeled T_3: If the binding proteins are increased, less T_3 binds to the resin, and if the proteins are decreased, more T_3 binds to the resin. The result, which is expressed as the percent of labeled T_3 bound to the resin, therefore, is a measure of the unoccupied binding sites on the patient's thyroid hormone-binding proteins.

    b. The T_3 resin uptake is elevated in hyperthyroidism. There is increased thyroid hormone in the blood; therefore, there is increased hormone bound to protein; therefore, there are fewer unoccupied binding sites; and, therefore, there is increased labeled T_3 binding to resin. Conversely, the T_3 resin uptake is decreased in hypothyroidism. In both instances the T_3 resin uptake varies directly with changes in the total T_4 and total T_3 concentrations and confirms the diagnosis suggested by the total T_4 and total T_3 levels.

    c. However, if the levels of total T_4, total T_3, or both are raised or lowered because of abnormalities of the binding proteins, rather than hypothyroidism or hyperthyroidism, the T_3 resin uptake will change in the opposite direction (i.e., when binding protein is increased, there is an increase in the total T_4 concentration; when there is increased binding protein, there is an increase in unoccupied binding sites and, therefore, decreased T_3 resin uptake).

4. Free thyroxine index

    a. If the total T_4 level and T_3 resin uptake are known, an index can be calculated that estimates the free T_4 level. The patient's T_3 resin uptake is divided by the average normal T_3 resin uptake, and the total T_4 is multiplied by this fraction. The result, which is called the free T_4 index, has approximately the same normal range as the total concentration of T_4. This process takes into consideration the effects of abnormalities of thyroid hormone-binding proteins on the total T_4 measurement.

    b. Example. A patient has a total T_4 of 15.0 mcg/dl (normal = 4.5–12.5). If the T_3 resin uptake is 45%, the free T_4 index equals 45% divided by 30% (which is the average normal uptake) multiplied by 15.0, or 22.5. This result suggests a diagnosis of hyperthyroidism. If the T_3 resin uptake is 15%, the free T_4 index is 7.5 ($15/30 \times 15.0$), suggesting that the patient is euthyroid but has an increased level of T_4-binding proteins.

5. Serum TSH measurement is a very sensitive test in the diagnosis of primary hypothyroidism. The serum concentration of TSH is measured by radioimmunoassay, and in a case of hypothyroidism it is elevated even before thyroid hormone levels fall below normal. Current methods may not distinguish between low levels and low-normal levels of TSH and are, therefore, not useful in the diagnosis of hyperthyroidism, in which TSH is suppressed. (New ultrasensitive TSH assays are being introduced that may prove useful in the diagnosis of both hypothyroidism and hyperthyroidism).

6. The uptake of radioactive iodine by the thyroid gland 24 hours after administration is increased in hyperthyroidism and decreased in hypothyroidism. This test is especially useful in detecting forms of hyperthyroidism in which the thyroid gland itself is not synthesizing excess hormone; that is, the hyperthyroidism associated with exogenous thyroid hormone administration, subacute thyroiditis, and ectopic hormone production (e.g., caused by struma ovarii). In these situations, blood hormone levels are high, but the radioactive iodine uptake is low.

B. Hypothyroidism

  1. Etiology

    a. Chronic thyroiditis [Hashimoto's disease] (see section II D 2) is the most common cause of spontaneous hypothyroidism in the United States.

Table 9-3. Symptoms of Hypothyroidism

Weakness, lethargy, and fatigue ("slowing down")
Dry skin and coarse hair
Puffy eyelids, face, and hands; swollen legs
Cold intolerance
Constipation
Weight gain
Hoarseness
Menorrhagia
Hearing loss

  b. Idiopathic atrophy of the thyroid is also common. Antithyroid antibodies are frequently present. This may represent an atrophic form of chronic thyroiditis.

  c. Hypothyroidism frequently develops following the treatment of Graves' disease, and the prevalence may approach 50% in patients treated with radioactive iodine. However, hypothyroidism also may occur after Graves' disease is treated by subtotal thyroidectomy or antithyroid drugs.

  d. Secondary hypothyroidism is caused by any of the conditions that may affect the hypothalamic-pituitary axis and cause hypopituitarism (see section I A 2 a).

  e. Less common causes of hypothyroidism include congenital athyreosis, congenital biochemical defects that prevent thyroid hormone production, and insensitivity of the tissues to thyroid hormone. Iodine deficiency is an uncommon cause of hypothyroidism in most highly developed countries, but it is common in some areas of the world.

2. Clinical features

  a. Symptoms (Table 9-3)

   (1) As metabolism slows because of the lessened effects of thyroid hormone on tissues, the patient may experience **weakness**, **lethargy**, **sleepiness and fatigue**, and **slowness of speech and thought**.

   (2) A **puffy appearance**, **constipation**, and a **constant feeling of cold** are common.

   (3) Slight-to-moderate **weight gain** reflects the decreased metabolism, but massive weight gain does not occur since appetite tends to be diminished.

   (4) Edema of the larynx and middle ear may cause **voice changes and hearing loss** in severe cases.

   (5) Excess and **irregular menstrual bleeding** may be associated with anovulatory cycles.

  b. Physical findings (Table 9-4)

   (1) **Puffiness** and **nonpitting edema** are caused by the accumulation of mucinous mucopolysaccharide-rich material in the tissues. The term **myxedema** describes this phenomenon and is sometimes used synonymously with severe hypothyroidism.

   (2) The characteristic puffy, dull appearance and the **slow return phase of** the Achilles and other **deep tendon reflexes** are perhaps the most helpful physical findings in suggesting the diagnosis.

  c. Effects on organ systems. All organ systems are affected, and some of the most important changes are listed in Table 9-5.

  d. Cretinism

   (1) Severe **hypothyroidism beginning in infancy** is called cretinism and is marked by mental retardation and impairment of physical growth and development.

   (2) Short limbs and a large head, with a broad, flat nose, widely set eyes, and a large tongue, characterize this form of dwarfism.

   (3) Epiphyseal dysgenesis, with abnormalities of the ossification centers, affects the femoral and humeral heads and other parts of the skeleton.

   (4) Early recognition and treatment prevents the otherwise irreversible mental and physical impairment.

Table 9-4. Physical Findings in Hypothyroidism

Thickened, puffy features
Yellowish, dry skin
Nonpitting edema
Hypothermia
Bradycardia
Slow return of deep tendon reflexes
Loss of lateral portion of eyebrows

Table 9-5. Effects of Hypothyroidism on Organ Systems

Cardiovascular system
  Decrease in cardiac output
  Pericardial effusion
Respiratory system
  Hypoventilation
  Pleural effusion
Gastrointestinal tract
  Constipation
Nervous system
  Decreased mental function
  Psychiatric changes
Blood
  Normochromic normocytic anemia

    e. Myxedema coma
      (1) Severe hypothyroidism, if untreated, may eventually lead to this serious condition, either gradually (over a period of years) or more acutely in response to precipitating factors such as infection or exposure to cold.
      (2) Hypothermia, hypoglycemia, shock, hypoventilation, and ileus may be present in myxedema coma in addition to the severely depressed state of consciousness.
      (3) The mortality rate is 50%–75%.

  3. Diagnosis
    a. Severe cases are suggested by the characteristic **symptoms and physical findings**; however, mild cases may escape detection unless laboratory tests are performed. Routine laboratory screening is especially recommended for newborns and elderly individuals with nonspecific complaints.
    b. Abnormal laboratory studies in hypothyroidism include:
      (1) Decreased serum concentration of total T_4
      (2) Decreased serum concentration of total T_3
      (3) Decreased T_3 resin uptake
      (4) Decreased free T_4 index
      (5) Increased serum concentration of TSH (in primary hypothyroidism)
      (6) Decreased radioactive iodine uptake

  4. Therapy
    a. Thyroid hormone preparations. Thyroid extract derived from animal sources and synthetic preparations containing both T_4 and T_3 have been used in the past and are still available. However, synthetic L-thyroxine sodium (Synthroid and Levothroid) is the agent of choice. The administered T_4 is slowly converted to T_3, and the proportions of circulating T_4 and T_3 approximate those of euthyroid individuals. The peaks and valleys of blood T_3 levels, which are seen when exogenous T_3 is given, are avoided.
    b. Initiation of treatment
      (1) Patients with severe hypothyroidism (myxedema) have an increased sensitivity to thyroid hormone and are at risk for acute cardiovascular and other complications if the hypothyroidism is corrected too quickly. Therefore, these patients are given a very small dose of thyroid hormone initially (i.e., 0.025 mg of L-thyroxine), which is increased to a full maintenance dose over a 6- to 12-week period.
      (2) Patients with less severe hypothyroidism may be started on a slightly higher dose (0.05 mg of L-thyroxine) and advanced to a full replacement dose more quickly (e.g., the dose may be raised to 0.1 mg in 2 weeks and to 0.125 mg or 0.15 mg in another 2 weeks).
    c. Maintenance therapy. Most patients require 0.1–0.15 mg of L-thyroxine daily. When this dose is tolerated and symptoms of hypothyroidism have resolved, blood TSH and thyroid hormone levels in the normal range indicate that enough hormone is being given. Normal blood concentrations of total T_4 and total T_3 indicate that the replacement dose is not excessive. Further blood tests and dosage adjustments are needed only occasionally.
    d. Myxedema coma has a high mortality rate and **must be treated rapidly**, despite the risk of sudden hormone replacement. L-thyroxine is given intravenously as a 0.5 mg bolus injection, and regular maintenance doses of L-thyroxine are then given daily. Ancillary treatment includes adrenal corticosteroids and respiratory support.

C. Hyperthyroidism

  1. Etiology
    a. Graves' disease (diffuse toxic goiter) is the most common cause of hyperthyroidism. It is

an autoimmune disorder in which an abnormal immunoglobulin G (thyroid stimulating immunoglobulin) binds to receptors for TSH on the thyroid follicular cells, causing diffuse enlargement of the gland and stimulation of thyroid hormone production. Graves' disease is most common in young women, although others may be affected.

b. Plummer's disease (nodular toxic goiter) is less common than Graves' disease and usually affects older individuals. Discrete areas of the thyroid function autonomously, for unknown reasons, secreting excessive amounts of thyroid hormone. The pathognomonic feature is the presence of unaffected thyroid tissue, the function of which is suppressed by the high thyroid hormone levels and consequent TSH suppression but which can be shown to concentrate radioactive iodine after TSH injection.

c. Subacute thyroiditis (see section II D 1) may cause transient hyperthyroidism.

d. Factitious hyperthyroidism may be caused by surreptitious ingestion of thyroid hormone by patients. Inadvertent administration of excessive doses of the hormone by physicians may have the same result.

e. Rare causes of hyperthyroidism include excess TSH production by **pituitary tumors, teratomas of the ovary** that produce thyroid hormone (**struma ovarii**), and overproduction of hormone by the thyroid gland following iodine ingestion, which is called **jodbasedow**.

2. Clinical features. Thyroid hormone increases oxygen consumption by tissues, raising heat production and energy metabolism. It interacts with the sympathetic nervous system in a way that seems to increase tissue sensitivity to catecholamines and adrenergic stimuli. It affects protein, fat, carbohydrate, and vitamin metabolism. These and other actions lead to profound changes in many organ systems when hormone excess is present.

a. Metabolic changes include an elevated **basal metabolic rate** and **weight loss**, despite increased appetite and food intake. **Sweating** and **heat intolerance** reflect the increased heat production.

b. The **cardiovascular system** is affected. The heart rate is increased; **sinus tachycardia** is common, with rates of 120 beats per minute or higher in severe cases. Systolic blood pressure tends to be elevated and diastolic blood pressure decreased, with a **wide pulse pressure**. Myocardial excitability is increased, and arrhythmias such as **atrial fibrillation** and **premature ventricular contractions** may occur.

c. Gastrointestinal symptoms of loose stools or **diarrhea** are common.

d. The **skin is warm and moist** because of peripheral vasodilatation and increased sweating. **Fine, silky hair** is characteristic.

e. CNS effects include **emotional lability, restlessness,** and **fine tremor.**

f. Muscle weakness and **fatigue** are common.

g. Ophthalmopathy. Stare and **lid lag** (i.e., slow closing of the upper lid when the eye moves downward, revealing sclera between the lid and cornea) may occur in any form of hyperthyroidism. True thyroid exophthalmos, however, is seen only in Graves' disease, occurring in about 50% of cases. The eye is pushed forward because of mucinous and cellular **infiltration of the extraocular muscles.** There is **inflammation of the conjunctiva** and surrounding tissues. The patient may complain of **tearing, eye irritation, pain,** and **double vision.** In severe cases vision may be threatened.

h. Thyroid storm is a sudden exacerbation of the signs and symptoms of hyperthyroidism. It may be precipitated by intercurrent illness, trauma, surgery, or childbirth. Marked fever, tachycardia, and agitation are present and may progress to stupor and coma, with vascular collapse. The mortality rate is high.

3. Diagnosis

a. Presenting symptoms of weight loss, nervousness, palpitations, muscle weakness, and diarrhea are characteristic of hyperthyroidism.

b. Many patients have a **family history** of thyroid disease.

c. Physical examination often reveals a fidgety, hyperkinetic patient with warm, moist skin, fine, silky hair, and a fine tremor of the hands.

(1) The eyes may be prominent, with retraction of the upper lid and a staring appearance.

(2) The thyroid is enlarged in most cases: In Graves' disease the enlargement is uniform, and a bruit may be heard over the gland; in Plummer's disease one or more nodular areas are usually felt.

(3) The heart rate is rapid.

(4) The return phase of the deep tendon reflexes is brisk.

d. Laboratory studies show an increase in the serum concentration of total T_4, the serum concentration of total T_3, and the T_3 resin uptake. The radioactive iodine uptake is high.

e. The **thyrotropin-releasing hormone (TRH) test** is useful in the diagnosis of doubtful cases. An injection of TRH is followed in 30–60 minutes by a rise in the serum level of TSH. A flat response (i.e., failure of TSH to rise), is a very sensitive indicator of hyperthyrodism.

4. Therapy. The adrenergic manifestations of hyperthyroidism, such as the sweating, tachycardia, and tremor, may be diminished by β**-blocking drugs.** These drugs do not affect thyroid function but provide symptomatic relief until treatment is definitive. Three methods for the treatment of Graves' disease are in common use: **antithyroid drugs, subtotal thyroidectomy,** and **radioactive iodine.**

　　a. Antithyroid drugs

　　　　(1) Mechanism of action. Methimazole and **propylthiouracil (PTU)** inhibit the oxidation of iodide and the coupling of iodotyrosines, thus decreasing the synthesis of thyroid hormone. PTU, in addition, decreases the conversion of T_4 to T_3 in peripheral tissues.

　　　　(2) Medical treatment of Graves' disease. Full doses (i.e., 30–80 mg of methimazole or 300–600 mg of PTU) are given daily until the patient is euthyroid. Although blockade of hormone synthesis is rapid, clinical improvement occurs only after a few weeks or months, because a large pool of stored hormone continues to be released from the thyroid. The dose is then tapered to the lowest dose that maintains euthyroidism, and the drug is continued for 1–1½ years. Treatment is then discontinued in the hope that a lasting or permanent remission has occurred.

　　　　(3) Drug toxicity

　　　　　　(a) A **skin rash** or joint pains occur in 3%–5% of patients, necessitating a switch to the alternative drug.

　　　　　　(b) Agranulocytosis occurs in less than 0.5% of patients, but it is life threatening. To detect the complication early, patients are instructed to stop the drug immediately if fever, sore throat, mouth ulcers, or other unexplained symptoms occur. Treatment is resumed only after examination shows the white blood cell count to be normal.

　　　　(4) Advantages of antithyroid drugs

　　　　　　(a) Hospitalization, surgery, and anesthesia are avoided.

　　　　　　(b) There is less likelihood of the occurrence of post-treatment hypothyroidism than in patients treated with radioactive iodine.

　　　　(5) Disadvantages of antithyroid drugs

　　　　　　(a) Permanent remission occurs in fewer than 50% of patients treated.

　　　　　　(b) Successful treatment is dependent on patient compliance, which is less of a problem when treatment is by means of surgery or therapy with radioactive iodine.

　　b. Subtotal thyroidectomy

　　　　(1) Preparation for surgery. Operation on a thyrotoxic patient produces the risk of thyroid storm; therefore, patients are treated with antithyroid drugs long enough to return them to a euthyroid state before surgery.

　　　　(2) Advantages of surgery

　　　　　　(a) Cure of hyperthyroidism is rapid.

　　　　　　(b) The success rate is high; most patients are cured, and fewer become hypothyroid after surgery than after treatment with radioactive iodine.

　　　　　　(c) Patient compliance is required for a shorter period of time than it is in prolonged antithyroid drug treatment.

　　　　(3) Disadvantages of surgery

　　　　　　(a) The patient must be hospitalized, and surgical and anesthetic risks are incurred.

　　　　　　(b) Surgical complications include hypoparathyroidism and recurrent laryngeal nerve paralysis.

　　c. Radioactive iodine

　　　　(1) Method of treatment. A single dose of iodine 131 (^{131}I) causes a decrease in function and size of the thyroid gland over a period of 6–12 weeks. About 75% of patients with Graves' disease are made euthyroid by a single dose; those who are still thyrotoxic after 12 weeks are given a second dose. Additional doses can be given if needed. Eventually almost all patients are cured in this way.

　　　　(2) Risks

　　　　　　(a) Hypothyroidism is present in about 10% of treated patients after 1 year and continues to develop at a rate of 2%–3% each year. After 10–15 years, up to 50% of treated patients are hypothyroid. This complication is easily treated, however, with a single daily dose of L-thyroxine sodium.

　　　　　　(b) No increase in the risk for leukemia, thyroid cancer, or other malignancies has been found in patients treated with radioactive iodine. However, concern about possible slight genetic effects, comparable in magnitude to the effects of a barium enema or intravenous urography, argue against the use of this treatment in women who are likely to bear children in the future.

　　　　(3) Advantages of radioactive iodine

　　　　　　(a) Hospitalization, surgery, and anesthesia are avoided.

　　　　　　(b) The rate of cure approaches 100%.

　　　　　　(c) Little patient compliance is required.

(4) Disadvantages of radioactive iodine
    (a) Multiple treatments may be needed.
    (b) There is a slight risk of genetic effects in future offspring.
    (c) Hypothyroidism, the treatment of which requires long-term patient compliance, is a common sequela.
d. Choice of therapy
    (1) Radioactive iodine is the treatment of choice for most patients over 30–40 years of age.
    (2) In younger patients, the choice is more difficult. If the clinical manifestations are mild, the thyroid hormone levels slightly to moderately elevated, and the thyroid only moderately enlarged, a trial of antithyroid drugs is reasonable, since patients with mild disease have a better chance for a lasting remission.
    (3) Surgery is a better choice for patients with large goiters and severe disease and for patients who are unwilling to take antithyroid drugs for a prolonged period.
    (4) Radioactive iodine treatment may be considered even in young patients if there are reasons to avoid surgery or drugs.
e. Treatment of Plummer's disease. Since antithyroid drug therapy does not lead to permanent remission in patients with Plummer's disease, the options for treatment are surgery and radioactive iodine.
    (1) Thyroidectomy or removal of a hyperfunctioning nodule rapidly cures the hyperthyroidism and relieves symptoms of pressure or tracheal or esophageal obstruction that may be caused by a large goiter.
    (2) Radioactive iodine treatment requires much larger doses in patients with Plummer's disease than in patients with Graves' disease because the affected thyroid cells are relatively radioresistant. However, since the unaffected thyroid cells are functionally suppressed, they do not trap ^{131}I and they are spared the effects of radiation. Hypothyroidism following radioactive iodine treatment is, therefore, less common in Plummer's disease.
f. Treatment of thyroid storm
    (1) The mainstay of treatment is iodine, which acts within 24 hours by inhibiting the release of thyroid hormone. Sodium iodide is given in an intravenous dose of 1–2 g over 24 hours, or potassium iodide may be given orally.
    (2) Antithyroid drugs are given, but because they block hormone synthesis without inhibiting the release of preformed hormone, their effect is less rapid.
    (3) Beta-blockers and adrenal corticosteroids are also used.

D. Thyroiditis

  1. Subacute thyroiditis (also called granulomatous thyroiditis and de Quervain's thyroiditis)
    a. Etiology. The cause of subacute thyroiditis is generally considered to be **viral**: Mumps and coxsackievirus, among others, have been suspected.
    b. Clinical features
      (1) There may be a prodrome, lasting 1 or 2 weeks, of malaise, upper respiratory symptoms, and fever. Then the thyroid gland becomes enlarged, firm, and tender, with pain radiating to the ears, neck, or arms.
      (2) Hyperthyroidism may occur, due to thyroid hormone leaking from damaged follicles into the circulation.
      (3) Disease course. The thyroid pain and hyperthyroidism subside in a few weeks or months. The gland usually returns to normal size; if enlargement persists, chronic thyroiditis should be suspected.

    c. Diagnosis
      (1) The disease is suspected when the thyroid becomes acutely swollen, tender, and painful, especially if symptoms of hyperthyroidism are present.
      (2) It is confirmed by finding a very **low radioactive iodine uptake in the face of high serum T_4 and T_3 levels.** The radioactive iodine uptake is low because the follicular cells are injured and unable to trap iodine and because the high levels of circulating thyroid hormone suppress TSH.
    d. Therapy. Treatment is **symptomatic**, since the disease is self-limited. Aspirin, nonsteroidal anti-inflammatory drugs, and adrenal corticosteroids (in severe cases) relieve the pain and tenderness. Beta-blocking drugs can be used to relieve the symptoms of hyperthyroidism.

  2. Chronic thyroiditis (Hashimoto's thyroiditis)
    a. Etiology. Chronic thyroiditis is a common disorder that mainly affects women. Antithyroid antibodies are present in the majority of patients. The disease is considered to be **autoimmune**.
    b. Clinical features
      (1) Autoimmune damage to the thyroid gland leads to lymphocytic infiltration, fibrosis,

and a weakened ability to produce hormone. These changes result in **thyroid enlargement**, the main clinical manifestation.

(2) **Hypothyroidism** is present in about 20% of patients when the disease is first diagnosed, and it may develop later in additional patients.

(3) Pain and tenderness of the gland sometimes occur, as in subacute thyroiditis.

c. **Diagnosis**

(1) The diagnosis is suspected in any patient with a firm, nontoxic goiter; a high titer of antithyroglobulin antibodies, antimicrosomal antibodies, or both is confirmatory.

(2) Thyroid function tests are usually normal unless the patient has hypothyroidism.

d. **Therapy.** Treatment with L-thyroxine sodium often decreases the size of the goiter and is therefore useful even in patients with normal thyroid function. The presence of hypothyroidism, of course, makes this treatment mandatory.

3. Painless thyroiditis (also called silent thyroiditis and lymphocytic thyroiditis with spontaneously resolving hyperthyroidism)

a. Painless thyroiditis is a syndrome that in some ways resembles subacute thyroiditis and in other ways resembles chronic thyroiditis.

b. **Clinical features**

(1) Transient, self-limited hyperthyroidism occurs, often with enlargement of the thyroid gland, and the radioactive iodine uptake is low, as it is in subacute thyroiditis. Thyroid pain and tenderness are absent, however.

(2) There is lymphocytic infiltration of the thyroid, as there is in chronic thyroiditis, and although antithyroid antibodies may be present, the titers are lower than they are in chronic thyroiditis.

(3) The important feature of this syndrome is the **self-limited nature of the hyperthyroidism**. In the absence of thyroid pain to suggest thyroiditis, this condition could easily be mistaken for Graves' disease and inappropriate treatment could be given. The low radioactive iodine uptake is the most useful finding in distinguishing painless thyroiditis from Graves' disease.

4. Rare forms of thyroiditis

a. **Suppurative thyroiditis** is caused by pyogenic bacterial infection. It is treated by antibiotics and surgical drainage, if necessary.

b. In **Riedel's struma** (fibrous thyroiditis) fibrous connective tissue replaces normal thyroid tissue and infiltrates surrounding structures. Surgery is indicated to exclude cancer and to relieve tracheal compression.

E. Thyroid cancer

1. Epidemiology

a. Thyroid cancer is common: It is found at autopsy in about 5% of patients with no known thyroid disease. However, death due to thyroid cancer is very uncommon—approximately 1200 individuals die from it each year in the United States.

b. These contradictory observations are explained best by the behavior of thyroid cancer. It is usually indolent, tending to remain localized to the thyroid for many years, which is the reason for the low mortality rate.

2. Etiology

a. **Radiotherapy.** There is an increased incidence of thyroid cancer in individuals who received x-ray therapy to the neck (for enlarged thymus, enlarged tonsils, and so forth) in childhood and in atomic-bomb survivors.

b. **Genetic factors.** One form of thyroid cancer, medullary carcinoma, may be familial.

c. **TSH** can induce thyroid cancer in animals, and many human thyroid cancers are dependent on TSH stimulation.

3. Types. Thyroid cancer may present as a solitary thyroid nodule or, less commonly, as multiple nodules or a mass in the neck. These tumors occasionally cause hoarseness, symptoms of tracheal or esophageal compression such as dyspnea or dysphagia, or pain.

a. **Papillary carcinoma**, which accounts for 60% of all thyroid cancer, affects the youngest age group: 50% of patients are less than 40 years of age. The neoplasm consists of columnar cells in folds (the papillae). It tends to grow slowly, often remaining localized to the thyroid for years, and eventually it spreads via the lymphatic system to other parts of the thyroid and to regional nodes. There are few recurrences after treatment, especially in young patients with small primary tumors.

b. **Follicular carcinoma**, which is 25% of all thyroid cancer, histologically may resemble normal thyroid tissue. It often functions like normal thyroid tissue, trapping iodide in a TSH-dependent fashion. It is more malignant than papillary cancer and often spreads to bone, the lungs, and the liver. The 10-year survival rate is 50%.

    c. Medullary carcinoma accounts for 5% of all thyroid cancer, and it arises from the parafollicular cells (or C cells) of the thyroid. It has a hyalin stroma, which may stain for amyloid. About 20% of these carcinomas are familial. This tumor often produces calcitonin and occasionally produces other hormones. It is more malignant than follicular carcinoma, with both local lymphatic and distant hematogenous spread.

    d. Anaplastic carcinoma, which is 10% of thyroid cancer, affects older patients and is highly malignant. It invades rapidly, metastasizes widely, and usually causes death within a few months.

  4. Therapy. Papillary, follicular, and medullary carcinoma are usually treated with a combination of surgery, suppression with thyroid hormone, and radioactive iodine. Anaplastic carcinoma is generally treated palliatively. It may require surgery to relieve obstruction; chemotherapy may delay death.

    a. Surgery

      (1) Papillary carcinoma, when small and limited to a single area of the thyroid, is often treated by removal of the involved lobe and the isthmus.

      (2) Follicular carcinoma and more extensive papillary tumors are usually treated by near-total thyroidectomy: Just enough tissue is left in association with the posterior capsule to spare the parathyroid glands. This more extensive procedure is more likely to be complicated by hypoparathyroidism, but it is followed by less tumor recurrence.

    b. Suppression therapy. Because many thyroid cancers are dependent on TSH stimulation, TSH should be suppressed with the highest dose of L-thyroxine that does not cause hyperthyroidism. This treatment is continued indefinitely.

    c. Radioactive iodine therapy. Follicular cancers often accumulate radioactive iodine, and many papillary cancers contain some follicular elements. A radioactive iodine scan in a patient whose normal thyroid tissue has been removed surgically may show functioning metastases that can be ablated with ^{131}I. In addition, radioactive iodine can be used to ablate any normal thyroid tissue that remains after near-total thyroidectomy, allowing subsequent scans to indicate metastatic tumor.

F. Thyroid nodules are present in 1% of individuals in their twenties and in 5% of individuals in their sixties; cancer is found in 10%–20% of the nodules that are investigated. The goal of management is surgical removal of those nodules with a high probability of malignancy and careful observation of the others, usually with attempted suppression by L-thyroxine.

  1. Pathology. Thyroid nodules may be true adenomas, cysts, localized areas of chronic thyroiditis, colloid nodules, hemorrhagic necrotic tissue, or carcinoma.

  2. Diagnosis

    a. Risk assessment

      (1) X-ray treatment of the head or neck in childhood is associated with an increased prevalence of thyroid nodules and thyroid cancer in adult life.

      (2) Sex. A higher percentage of nodules are malignant in men than in women (although nodules are much more common in women).

      (3) Age. A higher percentage of nodules are malignant in younger individuals (although nodules are much more common in older individuals). In children, 50% of nodules are malignant.

      (4) Disease course. Malignancy is suggested by recent growth of the nodule or by continuing growth despite suppressive therapy with L-thyroxine. Malignancy is less likely if the nodule disappears after aspiration of cyst fluid, if the nodule is visible as a "warm" or "hot" spot on scintiscan (i.e., as demonstrated by its uptake of radioactive iodine), or if the nodule shrinks with suppressive therapy.

      (5) Physical examination. Malignancy is suggested when the nodule is fixed in place, and there is no movement on swallowing. It is suggested by an unusually firm or hard consistency or irregularity of the nodule or by regional lymph node enlargement. Malignancy is less likely if there are multiple nodules or if the nodule is less than 1 cm in diameter.

    b. Laboratory evaluation

      (1) Radioactive iodine thyroid scintiscanning will identify the nodule as "hot," "warm," or "cold." Since most cancers appear on scan as cold areas, only cold nodules are considered to have a significant risk for malignancy. Seventy percent of all nodules are cold, however, and most of these are benign. Therefore, scanning may indicate a greatly reduced risk of malignancy in a nodule that is warm or hot, but it does not yield much additional information on the risk of malignancy in a nodule that is cold.

      (2) Fine-needle aspiration biopsy is safe, and it is easily done as an office procedure. Cells, not sections of tissue, are obtained and must be evaluated by a skilled cytopathologist. The overall results and predictive values are shown in Table 9-6.

Table 9-6. Results of Fine-Needle Aspiration Biopsy of Thyroid Nodules

Cytologic Findings	% of Nodules	% Positive for Cancer
Benign	61	2.5
Equivocal	24	15
Malignant	15	97

Note.—Adapted from Ashcraft MW, Solomon DH: The thyroid nodule. *Ann Intern Med* 96:221–232, 1982.

3. Therapy
 a. Surgical removal of the nodule is indicated if:
  (1) The history and physical examination raise a suspicion of cancer **or**
  (2) The cytologic findings are equivocal or malignant **or**
  (3) The nodule grows despite suppressive therapy with L-thyroxine
 b. Careful long-term observation of the nodule, with suppressive L-thyroxine therapy, is indicated if:
  (1) There are no suspicious findings in the history or on physical examination **and**
  (2) The cytologic findings are benign
 c. Finding the nodule to be functioning (i.e., "warm" or "hot") on scintiscan further supports a decision for conservative management.

III. DISORDERS OF THE PARATHYROID GLANDS

A. Primary hyperparathyroidism and hypercalcemia. Primary hyperparathyroidism is the result of oversecretion of parathyroid hormone (PTH), which in turn causes hypercalcemia. When primary hyperparathyroidism was first recognized in the early 1920s, patients had severe bone disease, recurrent urinary calculi, and systemic illness caused by marked hypercalcemia. Now the disease is diagnosed much earlier, and as a result, most cases are less severe.

1. Epidemiology
 a. Primary hyperparathyroidism is common, affecting about 1 individual in every 1000 who are screened.
 b. The disease is especially common in middle-aged and elderly women.

2. Etiology
 a. A single **parathyroid adenoma** causes 80%–90% of cases, and **hyperplasia** of all four glands causes 10%–20% of cases of primary hyperparathyroidism. Parathyroid carcinoma is a rare cause.
 b. Predisposing factors
  (1) Although most cases seem to arise without a cause, a history of radiation to the neck is present in 10% or more of patients.
  (2) Familial occurrence of parathyroid hyperplasia and of the syndrome of multiple endocrine neoplasia (MEN), which often involves parathyroid adenomas or hyperplasia, indicates that genetic factors may be important.

3. Pathophysiology. PTH is important in maintaining normal calcium homeostasis. As shown in Figure 9-1, PTH raises the level of serum calcium by its stimulating effect on vitamin D metabolism (which is important for gastrointestinal absorption of calcium), its action on renal calcium and renal phosphate handling (i.e., it increases the tubular reabsorption of calcium and inhibits the tubular reabsorption of phosphate), and its effect on bone reabsorption (i.e., it promotes the movement of calcium from the bone). A fall in the circulating level of ionized calcium stimulates PTH production, which then acts to raise the calcium level back to normal; an increase in the circulating level of ionized calcium inhibits PTH production. However, a parathyroid adenoma may function autonomously, producing excessive PTH despite high concentrations of serum calcium and causing the abnormalities of primary hyperparathyroidism.

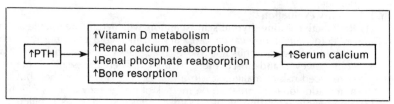

Figure 9-1. Actions of parathyroid hormone (PTH) in maintaining normal calcium homeostasis.

4. **Clinical features.** The serum calcium level is measured routinely in multichannel screening tests; this leads to early diagnosis of primary hyperparathyroidism. The disease commonly presents as mild asymptomatic hypercalcemia, although occasionally patients are seen with the classical findings of advanced kidney and bone disease. Patients with serum calcium levels higher than 11 or 12 mg/dl often have gastrointestinal symptoms, neurologic symptoms, or both.

   a. **Renal symptoms.** Although PTH increases renal calcium reabsorption, the hypercalcemia and resulting increased glomerular filtration of calcium commonly lead to **hypercalciuria**, which in turn may cause the formation of **urinary calculi**. Chronic hypercalcemia may cause deposition of calcium within the renal parenchyma (nephrocalcinosis), with eventual **renal failure**.

   b. **Skeletal symptoms.** PTH excess increases the rate of osteoclastic bone resorption and can lead to the disorder of bone metabolism called **osteitis fibrosa cystica**.

      (1) Symptoms include bone pain, fractures, and areas of swelling and deformity localized to involved bones.

      (2) There are areas of **demineralization** in the skeleton. In severe cases there may be **bone cysts** and "**brown tumors**," which are localized lesions consisting of proliferating osteoclasts, osteoblasts, and fibrous tissue.

      (3) X-rays may show **generalized osteopenia**, with demineralization of the skull and other areas. **Subperiosteal resorption** of bone occurs in the phalanges and distal portions of the clavicles. Loss of the lamina dura around the teeth is characteristic.

   c. **Gastrointestinal symptoms** related to the hypercalcemia of hyperparathyroidism include anorexia, weight loss, constipation, nausea and vomiting, and abdominal pain. There may be an increased incidence of peptic ulcer disease and pancreatitis in patients with hyperparathyroidism.

   d. **Neurologic manifestations** are also related to the hypercalcemia of hyperparathyroidism. Emotional changes and abnormal mentation may occur. Fatigue and muscle weakness are common.

5. **Diagnosis**

   a. **Laboratory findings**

      (1) **Blood chemistry. Elevation of the serum calcium level is the hallmark of primary hyperparathyroidism.** The serum phosphate level is lowered in many but not all cases. Since the serum chloride level tends to be increased (because of PTH-induced bicarbonaturia), the serum chloride-to-phosphate ratio is usually elevated (> 33); this finding is more consistent than that of hypophosphatemia. The serum alkaline phosphatase level is elevated only in patients with significant bone disease.

      (2) **Urine chemistry. Hypercalciuria** is common, but because of the calcium-reabsorbing action of PTH, about one-third of patients have normal urine calcium levels. **Nephrogenous cyclic adenosine 3′,5′-monophosphate (cAMP)**, which is the urinary cAMP excretion minus the cAMP calculated to have been filtered at the glomeruli, is a good index of PTH action on the renal tubules, and it is increased in hyperparathyroidism.

   b. **PTH assay.** The measurement of blood concentrations of PTH by radioimmunoassay is technically difficult, and results must be interpreted with caution. A definitely elevated PTH level in the presence of hypercalcemia is strong evidence for primary hyperparathyroidism, since other causes of calcium elevation tend to suppress PTH levels. However, the assay is often insensitive and may fail to show PTH elevation in patients with parathyroid adenomas; a negative test is not conclusive evidence against the diagnosis of primary hyperparathyroidism.

   c. **Diagnostic imaging.** Two noninvasive techniques, **ultrasonography** and **CT scanning**, may demonstrate parathyroid adenomas in more than 50% of all cases. A much more difficult procedure is **selective venous catheterization** in which blood samples are taken from veins draining various areas of the neck. A marked increase in PTH concentration suggests the location of the adenoma. This procedure is done in patients facing a second operation following an unsuccessful neck exploration.

6. **Differential diagnosis.** Causes of hypercalcemia are shown in Table 9-7.

   a. **Tumors**

      (1) **Malignant tumors with bone metastases** cause hypercalcemia through an increase in bone resorption due to local effects and sometimes through locally acting humoral substances (such as osteoclast activating factor) produced by the metastases.

      (2) **Tumors that cause hypercalcemia in the absence of bone metastases** are believed to produce a humoral factor that acts like PTH, may bind to PTH receptors, but is not measured by the PTH radioimmunoassay. Since this humoral factor may produce biochemical effects like those of PTH, including hypophosphatemia and increased amounts of urinary nephrogenous cAMP, differentiation from primary hyperparathy-

Table 9-7. Causes of Hypercalcemia

Primary hyperparathyroidism
Malignancy
  With bone metastases (e.g., breast cancer, myeloma, lymphoma)
  Without bone metastases (e.g., hypernephroma; pancreatic cancer; squamous cell carcinoma of the lung, cervix, and esophagus; head and neck tumors)
Sarcoidosis
Familial hypocalciuric hypercalcemia
Hypervitaminosis D
Milk-alkali syndrome
Hyperthyroidism
Thiazide therapy
Immobilization

roidism may be difficult unless PTH levels are clearly elevated or the malignancy can be diagnosed on clinical grounds.

b. Sarcoidosis may cause hypercalcemia because of production of 1,25-dihydroxyvitamin D_3 by granulomatous tissue. If no other findings indicate the presence of sarcoidosis, and the PTH concentration is not elevated, a therapeutic trial may be helpful: Serum calcium level will fall within 1 week of the start of glucocorticoid administration (e.g., 40 mg prednisone daily) in most cases of sarcoidosis, but it will be unaffected in most cases of primary hyperparathyroidism.

c. Familial hypocalciuric hypercalcemia is a poorly understood autosomal dominant disorder in which mild-to-moderate hypercalcemia is present but complications such as the formation of urinary calculi and renal failure rarely occur. PTH levels are normal or mildly elevated and the parathyroid glands may be hyperplastic, but subtotal parathyroidectomy does not cure the hypercalcemia. Diagnostic clues are the familial occurrence and the low (rather than high) urinary calcium excretion. Since surgical treatment is not beneficial and is not recommended, this condition should be ruled out in patients with apparent primary hyperparathyroidism.

d. Vitamin D intoxication, which is usually seen in patients receiving pharmacologic doses of the vitamin for the treatment of hypoparathyroidism, results in hypercalcemia. The diagnosis should be apparent from the patient's history. If a sufficiently rapid fall in serum calcium levels does not result when vitamin D ingestion is stopped, glucocorticoids should be given. Glucocorticoids inhibit the action of vitamin D on intestinal calcium absorption and rapidly lower serum calcium levels.

e. The **milk-alkali syndrome** is caused by the ingestion of large quantities of calcium and absorbable alkali, and it is characterized by hypercalcemia, systemic alkalosis, and renal damage due to nephrocalcinosis. The ingestion of more than 5 g of calcium carbonate (or 2 g of elemental calcium) daily, which is about double the dose usually recommended for the prevention or treatment of osteoporosis, would be necessary before the risk of developing this syndrome is introduced.

f. Other causes of hypercalcemia

  (1) Hypercalcemia may occur in **hyperthyroidism**, due to increased bone turnover. The diagnosis should be obvious because the hyperthyroidism, not the hypercalcemia, is the presenting complaint.

  (2) Thiazide diuretics decrease urinary calcium excretion but rarely cause hypercalcemia; they should be avoided, however, in patients with hyperparathyroidism.

  (3) Prolonged **immobilization** may lead to hypercalcemia because of continuing bone resorption in the absence of normal postural stimuli for bone formation. This problem is particularly common in children who are confined to bed for long periods of time (e.g., due to the use of a total body cast for the treatment of multiple traumatic fractures).

  (4) Paget's disease. Increased bone turnover and localized bone tumors due to defective regulation of bone metabolism in this condition may produce hypercalcemia.

  (5) Recovery from acute renal failure. Patients may develop a syndrome of hypercalcemia during the recovery period following rhabdomyolysis and acute renal failure. During the first 2–3 days following muscle injury, the initial muscle damage leads to local calcium and phosphate deposition. When renal function returns to normal, calcium and phosphate exit from sites of muscle damage and enter the circulation to produce hypercalcemia. This defect typically occurs 2–3 weeks following the acute muscle injury.

7. Therapy

a. Surgery

  (1) When the diagnosis of primary hyperparathyroidism is made with confidence, surgical exploration of the neck is usually undertaken.

    (a) In most cases a single adenoma is found and removed.
    (b) If parathyroid hyperplasia is found, the surgeon may remove three glands and part
        of the fourth, or the surgeon may remove all parathyroid tissue and transplant a
        portion to the muscles of the forearm, from which the removal of additional
        parathyroid tissue may easily be accomplished if necessary.
  (2) About 10% of initial neck explorations fail to reveal abnormal parathyroid tissue. The
      patient is then reevaluated, and additional invasive and noninvasive localizing pro-
      cedures are considered before a second operation is performed.
  (3) Postoperative course. Transient hypocalcemia is common after the removal of a para-
      thyroid adenoma because the remaining normal glands are likely to have been sup-
      pressed by long-standing hypercalcemia. Patients usually recover within a few weeks.
      In patients who are occasionally encountered with severe bone disease, marked intrac-
      table hypocalcemia may persist for several months, because when the excess PTH
      stimulus is suddenly removed, the demineralized bone becomes avid for calcium (the
      "hungry bones" syndrome).
  (4) Whether patients with mild asymptomatic hypercalcemia should be operated on is
      open to question. Asymptomatic patients with serum calcium levels no higher than
      11.0 mg/dl very often have no progression of their disease over periods of 10 years or
      more. Many physicians recommend following such patients closely and operating only
      if the calcium level rises or if the patient develops renal or skeletal symptoms or other
      manifestations of severer disease.
  b. Medical treatment is used if surgery is contraindicated by other illnesses or is refused by
    the patient or if surgery is unsuccessful.
    (1) Increased fluid intake and activity help to minimize hypercalcemia.
    (2) Oral phosphate in doses of 1–2 g often lowers the serum calcium level. The main com-
        plication, extraskeletal calcification, is very uncommon if this dose is not exceeded.
    (3) Estrogen may lower mildly elevated serum calcium levels to normal, apparently by de-
        creasing bone turnover. Since two-thirds of cases of primary hyperparathyroidism oc-
        cur in postmenopausal women, in whom estrogen administraton may be considered to
        be physiologic hormone replacement, this treatment is often useful.
  c. Emergency treatment of hypercalcemia is necessary if the calcium level rises to very high
    levels (higher than 13–15 mg/dl) before the adenoma can be removed or if surgical treat-
    ment is refused or is unsuccessful. Hypercalcemia that is caused by diseases other than hy-
    perparathyroidism, such as hypercalcemia due to malignancy, also may be treated by the
    methods that follow.
    (1) Hydration, sodium diuresis. Five to ten liters of intravenous saline daily, with large
        doses of furosemide, will increase renal calcium excretion and reduce serum calcium
        levels.
    (2) Phosphate administration is a rapid and effective way to lower serum calcium levels,
        but calcium phosphate deposition in extraskeletal tissues is a risk. Phosphate in a dose
        of 50 mmol (1.5 g of phosphorus) is given intravenously over 6–8 hours.
    (3) Plicamycin (formerly called mithramycin) is an antineoplastic agent that lowers serum
        calcium levels by inhibiting osteoclastic bone resorption. A single dose of 25 μg/kg ad-
        ministered intravenously over 4–6 hours may lower the serum calcium levels for sever-
        al days. This drug is commonly used in treating hypercalcemia due to malignancy.
    (4) Calcitonin lowers serum calcium levels by inhibiting bone resorption. It is less effective
        than either phosphate or mithramycin, and resistance to its action often develops
        within a few days.
    (5) Glucocorticoids lower serum calcium levels in patients with sarcoidosis and vitamin D
        intoxication and sometimes in patients with myeloma and hematologic malignancy.
        However, they do not lower serum calcium levels in hyperparathyroidism.

B. Hypoparathyroidism and hypocalcemia

  1. Etiology
    a. Surgical removal of the parathyroid glands is the common cause of hypoparathyroidism.
      This may be an unavoidable result of radical neck dissection for cancer or a rare complica-
      tion of subtotal thyroidectomy. Temporary hypoparathyroidism following neck surgery is
      not uncommon and perhaps is due to ischemic injury to the glands; however, recovery
      usually occurs in a few weeks or months.
    b. Idiopathic hypoparathyroidism is much less common. It is usually diagnosed in child-
      hood, may be familial, and is sometimes associated with adrenal insufficiency and muco-
      cutaneous candidiasis.

  2. Pathophysiology. PTH deficiency leads to hypocalcemia, the hallmark of hypoparathyroid-

ism, through the same mechanisms by which increased secretion of PTH causes hypercalcemia (see section III A 3). In addition, the decreased renal phosphate clearance leads to **hyperphosphatemia**, which is present in most cases of hypoparathyroidism.

3. **Clinical features and diagnosis.** Hypocalcemia produces acute symptoms related to increased neuromuscular irritability. In addition, long-term changes may occur as a result of effects on ectodermal tissues and ectopic calcium deposition.
   a. **Symptoms and signs**
      (1) **Latent tetany**
         (a) Mild hypocalcemia may cause **muscular fatigue and weakness** as well as **numbness** and tingling around the mouth and in the hands and feet.
         (b) **Chvostek's sign** may be positive: A tap over the facial nerve in front of the ear elicits a contraction of the facial muscles and upper lip. (Chvostek's sign, however, may be positive in 10% of normal individuals.)
         (c) **Trousseau's sign** may be positive: Inflation of a blood pressure cuff on the arm to a pressure higher than the patient's systolic pressure for 3 minutes elicits carpal spasm (i.e., flexion of the metacarpophalangeal joints and extension of the interphalangeal joints, with drawing together of the fingers and adduction of the thumb).
      (2) **Overt tetany.** Severer hypocalcemia causes **twitching and cramps of the muscles** with **carpopedal spasm. Laryngeal stridor** and **seizures** may occur in severe cases.
      (3) **Long-term effects of hypocalcemia**
         (a) **Ectodermal changes** include atrophy, brittleness, and ridging of the nails, dryness and scaling of the skin, and enamel defects and hypoplasia of the teeth.
         (b) **Calcification of the basal ganglia** may occur, and it is occasionally associated with parkinsonian signs and symptoms.
         (c) **Calcification of the lens may lead to cataract formation.**
   b. **Laboratory abnormalities. Hypocalcemia** and **hyperphosphatemia** are consistently present in hypoparathyroidism. PTH levels, of course, are low, but clinical assays may not be sensitive enough to distinguish between low and normal levels.

4. **Differential diagnosis**
   a. **Pseudohypoparathyroidism**
      (1) Pseudohypoparathyroidism is a hereditary disease with two distinct areas of clinical expression.
         (a) **Calcium metabolism is abnormal** because of end-organ resistance to the action of PTH; that is, the kidney and bone cannot respond to PTH, even though its concentration in the serum is normal or increased. The result is hypocalcemia and hyperphosphatemia, as are seen in true hypoparathyroidism.
         (b) **Developmental and skeletal abnormalities (Albright's hereditary osteodystrophy)** are present. The most common abnormalities are short stature, shortening of the metacarpal and metatarsal bones, and mental deficiency. (The skeletal abnormalities sometimes occur in the absence of any disorder of calcium metabolism; this has been called "pseudopseudohypoparathyroidism.")
      (2) If Albright's hereditary osteodystrophy is not present and if hypocalcemia is not clearly postsurgical in its onset, the differentiation between true hypoparathyroidism and pseudohypoparathyroidism may depend on laboratory tests.
         (a) PTH levels may be sufficiently elevated in pseudohypoparathyroidism to distinguish the syndrome clearly from hypoparathyroidism.
         (b) Injection of PTH is followed promptly by increased urine concentrations of phosphate and cAMP and, within 1 or 2 days, by an increase in serum calcium in patients with hypoparathyroidism. No response occurs in patients with pseudohypoparathyroidism.
   b. **Hypoalbuminemia** causes a decrease in the fraction of serum calcium that is bound to protein and, therefore, a decrease in total serum calcium; since the ionized fraction of serum calcium remains normal, however, there are no clinical manifestations of calcium deficiency. This should not be considered a form of true hypocalcemia. For each decrement in serum albumin of 1 g/L, the serum calcium is expected to fall about 0.8 mg/dl.
   c. **Renal failure.** Hypocalcemia in renal failure is caused by many factors. These include renal phosphate retention (with resultant hyperphosphatemia), reduced production of 1,25-dihydroxyvitamin D_3 by the diseased kidneys, and bone resistance to the calcemic action of PTH.
   d. **Malabsorption** associated with gastrointestinal disease may lead to inadequate calcium absorption and consequent hypocalcemia.
   e. **Vitamin D deficiency** or resistance to the actions of vitamin D may cause hypocalcemia through decreased gastrointestinal absorption of calcium.

f. Acute pancreatitis may lead to intra-abdominal precipitation of calcium soaps in areas of fat necrosis. Whether or not this explains the hypocalcemia that is sometimes seen in patients with acute pancreatitis is uncertain.

g. Osteoblastic metastasis of prostate, breast, or lung cancer may produce hypocalcemia, presumably due to rapid bone uptake of calcium.

h. Hypomagnesemia has two effects that lead to hypocalcemia: It decreases production of PTH, and it inhibits the actions of PTH and vitamin D on bone.

5. Therapy

  a. Hypoparathyroidism. PTH is neither practical nor available for long-term therapy. Instead, treatment with **supplemental calcium**, combined **with vitamin D** to enhance its absorption, is effective in correcting the hypocalcemia and hyperphosphatemia of hypoparathyroidism, even in cases caused by end-organ unresponsiveness to PTH (e.g., pseudohypoparathyroidism).

  (1) Calcium supplementation. Usually 1–2 g of elemental calcium are given daily. Commonly used preparations include calcium gluconate (each 1-g tablet contains 90 mg of elemental calcium), calcium carbonate (each tablet of Os-Cal 500 contains 500 mg of calcium), and calcium glubionate (each tablespoon of Neo-Calglucon contains 345 mg of calcium). The calcium is given in 3 or 4 divided doses. The dose can easily be raised or lowered to regulate serum calcium levels.

  (2) Vitamin D

   (a) Calciferol. For years **vitamin D$_2$ (ergocalciferol)** has been the standard vitamin D preparation used in the treatment of hypoparathyroidism. Since it must be converted to 1,25-dihydroxyvitamin D$_3$ to gain full activity, a conversion that is greatly inhibited in the absence of PTH, very large doses must be given. The average daily dose is 50,000 units, with a range of 25,000–150,000 units, although the recommended dietary allowance is only 200–400 units. The onset of action is slow (1–2 weeks), and the effect may persist for months after administration is stopped.

   (b) Calcitriol. The main advantage of **1,25-dihydroxyvitamin D$_3$ (calcitriol)** over vitamin D$_2$ is the faster onset and cessation of action, which may lead to more precise control of blood calcium levels. However, it is considerably more expensive than vitamin D$_2$, and most patients can be treated without difficulty with vitamin D$_2$. Calcitriol is given in doses of 0.25–2.0 μg/day.

  b. Treatment of acute **hypocalcemia**, which may occur shortly after parathyroid resection and may cause severe tetanic symptoms, consists of intravenous calcium administration. Ten percent calcium gluconate in a dose of 1–2 g is given intravenously over a period of about 10 minutes, followed by slow infusion of another g of calcium gluconate over the next 6–8 hours.

IV. DISORDERS OF GLUCOSE HOMEOSTASIS

A. Diabetes mellitus is characterized by hyperglycemia and other metabolic derangements that are **caused by inadequate action of insulin** on body tissues, either because of reduced circulating levels of insulin or resistance of target tissues to its actions. Because of the prevalence and importance of certain complications, diabetes may be considered to be a **syndrome** consisting of metabolic abnormalities, microvascular disease (i.e., retinopathy and nephropathy), large vessel disease (i.e., accelerated atherosclerosis), and peripheral and autonomic neuropathy.

1. Classification. In general, diabetes mellitus is divided into two categories—**type I or insulin-dependent diabetes** (which is also called juvenile-onset diabetes) and **type II or noninsulin-dependent diabetes** (which is also called maturity-onset diabetes). In addition, there are syndromes that overlap these two categories, which are related to the severity or stage of the disease—impaired glucose tolerance, gestational diabetes, previous abnormality of glucose tolerance, potential abnormality of glucose tolerance, and diabetes associated with certain other diseases.

  a. Type I diabetes (Table 9-8) affects about 10% of diabetic patients. "Dependence" on insulin means not only that insulin is needed for optimal control of blood glucose, which also may be true for type II disease, but that **without exogenous insulin the patient is prone to develop ketoacidosis.**

  (1) This is thought to reflect a complete or almost complete absence of insulin in these patients, in contrast to the partial lack of insulin or the resistance to insulin characteristic of type II patients.

  (2) Other key features of type I diabetes are its occurrence in children and young adults and its occurrence in individuals who are lean rather than obese.

  b. Type II diabetes (see Table 9-8) commonly affects older, overweight individuals.

  (1) Since some insulin is produced by these patients, **ketoacidosis does not occur.**

Table 9-8. Major Types of Primary Diabetes Mellitus

	Type I* Diabetes Mellitus	Type II† Diabetes Mellitus
Prevalence	0.2%–0.5%; male = female	2%–4%; female > male
Age at onset	Usually < 25 years	Usually > 40 years
Genetics	< 10% of first-degree relatives affected; 50% occurrence in identical twins	> 20% of first-degree relatives affected; 90%–100% occurrence in identical twins
HLA	Associated with HLA-B8, B15, DR3, DR4	None
Autoimmunity	Increased prevalence of autoantibodies to islet cells and other tissues	None
Body build	Usually lean	Usually obese—80% are > 15% above ideal weight
Metabolism	Ketosis-prone; absent insulin production	Ketosis-resistant; insulin levels may be high, normal, or low
Treatment	Insulin	Weight loss; possibly an oral agent (e.g., a sulfonylurea) or insulin

*Type I diabetes mellitus is also called insulin-dependent diabetes and juvenile-onset diabetes.
†Type II diabetes mellitus is also called noninsulin-dependent diabetes and maturity-onset diabetes.

     (2) Insulin therapy may be necessary, however, to prevent severe hyperglycemia.
  c. Related syndromes
    (1) Impaired glucose tolerance. This is a disorder of glucose metabolism in which blood glucose levels are higher than those of normal individuals and lower than those of diabetic patients. Impaired glucose tolerance increases the patient's risk for the macrovascular complications of diabetes (i.e., atherosclerosis) but not for the microvascular complications. Although affected individuals have an increased risk of developing diabetes, most do not develop the disease.
    (2) Gestational diabetes. Diabetes or impaired glucose tolerance develops in 2%–3% of pregnant, previously nondiabetic women, most often in the last trimester of the pregnancy. Beta-cell reserve is apparently inadequate for the increased insulin requirements of pregnancy. Careful screening for gestational diabetes and intensive treatment are essential because of an increased risk of neonatal morbidity. The glucose tolerance of most patients returns to normal within a few weeks following delivery, although many patients develop diabetes within 5–15 years.
    (3) Previous abnormality of glucose tolerance. This is a characteristic of individuals with normal glucose levels who formerly were glucose intolerant or diabetic because of pregnancy, illness, obesity, or drugs.
    (4) Potential abnormality of glucose tolerance. This is characteristic of individuals with an increased risk of future diabetes because of a history of having had large babies (over 9 pounds), the presence of diabetes in an identical twin, or similar factors.
    (5) Diabetes or impaired glucose tolerance **may occur secondary to** certain diseases that affect the production or action of insulin, such as **chronic pancreatitis, Cushing's syndrome, acromegaly, insulin receptor abnormalities,** and others.

  2. Etiology. The cause of diabetes mellitus is unknown. Many etiologic factors are suspected, however, with major differences between those factors that are etiologic for type I and type II diabetes.
    a. Type I diabetes
      (1) Etiologic factors
        (a) Genetic factors
          (i) Fifty percent of identical twins of patients with type I diabetes are diabetic.
          (ii) There is a strong association between type I diabetes and certain human leukocyte antigens [HLA antigens] (see Table 9-8).
        (b) Autoimmune factors
          (i) Antibodies to islet-cell antigens are commonly present in diabetic patients shortly after the disease is diagnosed, although they usually disappear within a few years.
          (ii) Antibodies against other tissues, such as antithyroid antibodies, also are increased in prevalence.

(c) **Environmental factors** are suggested by the fact that concordance rate for diabetes in identical twins is 50% rather than 100%, which would be the rate predicted if the disease was totally genetic. Also, seasonal occurrence has been observed, with an increased diagnosis of new cases in the fall and winter.

(2) How these factors interact to cause diabetes is speculative. For example, a viral infection may trigger beta-cell destruction in an individual with genetically determined susceptibility to such an infection and to autoimmune reactivity to islet-cell antigens.

b. **Type II diabetes**

(1) **Genetic factors** are even more important etiologically in type II than in type I diabetes. There is a 90%–100% concordance rate for diabetes in identical twins.

(2) **Obesity** is of major importance—80% of patients are more than 15% above their ideal weight. Obesity is associated with resistance to the action of insulin both in diabetic and nondiabetic individuals; this resistance may be caused partly by decreased numbers of insulin receptors and partly by abnormal insulin action beyond the receptor.

(3) Genetically susceptible individuals may be unable to sustain the increased insulin production needed to maintain carbohydrate homeostasis in the face of insulin resistance, with resulting diabetes.

3. **Pathophysiology**

a. **Levels of insulin**

(1) In **type I diabetes** some insulin may be produced for a few years after the disease is diagnosed, but insulin production eventually ceases totally.

(2) In **type II diabetes** insulin levels vary and often are similar to the levels of nondiabetic individuals of similar weight. However, these insulin levels are not normal but are low, when considered in relation to the elevated blood glucose concentrations of the diabetic patient, and they reflect a decrease in beta-cell sensitivity to glucose.

b. **Consequences of impaired insulin action**

(1) **Hyperglycemia.** Insulin increases the synthesis of glycogen in the liver and in muscle and increases the uptake of glucose in muscle and adipose tissue. In the absence of adequate insulin action, hepatic glucose production increases (with increased glycogenolysis and increased gluconeogenesis) and peripheral glucose utilization falls. The result is hyperglycemia.

(2) **Other metabolic derangements**

(a) Insulin normally acts as an anabolic, storage-promoting agent. It stimulates fatty acid formation from glucose and esterification of fatty acids to form triglycerides, and it stimulates amino acid storage as protein.

(b) Inadequate insulin action on target tissues causes inadequate disposal of ingested nutrients and excessive consumption of endogenous metabolic fuels. Blood fatty acids and lipids are increased because of decreased lipogenesis and increased lipolysis; blood amino acids are increased because of decreased protein synthesis and increased catabolism of muscle protein.

c. **Levels of other hormones**

(1) **Glucagon** levels are often elevated in diabetic patients, which may contribute to the hyperglycemia through glucagon's action in stimulating glycogenolysis and thus increasing glucose levels.

(2) **Epinephrine, cortisol, and GH** levels may be increased during periods of stress or poor diabetic control. This may contribute to the hyperglycemia through the anti-insulin effect and diabetogenic action of these hormones.

4. **Clinical features**

a. **Polyuria and polydipsia.** The most common symptom of hyperglycemia is increased urine volume, which is caused by the glucose-induced osmotic diuresis. Increased fluid intake is a response to the resulting dehydration and thirst.

b. **Weight loss** results from the loss of glucose in the urine and the catabolic effects of the decrease in insulin action, despite increased food intake. Generalized weakness also reflects the metabolic derangements.

c. **Infections of the skin, vulva, and urinary tract** are especially common in uncontrolled diabetes because hyperglycemia decreases resistance to infection.

d. **Blurring of vision** is caused by changes in the shape and refractive qualities of the lens that result from hyperglycemia-induced osmotic alterations.

5. **Diagnosis.** Diabetes mellitus is often suspected because of typical clinical manifestations, such as polyuria and unexplained weight loss; however, a definitive diagnosis is based on elevated **blood glucose levels**.

a. **Fasting serum glucose levels** that are persistently higher than 140 mg/dl are diagnostic of diabetes.

    b. Postprandial glucose levels may be measured 2 hours after a standard meal or after a 75-g glucose load. Values of 140 mg/dl or higher suggest impaired glucose tolerance, and values of 200 mg/dl or higher suggest diabetes. This measurement is more sensitive than a measurement of fasting glucose levels since the ability to return blood glucose to normal 2 hours after a meal is usually lost earlier than the ability to maintain a normal fasting glucose level.

    c. A **glucose tolerance test** is seldom needed to diagnose diabetes if one or both of the above glucose measurements have been taken. However, the glucose tolerance test is the diagnostic standard in questionable cases.

        (1) After at least 3 days of a normal diet, which includes a minimum of 150 g of carbohydrate, the patient ingests a 75-g glucose load. Serum glucose levels are measured at 0, 30, 60, 90, and 120 minutes.

        (2) The criteria for the diagnosis of impaired glucose tolerance and diabetes mellitus are shown in Table 9-9.

    d. Glycosylated hemoglobin measurements

        (1) The free amino acid groups of hemoglobin and other body proteins combine with glucose to form a reversible compound (Schiff base), which can then become a stable glycosylated protein (Amadori rearrangement). The extent of this nonenzymatic glycosylation is dependent on the concentration of glucose in blood; that is, the percent of hemoglobin that is glycosylated depends on the blood glucose levels that were present during the life span of the currently circulating red blood cells.

        (2) The glycosylated hemoglobin level, therefore, reflects the degree of hyperglycemia during the preceding 6–12 weeks, and it may be useful in estimating the average ability to control serum glucose levels during this time.

    e. Urine glucose levels. Glucose appears in the urine only when the renal threshold of about 180 mg/dl is exceeded. This threshold varies widely and tends to rise with age. Urine glucose measurement is, therefore, a very insensitive and unreliable test for diabetes. However, it can be a rough guide to the presence or absence of marked hyperglycemia and may be of use in the day-to-day management of diabetes.

  6. Acute complications of diabetes. Diabetic ketoacidosis, hyperosmolar nonketotic coma, and hypoglycemic coma are acute, life-threatening complications of diabetes mellitus; they cause rapid mental and physical deterioration and require prompt treatment. Since each of these complications may present with an alteration in mental status that often progresses to coma and since each of these conditions requires different treatment, accurate diagnosis is essential.

    a. Diabetic ketoacidosis occurs in an insulin-dependent diabetic patient whose circulating insulin is insufficient to allow glucose utilization by peripheral tissues and to inhibit glucose production and tissue catabolism. Increased levels of glucagon and hormones that increase in response to stress (i.e., epinephrine, norepinephrine, cortisol, and GH) contribute to the metabolic derangements.

        (1) Precipitating factors. Ketoacidosis may occur after several days of worsening diabetic control or may appear suddenly within a few hours. Precipitating factors include any event that decreases insulin availability or causes stress that increases the need for insulin. Common factors are the omission of insulin doses, infections, injuries, emotional stress, excessive alcohol ingestion, and intercurrent illness.

        (2) Pathophysiology

            (a) Hyperglycemia. Insufficient insulin reduces the peripheral utilization of glucose and, together with glucagon excess, increases hepatic production of glucose through the stimulation of gluconeogenesis and glycogenolysis and the inhibition of glycolysis. Protein breakdown in peripheral tissues provides a flow of amino acids to the liver as substrate for gluconeogenesis. Hyperglycemia is the result.

            (b) Osmotic diuresis results from the elevated serum glucose (and ketone) levels and produces **hypovolemia, dehydration**, and **loss of sodium, potassium, phosphate, and other substances in the urine**. Volume depletion stimulates catecholamine

Table 9-9. Glucose Tolerance Test

Test Results	Fasting Glucose Level (mg/dl)	Maximum Level at 30, 60, or 90 Minutes (mg/dl)	Level at 120 Minutes (mg/dl)
Normal	< 115	< 200	< 140
Impaired glucose tolerance	115–139	≥ 200	140–199
Diabetes mellitus	≥ 140	≥ 200	≥ 200

release, which further opposes insulin action in the liver and contributes to lipolysis.

(c) **Ketogenesis.** The lipolysis that results from insulin lack and catecholamine excess mobilizes free fatty acids from their stores in adipose tissue. Instead of reesterifying the incoming fatty acids to form triglycerides, the liver shifts its metabolic pathways toward the production of ketone bodies.

  (i) Glucagon increases the hepatic level of carnitine, which enables fatty acids to enter the mitochondria, where they undergo β-oxidation to ketone bodies.

  (ii) Also, glucagon decreases the hepatic content of malonyl coenzyme A (CoA), an inhibitor of fatty acid oxidation.

(d) **Acidosis.** The increased hepatic production of ketone bodies (acetoacetate and β-hydroxybutyrate) exceeds the body's ability to metabolize or excrete them. Their hydrogen ions are buffered by bicarbonate, leading to a fall in serum bicarbonate and pH. Arterial carbon dioxide tension (PCO_2) also falls because of ventilatory compensation. The anion gap increases because of the elevated plasma levels of acetoacetate and β-hydroxybutyrate. The result is metabolic acidosis that is associated with an increased anion gap.

(3) Clinical features and diagnosis

  (a) **Physical findings**

   (i) Patients with diabetic ketoacidosis have **rapid, deep breathing (Kussmaul's respiration)**, which is an effort to compensate for metabolic acidosis by increasing carbon dioxide excretion.

   (ii) An **odor of acetone** is often detected on the breath.

   (iii) Marked dehydration is common, with **dry skin and mucous membranes** and **poor skin turgor**.

   (iv) **Clouding of consciousness** is present in most cases, and about 10% of patients are **comatose**.

  (b) **Laboratory abnormalities**

   (i) **Hyperglycemia.** Serum glucose levels in ketoacidosis may be only slightly increased, but more often they are markedly elevated, averaging about 500 mg/dl. Renal function affects the degree of hyperglycemia: Glucose levels are greatly elevated only when urinary excretion of glucose is limited by volume depletion or renal abnormalities.

   (ii) **Hyperketonemia.** Serum levels of acetoacetate, acetone, and β-hydroxybutyrate are greatly increased. The agent nitroprusside, in the form of tablets or reagent strips, is commonly used to measure serum and urine ketone bodies. It reacts only with acetoacetate. If the other ketone bodies are increased to a much greater or much lesser extent than acetoacetate, the results of the test may be misleading.

   (iii) **Metabolic acidosis** is indicated by a **low serum bicarbonate** level (usually below 10 mmol/L) and a **low blood pH**. The anion gap is increased.

   (iv) Urinary levels of glucose and ketone bodies are increased. The diagnosis of diabetic ketoacidosis can be made rapidly if marked **glycosuria** and **ketonuria** are present.

   (v) **Other laboratory findings.** Serum potassium concentration may be increased initially because of potassium ion movement from the intracellular to the extracellular space in metabolic acidosis. Later the serum potassium level is low because of both renal losses and the movement of potassium ions back into cells as the acidosis is corrected. Serum sodium concentration tends to be low, mainly because of dilution as the osmotic effect of the hyperglycemia increases extracellular water. Serum osmolality is high, usually above 300 mOsm/kg.

(4) Therapy. The treatment of diabetic ketoacidosis has four main components.

  (a) **Insulin** is administered to increase the utilization of glucose in the tissues, to inhibit the flow of fatty acids and amino acids from the periphery, and to counter the effects of glucagon on the liver.

   (i) **Route of administration.** If volume depletion and vascular collapse are present, poor tissue perfusion may impair the absorption of intramuscular or subcutaneous insulin, and the intravenous route should be used.

   (ii) **Dosage.** A priming dose of 0.1 U/kg of regular insulin is given intravenously and is followed by the infusion of 0.1 U/kg/hr or about 5–10 U/hr. Similar doses may be given intramuscularly if the blood pressure is normal and tissue perfusion seems adequate. Much higher doses were used in the past, and many physicians still advocate their use. If the serum glucose level does not fall (75–100 mg/dl/hr), the serum level of ketone bodies does not fall, and serum pH does not rise in a few hours, larger doses of insulin (50–100 U/1–2 hr) must be given.

(iii) After the acidosis and hyperglycemia have resolved and the urine has become free of ketone bodies, treatment with intermediate-acting insulin is resumed.

(b) **Fluid replacement** corrects the dehydration caused by glucose-induced osmotic diuresis. The fluid deficit in patients with diabetic ketoacidosis averages 3–5 L, which must be promptly replaced.

(i) About 1 L of normal saline is given each hour for the first 2 hours, and then half normal saline is given at a slower rate. When the serum glucose level falls to 200–300 mg/dl, 5% or 10% glucose is infused to prevent hypoglycemia.

(ii) Fluid replacement lowers serum glucose levels, even without insulin, by increasing urine flow and hence glycosuria and by decreasing the levels of catecholamines and cortisol, which were increased by the stimulus of volume depletion.

(c) **Minerals and electrolytes must be replaced** because they are lost via osmotic diuresis.

(i) **Potassium.** Body stores of potassium are low and must be replaced. If initial serum potassium levels are elevated (due to severe acidosis), replacement is delayed; when the levels become normal or low, after therapy has been initiated, potassium chloride is infused at a rate of 20–40 mmol/hr.

(ii) **Phosphate** is administered if serum phosphate levels are very low; about 10 mmol/hr, for a total of 40–60 mmol, are given.

(iii) **Bicarbonate** is given only if the arterial pH falls below 7.1 in order to maintain the pH above that level. Since diabetic ketoacidosis will be corrected by fluids and insulin, excessive administration of bicarbonate may result in rebound alkalosis. Some physicians recommend bicarbonate administration only if the pH falls below 6.9.

(d) **Treatment of precipitating factors and complications**

(i) Urinary tract infections as well as other infections must be pursued and treated.

(ii) Meningitis, stroke, and myocardial infarction may escape detection in a patient whose sensorium is clouded by ketoacidosis.

(iii) Nasogastric aspiration should be performed if the patient is unconscious and has been vomiting or has gastric dilatation.

(iv) Blood or plasma expanders should be given if hypotension persists despite fluid replacement.

b. **Hyperosmolar nonketotic coma** is much less common than ketoacidosis, but it has a much higher mortality rate. It occurs mainly in elderly patients with type II diabetes, often previously undiagnosed.

(1) **Pathophysiology.** Often a precipitating factor, such as infection, increased glucose ingestion, omission of insulin, or intercurrent illness, causes increasing hyperglycemia over a period of a few days or weeks. Osmotic diuresis, without adequate fluid intake, causes dehydration and progressive decline in mental status. Ketoacidosis is mild or absent, presumably because enough insulin is present to inhibit hepatic ketogenesis.

(2) **Clinical features.** The **hyperglycemia** tends to be more marked than it is in ketoacidosis, with plasma glucose concentrations typically about 1000 mg/dl. In the absence of ketoacidosis, the osmotic diuresis continues longer before diagnosis and produces severer dehydration. **Serum osmolality** is very high, averaging about 360 mOsm/kg. The dehydration may cause **mental obtundation, siezures, and focal neurologic signs**.

(3) **Therapy** is similar to that for diabetic ketoacidosis: Fluid replacement and reversal of the hyperglycemia with insulin are the main goals. Fluid replacement in elderly patients with cardiovascular disease requires care to avoid volume expansion, which might precipitate heart failure.

c. **Hypoglycemic coma** must be rapidly differentiated from diabetic ketoacidosis and hyperosmolar nonketotic coma, since therapy is obviously quite different.

(1) The **etiology** of hypoglycemia in insulin-treated diabetic patients ("insulin shock") includes excessive insulin dosage, delay in the ingestion of a meal, and excessive physical activity. Sulfonylureas may cause hypoglycemic reactions, but much less often than insulin.

(2) **Clinical features.** Hypoglycemia produces symptoms through two mechanisms.

(a) A fall in the serum glucose concentration stimulates catecholamine production and sympathetic nervous system outflow. **Adrenergic stimulation** then causes sweating, tachycardia, palpitations, tremulousness, and muscular weakness.

(b) Prolonged hypoglycemia deprives the CNS of its main source of fuel, glucose. **CNS symptoms** of hypoglycemia usually occur later than the adrenergic symptoms, and they are potentially more serious. Mental changes may progress from somnolence and confusion to coma. Headache, slurred speech, focal neurologic signs, and seizures may occur.

(3) The **diagnosis** of hypoglycemia is obvious if symptoms of sweating, palpitation, and tremulousness occur at the time of peak action of a recent insulin dose. Patients learn to recognize this reaction and treat it by drinking orange juice or eating candy. However, less obvious is the cause of coma in a diabetic patient brought to the emergency room. Clues that suggest hypoglycemia rather than ketoacidosis are the history of a missed meal or unusually vigorous exercise, the finding of profuse sweating rather than dehydration, and the absence of Kussmaul's respiration. A fingerstick blood glucose determination is useful for rapid confirmation of hypoglycemia.

(4) Therapy

(a) A patient who is unable to take glucose orally is given 50 ml of **50% glucose intravenously** over 3–5 minutes, followed by a constant infusion of 5% or 10% glucose. Some patients regain consciousness immediately, others more slowly. Glucose infusion may have to be maintained during the expected duration of action of the insulin or oral agent responsible for the hypoglycemia. If the hypoglycemia is caused by **chlorpropamide**, this may be several days.

(b) An intramuscular injection of 1 mg of **glucagon** may raise the serum glucose level rapidly, allowing the patient to regain consciousness and take oral glucose. Teaching a patient's family members to inject glucagon may decrease the frequency of emergency room visits.

(c) Following an episode of insulin-induced hypoglycemia, the insulin dosage, diet, or both should be readjusted to prevent subsequent attacks.

7. Chronic complications of diabetes. Patients with diabetes frequently develop microvascular disorders involving the small blood vessels of the eye, kidney, and muscle; macrovascular disease, that is, atherosclerotic disease of the medium and large vessels; and diabetic neuropathy, that is, abnormalities of the peripheral and autonomic nervous systems.

a. Pathogenesis. A major unresolved question is whether the complications of diabetes, especially those involving small vessels, are related to the degree of hyperglycemia or to genetic factors independent of glucose levels. How intensively the hyperglycemia should be treated depends largely on the value of improved glucose control in the prevention of diabetic complications when weighed against the potential damage of hypoglycemia.

(1) Genetic influences are suggested by the finding of thickened muscle capillary basement membranes in nondiabetic relatives of diabetic patients and by a relationship between HLA haplotype and microvascular complications. Furthermore, retinopathy and nephropathy are rare in patients who are not genetically predisposed but who develop diabetes secondary to chronic pancreatitis.

(2) Metabolic influences are suggested by changes in tubular and glomerular basement membranes of normal kidneys that are transplanted into diabetic patients. Improved glucose control has reduced the width of muscle capillary basement membranes (but usually has not lessened retinal and renal abnormalities). Several possible mechanisms through which elevated glucose levels might cause microvascular complications have been proposed.

(a) Nonenzymatic glycosylation of proteins in the lens of the eye and in capillary basement membranes, similar to the process that produces glycosylated hemoglobin, may produce abnormalities that are related to the blood glucose levels.

(b) When glucose levels are elevated, the enzyme aldose reductase converts glucose to sorbitol, which may cause damage in nerve cells, the lens of the eye, and renal tissue.

(3) Consideration of these and many other observations suggests that both genetic and metabolic factors affect the development of the microvascular complications of diabetes.

b. Diabetic retinopathy is directly related to the duration and severity of diabetes. Prevalence increases from 3% at the time diabetes is diagnosed to 20%–45% after 10 years. Twenty percent of new cases of blindness in adults are caused by diabetes.

(1) Types

(a) Background (simple, nonproliferative) retinopathy makes up 90%–95% of all cases. Increased capillary permeability, vascular occlusion, and weakness of supporting structures lead to the findings on funduscopic examination of venous dilatation, exudates, hemorrhages, and microaneurysms.

(b) Proliferative retinopathy makes up 5%–10% of all cases. New vessels form on the surface of the retina (neovascularization) and may grow into the vitreous body of the eye. Preretinal or vitreous hemorrhage may lead to clot retraction and scar formation, with retinal detachment. Vitreous hemorrhage may cause sudden blindness.

(2) Therapy
  (a) Background retinopathy is less likely to progress if diabetic control is good.
  (b) Proliferative retinopathy may be treated with laser-beam photocoagulation, which is effective in obliterating new vessels.
c. Diabetic nephropathy. The renal lesion that is specific for diabetes is **intercapillary glomerulosclerosis (Kimmelstiel-Wilson syndrome).** Other renal diseases associated with diabetes are papillary necrosis, chronic interstitial nephritis, and arteriosclerotic disease.
  (1) Incidence. Most patients with type I diabetes and about one-third of patients with type II diabetes develop significant renal disease. Nearly all patients with severe glomerulosclerosis also have retinopathy.
  (2) Pathology. The pathologic features of diabetic glomerulosclerosis are an increase in the mesangial matrix and increased width of the glomerular basement membrane, hyaline arteriosclerosis of the afferent and efferent arterioles, and IgG and albumin deposits lining the tubular and glomerular basement membranes. Diabetic kidneys tend to be large, even when end-stage renal disease is present.
  (3) Clinical features
    (a) The first manifestation is usually **proteinuria**, which often progresses to the **nephrotic syndrome**.
    (b) When renal failure occurs, the progression to **end-stage renal disease** is rapid; transplantation or dialysis usually becomes necessary within 3 years.
d. Atherosclerosis. The incidence of atherosclerosis is considerably increased in diabetic patients; that is, **diabetes**, like hypertension, smoking, hyperlipidemia, obesity, and a positive family history, **is a major risk factor for the development of atherosclerosis.** Whether this is a result of hyperglycemia itself, is due to genetic factors, or is due to associated increased prevalence of other risk factors for atherosclerosis, such as hypertension and hyperlipidemia, is not known.
  (1) Coronary artery disease is twice as common in diabetic patients compared to nondiabetic patients. Small vessel disease may contribute to myocardial ischemia.
  (2) Peripheral vascular disease is common in diabetic patients, and it is most likely to affect the legs and feet. Small vessel disease may play a major role: Ischemic changes in a foot with a normal pedal pulse on examination is typical of diabetes. Foot infections, poorly healing ulcers, and eventual gangrene, resulting in amputation, are frequent complications.
e. Diabetic neuropathy is common. Older patients with a relatively long history of diabetes and severe hyperglycemia have an increased incidence of the disease. Accumulation of sorbitol within Schwann cells, with subsequent cell damage, may play a causative role. Slowing of nerve conduction velocity occurs, with changes in Schwann cell function and eventual segmental demyelination.
  (1) Types
    (a) Peripheral polyneuropathy is the most common syndrome. Distal, bilateral sensory changes predominate. Symptoms include paresthesias and pain of the feet. There are findings of decreased reflexes, loss of vibration sense, and loss of pain sensation. Less often, weakness occurs, as does upper extremity involvement.
    (b) Autonomic neuropathy is less common than peripheral polyneuropathy, but usually it is seen in patients who have peripheral polyneuropathy. **Postural hypotension** is the chief manifestation. Other clinically important problems are **sexual impotence** in diabetic men and **urinary retention** with abnormal bladder function. Abnormal gastrointestinal motility may result in **delayed gastric emptying (diabetic gastroparesis)**, constipation, and diarrhea. The adrenergic symptoms of hypoglycemia may be decreased or absent, leading to delayed recognition and treatment of insulin reactions.
    (c) Less common forms of diabetic neuropathy are **radiculopathy**, causing lancinating pain in a single dermatome, and mononeuropathy, involving cranial nerves or proximal motor nerves.
  (2) Therapy. Treatment is symptomatic. Improved diabetic control may lessen the symptoms of peripheral polyneuropathy.

8. Treatment of diabetes
  a. Goals of treatment
    (1) Control of symptoms. The polyuria, weight loss, increased incidence of infections, blurring of vision, and other symptoms of diabetes are related to the hyperglycemia. Return of serum glucose levels to normal brings relief of these symptoms.
    (2) Prevention of acute complications. Diabetic ketoacidosis and nonketotic hyperglycemic coma are prevented by careful management of diabetes.
    (3) Prevention of long-term complications. If scrupulous control of blood glucose levels

prevents the complications of retinopathy, nephropathy, and neuropathy, then intensive insulin therapy may be worth the added inconvenience and the risk of hypoglycemia; if not, perhaps the glucose concentrations need to be lowered only enough to relieve symptoms and prevent ketoacidosis. This is an area of controversy.

b. Diet. Before insulin was available, severe restriction of carbohydrate intake was necessary to prolong life in type I diabetes. In patients receiving insulin, the regularity and timing of carbohydrate intake may be more important than the quantity. Many physicians believe it is equally important to avoid excessive fat intake, which increases the risk of atherosclerosis. Currently, seeking to balance these considerations, it is recommended that protein should be 20%, carbohydrate 50%, and fat 30% of caloric intake.

(1) Type I diabetes. The chief goals of dietary treatment are to provide adequate calories for growth and exercise and to insure day-to-day regularity of food intake so that the availability of insulin is coordinated with carbohydrate intake.

(2) Type II diabetes. The chief goal in most cases is to attain the patient's ideal weight by means of caloric restriction and regular exercise. Since many patients will become normoglycemic with diet alone, if significant weight loss is achieved, initial treatment should emphasize the importance of diet. Unfortunately, the majority of patients are not able to lose enough weight to control glucose levels through diet alone.

(3) Diet calculation

(a) The ideal body weight should be estimated.

(i) For men, the allowance is 106 pounds for the first 5 feet in height, and 6 pounds for each additional inch.

(ii) For women, the allowance is 100 pounds for the first 5 feet in height, and 5 pounds for each additional inch.

(iii) For heavy-framed individuals, 5–15 pounds may be added.

(b) The total daily caloric requirement should be determined. The ideal body weight should be converted to kg by dividing the number of pounds by 2.2. The data in Table 9-10 can then be used to determine the daily caloric need, which will vary with the patient's activity level and need to gain or lose weight.

(c) The protein, carbohydrate, and fat intake should be determined by calculating 20% of the total calories as protein (4 kcal/g), 50% as carbohydrate (4 kcal/g), and the remaining 30% as fat (9 kcal/g).

(d) The total food intake should be divided into meals. For the average person, two-sevenths of the total should be eaten at breakfast, at lunch, and at dinner, and one-seventh should be eaten at bedtime. Food exchange lists are available to aid in apportioning the food components to each meal.

(e) Additional suggestions

(i) Increased intake of polyunsaturated fats and reduced intake of saturated fats is desirable. Cholesterol intake should not exceed 300–500 mg/day.

(ii) For a balanced amino acid content, 50% of protein should be derived from the meat exchange list.

(iii) Increased fiber intake, in the form of unprocessed bran, cereals, fruits, and vegetables, may lower blood glucose levels and decrease the need for insulin.

c. Oral hypoglycemic agents are sulfonylurea derivatives that reduce serum glucose levels in patients with type II diabetes. They are often used in patients with mild-to-moderate diabetes whose glucose levels are not controlled by diet alone. Currently available agents are listed in Table 9-11.

(1) Pharmacology

(a) Metabolism. The oral hypoglycemic agents are readily absorbed and are metabolized in the liver.

(i) Chlorpropamide undergoes very little metabolic alteration and is excreted largely unchanged in the urine; therefore, renal failure causes accumulation of active drug.

Table 9-10. Daily Caloric Requirement*

Habitus	Activity Level		
	Sedentary	Moderately Active	Very Active
Obese	20–25	30	35
Normal	30	35	40
Underweight	35	40	45–50

*Calories (kcal) required per kg of ideal body weight per day.

Table 9-11. Oral Hypoglycemic Agents

Drug	Duration of Action (hours)	Usual Starting Dose (mg)	Daily Dose Range (mg)
Tolbutamide	6–12	1000–2000 in 1 or 2 doses	500–3000
Tolazamide	12–24	100–250 in 1 dose	100–1000
Acetohexamide	12–24	250 in 1 dose	250–2000
Chlorpropamide	60–90	250 in 1 dose	100–750
Glyburide	24	2.5–5 in 1 dose	1.25–20
Glipizide	24	5 in 1 dose	2.5–40

      (ii) The active metabolite of acetohexamide is also retained in patients with renal failure.

     (iii) Liver disease may increase the hypoglycemic effects of tolbutamide and tolazamide.

     (iv) Drugs such as salicylates, sulfonamides, warfarin, and phenytoin may increase free sulfonylurea levels in the blood by displacing them from binding to albumin or by inhibiting their metabolism, thus increasing the risk for hypoglycemia.

   (b) Mode of action

      (i) The acute effect of these agents is to increase insulin output by the beta cells.

     (ii) With long-term use, they also appear to increase the action of insulin on peripheral tissues, perhaps through an effect on insulin receptors or through postreceptor mechanisms.

(2) Clinical use

   (a) The patients most likely to respond to oral agents are those with type II diabetes of recent onset, who have not required insulin in the past or who have needed less than 20 units daily.

   (b) After it is evident that therapy via diet alone will not be sufficient, an oral agent may be prescribed. A low dose is given initially and is increased at intervals of about 1 week until good glucose control is achieved or maximal recommended dosage is reached.

   (c) If oral agents are not effective (primary failure), insulin therapy must be initiated. Oral agents may produce satisfactory glycemic control for months or years, with secondary failure eventually occurring for unknown reasons.

(3) Side effects

   (a) Hypoglycemia may result from excessive dosage, interaction with drugs that potentiate the action of sulfonylureas, renal or hepatic disease, or inadequate food intake. Prolonged duration of the hypoglycemia, which is associated especially with chlorpropamide, may necessitate hospitalization and continuous intravenous glucose infusion over a period of several days.

   (b) Sensitivity to alcohol, with reactions similar to those seen with disulfiram, may occur, especially in association with chlorpropamide.

   (c) Hyponatremia may result from the action of chlorpropamide (and, less commonly, other agents) potentiating the effect of ADH on the renal tubules.

   (d) In one large study, there was an increased rate of **mortality from cardiovascular disease** in patients treated with tolbutamide. The results of this study are controversial but have led some physicians to question the use of this class of drugs.

   (e) Rare side effects include skin reactions, gastrointestinal symptoms, and bone marrow depression.

(4) Choice of agent. Glipizide and glyburide, which are newer agents, do not cause the alcohol intolerance and hyponatremia that are occasionally associated with older drugs. For the most part, however, none of the sulfonylureas has any definite advantage over the others.

 d. Insulin

  (1) Indications

   (a) Patients with type I diabetes are, by definition, dependent on insulin treatment.

(b) Insulin is indicated in type II patients in whom satisfactory control of blood glucose levels is not obtained with diet and oral hypoglycemic drugs. Patients who are usually well controlled with oral agents may require insulin temporarily during times of stress or illness or after surgery.

(c) Gestational diabetes that is not controlled by diet should be treated with insulin.

(2) Insulin preparations

(a) Most insulin is produced from pork and beef pancreas. Recently human insulin has been prepared by recombinant DNA technology. Beef insulin differs from human insulin in three amino acid residues, and pork insulin differs from human insulin in one amino acid residue.

(b) Conventional insulins have 10–50 parts per million of proinsulin as a contaminant; highly purified insulins have less than 10 parts per million.

(c) Insulin preparations are available with rapid (regular insulin), intermediate, and long durations of action (Table 9-12).

(3) Evaluation of glucose control

(a) Patients treated with insulin may have blood sugar determinations every week or every several weeks if their glucose control is stable, or determinations may be made several times daily if glucose levels are unstable or if the insulin dose is being adjusted. In hospitalized patients and in patients who learn to measure their blood sugar levels at home, glucose levels are commonly measured before breakfast and at one or more additional times daily, for example at 4 P.M., at bedtime, or before each meal. Home monitoring is done using test strips (e.g., Dextrostix) with or without a meter (e.g., Glucometer). Checking urine glucose concentrations one or more times daily is simpler, but it is much less accurate.

(b) Fasting serum glucose levels below 140 mg/dl and 2-hour postprandial glucose levels below 200 mg/dl are considered to be satisfactory in most patients. Lower glucose levels are the aim in pregnant women and in patients who are well motivated to achieve optimal control. In patients with widely fluctuating glucose levels and frequent hypoglycemia (so-called "brittle" diabetes) and often in insulin-resistant patients, higher glucose levels may have to be tolerated.

(4) Insulin regimens

(a) Single dose of intermediate-acting insulin. The simplest regimen, and the most commonly used, is a single dose of an intermediate-acting insulin daily before breakfast. An initial dose of 10–20 units of NPH or Lente insulin is given, and its effect on blood and urine glucose levels is observed. The dose can be raised by 4–10 units every few days.

(b) Split dose of intermediate-acting insulin. If a single morning dose of NPH or Lente insulin produces a good afternoon glucose level but fails to maintain control until the next morning, an evening dose can be added. About two-thirds of the daily dose is given before breakfast, and one-third is given before dinner. The morning dose is adjusted according to the afternoon glucose level, and the evening dose is adjusted according to the fasting glucose level.

(c) Combined intermediate–regular (fast-acting) insulin. If the glucose level is elevated in late morning, 4–10 units of regular insulin can be added to the morning

Table 9-12. Insulin Preparations and their Usual Onset, Peak, and Duration of Action

Types of Insulin Preparations	Onset of Action (hours)	Peak Effect (hours)*	Duration of Action (hours)*
Fast-acting			
Regular	1/2–1	2–3	6
Semilente	1/2–1	3–6	12
Intermediate-acting			
NPH†	1–2	6–12	14–24
Lente	1–4	8–14	18–24
Long-acting			
PZI‡	4–8	16–24	36
Ultralente	4–8	20–30	36

*Peak action may be delayed and duration of action prolonged after months or years of insulin therapy.

†NPH = isophane insulin suspension.

‡PZI = protamine zinc insulin.

dose of intermediate-acting insulin. If the glucose level is high in late evening, regular insulin can be added to the evening dose of intermediate-acting insulin. The dose of intermediate-acting insulin may have to be lowered slightly when regular insulin is added.

(d) **Intensive insulin therapy**

(i) **Multiple injections.** In patients with unstable diabetes, the rise in blood sugar levels after meals may best be controlled by a dose of regular insulin before each meal. Basal insulin requirements may be supplied by a single dose of intermediate- or long-acting insulin each morning. Frequent home glucose measurements allow the adjustment of each dose and the addition of extra doses when necessary.

(ii) **Portable infusion pump.** The closest control of serum glucose levels is achieved by the constant infusion of regular insulin through a needle placed subcutaneously in the abdominal wall or thigh. A basal rate of about 12.5–15 mU/kg/hr is supplemented with pulse doses 15–30 minutes before each meal. The benefit of tighter glucose control with intensive therapy must be balanced against the increased risk of hypoglycemia and the incovenience of the portable pump.

(5) **Factors affecting insulin requirements**

(a) **Intercurrent illness or** other **stress** may increase insulin needs, perhaps because of increased levels of catecholamines. A temporary increase in the dosage of intermediate-acting insulin or supplementary doses of regular insulin may be needed.

(b) **Exercise** increases glucose utilization and may cause hypoglycemia unless the insulin dose is reduced or extra carbohydrate is ingested.

(c) **Somogyi effect.** Insulin-induced hypoglycemia causes release of counter-regulatory hormones such as epinephrine and glucagon, which may then cause rebound hyperglycemia. If the cause for this hyperglycemia is not recognized, the insulin dose may be increased, leading to even more severe hypoglycemia. Hypoglycemia during the hours of sleep may be an unrecognized cause of increased morning fasting glucose levels; if this is found to be the case, a decrease in the insulin dose may correct the morning hyperglycemia.

(6) **Complications of insulin therapy**

(a) **Local allergy.** Red, itchy lumps may form at the injection site minutes or hours after an insulin dose. This tends to occur within a few weeks of initial insulin treatment and usually resolves in a few weeks or months. Switching to more purified insulin or adding small amounts of diphenhydramine or dexamethasone to the insulin injection may be helpful.

(b) **Systemic allergy.** Generalized urticaria, angioedema, and anaphylaxis are rare but life-threatening reactions to insulin. Since a ketosis-prone patient cannot survive without insulin, he or she must be hospitalized and insulin desensitization must be performed. An initial intradermal dose of 1/10,000 unit of insulin is given and is increased every 30 minutes.

(c) **Antibody-mediated insulin resistance** is caused by IgG insulin-binding antibodies in the serum. Insulin resistance is often defined as a need for more than 200 units daily, and it is more common in patients who have been exposed to insulin intermittently. Antibody-mediated resistance is often self-limited, resolving within 6 months. Treatment consists of switching to purified pork or human insulin and cautious use of glucocorticoids if necessary (too sudden release of antibody-bound insulin in response to steroid therapy may cause hypoglycemia).

(d) **Lipodystrophy**

(i) **Lipohypertrophy.** Local swellings, composed of fibrous and fatty tissue, may occur at insulin injection sites, perhaps because of a local lipogenic effect of insulin on the fat cells. The swellings may regress if purified insulin is used and the site of lipohypertrophy is avoided.

(ii) **Lipoatrophy.** Pits may form at injection sites due to the disappearance of subcutaneous fat. These may slowly disappear if purified pork or human insulin is injected into the perimeter of the atrophic area.

B. **Hypoglycemia.** It is not possible to give a simple definition of hypoglycemia. Glucose levels below 45 or 55 mg/dl may be associated with hypoglycemic symptoms, but some normal individuals have glucose levels lower than this without symptoms after several days of fasting or several hours after a glucose load, with resultant excessive secretion of insulin. If the diagnosis is in doubt, it should be based on **Whipple's triad**: symptoms of hypoglycemia; low serum glucose levels; and relief of the symptoms when normoglycemia is restored.

1. Insulinomas are rare tumors that arise from the beta cells of the islets of Langerhans. Most are single, benign adenomas, but about 10% of these tumors are multiple, and 10% are malignant. They occur with equal frequency in the head, the body, and the tail of the pancreas. Beta-cell hyperplasia may occasionally produce a similar syndrome.

  a. Clinical features. These tumors produce excessive quantities of insulin, leading to **fasting hypoglycemia** (i.e., a category of hypoglycemia in which the lowest levels of serum glucose and the severest symptoms occur after prolonged periods without food intake). Symptoms are most likely to occur in the early morning or late afternoon or after fasting or exercise. The symptoms of hypoglycemia are the same as those that result from insulin overdose in diabetic patients (see section IV A 6 c). Patients may gain weight before the diagnosis is made because they learn to relieve or avoid hypoglycemic symptoms by frequent snacking on carbohydrates.

  b. Diagnosis

    (1) An elevated serum insulin concentration at a time when the glucose level is low is strong evidence for the presence of an insulinoma, if an exogenous insulin source is excluded. In normal individuals, insulin levels fall as glucose levels fall, and insulin levels become undetectable at glucose levels below 30 mg/dl. If the serum glucose concentration is less than 45 mg/dl, an insulin level higher than 10 μU/ml is abnormal.

    (2) A **prolonged fast**, extending for 24–72 hours, may be necessary to demonstrate fasting hypoglycemia with inappropriately high insulin levels.

    (3) C-peptide suppression test. If prolonged fasting does not produce hypoglycemia but an insulinoma is still suspected, hypoglycemia can be induced with the administration of exogenous regular insulin (0.1 U/kg intravenously over 1 hour). The induced hypoglycemia suppresses endogenous insulin production in a normal individual but fails to suppress the autonomous insulin production by an insulinoma. Serum insulin measurement cannot be used to evaluate endogenous insulin production since the injected insulin would be measured as well. However, C peptide, which is separated from the proinsulin molecule when the latter is cleaved to form insulin, can be measured. Since C peptide is not present in injected insulin, its concentration in serum reflects endogenous insulin production. A level of C peptide that is greater than 1.2 ng/ml after an insulin infusion suggests the autonomous insulin production of an insulinoma.

    (4) Proinsulin, the large precursor molecule of insulin, is produced in increased amounts by insulinomas. Proinsulin normally makes up 5%–20% of the total insulin in blood that is measured by radioimmunoassay; in patients with an insulinoma, proinsulin usually exceeds 25%.

    (5) Diagnostic imaging. CT, ultrasonography, and selective arteriography may be used in an attempt to identify and localize an insulinoma. These tumors may be quite small, however, averaging 1–2 cm, and they often cannot be visualized.

  c. Therapy

    (1) Surgical removal of an adenoma or partial pancreatectomy for mutiple adenomas or beta-cell hyperplasia is the treatment of choice.

    (2) Medical treatment is reserved for patients whose tumors cannot be completely removed because of metastatic disease or other reasons.

      (a) Diazoxide inhibits the release of insulin from beta cells. A dose of 200 mg daily, which can be raised as high as 800 mg if necessary, can prevent hypoglycemia in patients with an inoperable insulinoma.

      (b) Streptozotocin is an antibiotic that specifically destroys beta cells. It is used to treat malignant beta-cell tumors.

2. Factitious hypoglycemia is caused by the surreptitious self-administration of insulin or an oral hypoglycemic drug, most often by an individual who is familiar with health care, such as a nurse or medical technologist, or by a diabetic or relative of a diabetic. Differentiation from hypoglycemia caused by an insulinoma may depend on special studies.

  a. Serum C-peptide measurement indicates the source of insulin secretion [see section IV B 1 b (3)]. The low glucose and high insulin levels that are pathognomonic of an insulinoma should be accompanied by increased C-peptide levels; if the latter is **low**, indicating an **exogenous** source of the high insulin concentration, the disease is factitious.

  b. Ingestion of a sulfonylurea, however, will stimulate endogenous insulin production and the C-peptide level will be high; therefore, **screening of blood or urine for sulfonylureas** is also needed to rule out factitious disease.

3. Extrapancreatic tumors may cause hypoglycemia. These usually are large, intra-abdominal tumors, most often of mesenchymal origin (e.g., fibrosarcoma), although they may be hepatic carcinomas or other tumors. The mechanism of hypoglycemia is poorly understood; increased utilization of glucose by some tumors and production by others of an insulin-like substance have been observed.

4. Ethanol-induced hypoglycemia occurs in patients whose glycogen stores are depleted because of inadequate recent food intake, usually 12–24 hours after a bout of heavy drinking. The oxidation of ethanol to acetaldehyde and acetate generates NADH and decreases the availability of NAD, which is needed for gluconeogenesis. When neither glycogenolysis nor gluconeogenesis is available to maintain hepatic glucose production in the fasting state, hypoglycemia results. Prompt recognition with glucose administration is essential since the mortality rate is higher than 10%.

5. **Liver disease** may result in impairment of glycogenolysis and gluconeogenesis sufficient to cause fasting hypoglycemia. This is seen in fulminant viral hepatitis or acute toxic liver disease but not in the usual, less severe, cases of cirrhosis or hepatitis.

6. **Other causes of fasting hypoglycemia** include cortisol deficiency, GH deficiency, or both, which may occur in **adrenal insufficiency** or **hypopituitarism**. Hypoglycemia may occur in patients with **renal failure** and **heart failure**; however, the causes are poorly understood.

7. **Reactive hypoglycemia.** Insulinoma and the other conditions discussed above produce hypoglycemia most commonly in the fasting state. Another, smaller group of disorders cause hypoglycemia a few hours after the ingestion of carbohydrates, thus the term reactive hypoglycemia.

   a. **Alimentary hypoglycemia** occurs in patients who have had a gastrectomy or other surgical procedure that leads to abnormally rapid movement of food into the small bowel. Rapid absorption of carbohydrate stimulates excessive insulin secretion, causing hypoglycemia several hours after a meal.

   b. **Reactive hypoglycemia of diabetes.** Patients with early diabetes occasionally have a late but excessive release of insulin after a carbohydrate-containing meal. The glucose level is elevated at 2 hours but then sinks to hypoglycemic levels between 3 and 5 hours after the meal.

   c. **"Functional" hypoglycemia**, although commonly diagnosed in patients with chronic fatigue and anxiety, is probably a rare condition.

      (1) **Clinical features**

         (a) Hypoglycemia, with adrenergic symptoms such as sweating and palpitations, occurs 2–5 hours after a carbohydrate-rich meal, presumably because of increased insulin production or insulin sensitivity.

         (b) Hypoglycemia is not a cause of chronic fatigue, depression, and lack of energy.

      (2) **Diagnosis**

         (a) The overdiagnosis of functional hypoglycemia stems in part from misinterpretation of the 5-hour glucose tolerance test. One in four normal individuals has a serum glucose level below 50 mg/dl 3–5 hours after the nonphysiologic stimulus of 75–100 g of glucose, and some normal individuals have levels below 35 mg/dl, without symptoms. These responses do not prove functional hypoglycemia.

         (b) The diagnosis depends on finding hypoglycemia that coincides with the patient's typical symptoms and on finding relief of symptoms by carbohydrate ingestion.

      (3) **Therapy** consists of eating four to six small meals daily that are low in carbohydrate and high in protein.

V. DISORDERS OF THE ADRENAL GLAND

A. General considerations

1. Diseases of the **adrenal cortex** are caused by the excessive production of cortisol (**Cushing's syndrome**), aldosterone (**primary aldosteronism**), and adrenal androgens (**congenital adrenal hyperplasia**) and by inadequate production of cortisol and aldosterone (**Addison's disease**).

2. Loss of the **adrenal medulla** does not cause illness, but **catecholamine overproduction by a pheochromocytoma** (a tumor of the adrenal medulla) causes a characteristic hypertensive syndrome.

B. Cushing's syndrome is caused by excessive concentrations of cortisol in the circulation. It is considerably more common in women than in men.

1. **Etiology**

   a. The most common cause of spontaneous Cushing's syndrome is **bilateral adrenal hyperplasia** (which is also known as **Cushing's disease**).* Bilateral adrenal hyperplasia is due to increased pituitary secretion of ACTH. Whether the primary defect originates in the hypo-

---

*Excess production of ACTH by the pituitary gland is **Cushing's disease**. **Cushing's syndrome** is a nonspecific designation that is associated with increased glucocorticoid levels from any origin.

thalamus (through elaboration of excessive corticotropin releasing factor) or in the pituitary gland is uncertain. Pituitary tumors that are large enough to be seen on skull x-ray, which are usually chromophobic adenomas, are present in about 10% of these patients, and smaller basophilic adenomas are found in more than 50%.

b. Adrenal adenomas and adrenal carcinomas may cause Cushing's syndrome.

c. Ectopic ACTH production by tumors, such as oat cell carcinoma of the lung, carcinoma of the pancreas, bronchial adenoma, and others, causes adrenal hyperplasia and Cushing's syndrome.

d. Iatrogenic Cushing's syndrome is seen more often than the spontaneously occurring syndrome. It is an expected complication in patients receiving long-term glucocorticoid treatment for asthma, arthritis, and other conditions.

2. Clinical features

a. Central obesity is caused by the effect of excess cortisol secretion on fat distribution. Fat accumulates in the face, neck, and trunk, while the limbs remain thin. The "**moon face**," "**buffalo hump**" (cervical fat pad), and **supraclavicular fat pads** contribute to the cushingoid appearance of affected individuals.

b. Hypertension results from the vascular effects of cortisol as well as other actions of the hormone, including sodium retention.

c. Decreased glucose tolerance is common; 20% of patients have overt diabetes. This is a result of the increased hepatic gluconeogenesis and decreased peripheral glucose utilization caused by elevated levels of cortisol.

d. Symptoms of androgen excess (e.g., oligomenorrhea, hirsutism, and acne) may occur in women with Cushing's disease because of stimulation by ACTH of adrenal androgen production.

e. Purple striae are linear marks on the abdomen, where the thin, wasted skin is stretched by underlying fat.

f. Muscle wasting and weakness reflect the catabolic effects of cortisol on muscle protein.

g. Osteoporosis is a frequent result of cortisol excess. It is caused by increased bone catabolism and perhaps by the inhibitory effects of cortisol on collagen synthesis and calcium absorption.

h. Susceptibility to bruising is probably caused by enhanced capillary fragility.

i. Psychiatric disturbances, especially depression, are frequent results of cortisol excess.

j. Growth retardation in children may be severe.

3. Diagnosis

a. The **overnight dexamethasone suppression test** is recommended as an initial screening procedure for any patient suspected of having Cushing's syndrome. The patient takes 1.0 mg of dexamethasone orally at 11 P.M., and the serum cortisol level is measured at 8 A.M. the following morning.

(1) Most individuals demonstrate normal suppression of ACTH and cortisol by the dexamethasone, and their serum cortisol level is less than 5 μg/dl. Since this test is very sensitive, the diagnosis need not be considered further in these cases.

(2) Patients with Cushing's syndrome will have cortisol levels greater than 5 μg/dl and usually greater than 10 μg/dl. This result indicates that further study is needed. (The test is not very specific; mental or physical stress may produce a false-positive result.)

b. The **standard dexamethasone suppression test** is the most relied-upon biochemical test for Cushing's syndrome, although false-positive and false-negative results are not rare. The suppressibility of the hypothalamic-pituitary-adrenal axis is tested by the administration of dexamethasone in both low and high doses, each for 2 days, with measurement of the serum cortisol concentration and the urinary 17-hydroxycorticosteroid level on the second day of each dose level (Table 9-13).

(1) The pattern of response is useful:

(a) To distinguish normal individuals from those with Cushing's syndrome

(b) To separate patients with Cushing's disease from those with adrenal tumors or ectopic ACTH production

(2) Patients with Cushing's disease behave as though their feedback response to glucocorticoids is intact but set at a higher than normal level; they respond to high but not to low doses of dexamethasone. Patients with adrenal tumors and ectopic ACTH secretion produce corticoids autonomously, without suppression even by high doses of dexamethasone.

c. ACTH measurement may help to differentiate the causes of Cushing's syndrome.

(1) ACTH levels are usually high-normal or slightly elevated in patients with Cushing's disease and may be markedly elevated in patients with ectopic ACTH production.

(2) When an autonomously functioning adrenal tumor is the source of excess cortisol secretion, pituitary secretion of ACTH is suppressed due to the excessive cortisol production, and the ACTH level is extremely low or undetectable.

Table 9-13A. Standard Dexamethasone Suppression Test: Method

Day	Dosage (Dexamethasone)	Measurements
1	None (baseline)	24-hour urinary 17-hydroxycortico-steroid and 4 P.M. serum cortisol levels
2,3	Low-dose (0.5 mg every 6 hours)	Repeat measurements on day 3
4,5	High-dose (2.0 mg every 6 hours)	Repeat measurements on day 5

Table 9-13B. Standard Dexamethasone Suppression Test: Response

Test Results	Suppression with Low Dose*	Suppression with High Dose[†]
Normal	Yes	Yes
Cushing's disease	No	Yes
Adrenal tumor or ectopic ACTH production	No	No

*17-hydroxycorticosteroid excretion < 3 mg/24 hr; serum cortisol level < 5 μg/dl.
[†] > 50% fall in 17-hydroxycorticosteroid baseline levels; serum cortisol level < 10 μg/dl.

d. Laboratory findings
   (1) The **serum cortisol** level in normal individuals is highest in early morning and falls throughout the day, reaching a low point at about midnight. Although the morning level may be increased in patients with Cushing's syndrome, a loss of the normal diurnal variation and an increase in the evening level are more consistent findings.
   (2) The **24-hour urinary free cortisol** excretion rate is increased in most patients with Cushing's syndrome. However, because serum and urine cortisol levels may be increased by mental or physical stress and are not always raised above the normal range in patients with Cushing's syndrome, a single random measurement is not very useful in screening for this disease.
   (3) **Nonspecific laboratory abnormalities** include leukocytosis, with a relatively low percentage of lymphocytes and eosinophils, and an elevation in the serum glucose level.
e. Radiographic findings
   (1) **Skull x-rays reveal** enlargement of the sella turcica in the 10% of patients with Cushing's syndrome who have **macroadenomas**.
   (2) **CT scans with injection of contrast medium show microadenomas** in many of the remaining patients.
   (3) **CT scans of the adrenal gland** reveal most adrenal tumors. Uniform enlargement of both adrenal glands suggests an ACTH-dependent form of Cushing's syndrome, either Cushing's disease or the ectopic ACTH syndrome.

4. Therapy
   a. Adrenal adenomas can usually be resected completely, with cure of the disease. Cortisol replacement is needed for a number of months postoperatively, until the remaining normal adrenal tissue, suppressed by the previous high cortisol levels, regains its ability to produce cortisol.
   b. Adrenal carcinoma is often inoperable when first diagnosed due to metastases, usually to the liver and the lungs, and prolonged survival is uncommon. Mitotane, metyrapone, and aminoglutethimide are drugs that block adrenal steroid production, and they may relieve the manifestations of excess cortisol production in patients with inoperable adrenal carcinoma.
   c. The **ectopic ACTH syndrome** can be cured by removal of the tumor, but this is not possible in most cases. The tumor causing the syndrome is usually the main problem rather than the Cushing's syndrome itself.
   d. Cushing's disease may be treated in several ways.
      (1) Pituitary irradiation is effective in many children, but it cures less than one-third of adult patients; the reason for the difference in response between children and adults is not clear.
      (2) Bilateral adrenalectomy cures Cushing's disease, but leaves the patient with **Addison's disease** and the need for lifelong steroid replacement. Also, adrenalectomy is

sometimes followed by the development of **Nelson's syndrome**, in which a pituitary adenoma undergoes rapid growth, perhaps because it is no longer inhibited by above-normal levels of cortisol.

(3) Transsphenoidal pituitary surgery is the treatment of choice. Even when tumors cannot be seen on CT scan, transsphenoidal exploration may disclose a microadenoma. Surgery is successful in 50%–95% of cases and is followed by normal pituitary and adrenal function as well as cure of Cushing's disease.

C. Adrenal insufficiency (Addison's disease)

1. Etiology

a. Primary adrenal insufficiency

(1) Idiopathic atrophy of the adrenal cortex, due to an autoimmune process, is the most common cause of adrenal insufficiency.

(2) Tuberculosis may involve the adrenal glands, with destruction of both cortices and medullae.

(3) Iatrogenic causes

(a) Bilateral adrenalectomy for Cushing's disease or as palliative treatment of metastatic breast cancer results in adrenal insufficiency.

(b) Adrenal suppression following prolonged steroid therapy may persist for up to 1 year or longer.

(4) Less common causes of adrenal destruction include **amyloidosis, fungal infections, syphilis, bilateral adrenal hemorrhage** (especially in patients receiving anticoagulants), and **metastatic malignancy. Acquired immune deficiency syndrome (AIDS)** sometimes leads to adrenal insufficiency through cytomegalovirus and other infections of the adrenal glands.

b. Secondary adrenal insufficiency is due to pituitary disease and results from any of the causes of hypopituitarism (see section I A 2 a).

2. Clinical features. The symptoms of adrenal insufficiency are caused by both cortisol and aldosterone deficiencies.

a. Cortisol deficiency

(1) Hyperpigmentation of the skin is caused by increased melanocyte-stimulating hormone (MSH) activity that accompanies the increased pituitary secretion of ACTH. The latter is a feedback response to the cortisol deficiency. Hyperpigmentation is most noticeable over exposed areas, on mucous membranes, and in skin creases and scars. [In secondary adrenal insufficiency (which is caused by pituitary disease) ACTH levels are low rather than elevated and hyperpigmentation is absent.]

(2) Hypotension, often orthostatic, is caused by the absence of cortisol's pressor effect on vascular tone and by a decrease in cardiac output.

(3) Gastrointestinal symptoms include anorexia, nausea and vomiting, and weight loss.

(4) Hypoglycemia is related to decreased cortisol-induced gluconeogenesis.

(5) Mental symptoms may include lethargy and confusion. Psychotic manifestations occur on occasion.

(6) Intolerance to stress. Patients who cannot increase their cortisol output in response to severe stress risk an acute exacerbation of the symptoms just discussed, with life-threatening vascular collapse.

b. Aldosterone deficiency*

(1) Sodium loss results from reduced aldosterone-mediated reabsorption of sodium in the distal renal tubules. **Hypovolemia, decreased cardiac output,** and **decreased renal blood flow with azotemia** as well as weakness, hypotension, and weight loss may be related to sodium depletion.

(2) Potassium retention caused by aldosterone deficiency may lead to **hyperkalemia** and **cardiac arrhythmias.**

3. Diagnosis

a. ACTH testing is needed for a definitive diagnosis. The normal adrenal gland sharply increases its output of cortisol in response to ACTH; absence of this response proves adrenal insufficiency.

(1) Short ACTH test. The serum level of cortisol is measured before and 30 minutes after an intravenous or intramuscular injection of 0.25 mg (25 units) of cosyntropin, a synthetic form of ACTH. The serum cortisol level should rise at least 7 μg/dl and should

---

*The renin-angiotensin system is not affected by secondary adrenal insufficiency, and since it, rather than ACTH, has primary control of aldosterone production, there is usually no deficiency of aldosterone in secondary adrenal insufficiency.

reach a level of 18 μg/dl or higher. Although this test is useful as an office procedure, it is less reliable than the standard ACTH test.

(2) Standard ACTH test

(a) ACTH in a dose of 25–40 units is given intravenously over 8 hours. The 24-hour urinary excretion rate of free cortisol or the 17-hydroxycorticosteroid excretion rate is measured the day before the infusion and on the day of the infusion. In addition, serum cortisol levels can be measured before the infusion is started and again after it has run for 6–8 hours. Dexamethasone in 0.5-mg doses every 6 hours may be given during the test to protect the patient against adrenal insufficiency.

(b) A normal response is a threefold to fivefold increase in urinary corticoid and a 15–40 μg/dl rise in serum cortisol level.

(c) If hypopituitarism is suspected, the ACTH infusion should be given daily for 4 or 5 days. A lack of response on the first or second day, followed by a stepwise increase and eventual normal response by the fourth or fifth day, is typical of secondary adrenal insufficiency; the adrenal tissue is suppressed by long-term ACTH deficiency, but it can be "primed" by daily stimulation.

b. Laboratory findings

(1) Nonspecific laboratory abnormalities may include **hyponatremia, hyperkalemia, hypoglycemia,** and an **increased eosinophil count** (glucocorticoids lower the eosinophil count). Chest x-ray may reveal a **small heart.**

(2) Plasma cortisol, urinary free cortisol, and **urinary 17-hydroxycorticosteroid levels are low.** Baseline levels, however, may overlap with the values in normal individuals.

4. Therapy

a. Glucocorticoid replacement is needed in all patients. The usual dose of cortisol is 20 mg orally each morning and 10 mg each evening. The dose must be raised at times of stress: Typical doses would be 40–60 mg daily during minor stress (e.g., common cold or dental extraction), 100 mg during moderate stress (e.g., influenza or minor surgery), and "stress doses" of 300 mg or more during severe stress (e.g., major surgery or a serious infection or injury).

b. Mineralocorticoid replacement is not required by all patients. Persistence of low blood pressure, weakness, and low serum sodium and high serum potassium levels indicates a need for mineralocorticoid treatment in addition to cortisol. **Fludrocortisone** is given in a daily dose of 0.05–0.2 mg.

5. Adrenal crisis (addisonian crisis) is an acute, life-threatening complication of Addison's disease in which the manifestations of adrenal insufficiency are greatly exaggerated.

a. Clinical features. Fever, vomiting, abdominal pain, altered mental status, and vascular collapse may occur in untreated Addison's disease or in a treated patient following acute stress if additional glucocorticoid replacement is not provided.

b. Therapy. Immediate intravenous administration of 100 mg of cortisol over 5–10 minutes should be followed by an additional 300 mg in the next 24 hours. Intravenous saline is also needed, and mineralocorticoid replacement should be provided if hypotension and volume depletion persist.

D. Primary aldosteronism

1. Etiology. Excessive adrenal production of aldosterone is usually caused by a single **small** (0.5–3 cm) **adrenal adenoma.** Less often (i.e., in 20%–40% of cases) there is bilateral hyperplasia of the adrenal cortex.

2. Clinical features. Aldosterone increases the reabsorption of sodium and the excretion of potassium and hydrogen ions in the distal renal tubules.

a. Sodium retention causes blood pressure elevation, which is the chief clinical manifestation of this syndrome. The amount of sodium and water that are retained is limited by compensatory mechanisms that increase renal sodium excretion in response to extracellular fluid volume expansion; sodium balance is restored after 1–2 kg of fluid have accumulated. Although this amount of volume expansion does not cause edema, the long-term increase in cardiac output, and perhaps other effects of mineralocorticoid excess, lead to hypertension.

b. Potassium loss causes hypokalemia, which may produce **muscle weakness, paresthesias,** and **tetany** in severe cases. **Hypokalemic nephropathy** may cause polyuria. **Metabolic alkalosis** is a result of the renal loss of potassium and hydrogen ions.

3. Diagnosis

a. Laboratory diagnosis of primary aldosteronism

(1) Hypokalemia in a hypertensive patient is often the clue that triggers the search for primary aldosteronism, although not all patients with aldosteronism have a low serum level of potassium.

(2) Aldosterone must be measured under standardized conditions because it is affected by sodium balance, diuretics, and other factors.

    (a) Diuretics and vasodilators must be discontinued at least 2 weeks before studies of aldosterone (and renin) are undertaken.

    (b) Random aldosterone measurements in patients with primary aldosteronism may overlap those of normal individuals; sodium loading may be necessary to differentiate the aldosterone levels in patients with primary aldosteronism (which are not suppressed by a sodium load) from the levels in normal individuals (which are suppressed by a sodium load). Two of the many ways that this procedure can be performed are as follows.

        (i) The **24-hour urinary aldosterone excretion rate** can be measured after the patient has ingested more than 150 mEq of sodium for at least 3 days. (This can be assured by giving sodium chloride tablets.) An elevated aldosterone level in a 24-hour urine sample that contains more than 150 mEq of sodium suggests primary aldosteronism. (Sodium loading may further lower serum levels of potassium; therefore, caution is necessary if the patient is hypokalemic.)

        (ii) **Plasma levels of aldosterone** can be measured after 2000 ml of normal saline have been infused over a period of 4 hours. Normally, the values are less than 8–10 ng/dl. Severe hypertension or congestive heart failure are contraindications to saline infusion.

(3) Plasma renin activity is the most useful indicator of whether elevated aldosterone production is primary or secondary.

    (a) Secondary aldosteronism is caused by conditions that originate outside the adrenal gland and that reduce the effective arterial blood volume, thus diminishing the pressure or tension sensed by the juxtaglomerular cells, which are associated with the stimulation of aldosterone secretion. Such conditions include heart failure, nephrosis, cirrhosis, volume depletion caused by diuretics, and renovascular disease. Decreased pressure on the juxtaglomerular cells stimulates renin release, which increases angiotensin II and, in turn, aldosterone. Thus, **the high aldosterone level is accompanied by increased renin activity**.

    (b) In **primary aldosteronism** the enhanced aldosterone production is caused by an adrenal abnormality, not by increased renin activity; the resulting volume expansion suppresses renin production. This combination of **increased aldosterone production and reduced renin activity can only be caused by primary aldosteronism**, and it is a reliable indicator of this diagnosis.

    (c) Suppression of renin activity is diagnosed with certainty only if levels remain low following manipulations that are known to stimulate renin in normal individuals, such as dietary sodium restriction, several hours of upright posture, or furosemide administration.

b. Adenoma versus hyperplasia. It is important to distinguish between aldosteronism that is due to an adenoma and aldosteronism that is due to hyperplasia because the distinction affects treatment, which is usually surgical in cases of adrenal adenoma and medical in bilateral hyperplasia.

    (1) The biochemical changes of aldosteronism—the hypokalemia, the increased aldosterone level, and the low renin activity—are more pronounced in cases caused by a unilateral adenoma than in cases caused by hyperplasia.

    (2) The plasma aldosterone concentration may be measured at 8 A.M., after 8 hours of recumbency, and again at noon, after 4 hours of ambulation.

        (a) Levels are higher after ambulation in normal subjects and in patients with bilateral hyperplasia, because renin and angiotensin are stimulated by the upright posture and sympathetic outflow.

        (b) However, patients with unilateral adrenal adenomas have a paradoxical fall in plasma aldosterone levels, presumably because when renin is profoundly suppressed aldosterone is influenced mainly by the diurnal fall in ACTH.

    (3) Adrenal vein aldosterone concentrations may be measured in blood samples obtained by selective catheterization. A very high level on one side indicates an adenoma; high levels on both sides indicate bilateral hyperplasia.

    (4) CT scans and **adrenal venography** sometimes reveal aldosterone-producing adenomas, but these tumors may be very small and often cannot be visualized.

4. Therapy

  a. Surgery

    (1) Removal of a unilateral adenoma results in cure of the hypertension in about 60% of cases and improvement in another 25%.

(2) In contrast, only 20%–50% of patients with bilateral hyperplasia are improved by surgery, even if bilateral adrenalectomy is performed. Medical treatment is preferable.

b. Medical treatment. Spironolactone inhibits the effects of aldosterone on the renal tubule. A dose of 200–400 mg daily corrects the hypokalemia and often corrects the hypertension.

E. Congenital adrenal hyperplasia

1. **Etiology and pathophysiology.** Congenital adrenal hyperplasia is caused by a defect in one of the enzymes that are necessary for the synthesis of cortisol. Cortisol deficiency stimulates ACTH, which causes hyperplasia of the adrenal cortex and overproduction of whatever ACTH-dependent steroids are not affected by the enzyme deficiency (mainly adrenal androgens).

2. **Clinical features**
   a. **Androgen excess** is caused by increased adrenal production of dehydroepiandrosterone, androstenedione, and testosterone.
      (1) If present during fetal development, this disorder may cause **ambiguous genitalia** in females. If androgen excess is manifested in the postnatal period, it may cause **virilization** in prepubertal girls or in young women.
      (2) In males the consequence of androgen excess during fetal development is macrogenitosomia. In the postnatal period, the consequence is **precocious puberty**.
   b. The cortisol deficit usually does not cause major clinical manifestations because the ACTH stimulation and adrenal hyperplasia maintain cortisol levels in the low-normal range, despite the enzyme deficiency.
   c. Other mainfestations occasionally occur, depending on the specific enzyme affected.
      (1) **21-Hydroxylase deficiency** accounts for 95% of cases of adrenal hyperplasia. In the mild (simple virilizing) form, only the androgen-excess symptoms are of importance. In the severe (salt-losing) form, the production of aldosterone is impaired as well as that of cortisol; mineralocorticoid deficiency leads to hyponatremia, hyperkalemia, dehydration, and hypotension.
      (2) In **11-hydroxylase deficiency** there is overproduction of deoxycorticosterone, a mineralocorticoid, as well as adrenal androgens. This causes hypertension through mechanisms that are similar to those causing hypertension in primary aldosteronism.
      (3) In **17-hydroxylase deficiency** there is overproduction of deoxycorticosterone and resulting hypertension. However, because 17-hydroxylase is necessary for sex steroid synthesis, there is androgen deficiency rather than excess and there is estrogen deficiency. This causes the development of ambiguous genitalia in males and primary amenorrhea in females.

3. **Diagnosis.** Concentrations of adrenal androgens and precursors of cortisol are increased in blood and urine. The most useful measurements are of **blood testosterone, androstenedione, dehydroepiandrosterone**, and **17-hydroxyprogesterone** (a cortisol precursor) as well as **urinary 17-ketosteroids** and **pregnanetriol** (a metabolite of 17-hydroxyprogesterone).

4. **Therapy**
   a. **Medical treatment. Cortisol** administration will suppress the overproduction of ACTH and adrenal androgens. In the salt-losing syndrome, mineralocorticoid replacement with fludrocortisone may be necessary.
   b. **Surgery.** Reconstructive surgery of the external genitalia in female infants is done in the first few years of life.

F. Pheochromocytoma is a tumor of **chromaffin cells**, the cells that synthesize and store catecholamines. Chromaffin cells are located mainly in the adrenal medulla, but they also are located in sympathetic ganglia and elsewhere. The cells in the adrenal medulla produce epinephrine and norepinephrine; the extra-adrenal chromaffin cells make only norepinephrine.

1. **Epidemiology**
   a. **Incidence.** Pheochromocytoma is a rare cause of hypertension. It is found in about 0.5% of patients with severe hypertension and in less than 0.05% of all hypertensive patients. However, because it may cause a dramatic and debilitating syndrome, often with fatal complications if undetected, diagnostic efforts and awareness are required out of proportion to its frequency of occurrence.
   b. **Familial occurrence.** Pheochromocytomas may occur sporadically or may occur as part of one of several familial syndromes.
      (1) **Multiple endocrine neoplasia, type II (Sipple's syndrome)** is characterized by multiple pheochromocytomas and medullary carcinoma of the thyroid; hyperparathyroidism is often present.

> **(2) Neurofibromatosis and von Hippel-Lindau disease** may be associated with pheochromocytoma.

2. **Pathology.** The majority of pheochromocytomas are single tumors of the adrenal medulla. However, 10%–20% are located outside of the adrenal gland, and 1%–3% are in the chest or neck. About 20% are multiple, and 10% are malignant.

3. **Clinical features.** The **manifestations of pheochromocytoma** (Table 9-14) are caused by increased levels of circulating catecholamines. Hypertension is paroxysmal in about half of the cases and is sustained in the rest. The diagnosis is often suggested by the **paroxysmal nature of the symptoms**. Attacks typically last less than 1 hour and may be precipitated by exercise, induction of anesthesia, urination (suggesting a pheochromocytoma of the bladder), or palpation of the abdomen. Other features that suggest the presence of a pheochromocytoma are **hyperglycemia, hypermetabolism,** and **postural hypotension** in a hypertensive patient.

4. **Diagnosis.** Pheochromocytoma is suspected far more often than it is diagnosed. Many patients with symptoms of catecholamine excess prove to have normal hormone levels.
   a. The levels of **urine catecholamines** and their metabolites are elevated in most confirmed cases. A screening test of the **24-hour urinary metanephrine excretion rate** may be the most useful, but tests of **urinary free catecholamine** (i.e., epinephrine and norepinephrine) and **vanillylmandelic acid** concentrations are also of value. Stressful illness can raise catecholamine levels twofold; greater than twofold elevations are more suggestive of pheochromocytoma.
   b. **Serum catecholamine levels** are quite variable and are more difficult to interpret than the 24-hour urine measurements.
   c. The **clonidine suppression test** is useful in patients with mild catecholamine elevation. Three hours after an oral dose of 0.3 mg of clonidine, the plasma level of norepinephrine is lowered into the normal range in most normal individuals but it remains elevated in patients with pheochromocytoma.
   d. **CT scans** of the abdomen detect as many as 90% of these tumors since they usually are greater than 1 cm in diameter.
   e. **Adrenal scanning** with ^{131}I iodobenzylguanidine is especially useful for localizing extra-adrenal tumors, but this procedure is not widely available.

5. **Therapy**
   a. **Medical treatment**
      (1) The α- and β-adrenergic blocking agents are useful for inoperable tumors and for preparation for surgery.
         (a) **Alpha-adrenergic blocking agents** relieve the hypertension and adrenergic symptoms.
            (i) **Phenoxybenzamine** is given orally, starting with 10 mg twice daily and increasing to 40 mg twice daily if necessary.
            (ii) **Phentolamine** can be given intravenously to treat acute severe elevations in blood pressure.
            (iii) **Prazosin** can also be given to produce sustained α-adrenergic blockade.
         (b) **Beta-adrenergic blocking agents** should not be used alone, since unopposed alpha-adrenergic stimulation may lead to exacerbation of the hypertension. Beta-blockers are sometimes useful in conjunction with alpha-blockers.
      (2) **Metyrosine,** which is an inhibitor of tyrosine hydroxylase, blocks the formation of norepinephrine and epinephrine and is an alternative agent for the relief of the symptoms of pheochromocytoma. It may be used if intolerance to the adrenergic blocking agents is a problem.
   b. **Surgery. Surgical removal of the pheochromocytoma is the treatment of choice.** Careful exploration of the adrenal gland and the periaortic sympathetic chain is performed.
      (1) **Complications** that frequently occur during and after surgery are extreme swings in blood pressure, cardiac arrhythmias, and shock. These are caused by the sudden re-

Table 9-14. Manifestations of Pheochromocytoma

Hypertension
Headache
Sweating
Palpitations
Nervousness
Weight loss

Note.—The adrenergic symptoms of hypertension, tremor, weakness, sweating, and palpitations may all occur paroxysmally due to variations in the function of the tumor.

moval of the source of excess catecholamine production and by the low blood volume that results from long-term constriction of the vascular compartment.

   (2) To prevent vascular instability during removal of a pheochromocytoma, patients are treated with α-blockers to maintain normal blood pressure for at least 1 week before surgery. Beta-blockers may be added for a few days before surgery, especially if tachycardia or another arrhythmia is present.

VI. FEMALE REPRODUCTIVE DISORDERS. Endocrine disorders that affect the female reproductive system usually cause menstrual abnormalities and include those disorders in which menarche does not occur (**primary amenorrhea**) and those disorders that cause cessation of menstrual periods after menarche (**secondary amenorrhea**). Androgen-excess syndromes are a common cause of reproductive abnormalities that also are considered in this section.

A. Primary amenorrhea (Table 9-15)

   1. Gonadal dysgenesis (Turner's syndrome) occurs in 1 in 2500–10,000 live female births.
      a. Etiology and pathophysiology. Gonadal dysgenesis is caused by a **chromosomal abnormality** that is not familial and is not related to the mother's age. Patients have a chromatin-negative buccal smear and a 45,X karyotype.
      b. Clinical features
         (1) **Ovaries fail to develop**; only bilateral streaks of connective tissue are present, without germ cells. Estrogen deficiency, caused by the absence of ovarian tissue, results in **sexual infantilism**, with absence of breast development and other secondary sexual characteristics, and increased levels of LH and FSH.
         (2) **Somatic abnormalities** are associated with the gonadal dysgenesis. Most patients are short, between 48 and 58 inches in height. Other features, present in varying numbers of patients, include a short, webbed neck, epicanthal folds, low-set ears, a shield-like chest with widely spaced nipples, cubitus valgus (wide carrying angle), and renal and cardiac abnormalities.
      c. Therapy
         (1) **Estrogen therapy** induces the development of secondary sexual characteristics. If estrogen is given cyclically with progesterone, regular menstrual bleeding will occur but fertility, of course, is not possible.
         (2) **Removal of streak gonads.** Gonadal dysgenesis may occur in patients with sex chromosome mosaicism in which one or more cell lines bear a Y chromosome. The frequency of gonadoblastoma and other gonadal tumors is increased in patients with these gonads, and their prophylactic removal is recommended.

   2. Testicular feminization syndrome. Patients with this syndrome are genetic males, with a 46,XY karyotype, but they have normal female external genitalia and are raised as girls.
      a. Pathogenesis. The basic defect is resistance of target tissues to the action of androgens. The fetal testes produce testosterone, but because the wolffian ducts and genital tissues cannot respond to testosterone, female differentiation of the external genitalia takes place. The fetal testes also produce mullerian duct inhibiting factor, which has its normal effect in inhibiting the mullerian anlage, and so the fallopian tubes, uterus, and upper vagina do not develop.
      b. Clinical features. The result is a phenotypic female with a vagina that ends in a blind pouch, hypoplastic male ducts instead of the fallopian tubes and uterus, and testes located in the abdomen, inguinal canal, or labia majora. Endogenous estrogen stimulates normal breast development at puberty. The condition is suspected when menarche fails to occur or when a testis is felt as an abdominal mass, which is explored.

Table 9-15. Causes of Primary Amenorrhea

Gonadal causes
Gonadal dysgenesis (Turner's syndrome)
Testicular feminization syndrome
Resistant ovary syndrome
Extragonadal causes
Hypopituitarism
Hypogonadotropic hypogonadism
Delayed menarche
Congenital adrenal hyperplasia
Abnormalities of the uterus or vagina

c. Therapy. The testes are prone to malignant degeneration and should be removed. Estrogen treatment is then given to maintain secondary sexual characteristics.

3. **Resistant ovary syndrome.** Inability of the ovaries to respond to normal or increased stimulation by gonadotropins may be a result of autoimmune destruction of the ovaries or other conditions.

4. **Hypogonadotropic hypogonadism**
   a. **Panhypopituitarism** due to destructive lesions of the hypothalamic-pituitary area (see section I A 2 a) causes primary or secondary amenorrhea, depending on whether the problem is prepubertal or postpubertal in onset.
   b. **Isolated gonadotropin deficiency** is most often caused by defective hypothalamic production of GnRH, usually of unknown etiology. In **Kallmann's syndrome** this defect is associated with anosmia.

5. **Delayed menarche** should be considered when menstrual periods have not begun by the age of 16 years. A diagnosis of delayed menarche, as opposed to that of primary amenorrhea, can only be made in retrospect, after spontaneous menstrual periods have begun. A family history of late pubertal development suggests that spontaneous menarche may yet be expected. If severe psychological stress is caused by the absence of sexual development, it may be necessary to give one or more 6-month courses of estrogen therapy, with long treatment-free periods to observe if spontaneous puberty will occur.

B. **Secondary amenorrhea** (Table 9-16)

1. **Hypothalamic** (also called "**psychogenic**," "**functional**," and "**idiopathic**") **amenorrhea** is the **most common form of nonphysiologic secondary amenorrhea**. Obvious psychological stress may or may not be present. LH and FSH levels are low in some cases and normal in others. If the hypothalamic releasing hormone GnRH is infused in physiologic fashion (pulse doses every 90–120 minutes), all abnormalities may be corrected: Ovarian follicles mature, ovulation takes place, a corpus luteum develops and functions, and pregnancy may occur. This supports the clinical impression that most cases of functional or idiopathic amenorrhea are caused by abnormal hypothalamic GnRH production.

2. **Malnutrition.** Menarche seems to occur when a critical body weight is reached, and menstruation often ceases when a woman whose menstrual cycle was previously normal falls below this critical weight, whether because of food deprivation, chronic illness, excessive dieting, or anorexia nervosa.

Table 9-16. Causes of Secondary Amenorrhea

Pregnancy

Menopause

Uterine causes
   Intrauterine synechiae (Asherman's syndrome)
   Hysterectomy

Hypothalamic-pituitary causes
   Hypopituitarism
   Hypothalamic ("psychogenic") amenorrhea
   Malnutrition, chronic illness
   Exercise
   Oral contraceptive discontinuation

Ovarian causes
   Primary ovarian failure ("premature menopause")
   Oophorectomy
   Radiotherapy, chemotherapy

Estrogen excess
   Ovarian tumors

Prolactin excess
   Pituitary tumors

Androgen excess
   Polycystic ovary syndrome
   Adrenal androgen overproduction
   Ovarian tumors

3. Exercise. Amenorrhea is present in up to 50% of female ballet dancers, runners, and athletes. Exercise-related weight loss is at least partially responsible; the risk of amenorrhea is much higher in women who have lost more than 10%–15% of their body weight. Levels of LH, FSH, and estrogen tend to be low, suggesting a hypothalamic abnormality.

4. "Post-pill amenorrhea" refers to a delay of more than 6 months in the return of menses after the discontinuation of oral contraceptive use. It occurs in fewer than 1% of pill users, and other causes of amenorrhea must be excluded before contraceptive use is blamed.

5. Primary ovarian failure ("premature menopause") is similar to normal menopause; that is, ovarian function declines, estrogen levels fall, and gonadotropin levels rise. However, primary ovarian failure occurs before the age of 40 years. Autoantibodies against ovarian antigens have been found in some cases.

6. Ovarian tumors such as granulosa-theca cell tumors may inhibit normal menstrual cycling by producing excessive quantities of estrogen.

7. Prolactin excess is a common cause of secondary amenorrhea (see section I A 4 b).

C. Androgen excess syndromes

1. The polycystic ovary syndrome (which is also called the Stein-Leventhal syndrome) is a disorder of unknown etiology that is characterized by a chronic lack of ovulation, associated with symptoms of androgen excess and often with obesity. It is present in 3%–7% of reproductive-age women.

a. Pathophysiology (Fig. 9-2)

(1) The ovary produces excess androgenic steroids, especially **androstenedione**. The androstenedione is converted to estrone, an estrogen, in fat and other peripheral tissues. The increased circulating and intraovarian levels of androstenedione and other androgens prevent the maturation of graafian follicles, causing **anovulation**.

(2) The increased circulating level of estrone has a positive feedback effect on pituitary production of LH and a negative effect on production of FSH. The **increased LH level** causes hyperplasia of ovarian thecal cells and stroma and increased androgen production. The **decreased FSH level** contributes to the lack of follicle maturation.

(3) Obesity may enhance the elevated levels of sex steroids by decreasing sex hormone–binding globulin, thus increasing the level of free testosterone, and by increasing the peripheral conversion of androstenedione to estrone.

(4) As a result of the **arrested follicle development**, the ovaries are enlarged, with thickened capsules and many small follicular cysts. Stromal and thecal hyperplasia is seen on microscopic examination.

(5) The initiating event in this cycle is uncertain, and it may not be the same in all cases. Some authorities believe that the basic abnormality is in the hypothalamic-pituitary axis, with constant (rather than cyclic) overproduction of LH; others believe that excess ovarian secretion of androgen is the primary event. Abnormalities of adrenal androgen production have been found in these patients, and some investigators believe that this may initiate the cycle; there are reports of disappearance of the polycystic ovary syndrome following the removal of an androgen-secreting adrenal adenoma.

b. Clinical features

(1) Infertility and menstrual abnormalities are the result of chronic anovulation. Most patients have amenorrhea or oligomenorrhea. The prolonged, noncyclic, unopposed estrogenic stimulation of the endometrium may cause functional bleeding and an increased risk of endometrial carcinoma.

(2) Androgen excess causes oiliness of the skin, acne, and hirsutism in the majority of

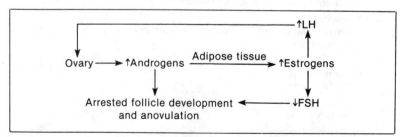

Figure 9-2. Pathogenesis of the polycystic ovary syndrome. The etiology of this syndrome is not known; however, an abnormality in the hypothalamic-pituitary axis and abnormalities in ovarian or adrenal androgen production have been theorized.

women with this syndrome. Signs of true virilization (i.e., deepening of the voice, enlargement of the clitoris, and so forth) are rare.

(3) **Obesity** is present in about 40% of patients.

c. **Laboratory findings**

(1) An **increased LH-to-FSH ratio** ($\geq$ 2.0) is a very useful diagnostic finding. The LH level is usually elevated, and the FSH level is in the low-normal range.

(2) **Serum testosterone and androstenedione** levels are usually elevated. Increased levels of the androgens of predominantly adrenal origin (i.e., dehydroepiandrosterone and dehydroepiandrosterone sulfate) are found to be increased less often.

(3) **Serum estrone levels** are usually high, and estradiol levels are normal.

d. **Therapy.** The two **main goals of treatment are the relief of symptoms of androgen excess and the induction of ovulation and fertility.** Treatment of the former (e.g., with birth-control pills) may preclude treatment of the latter; a clear view of therapeutic goals in each case is, therefore, essential.

(1) **Androgen excess.** Oral contraceptives, glucocorticoids, and spironolactone are used to treat the hirsutism and other symptoms associated with androgen excess. Some authorities advocate initial testing to determine whether androgen levels can be suppressed by contraceptives or by glucocorticoids, and others prefer a trial-and-error approach.

(a) **Estrogen-progestin combinations** decrease androgen levels by feedback inhibition of pituitary LH production and by stimulation of hepatic synthesis of sex hormone–binding globulin, which decreases the unbound fraction of testosterone.

(i) Side effects of fluid retention, nausea, and break-through bleeding may occur.

(ii) Potential complications, which are related to the estrogen dose and to cigarette use, include thrombophlebitis, myocardial infarction, and hypertension.

(b) **Glucocorticoids** decrease adrenal androgen production by suppressing ACTH; they may also lower ovarian androgen secretion, although the mechanism is unknown.

(i) Since ACTH production peaks in early morning, a bedtime dose of 0.5 mg of dexamethasone is recommended.

(ii) Potential undesired side effects are weight gain, depression, and suppression of the hypothalamic-pituitary-adrenal response to stress.

(c) **Spironolactone**, an aldosterone antagonist that is used mainly for its diuretic and antihypertensive properties, has additional actions that make it useful in the treatment of hirsutism: It decreases ovarian and adrenal synthesis of androgens, and it inhibits androgen binding to receptors in hair follicles and other target tissues. A dose of 100 mg once or twice daily is often effective.

(d) The effects of hormone therapy in diminishing the growth of unwanted facial and body hair are seldom dramatic and usually take place over a period of months. Mechanical methods of hair removal are usually needed as well; these include shaving, electrolysis, bleaching, chemical depilatories, and wax treatments.

(2) **Infertility**

(a) **Clomiphene citrate** blocks the binding of estrogen to receptors in target tissues. By blocking estrogen's negative feedback effects on the hypothalamus and pituitary gland, it stimulates LH and FSH production.

(i) If given on the fifth day through the ninth day following a menstrual period induced by progesterone, clomiphene citrate often stimulates follicle maturation and ovulation.

(ii) Ovulation can be induced with clomiphene citrate in about 80% of cases.

(b) **Human menopausal gonadotropin** has both FSH and LH bioactivity.

(i) It is injected daily until rising serum estrogen levels and ultrasonography of the ovary indicate that follicle maturation has occurred.

(ii) Then human chorionic gonadotropin, which has mainly LH activity, is injected to induce ovulation. The risk of ovarian hyperstimulation and of multiple gestation is high, and this therapy should be reserved for resistant cases of infertility.

(c) **GnRH**, when given intravenously or subcutaneously in pulse doses every 90–120 minutes, may induce ovulation without causing ovarian hyperstimulation. This is a promising new form of treatment.

(3) **Chronic anovulation and abnormal menstrual bleeding.** Unopposed noncyclic stimulation of the endometrium by estrogen may cause functional bleeding and may increase the risk of endometrial cancer. Persistent endometrial proliferation can be interrupted either with progestin treatment (e.g., Provera at 10 mg daily for 10 days every 1–3 months) or with cyclic estrogen-progestin therapy.

2. **Androgen-producing ovarian tumors** are rare. Arrhenoblastoma, the most common, makes

up less than 1% of solid ovarian tumors; others are hilar cell tumors, adrenal rest tumors, and granulosa cell tumors. Testosterone levels tend to be higher than those in the polycystic ovary syndrome, and virilization occurs more frequently. Androgen levels are not suppressed by treatment with glucocorticoids or estrogen-progestin combinations, as they often are in the polycystic ovary syndrome. Diagnosis depends on detection of the tumor by pelvic examination (the majority are palpable) and on diagnostic imaging techniques.

3. Hyperthecosis of the ovary is probably a severe form of the polycystic ovary syndrome, but the androgen excess is more evident. The diagnosis depends on the histologic finding of luteinized thecal and stromal cells. Medical treatment is not effective, and oophorectomy may be necessary.

4. Adrenal tumors, either adenomas or carcinomas, may produce excess androgens with or without excess cortisol. High levels of adrenal androgens (urinary 17-ketosteroids, serum dehydroepiandrosterone) that cannot be suppressed by dexamethasone suggest this diagnosis; 24-hour urinary 17-ketosteroids greater than 50–100 mg strongly suggest adrenal carcinoma.

5. Congenital adrenal hyperplasia is discussed in the section on disorders of the adrenal gland (see section V E).

6. Idiopathic hirsutism, or idiopathic androgen excess syndrome, is a poorly understood but common condition in which mild hirsutism and sometimes acne and menstrual irregularities occur in the absence of marked hormone abnormalities. Testosterone levels may be high-normal or slightly elevated, or there may be elevations in free testosterone (with decreased sex hormone-binding globulin) and adrenal androgens. Polycystic ovaries and LH and FSH abnormalities are absent. Whether the ovary or the adrenal gland is the source of mild androgen excess is unclear. Estrogen-progestin combinations, glucocorticoids, and spironolactone (see section VI C 1 d) sometimes decrease the androgen levels and the symptoms.

VII. MALE REPRODUCTIVE DISORDERS AND GYNECOMASTIA

A. Hypogonadism in the male affects two separate functions—the production of spermatozoa by the seminiferous tubules and the secretion of testosterone by the Leydig cells. The seminiferous tubule defect causes infertility; the testosterone deficiency leads to inadequate development and maintenance of secondary sexual characteristics.

1. Physical and developmental effects
   a. Before puberty, testicular failure prevents normal sexual development. The penis and testes remain small, and spermatozoa are absent. Facial and body hair is sparse. The voice remains high-pitched, and muscle mass and strength are diminished. Increased growth of long bones (because of delayed epiphyseal closure) produces the "eunuchoidal habitus," in which the arm span is more than 2 inches greater than the height, and the floor-to-pubic symphysis distance is more than 2 inches greater than the symphysis-to-crown distance.
   b. After puberty, loss of libido and sexual potency may be the first symptoms of testicular failure. Partial regression of secondary sex characteristics may occur gradually, with slowing of facial and body hair growth and decreased muscle mass.

2. Clinical syndromes
   a. Hypogonadotropic syndromes (Table 9-17). The causes of hypogonadism are divided into **disorders of the hypothalamic-pituitary axis (hypogonadotropic hypogonadism)** and **disorders that originate with testicular damage**, with consequent feedback stimulation of LH and FSH (**hypergonadotropic hypogonadism**).
      (1) Hypogonadotropic (secondary) hypogonadism is characterized by deficiency of LH and FSH, with resulting testosterone deficiency and eunuchoidism. **Kallmann's syndrome** is a form of hypogonadotropic hypogonadism that is associated with midline defects such as agenesis of the olfactory lobes, anosmia, and cleft palate. It is more common in men than in women. The basic hormonal defect is in the hypothalamus, rather than in the pituitary gland, which has been demonstrated by LH and FSH response to GnRH administration.
      (2) Delayed puberty is a retrospective diagnosis. Puberty may occur spontaneously up to about the age of 20 years; until this age, true hypogonadotropic hypogonadism cannot be diagnosed with certainty unless associated abnormalities such as anosmia are present. The diagnosis of delayed puberty is suggested by a family history of late maturation.
         (a) If delayed puberty is suspected, a course of therapy with low doses of testosterone can be initiated to induce pubertal changes; true puberty may be induced by this treatment.
         (b) Testosterone should be given for no more than 6 months at a time, with 6 months

Table 9-17. Causes of Hypogonadism in the Male

Hypogonadotropic syndromes
  Hypopituitarism
  Hypogonadotropic eunuchoidism
    Kallmann's syndrome
  Delayed puberty

Hypergonadotropic syndromes
  Klinefelter's syndrome
  Testicular agenesis
  Testicular injury
    Mumps orchitis
    Other infections (e.g., gonorrhea)
    Trauma
    Surgery
    Radiotherapy
    Cancer chemotherapy
  Cryptorchidism
  Myotonic dystrophy

between courses, to avoid causing epiphyseal closure and limitation of ultimate height and to allow recognition of the onset of spontaneous puberty, if it should occur.

  b. Hypergonadotropic syndromes (primary hypogonadism)

    (1) Klinefelter's syndrome, in which the presence of two or more X chromosomes cause congenital testicular damage, occurs in about 1 in 400 male births.

      (a) About 80% of patients have a **47,XXY karyotype**. The testes are small (less than 2 cm in length). There is hyalinization of the seminiferous tubules and **azoospermia**. Leydig cell function is variable. Testosterone levels are deficient and **eunuchoidism** is present in many but not all cases. **Gynecomastia** is present, and LH and FSH levels are elevated, even (for unknown reasons) in patients without testosterone deficiency. Mental deficiency is an associated finding in 25% of all patients.

      (b) The only available treatment is testosterone replacement in those patients who require it.

    (2) Testicular agenesis is recognized by failure of pubertal development and absence of testes in the scrotum or in the inguinal canals. Loss of the testes occurs after 7–14 weeks gestation, since absence of testicular hormones before this stage would result in a female phenotype.

    (3) Mumps orchitis affects mainly germinal cells; if the disease is bilateral, infertility may result, although this is uncommon. Testosterone production is usually unimpaired.

    (4) Cryptorchidism, especially if it is bilateral, may be associated with hypogonadism because the undescended testes are damaged by trauma or torsion. An association between hypogonadism and cryptorchidism may exist because the cryptorchidism is sometimes a consequence of an intrinsic abnormality in the testes. Treatment with human chorionic gonadotropin or GnRH may induce testicular descent in some cases.

    (5) Myotonic dystrophy is a syndrome consisting of myotonia, cataracts, and testicular atrophy.

  3. Therapy

    a. Testosterone deficiency. Although oral androgenic steroids are available, they do not provide fully virilizing blood levels of male homones. The usual treatment of male hypogonadism is the injection of 200–300 mg of a long-acting testosterone preparation (e.g., Delatestryl or Depo-Testosterone) every 2–3 weeks.

    b. Infertility. It is impossible to induce sperm production and fertility in individuals with primary testicular injury. In hypogonadotropic hypogonadism, it is sometimes possible to bring about spermatogenesis by providing the testes with adequate gonadotropic stimulation. This can be done either by injections three times per week of human chorionic gonadotropin (which has LH activity) and human menopausal gonadotropin (which has FSH activity) or by administration via portable infusion pump of pulse doses of GnRH every 90–120 minutes. Both of these methods are expensive and impractical for long-term use, but they have been used successfully in highly motivated men for the period of several months that is needed to induce spermatogenesis.

B. Gynecomastia is enlargement of the male breast. In true gynecomastia, firm, sometimes tender, glandular tissue is present. The disorders that cause gynecomastia are usually associated with increased levels of estrogens, decreased levels of androgens, or both.

1. **Pubertal gynecomastia.** At the age of 12–15 years, about two-thirds of normal boys have some degree of gynecomastia, usually a small, firm subareolar nodule that disappears in most cases within 1–2 years.
   a. In the occasional boy with persistent breast enlargement, **medical treatment with danazol**, a weak synthetic androgen that inhibits gonadotropin, may be tried.
   b. If this is ineffective, however, **reduction mammoplasty** must be considered if psychological stress is severe.

2. **Hypogonadism**, either primary (hypergonadotropic) or secondary (hypogonadotropic), may be associated with gynecomastia.

3. **Refeeding after a period of starvation** often leads to transient gynecomastia, which may last for several months. Renewed secretion of previously inhibited gonadotropins and sex steroids and decreased hormone inactivation by the starved liver may be contributing factors.

4. **Liver disease**, especially alcoholic cirrhosis, is a common cause of gynecomastia.
   a. Estrogen levels are increased because of accelerated conversion of androgenic precursors by peripheral tissues.
   b. Also, alcohol inhibits the testicular production of testosterone and the pituitary production of gonadotropins and increases hepatic metabolism of testosterone.

5. **Chronic renal failure** is associated with gynecomastia, especially after the start of hemodialysis. The refeeding phenomenon may play a role as may an increase in the ratio of estrogens to androgens in chronic renal failure.

6. **Drugs**
   a. **Estrogens**, commonly used to treat prostatic carcinoma, stimulate the breast directly.
   b. **Spironolactone**, **cimetidine**, and **digitalis** also produce gynecomastia. They are believed to inhibit androgen action by displacing dihydrotestosterone from its intracellular receptor.
   c. **Marijuana** binds to estrogen receptors and may cause gynecomastia through a direct estrogenic action.
   d. Other drugs that may cause this problem include **phenothiazines, tricyclic antidepressants, methyldopa, reserpine**, and **isoniazid**.

7. **Tumors** may cause gynecomastia.
   a. **Adrenal and testicular tumors** may cause gynecomastia through the production of estrogen.
   b. **Testicular choriocarcinomas** may cause gynecomastia through the secretion of chorionic gonadotropin, which stimulates testicular estrogen production.
   c. Other malignant tumors may cause the condition through the ectopic production of gonadotropins.

8. **Hyperthyroidism** increases the conversion of androgens to estrogens in the peripheral tissues and increases the circulating level of sex hormone–binding globulin, which raises the estrogen to androgen ratio. These hormonal changes may cause gynecomastia in men with hyperthyroidism.

VIII. METABOLIC BONE DISEASE.
The metabolic bone diseases are commonly classified into three main categories: osteomalacia, osteoporosis, and osteitis fibrosa cystica. Osteitis fibrosis cystica is discussed briefly in the section on hyperparathyroidism (see section III A 4 b).

A. Osteomalacia

1. **Definition.** Osteomalacia is a **skeletal abnormality** in which there is inadequate mineralization of bone matrix. In children this usually takes the form of **rickets**, caused by vitamin D deficiency. In adults, osteomalacia may be caused by many specific abnormalities of calcium, phosphorus, and vitamin D metabolism.

2. **Etiology**
   a. **Vitamin D deficiency**
      (1) Deficiency of vitamin D causes osteomalacia because its most active metabolite, 1,25-dihydroxyvitamin D_3, is essential for the absorption of calcium and phosphate from the gastrointestinal tract.
      (2) Deficiency of vitamin D is now rare in the United States; most Americans obtain the recommended dietary allowance of 200–400 units of vitamin D from fortified foods, especially dairy products. However, dietary deficiency may still occur because of poverty, food faddism, or eating disorders such as anorexia nervosa.
      (3) Exposure to sunlight converts 7-dehydrocholesterol in the skin to vitamin D_3, and this is

an important source of the vitamin. Absence of sunlight may contribute to vitamin D deficiency.

b. Abnormal metabolism of vitamin D

    (1) Liver disease, when far advanced, may cause osteomalacia by interfering with the normal hepatic conversion of vitamin D to 25-hydroxyvitamin D_3.

    (2) Anticonvulsant drugs, such as phenobarbital and phenytoin, if taken over a long period of time, may alter the metabolism of vitamin D by inducing hepatic microsomal enzymes. Osteomalacia and decreased serum levels of 25-hydroxyvitamin D_3 have been described in patients under long-term treatment with anticonvulsants.

    (3) Hereditary vitamin D-dependent rickets is a rare autosomal recessive disorder, which is thought to be caused by a congenital defect in the renal conversion of 25-hydroxyvitamin D_3 to 1,25-dihydroxyvitamin D_3, the most active metabolite. It responds to small, physiologic doses of 1,25-dihydroxyvitamin D_3, but only to very large, pharmacologic doses of 25-hydroxyvitamin D_3.

c. Renal abnormalities

    (1) Renal osteodystrophy may occur in patients with chronic renal failure of any cause. Both osteomalacia, caused by impaired renal production of 1,25-dihydroxyvitamin D_3, and osteitis fibrosa cystica, caused by the secondary hyperparathyroidism of renal failure, are present in varying degrees.

    (2) Familial vitamin D-resistant rickets is an X-linked dominant disorder in which osteomalacia is caused by excessive renal loss of phosphate. Very large doses of vitamin D must be given, along with phosphate, to raise the low serum phosphate level to normal.

    (3) In **Fanconi's syndrome**, renal tubular defects may lead to the loss of phosphate as well as calcium, glucose, and amino acids, with resulting osteomalacia.

d. Gastrointestinal disorders. Any disease or surgical procedure that leads to malabsorption and steatorrhea may reduce the absorption of calcium, phosphate, and vitamin D, and osteomalacia may result.

e. Tumors, such as hemangiopericytomas and giant cell tumors of bone, may produce a humoral substance that causes phosphaturia and osteomalacia; the syndrome (**"oncogenic osteomalacia"**) is cured by removal of the tumor.

3. Pathophysiology

    a. The **common defect** in the various diseases associated with osteomalacia is **the lack of calcium and phosphorus for mineralization of bone matrix**. Circulating phosphate levels are usually low, either because of decreased gastrointestinal absorption or excessive renal excretion. Calcium levels may be low, but they are often normal because of compensatory parathyroid hyperactivity.

    b. Rickets is caused by defective mineralization of bone before closure of the cartilagenous growth plates. Deformity occurs because of pressure on weakened growth plates and on the abnormally soft shafts of the long bones. After closure of the growth plates, only osteomalacia can occur, with defective mineralization of mature lamellar bone.

    c. Histologically, bone biopsy shows an excess of unmineralized bone matrix, which is seen as an increase in the volume and thickness of osteoid seams covering the bone surfaces.

4. Clinical features

    a. Pain and tenderness are common in affected areas of the skeleton, especially the spine, ribs, pelvis, and lower extremities.

    b. Muscle weakness is common, affecting particularly the proximal muscles of the legs.

    c. Skeletal deformities and fractures occur in severe cases.

        (1) The long bones may bow because of the softening of the skeleton.

        (2) Rickets in children is associated with widening of the epiphyses; swelling of the wrists, knees, ankles, and costochondral joints; bowlegs; and disturbances in growth.

5. Laboratory findings

    a. X-rays may show **decreased bone density** and coarsening of the trabecular pattern. **Looser's zones** are radiolucent bands that are perpendicular to the periosteal surface, caused by pseudofractures.

    b. Although laboratory abnormalities depend on the cause and the severity of the osteomalacia, they often include **low serum phosphate**, **low or normal serum calcium**, and **increased serum alkaline phosphatase** levels.

6. Therapy

    a. Treatment of the primary disorder is sometimes possible (e.g., correction of a bowel disorder causing malabsorption or removal of a tumor causing osteomalacia).

    b. Vitamin D is usually the mainstay of treatment.

        (1) In simple vitamin D deficiency, a physiologic dose of 400 units daily may be all that is needed.

(2) In vitamin D-resistant rickets, 50,000–100,000 units daily, or more, may be needed. The dose is adjusted to achieve healing of the bone lesions without inducing hypercalcemia, the main complication of excessive vitamin D administration.

B. Osteoporosis

1. Definition. Osteoporosis is a decrease in total bone volume or, simply, too little bone. The bone that is present is normal. The decrease in bone mass leads to an increased susceptibility to fractures. Both increased bone resorption and decreased bone formation have been observed.

2. Etiology
  a. Loss of bone mass at maturity
    (1) After reaching its peak in an individual about the age of 30–35 years, bone mass declines throughout the remaining years of life. A low total bone mass at maturity, a relatively rapid rate of bone loss, or both contribute to the development of "involutional" osteoporosis.
    (2) Genetic factors affect the bone mass at maturity.
      (a) Men and blacks have greater peak bone mass and less osteoporosis; women and individuals of northern European ancestry have less bone mass at maturity and more osteoporosis.
      (b) A familial tendency toward osteoporosis has been observed.
  b. Calcium deficiency. Evidence suggests that calcium intake in American women is less than is needed to maintain calcium balance. More than 75% of women over the age of 35 years fail to ingest the recommended daily allowance of 800 mg of calcium. Also, calcium absorption decreases in later life. The need to maintain normal serum levels of calcium may lead to increased bone resorption, through the action of PTH. (The effect of PTH on bone is to increase the rate of calcium and phosphate resorption, and when calcium levels are low, the secretion of PTH increases.)
  c. Hormone changes. When estrogen levels fall, whether because of ovarian disease, oophorectomy, or normal menopause, the rate of bone loss is accelerated. It is theorized that estrogen deficiency increases the sensitivity of bone to the action of PTH. The increased rate of bone loss persists for 3–7 years after menopause.

3. Classification
  a. Two types of osteoporosis have been described.
    (1) Postmenopausal osteoporosis mainly affects women within 15 years of menopause. The loss of trabecular bone is accelerated, and fractures of the vertebrae, which consist largely of trabecular bone, are common.
    (2) Senile osteoporosis affects men and women over the age of 75 years, causing loss of both cortical and trabecular bone. Fractures of the hip, which is largely cortical bone, occur as well as vertebral fractures.
  b. Secondary osteoporosis may be associated with glucocorticoid therapy or spontaneous Cushing's syndrome, malabsorption syndromes or malnutrition, multiple myeloma, prolonged immobilization, and other causes.

4. Clinical features
  a. Fractures
    (1) Vertebral compression fractures typically affect T8 to L3 and occur more commonly in women. They may cause acute back pain that persists for several months or may occur gradually and painlessly.
    (2) Hip fractures, characteristically in the neck and intertrochanteric regions of the femur, are common in both men and women over 65 years of age. Loss of function frequently results, and, because of complications, mortality rates may be as high as 20% within 1 year.
    (3) The **distal radius** and other areas may also be the site of fractures.
  b. Pain and deformity. Back pain may persist long after an episode of vertebral fracture because of spinal deformity and alteration of spinal mechanics. Several inches may be lost from height, and severe kyphosis may be the result of multiple vertebral fractures.

5. Diagnosis
  a. X-rays of the spine may reveal a decrease in bone density, with accentuation of the cortical outlines and prominence of the trabeculae.
    (1) However, about 30% of bone tissue must be lost before these abnormalities appear on plain x-ray.
    (2) Wedge-shaped deformities and compression fractures on spinal x-ray also suggest the diagnosis of osteoporosis.

    b. Quantitative CT and single and dual photon absorptiometry are more sensitive but often unavailable methods of quantitating bone density.

6. Therapy. Osteoporosis is prevented more effectively than it is treated. Therapeutic agents can slow the rate of bone loss but cannot restore bone mass that has been lost.

  a. Estrogen

    (1) An important means of preventing osteoporosis is the administration of estrogen after menopause. The decision to use menopausal estrogen replacement should be based on the benefits and risks of estrogen use in each individual patient.

      (a) There is a greater risk for osteoporosis and, therefore, greater potential benefit of estrogen use in an individual who:

        (i) Has a small stature and slender build

        (ii) Has a family history of osteoporosis

        (iii) Is white and of northern European ancestry

        (iv) Experienced early menopause

        (v) Smokes

      (b) Obese women have higher estrogen levels after menopause. This decreases their risk for osteoporosis.

      (c) The adverse effects of estrogen, which must be balanced against its benefits, are:

        (i) A fourfold to eightfold increase in the risk for endometrial cancer

        (ii) Increased risk that unscheduled uterine bleeding may occur and require gynecologic investigation

        (iii) Possible symptoms of nausea, breast tenderness, and fluid retention

        (iv) Increased risk for gallbladder disease and hypertension

      (d) Other benefits of estrogen therapy, such as the relief of menopausal symptoms, must of course be considered.

    (2) Treatment of osteoporosis

      (a) Once a patient is known to have osteoporosis, the benefit of estrogen treatment clearly outweighs the risk, provided that there are no major contraindications to estrogen use, such as breast or endometrial cancer, liver or gallbladder disease, or thromboembolic disease.

      (b) Estrogen has been shown to reduce the rate of vertebral, hip, and wrist fractures, even when started years after menopause.

    (3) Mode of administration

      (a) Estrogen can be given in relatively low doses, such as 0.625 mg of conjugated estrogens (Premarin) or 20 μg of ethinyl estradiol daily.

      (b) Many physicians believe that the cyclic administration of estrogen for 25 days each month, with the addition of a progestin [e.g., medroxyprogesterone acetate (Provera) in a dose of 5–10 mg] for the final 10 days will reduce the risk of uterine cancer. The use of progestins is controversial, however, since they may produce undesired effects, such as unfavorable changes in blood lipoprotein patterns.

  b. Calcium

    (1) Patients with osteoporosis should ingest at least 1000–1500 mg of elemental calcium daily. Since the average American takes in only about 500 mg in food, calcium supplements should be given. Calcium carbonate tablets (e.g., 500 mg of Os-Cal two or three times daily) are usually well tolerated. Exogenous calcium, like estrogen, reduces the rate of bone loss and the fracture rate in patients with osteoporosis.

    (2) Because of the safety of calcium supplementation and the prevalence of inadequate calcium intake, many authorities recommend calcium supplementation for all susceptible women, starting before menopause.

  c. Vitamin D, calcitonin, and **sodium fluoride** have been used to treat osteoporosis, but their efficacy is less certain than that of estrogen and calcium.

STUDY QUESTIONS

Directions: Each question below contains five suggested answers. Choose the **one best** response to each question.

1. Excessive production of aldosterone results in which of the following clinical features?

(A) Sodium depletion
(B) Acidosis
(C) Hypotension
(D) Potassium retention
(E) Plasma renin activity suppression

2. A young man with polyuria has a dehydration test. After fluid restriction, his maximum urine osmolality is 550 mOsm/kg and his plasma osmolality is 295 mOsm/kg. One hour after a subcutaneous injection of 5 units of aqueous vasopressin, his urine osmolality is 720 mOsm/kg. The likely diagnosis is

(A) no disease
(B) diabetes insipidus
(C) partial diabetes insipidus
(D) nephrogenic diabetes insipidus
(E) diabetes mellitus

3. Diabetic autonomic neuropathy is suggested by all of the following clinical manifestations EXCEPT

(A) hypertension
(B) impotence
(C) urinary retention
(D) gastroparesis
(E) decreased awareness of hypoglycemia

4. All of the following pathophysiologic features commonly are present in diabetic ketoacidosis EXCEPT

(A) decreased peripheral utilization of glucose
(B) increased protein catabolism
(C) decreased lipolysis
(D) osmotic diuresis
(E) increased anion gap

5. All of the following statements about thyroid storm are true EXCEPT

(A) iodine treatment often is effective within 24 hours
(B) surgery, infections, and childbirth may precipitate thyroid storm in a patient with Graves' disease
(C) antithyroid drugs such as propylthiouracil are useful in the treatment of thyroid storm
(D) propranolol and other β-blocking drugs are indicated in thyroid storm
(E) thyroid storm is associated with a sudden increase in thyroid hormone levels

Directions: Each question below contains four suggested answers of which **one or more** is correct. Choose the answer

A   if **1, 2, and 3** are correct
B   if **1 and 3** are correct
C   if **2 and 4** are correct
D   if **4** is correct
E   if **1, 2, 3, and 4** are correct

6. Clinical features associated with hyperparathyroidism include

(1) osteitis fibrosa cystica
(2) increased serum chloride-to-phosphate ratio
(3) urinary calculi
(4) calcification of the basal ganglia

7. Pheochromocytomas, which arise from the chromaffin cells, are

(1) part of Sipple's syndrome
(2) most often single tumors of the adrenal medulla
(3) rare causes of hypertension
(4) frequent causes of hypoglycemia

8. A 63-year-old woman develops unexplained shock that is unresponsive to pressor agents after a cholecystectomy. It is then learned that she had been taking her neighbor's prednisone tablets almost daily for several years because they helped relieve her arthritis. She recovers promptly after cortisol is given intravenously. This complication probably would not have occurred if

(1) she had not taken any prednisone for the past 3 months
(2) she had taken the prednisone for a total of no more than 1 or 2 weeks
(3) she had a normal response to an adrenocorticotropic hormone (ACTH) test before surgery
(4) the daily amount of prednisone she had taken was less than a physiologic dose (i.e., about 5 mg)

9. Pseudohypoparathyroidism is a hereditary disease with clinical manifestations that include

(1) no response of low serum calcium levels to vitamin D and oral calcium supplementation
(2) low serum levels of parathyroid hormone (PTH)
(3) exaggerated response of urinary cyclic adenosine 3',5'-monophosphate (cAMP) to PTH injection
(4) short stature

10. Estrogen therapy is associated with

(1) increased risk of uterine cancer
(2) decreased rate of bone loss after menopause
(3) increased risk of gallbladder disease
(4) relief of symptoms of hot flashes

11. Diabetic ketoacidosis is treated through insulin administration, fluid replacement, mineral and electrolyte replacement, and the management of precipitating factors and complications. The therapeutic approach includes

(1) low insulin doses (0.1 U/kg/hr), which usually are as effective as higher doses in reducing serum glucose levels
(2) glucose infusion to prevent hypoglycemia
(3) bicarbonate in the face of marked acidosis
(4) potassium replacement starting with the initial insulin dose

Directions: The groups of questions below consist of lettered choices followed by several numbered items. For each numbered item select the **one** lettered choice with which it is **most** closely associated. Each lettered choice may be used once, more than once, or not at all.

Questions 12–14

For each result of thyroid function tests, select the clinical condition with which it is most likely to be associated.

(A) Graves' disease
(B) Hypothyroidism
(C) Pregnancy
(D) Subacute thyroiditis
(E) Nontoxic goiter

12. Elevated serum thyroxine (T_4), low radioactive iodine uptake

13. Elevated serum T_4, low triiodothyronine (T_3) resin uptake

14. Elevated serum T_4, elevated radioactive iodine uptake

Questions 15–19

For each primary pathologic process, select the disease it is most likely to cause.

(A) Graves' disease
(B) Testicular feminization syndrome
(C) Addison's disease
(D) Hypopituitarism
(E) Acromegaly

15. Excessive production of hormone by an endocrine tumor

16. Destruction of an endocrine gland by tumor, infection, trauma, or infarction

17. Stimulation of an endocrine gland by autoimmune mechanisms

18. Destruction of an endocrine gland by autoimmune mechanisms

19. Impaired sensitivity of peripheral tissues to normal circulating levels of a hormone

Questions 20–23

A patient is suspected of having Cushing's disease. For diagnostic purposes, dexamethasone is given in a low dose (2 mg daily) for 2 days and a high dose (8 mg daily) for 2 days. For each change in urinary 17-hydroxycorticoids and urinary free cortisol levels, select the diagnosis it represents.

(A) Cushing's disease due to pituitary adrenocorticotropic hormone (ACTH) excess
(B) Cushing's syndrome due to an adrenal tumor
(C) Ectopic ACTH syndrome
(D) Adrenal insufficiency
(E) No adrenal disease

20. They fall distinctly with low-dose dexamethasone and high-dose dexamethasone

21. They do not change with low-dose dexamethasone but fall distinctly with high-dose dexamethasone

22. They do not fall with either low-dose or high-dose dexamethasone; the plasma ACTH level is elevated

23. They do not fall with either low-dose or high-dose dexamethasone; the plasma ACTH level is low

ANSWERS AND EXPLANATIONS

1. The answer is E. [*V D 2, 3 a (3)*] Excessive circulating levels of aldosterone increase the reabsorption of sodium, in exchange for potassium and hydrogen ions, in the distal tubules. The resulting expansion of extracellular fluid volume causes suppression of plasma renin activity and eventually causes hypertension. The loss of potassium and hydrogen ions causes a tendency toward metabolic alkalosis.

2. The answer is C. (*I B 1 c; Table 9-2*) The definite response by the patient to the injection of antidiuretic hormone (ADH) indicates that he did not produce maximally effective levels of ADH after fluid restriction, and, therefore, he has either partial or complete diabetes insipidus. The ability to achieve normal or near-normal urine concentration, however, indicates that the ADH deficit is only partial. The response to ADH rules out nephrogenic diabetes insipidus. Diabetes mellitus, another cause of polyuria, is diagnosed by blood and urine glucose levels rather than by studies of renal water handling.

3. The answer is A. [*IV A 7 e (1) (b)*] Postural hypotension, rather than hypertension, is a common finding in patients with diabetic autonomic neuropathy. Impotence, bladder dysfunction and urinary retention, and delayed gastric emptying also are common. Hypoglycemic reactions may become severe because the early adrenergic warning signals (e.g., sweating, tremor, and palpitations) may not be perceived by a patient with autonomic neuropathy.

4. The answer is C. [*IV A 6 a (2)*] Because of insufficient levels of insulin and excessive levels of glucagon, the peripheral tissue utilization of glucose is reduced. Protein catabolism is accelerated, increasing the flow of amino acids to the liver to be used in gluconeogenesis. Lipolysis is also accelerated, increasing the supply of free fatty acids that the liver can use in the production of ketone bodies. The high blood levels of glucose and ketone bodies cause an osmotic diuresis, and the circulating ketone bodies are unmeasured anions that raise the anion gap.

5. The answer is E. (*II C 2 h, 4 f*) Although any severe stress may precipitate thyroid storm, a marked change in hormone levels, compared with the levels prior to the onset of thyroid storm, has not been observed. Iodine, antithyroid drugs, and β-blocking agents are all indicated in the treatment of thyroid storm. Iodine inhibits the release of thyroid hormone, and antithyroid drugs block the synthesis of the hormone. Beta-blockers prevent many of the tissue effects of excessive hormone concentrations.

6. The answer is A (1, 2, 3). [*III A 4, 5, B 3 a (3) (b)*] Excessive circulating levels of parathyroid hormone (PTH) act on the skeleton to cause osteitis fibrosa cystica and on the renal tubules to cause phosphaturia and consequent hypophosphatemia. Chloride retention, along with the tendency to a low serum phosphate level, raises the chloride-to-phosphate ratio (> 33). Hypercalciuria increases the risk of urinary calculi. Calcification of the basal ganglia, however, is a result of long-standing hypocalcemia, which occurs in hypoparathyroidism and pseudohypoparathyroidism.

7. The answer is A (1, 2, 3). (*V F 1, 3*) Pheochromocytoma is a tumor of chromaffin cells, which are located primarily in the adrenal medulla. The syndrome of multiple endocrine neoplasia, type II, also known as Sipple's syndrome, consists of pheochromocytomas (often multiple), medullary carcinoma of the thyroid, and parathyroid disease. Sporadic pheochromocytomas are sometimes multiple and sometimes extra-adrenal, but most commonly they are single tumors arising in the adrenal medulla. Fewer than 0.5% of hypertensive patients have a pheochromocytoma. Catecholamines stimulate glycogenolysis, and serum glucose levels tend to be elevated in patients with pheochromocytomas.

8. The answer is C (2, 4). [*V C 1 a (3) (b)*] Recovery of the hypothalamic-pituitary-adrenal axis after prolonged suppression requires about 6–9 months on the average, although much earlier or much later recovery is not unusual. A physiologic (as opposed to pharmacologic) dose of prednisone is not likely to cause prolonged suppression nor is a course of treatment that lasts less than 2 weeks. A normal response to adrenocorticotropic hormone (ACTH) indicates recovery of the adrenal glands but does not prove that the hypothalamic-pituitary axis can respond normally to stressful stimuli.

9. The answer is D (4). (*III B 4 a*) The hypocalcemia in pseudohypoparathyroidism is caused by the failure of end-organ response to parathyroid hormone (PTH) but can be overcome by large doses of vitamin D and calcium. PTH levels tend to be elevated because the hypocalcemia stimulates parathyroid gland production of PTH. The renal refractoriness to PTH is demonstrated by the failure of injected PTH to stimulate urinary cyclic adenosine 3′,5′-monophosphate (cAMP) excretion. The associated somatic abnormalities are called Albright's hereditary osteodystrophy and include short stature and shortening of the metacarpal and metatarsal bones.

10. The answer is E (all). [*VIII B 7 a (1)*] The decision of whether to prescribe estrogen in postmenopausal women involves a consideration of the benefits and risks in each individual patient. Benefits include a decrease in the risk for osteoporosis and relief of symptoms due to estrogen deficiency, such as hot flashes and genital atrophy. Risks include an increase in the incidence of uterine cancer and gallbladder disease.

11. The answer is A (1, 2, 3). [*IV A 6 a (4) (a), (b), (c)*] Low doses of insulin are as effective as higher doses, except occasionally in patients with insulin resistance; if the glucose response is not adequate within a few hours, high-dose therapy should be started. Glucose infusion should be started when the serum glucose level has fallen to about 200–300 mg/dl to prevent hypoglycemia. Unless acidosis is severe (i.e., a pH less than 7.1), rebound alkalosis may occur if bicarbonate is given. Serum potassium levels may be elevated at first, due to potassium movement out of cells; potassium administration should be started only after adequate renal function is observed and the serum potassium level has fallen to low or normal levels.

12–14. The answers are: 12-D, 13-C, 14-A. [*II A 1 a, 3 c, C 3 d, D 1 c (2)*] In subacute thyroiditis, injured thyroid follicular cells release thyroid hormone, raising the blood level of thyroxine (T_4). Radioactive iodine uptake is low, however, because the injured follicular cells are unable to trap iodine normally. Also, thyroid-stimulating hormone (TSH) is suppressed by the increased level of circulating thyroid hormone, and this further reduces the radioactive iodine uptake.

The high estrogen levels in pregnancy cause increased production of thyroxine-binding globulin. This raises the serum level of total thyroxine and lowers the triiodothyronine (T_3) resin uptake. The patient remains euthyroid, however, since the serum free T_4 level remains normal.

In Graves' disease, the follicular cells trap increased amounts of iodine and produce increased amounts of thyroid hormone. Therefore, both the radioactive iodine uptake and the serum T_4 level are elevated. This combination of findings indicates hyperthyroidism, caused either by Graves' disease or by Plummer's disease.

15–19. The answers are: 15-E, 16-D, 17-A, 18-C, 19-B. (*I A 2 a, 3 a; II C 1 a; V C 1 a; VI A 2 a*) The usual cause of acromegaly is a growth hormone (GH)-secreting pituitary adenoma. Whether these adenomas arise de novo or are caused by excessive hypothalamic production of GH-releasing hormone is not known. Rarely, GH-releasing hormone production by an islet cell adenoma may cause acromegaly.

Pituitary tumors may compress normal tissue, impairing its function. Surgical removal of the tumor may further damage the hypothalamus and pituitary gland. Ischemic infarction at childbirth (Sheehan's syndrome) and various destructive, infectious, and granulomatous lesions also cause hypopituitarism.

Graves' disease is caused by abnormal stimulation of the thyroid gland by thyroid-stimulating immunoglobulin. This immunoglobulin G (IgG) antibody binds to receptors for thyroid-stimulating hormone (TSH). It then stimulates growth and hormone production by the thyroid follicular cells.

Addison's disease is most commonly caused by atrophy of the adrenal cortex. Anti-adrenal antibodies are often present. Other evidence of autoimmunity, such as antibodies against other tissues and the presence of other autoimmune diseases, also are common findings.

The testicular feminization syndrome results from the inability of tissues to respond to testosterone and other androgens. If not stimulated by androgens, the fetal external genitalia develop as female organs. Therefore, a genetic male infant with testes and normal male testosterone levels is born with female external genitalia and is considered to be a normal female.

20–23. The answers are: 20-E, 21-A, 22-C, 23-B. [*V B 3 b (2), c, d (2); Table 9-13*] Although basal cortisol levels may be increased by physical or emotional stress, even low doses of dexamethasone usually result in normal suppression in such cases.

The pituitary secretion of adrenocorticotropic hormone (ACTH) in Cushing's disease can be suppressed by dexamethasone or other glucocorticoids. Larger-than-normal doses of dexamethasone, however, are necessary for suppression.

The production of ACTH by oat cell carcinoma of the lung and other tumors is not suppressed by dexamethasone. Therefore, even high doses do not lower cortisol levels. The increased blood ACTH levels are helpful in distinguishing ectopic ACTH syndrome from adrenal tumors, in which ACTH (of pituitary origin) is suppressed.

Cortisol production by adrenal adenomas and carcinomas is autonomous; it is not under the control of pituitary ACTH. ACTH levels are, in fact, suppressed by the increased circulating cortisol. Therefore, even high doses of dexamethasone will not lower cortisol levels by suppressing pituitary excretion of ACTH.

Rheumatic Diseases

Douglas C. Conaway
Allen R. Myers

I. OSTEOARTHRITIS

A. Definition. Osteoarthritis, also called **degenerative joint disease**, is a common age-related deterioration of articular cartilage and underlying bone.

B. Etiology. Osteoarthritis has no single known cause. The factors listed below are believed to interact to cause varying degrees of articular damage in individual patients.

1. **Wear and tear.** Changes due to repetitive **microtrauma** in subchondral bone may impair its ability to absorb the longitudinal forces of joint impact loading, leading to cartilage degeneration.

2. **Aging**
   a. Although the number and function of chondrocytes are preserved in aging cartilage, proteoglycan aggregation may be diminished. This proteoglycan abnormality may impair the ability of articular cartilage to dissipate loading forces.
   b. Loosening or separation of the collagen network may occur with repetitive mechanical stress.

3. **Obesity** increases loading stress on weight-bearing joints, especially the knees.

4. **Genetic factors** appear to be important in the development of erosive osteoarthritis of the distal and proximal interphalangeal joints. This autosomal dominant variant is 10 times more common in women than in men.

5. **Inflammation.** Enzymatic breakdown of cartilage matrix proteins is more important in inflammatory joint diseases than in osteoarthritis. However, immunoglobulin and complement deposits have been found in superficial articular cartilage in osteoarthritis, suggesting that antigenic components of exposed cartilage can elicit a mild inflammatory response in osteoarthritis.

6. **Neuropathy.** Muscle tone around a joint modulates the forces of joint impact loading. If proprioceptive input to the joint is impaired, abnormal muscle tone may result in osteoarthritis by transferring abnormal forces to the joint.

7. **Deposition diseases** (e.g., hemochromatosis, ochronosis, Wilson's disease, and crystal deposition diseases) cause deposition of substances in the cartilage matrix, which can result in direct chondrocyte injury or can impair the ability of the matrix to dissipate loading forces.

C. Pathogenesis

1. **Initial insult.** The initial insults described above damage chondrocytes (leading to release of neutral proteases and collagenases and to degradation of the matrix) and stimulate replication of the remaining chondrocytes, which synthesize more proteoglycan. The opposing forces of cartilage breakdown and repair determine the rate of cartilage destruction.

2. **Progressive change.** With ongoing cartilage destruction, collagen is progressively altered. The cartilage swells, and proteoglycan concentration diminishes.

3. **Mechanical factors**
   a. With advancing disease, loss of proteoglycan leads to impairment of cartilage elasticity and transmission of increasingly abnormal forces to the chondrocytes.
   b. Since subchondral bone also is important in dissipating loading forces, the subchondral eburnation (bone sclerosis) that occurs in osteoarthritis also causes transmission of increased joint loading forces to chondrocytes.

D. Pathology

1. **Cartilage changes**
   a. Early in osteoarthritis, cartilage **changes in color** from blue to yellow due to loss of proteoglycan.
   b. Localized areas of **softening** are the earliest pathologic changes in osteoarthritis.
   c. Superficial **chipping and flaking** of cartilage signify more advanced disease.
   d. Vertical **fibrillations** in the cartilage indicate further progression.
   e. Focal and later confluent **erosions** eventually progress to full-thickness cartilage loss if healing forces are overwhelmed by destructive forces.

2. **Bone changes**
   a. **New bone formation** can occur under the cartilage (seen as **eburnation** on x-ray) or at the joint margin (seen as osteophytic **spurs** on x-ray).
   b. **Subchondral cysts.** Large pseudocystic areas can form in the juxta-articular bone, presumably due to transmission of increased mechanical forces to bone and to impaired perfusion due to subchondral microfractures.

E. Classification

1. **Primary osteoarthritis** has no underlying cause for joint damage.
   a. **Primary generalized osteoarthritis** occurs predominantly in middle-aged, postmenopausal women and is characterized by prominent involvement of the distal and proximal interphalangeal joints and the first carpometacarpal joints. Knees, hips, and first metatarsophalangeal joints often are involved as well. These cases may represent a form of ordinary osteoarthritis that involves more joints in a more severe fashion.
   b. **Erosive osteoarthritis** also occurs predominantly in middle-aged, postmenopausal women and typically affects the distal and proximal interphalangeal joints of the hand as well as the zygapophyseal joints of the cervical spine. Many cases exhibit autosomal dominant, sex-influenced characteristics. Episodic tenderness, swelling, and redness occur. Characteristic radiographic abnormalities include bone erosions and ankylosis, which are unusual in other types of osteoarthritis.

2. **Secondary osteoarthritis** exhibits an underlying cause for degenerative joint disease.
   a. **Mechanical abnormalities**
      (1) **Congenital or developmental defects**
         (a) In **congenital hip dysplasia**, the acetabulum fails to develop fully, and a shallow cavity exists. The hip usually dislocates and causes limping during childhood, although in some cases this does not occur until adolescence or adulthood. Subtle dysplasia may be an important cause of hip osteoarthritis in the adult.
         (b) **Slipped capital femoral epiphysis** typically becomes symptomatic at age 10 to 15. Although most patients have groin pain or limp, some remain asymptomatic until osteoarthritis develops in middle age.
         (c) **Legg-Calvé-Perthes disease**, or avascular necrosis of the capital femoral epiphysis, typically occurs between the ages of 4 and 8. Interruption of the blood supply to the femoral head causes bone necrosis and eventual remodeling, with deformity that can lead to osteoarthritis.
      (2) **Fractures or other traumatic events** that distort joint anatomy lead to progressive wear and tear of cartilage.
      (3) **Loose bodies.** Segments of articular cartilage, with or without underlying bone, may break off and traumatize the joint surface, leading to osteoarthritis. This may occur in osteochondritis dissecans and osteochondromatosis.
   b. **Postinflammatory disorders.** Destruction of cartilage matrix by inflammatory processes (e.g., rheumatoid arthritis and infectious arthritis) also seems to accelerate degenerative changes in involved joints.
   c. **Metabolic disorders**
      (1) **Ochronosis.** In this disorder, homogentisic acid is deposited in hyaline cartilage and in the nucleus pulposus of the intervertebral disks as a result of homogentisic acid oxidase deficiency. Homogentisic acid may be toxic to chondrocytes or may interfere with normal cartilage elasticity. The large joints (e.g., knees, hips, and shoulders) and intervertebral disks are symptomatically affected; the small joints of the hands and feet are spared.
      (2) **Calcium pyrophosphate dihydrate (CPPD) deposition** in cartilage may be a primary factor leading to joint damage in osteoarthritis, or it may be merely a manifestation of the disease. Degenerative knee disease is the common finding (with **chondrocalcinosis** on x-ray), but wrist, metacarpophalangeal joint, hip, shoulder, elbow, and ankle involvement also are common.

(3) Wilson's disease is a disorder of copper metabolism characterized by excessive copper deposition in tissues. Adult patients can manifest a variant of osteoarthritis involving the metacarpophalangeal joints, wrists, knees, shoulders, and hips. CPPD crystals are found in articular cartilage in some patients; copper levels in joint tissue are not elevated.

(4) Hemochromatosis. Patients with this "iron overload" disease can have a characteristic arthropathy involving degenerative changes of the metacarpophalangeal joints, wrists, knees, hips, and shoulders. CPPD crystals often are present in articular cartilage. Conceivably, the presence of iron in synovial lining cells could modulate CPPD deposition via pyrophosphatase inhibition.

d. Neuropathic joint disorders. Abnormal forces can be transferred to the joint if its proprioceptive input is impaired, and progressive osteoarthritis due to repeated microtraumatic episodes may ensue. Typical associated diseases are syphilis, diabetes mellitus, syringomyelia, and other central or peripheral nervous system disorders.

e. Osteonecrosis. Avascular necrosis in the subchondral bone can lead to collapse of the articular surface, with consequent surface irregularities leading to osteoarthritis.

f. Hemophilia. Repeated hemarthroses may lead to synovial hemosiderosis, synovial lining cell proliferation, and collagenase production with consequent cartilage damage.

g. Paget's disease. The deformation caused by bone remodeling in Paget's disease can lead to mechanical incongruities and osteoarthritis.

h. Acromegaly. Cartilage proliferation with resultant fissuring and mechanical incongruities predisposes to premature osteoarthritis.

F. Clinical features

1. **Symptoms** of osteoarthritis vary with the joint involved and the severity of the disease.
   a. Pain. Most patients experience the gradual onset of a deep, aching pain, which worsens with activity and is relieved by rest. With more severe disease, pain can occur even at rest and interfere with sleep.
   b. Morning stiffness in osteoarthritis is brief (less than 30 minutes) in contrast to that occurring in inflammatory rheumatic conditions, which may be much longer.
   c. Gelling phenomenon refers to the sensation of renewed stiffness in osteoarthritic joints after prolonged inactivity.
   d. Tenderness. Mild or moderate tenderness can be present in joints.
   e. Painful range of motion in large joints (e.g., knees and hips) is the equivalent of tenderness in small joints.

2. **Signs**
   a. Crepitus (i.e., a grinding sound or sensation) can be felt and sometimes heard when a joint is put through full range of motion. Crepitus is due to surface incongruities in the joint.
   b. Warmth. Involved joints usually are cool but can feel warm with flare-ups of disease activity.
   c. Joint enlargement. Soft tissue swelling may occur if an effusion is present. More commonly, bone enlargement occurs in the form of osteophytes.
   d. Deformity. Varus (medial) or **valgus** (lateral) **angulation** of joints can occur late in the disease. Gross bone enlargement and joint subluxation also can occur in severe disease.
      (1) Heberden's nodes specifically refer to enlargement of the distal interphalangeal joints of the hand.
      (2) Bouchard's nodes specifically refer to enlargement of the proximal interphalangeal joints of the hand.

G. Diagnosis of osteoarthritis is made on the basis of the patient history combined with physical, laboratory, and radiographic findings.

1. **Joint involvement.** Joints typically involved include the distal and proximal interphalangeal and the first carpometacarpal joints of the hands. Also, knees, hips, and first metatarsophalangeal joints as well as cervical and lumbar spine facet joints may be involved in primary osteoarthritis. Involvement of other joints with typical findings suggests a secondary cause of osteoarthritis.

2. **Laboratory findings**
   a. Hematologic findings generally are normal, including the erythrocyte sedimentation rate.
   b. Synovial fluid findings. Typical osteoarthritic synovial fluid is slightly turbid, with a white cell count that is only mildly inflammatory (i.e., < 2000 cells/mm³ and < 25% neutrophils). It contains no crystals and demonstrates a good mucin clot. The mucin clot test is a gross test for the integrity of hyaluronate in synovial fluid. When a small amount of noninflammatory fluid is added to acetic acid, the highly polymerized, intact hyaluronate forms

a firm ("good") mucin clot. In contrast, the fragmented hyaluronate of inflammatory effusions gives a poor mucin clot.

3. **Radiographic findings**
   a. **Findings typically present** include:
      (1) Joint space narrowing (due to loss of cartilage)
      (2) Subchondral eburnation (due to periarticular new bone formation)
      (3) Marginal osteophytes
      (4) Subchondral cysts
   b. **Findings typically absent** include:
      (1) Periarticular osteopenia
      (2) Marginal erosions (except in the distal and proximal interphalangeal joints in the erosive osteoarthritis variant)
   c. **Clinical correlates**
      (1) **Comparison views.** Obtaining x-rays of the contralateral joint can be helpful.
      (2) **Standing views** best demonstrate the amount of cartilage loss in knees.

4. **Differential diagnosis**
   a. **Absence of periarticular abnormality.** Patients may complain of pain in a joint yet have involvement of a periarticular structure such as a tendon, ligament, or bursa as the real cause of symptoms.
   b. **Absence of inflammatory rheumatic disease.** Systemic complaints (e.g., anorexia, weight loss, fatigue, and fever), prominent morning stiffness, and stigmata of inflammatory rheumatic diseases should be sought.

H. Therapy

1. **Joint conservation and weight reduction.** Joint overuse or repetitive trauma must be avoided. A midday rest period may be helpful. Weight loss may be beneficial in arthritis of weight-bearing joints such as the knees.

2. **Supports**
   a. A **knee cage or brace** sometimes is used when knee ligamentous instability coexists with osteoarthritis.
   b. A **soft cervical collar** may be used for symptomatic flare-ups of cervical spine osteoarthritis.
   c. A **lumbar corset** (back brace) sometimes is used to buttress sagging abdominal or back muscles.
   d. A **cane** may be helpful in supporting a patient with unilateral hip or knee osteoarthritis.

3. **Exercise.** Isometric strengthening of supporting muscles around joints may be helpful (e.g., quadriceps-setting exercises in knee arthritis). Swimming is the best form of aerobic exercise for a patient with osteoarthritis of the hips or knees; running should be avoided by these patients.

4. **Analgesia**
   a. **Moist heat** or heating pads often can temporarily lessen the pain of osteoarthritis.
   b. **Transcutaneous nerve stimulation** can modulate pain receptor input from the periphery to the spinal neurons, particularly in the chronic pain of lumbar or cervical spine osteoarthritis.
   c. **Drugs**
      (1) Pain relief with low-to-moderate doses of acetaminophen, aspirin, or other **nonsteroidal anti-inflammatory drugs** may be useful.
      (2) **Narcotics** should be avoided, although propoxyphene may be useful in severe cases for management of pain associated with flare-ups of disease activity.
      (3) Oral **corticosteroids** have no place in the management of osteoarthritis. Occasional intra-articular injections of corticosteroids may be of temporary benefit in flare-ups, but there must be concern for possible acceleration of the disease process by the steroid. Injection into periarticular areas (e.g., tendon sheaths or bursae) is preferable if these structures are inflamed.

5. **Surgery.** In advanced disease of the knee or hip, total **joint replacement** can be dramatically effective in alleviating pain and restoring function. **Angulation osteotomy** is still performed in osteoarthritis of the knee to treat unicompartmental disease.

II. CRYSTAL-RELATED JOINT DISEASES

A. Gout

1. **Definition.** Gout is the name given to a group of disorders of purine metabolism, which are

characterized by serum uric acid elevation (**hyperuricemia**) **and urate deposition** in articular or extra-articular tissues. Elevation of serum uric acid alone is not sufficient for the diagnosis of gout; in fact, only 10% of patients with hyperuricemia develop gout. Some unknown factor seems to predispose to urate deposition and articular inflammation in the setting of sustained hyperuricemia.

2. **Etiologic classification of hyperuricemia.** All gouty syndromes are characterized by either episodic or constant elevation of serum uric acid concentration above 7 mg/dl. Patients with elevated serum uric acid can be classified as **overproducers** or **underexcreters** of uric acid, depending on the amount of uric acid excreted during a 24-hour period.

   a. **Overproducers**, who comprise about 10% of the gout population, excrete more than 750–1000 mg of uric acid per day on an unrestricted diet. These patients synthesize greater than normal amounts of uric acid de novo from intermediates or via breakdown of purine bases from nucleic acids. The defect causing uric acid overproduction may be primary or secondary; in some cases, the mechanism is unknown.

      (1) **Primary overproduction hyperuricemia** is associated with specific enzymatic defects, including:

         (a) Hypoxanthine-guanine phosphoribosyl transferase (HGPRT) deficiency or absence

         (b) Phosphoribosyl-1-pyrophosphate synthetase overactivity

      (2) **Secondary overproduction hyperuricemia** most often is associated with increased nucleic acid turnover that occurs due to other conditions or diseases, including:

         (a) Myeloproliferative disorders

         (b) Lymphoproliferative disorders

         (c) Hemolytic anemias

         (d) Hemoglobinopathies

         (e) Psoriasis

         (f) Cancer chemotherapy

         (g) Alcohol abuse (one effect of alcohol is to increase uric acid synthesis by increasing adenine nucleotide turnover)

   b. **Underexcreters**, who comprise about 90% of the gout population, excrete less than 700 mg of uric acid per day. This group includes patients with combined defects, since overproducers of uric acid also may be underexcreters. The decreased renal excretion of uric acid is the basis for hyperuricemia in these patients. This may be due to:

      (1) **Renal diseases**, such as chronic renal failure (decreased renal functional mass) and lead nephropathy (lead toxicity is presumed to cause a tubular defect in uric acid handling)

      (2) **Endocrine disorders** (e.g., hyperparathyroidism, hypoparathyroidism, and pseudohypoparathyroidism), which are associated with uric acid underexcretion for unknown reasons

      (3) **Drug effects**, as occur with:

         (a) Diuretics (volume depletion and consequent increased tubular reabsorption of uric acid with possible decreased tubular secretion of uric acid)

         (b) Alcohol (decreased uric acid excretion due to increased synthesis of lactate, which competes with urate for tubular secretion)

         (c) Pyrazinamide (decreased tubular secretion of uric acid)

         (d) Low-dose aspirin (decreased tubular secretion of uric acid)

      (4) **Volume depletion states** (increased tubular reabsorption of uric acid), such as:

         (a) Adrenal insufficiency

         (b) Nephrogenic diabetes insipidus

      (5) **Organic acid accumulation** (ketones and lactate compete with urate for tubular secretion)

3. **Associated conditions**

   a. **Obesity.** Serum uric acid level rises with body weight. Gout is significantly more common in individuals who are more than 15% overweight.

   b. **Diabetes mellitus.** Impaired glucose tolerance is common in gout and may be a function of obesity.

   c. **Hypertension** is common in patients with gout, but no independent correlation exists between blood pressure and serum uric acid level. Obesity probably is responsible for a high rate of hypertension in patients with gout.

   d. **Hyperlipidemias**, namely types II and IV, are common in gout; however, diet, alcohol intake, and body weight seem to be more important associations in these patients.

   e. **Atherosclerosis.** Death in patients with gout is commonly due to cardiovascular or cerebrovascular diseases. However, the above-mentioned risk factors that commonly occur in gout patients seem to explain the tendency for accelerated atherogenesis.

   f. **Avascular necrosis** of the femoral head occurs more commonly in gout patients than in normal individuals. The association may be explained partly by the presence of related risk factors (i.e., chronic alcoholism and hyperlipidemias).

4. **Clinical stages of gout**
   a. **Asymptomatic hyperuricemia** is the stage that is characterized by an increased serum uric acid level in the absence of clinical evidence of deposition disease (i.e., arthritis, tophi, nephropathy, or uric acid stones).
      (1) The **risk of acute gouty arthritis or nephrolithiasis** increases as the serum uric acid concentration increases. However, most patients do not develop either of these conditions. Hyperuricemia occasionally can lead to urate deposition in the interstitium of the kidney—a condition called **urate nephropathy** [see section II A 4 e (1)].
      (2) The **risk of uric acid stone formation** in patients with hyperuricemia is most closely related to a urinary uric acid excretion of greater than 1000 mg/day. This group of patients also is at risk for **acute obstructive uropathy**, a form of acute renal failure that can develop due to sudden increases in serum uric acid levels, with subsequent precipitation of uric acid crystals in the collecting tubules and ureters [see section II A 4 e (2)].
      (3) **Therapy.** In general, patients who do not have evidence of urate deposition do not require treatment. Secondary causes of hyperuricemia (e.g., medications, obesity, alcohol intake, and other disease) should be altered if possible.
   b. **Acute gouty arthritis**—the second stage and primary manifestation of gout—is an extremely painful and acute-onset arthritis.
      (1) **Typical patient.** Most patients (80%–90%) are middle-aged or elderly men who have had sustained asymptomatic hyperuricemia for 20–30 years before the first attack. Women seem to be spared until menopause, perhaps via an estrogen effect on uric acid clearance. Onset of acute gouty arthritis in the teens or twenties is unusual and most often associated with a primary or secondary cause of uric acid overproduction.
      (2) **Typical attack**
         (a) A monoarticular, lower extremity presentation is most common, with 50% of patients experiencing their first attack in the first metatarsophalangeal joint (called **podagra**). Many attacks occur suddenly at night, with rapid evolution of joint erythema, swelling, tenderness, and warmth. Intense joint inflammation can extend into the soft tissues and mimic cellulitis or phlebitis. Fever can occur in particularly severe attacks.
         (b) Attacks usually resolve in a few days, although some can extend over several weeks. The joint usually returns to normal between attacks. Polyarticular involvement can occur in some cases, and a typical progression from monoarticular to polyarticular involvement occurs by extension to adjacent joints.
      (3) **Pathogenesis of acute attacks**
         (a) Sustained hyperuricemia leads to the development of **microtophi** (i.e., small crystal aggregates) in the synovial membrane and cartilage.
         (b) Through an unknown mechanism, microtophi are disrupted and crystals are released into the joint space. (Trauma, joint temperature changes, and fluctuations in serum or synovial fluid uric acid concentration are potential initiators of this process.)
         (c) Urate crystals are coated by immunoglobulins, which enhance phagocytosis by neutrophils.
         (d) Phagosomes in the crystal-containing neutrophils fuse with lysosomes, and the lysosomal enzymes digest the protein coating of the crystals. The naked crystals then apparently disrupt the phagosomal membranes.
         (e) Neutrophils are damaged by the crystals, and lysosomal enzymes are released into synovial fluid, potentiating inflammation.
         (f) Inflammatory mediators such as interleukin 1 can be released from synovial macrophages exposed to uric acid crystals and may be responsible for extension of inflammation to other joints and into soft tissues.
      (4) **Diagnosis of acute gout**
         (a) **Laboratory findings**
            (i) **Serum findings.** The serum uric acid value often is not helpful in the clinical diagnosis of acute gout. Serum uric acid concentration is normal in at least 10% of patients at the time of an acute attack, and an elevated serum uric acid level is not at all specific for acute gout.
            (ii) **Synovial fluid findings.** The demonstration of urate crystals, especially intracellular crystals, in synovial fluid is diagnostic. These crystals characteristically are needle-shaped and negatively birefringent in red-compensated, polarized light, and they may be present in neutrophils during an acute attack. Synovial fluid white cell counts of 10,000–60,000/mm³ (predominantly neutrophils) also are common in acute attacks.

        (iii) Hematologic findings. Leukocytosis (i.e., white cell count of 10,000–15,000/mm³) is common, and the erythrocyte sedimentation rate commonly is moderately elevated as an acute phase response.

    (b) Radiographic findings. In the initial attacks of gout, only soft tissue swelling is seen in radiographs of involved joints.

    (c) Colchicine trial. In a typical clinical setting (i.e., a middle-aged man with an acute attack of podagra), a good clinical response to colchicine treatment is reasonably specific for acute gout. Other forms of acute arthritis can respond to colchicine (e.g., sarcoid arthropathy and pseudogout); therefore, this trial may not be as specific in less typical presentations.

(5) Therapy for acute gouty arthritis. Drug treatment of the acute attack is most effective when started very early after symptoms begin. As with any inflammatory arthritis, rest or immobilization of the involved joint is an important adjunct to treatment.

    (a) Colchicine

        (i) Oral colchicine can be used when the diagnosis of gout is uncertain, because marked clinical improvement is relatively specific for gout. A 0.6-mg dose is given hourly until clinical improvement occurs or symptoms of gastrointestinal toxicity (i.e., nausea, vomiting, and diarrhea) intervene. A maximum of 6 mg should be used in this type of trial. It is common for side effects to occur before or simultaneously with relief.

        (ii) Intravenous colchicine also can be given to treat acute attacks. A 2-mg dose is given in 20 ml of normal saline over 20 minutes; 1-mg doses can be given twice, at 6-hour intervals, if relief has not occurred. The incidence of gastrointestinal side effects is much lower with the intravenous preparation, but local extravasation can cause necrosis, and bone marrow suppression can occur with high doses. These risks are minimized with maintenance of a secure intravenous line, avoidance of colchicine in neutropenic patients, and administration of lower dosages in patients with liver or renal diseases that might impair colchicine excretion.

    (b) Nonsteroidal anti-inflammatory drugs

        (i) Indomethacin is the prototypical drug of this category and the one usually selected when the diagnosis of gout is secure and contraindications to the drug are not present. An initial dose of 50–75 mg is followed by 50 mg every 6 hours to a maximum of 200 mg in the first 24 hours. The dosage typically is decreased to 150 mg in the next 24 hours, with further decrease instituted according to clinical response.

        (ii) Newer nonsteroidal agents (e.g., naproxen, sulindac, ibuprofen, and piroxicam) also have been used successfully. All are to be avoided in the setting of active peptic ulcer disease, gastrointestinal bleeding, and inflammatory bowel disease and when renal prostaglandin synthesis is important in preserving tissue perfusion (as in congestive heart failure and renal insufficiency).

    (c) Corticosteroids. Intra-articular injections of corticosteroids can be used to treat acute gout of a single joint, particularly when the use of other agents is contraindicated.

    (d) Drugs that alter serum uric acid concentrations should be avoided during acute attacks, because raising or lowering serum uric acid can prolong attacks. In patients already taking such drugs (e.g., allopurinol or probenecid), the dosage should not be altered.

c. Intercritical gout refers to the third stage of gout, which is an asymptomatic period after the initial attack that may be interrupted by new acute attacks.

(1) Recurrence of monoarticular attacks. About 7% of patients never experience a new attack of acute gouty arthritis after the first episode. However, 62% experience a recurrence within 1 year. Typically, the patient is asymptomatic between attacks, but attacks eventually become more frequent and abate more gradually if urate deposition remains untreated over time.

(2) Progression to polyarticular attacks. Attacks tend to become polyarticular and more severe over time. Some patients develop a chronic inflammatory arthritis without asymptomatic intervals—a condition that may be difficult to distinguish from rheumatoid arthritis.

(3) Progression to chronic tophaceous gout typically occurs over a 10- to 20-year period of untreated urate deposition.

(4) Radiographic changes. Radiographs most often show the soft tissue swelling of acute attacks, although cartilage loss or marginal erosions can occur with repeated attacks.

(5) Prophylaxis for recurrent attack

    (a) Colchicine, in 0.6-mg doses given two or three times daily, is used to prevent recurrences. Maintenance colchicine usually is continued for 6 months to 1 year after a satisfactory reduction in serum uric acid levels has been achieved.

(b) **Indomethacin** in 25-mg doses given twice daily, can be used for patients who cannot tolerate colchicine.

(c) **Dietary restrictions.** Large purine loads and alcohol overindulgence may precipitate acute attacks by causing fluctuations in serum uric acid. Patients prone to such attacks should avoid such precipitants.

(d) **Drug restrictions.** Intermittent salicylate use or institution of thiazide treatment causes fluctuations in uric acid excretion and serum uric acid levels and may precipitate an acute gouty attack.

d. **Chronic tophaceous gout** develops in the untreated patient and is the final stage of gout. The **tophus** is a collection of urate crystal masses surrounded by inflammatory cells and variable fibrosis.

(1) **Typical locations of tophaceous deposits**

(a) The **pinna** of the external ear is the classic site of tophus development, although deposition here is uncommon.

(b) Other common locations are the surfaces of chronically involved joints and subchondral bone as well as extensor surfaces of the forearms, olecranon bursae, and the infrapatellar and Achilles tendons.

(2) **Pathogenesis of tophaceous gout**

(a) Although microtophi may form in joints early in the urate deposition phase, aggregates that are large enough to be palpable or to cause anatomic deformities take years to develop. The rate of tophus formation is directly related to the severity and duration of hyperuricemia in gout patients. Tophi do not occur in patients with asymptomatic hyperuricemia.

(b) Erosion of cartilage and adjacent subchondral bone occurs due to displacement of normal tissue by the tophus and by the inflammatory reaction to it.

(3) **Diagnosis of tophaceous gout**

(a) **Physical appearance.** Tophi are firm, moveable, and cream-colored or yellowish in appearance if superficially located. If they ulcerate, a chalky material is extruded.

(b) **Radiographic findings.** Tophaceous deposits appear as well-defined, large erosions (**punched-out erosions**) of the subchondral bone. These erosions are most common at the first metatarsophalangeal joint and at the bases and heads of phalanges; however, any articulation can be affected. Typical gouty erosions have an **overhanging edge** of subchondral new bone formation. Periarticular osteopenia is absent.

(c) **Aspiration.** Tophi can be aspirated and crystals demonstrated by polarized microscopy.

(d) **Biopsy.** If aspiration is not successful, biopsy of a lesion may be necessary to differentiate a tophus from a rheumatoid nodule [see section III F 3 b (1)]. Specimens must be fixed in alcohol, since formalin dissolves urate.

(4) **Therapy for chronic gout** revolves around the control of hyperuricemia. Lifelong treatment usually is begun after the first attack of acute gout, to prevent the otherwise high incidence of tophaceous and joint destructive changes that occur in gout patients who are not treated with uric acid–lowering drugs. (Possible prevention of renal calculi is an additional benefit.) Drugs that increase renal uric acid excretion (**uricosuric drugs**) or that decrease uric acid production (**xanthine oxidase inhibitors**) are available. The therapeutic aim with either type of drug is to decrease serum uric acid level below 7 mg/dl, because concentrations above this level allow saturation of extracellular fluid and consequent urate deposition in tissues. Patients who have had acute attacks should receive prophylactic agents (e.g., colchicine or indomethacin) for several weeks before beginning drug treatment to lower serum uric acid.

(a) **Uricosuric drugs** include probenecid and sulfinpyrazone.

(i) **Indications.** These drugs can be used in patients who excrete less than 700 mg of uric acid daily, who have normal renal function, and who have no history of urinary stones.

(ii) **Administration.** Drug dosages are increased at weekly intervals until satisfactory reduction of serum uric acid is achieved. Probenecid is given twice daily, with doses starting at 250 mg and increasing to a total dose of 750 mg. Sulfinpyrazone also is given in divided doses, starting at 100 mg and increasing to a total daily dose of 400 mg, if necessary.

(iii) **Disadvantages.** These drugs are reasonably safe. However, disadvantages include twice-daily dosing, salicylate interference with drug effect, and possible urinary uric acid precipitation.

(b) **Xanthine oxidase inhibitors** include allopurinol, which is an analog of hypoxanthine. In addition to inhibiting de novo uric acid synthesis, allopurinol competitively inhibits xanthine oxidase via enzymatic conversion to oxypurinol.

    (i) Indications. Allopurinol clearly is preferable to uricosuric drugs in patients who excrete more than 1000 mg of uric acid per day, have a history of nephrolithiasis, or have abnormal renal function (uricosurics are less effective at creatinine clearances below 30–50 ml/min). Other indications include tophaceous gout, allergy to uricosurics and failure of uricosurics to reduce serum uric acid level below 7 mg/dl.

    (ii) Administration. Allopurinol is begun in daily doses of 100 mg and increased at weekly intervals to reduce the serum uric acid level below 7 mg/dl. Most patients require 300 mg/day; however, some require as much as 600 mg/day to control the serum uric acid level.

    (iii) Toxicity. Caution must be taken when using allopurinol in renal failure, because the incidence of **allopurinol toxicity syndrome** rises with the serum concentration of its metabolite, oxypurinol. Dosage reductions to 100–150 mg/day are important in moderate-to-severe renal failure, even if serum uric acid concentrations of 7 mg/dl are not achievable. Other toxic reactions can occur with this medication, including skin rash, bone marrow suppression, vasculitis, and hepatitis. Lastly, dosages of 6-mercaptopurine and azathioprine must be reduced because allopurinol potentiates their purine antagonism.

  (c) Nonpharmacologic intervention

    (i) Weight reduction. Gradual weight reduction usually helps to lower serum uric acid level and can be an adjunctive control measure if feasible.

    (ii) Dietary restrictions. Severe reduction in dietary protein intake usually is unnecessary, but avoidance of foods very high in purine content is desirable. Anchovies and organ meats are important examples.

    (iii) Alcohol restrictions. Chronic alcohol use can stimulate purine production, and patients not responding to drug treatment of elevated serum uric acid should avoid overuse of alcohol.

e. Renal disease may arise at any stage of gout, but nephrolithiasis is the only common clinical presentation of renal involvement.

  (1) Urate nephropathy. In some patients with long-standing gout, tophi have been found at autopsy in the renal interstitium and uric acid deposits found in the renal tubules. (**Pyelonephritis** also can occur in these patients, but the most common renal lesion is **nephrosclerosis** associated with uncontrolled hypertension.)

    (a) Etiology and pathogenesis

      (i) Nephrosclerosis of uncontrolled hypertension is the most common cause of reduced creatinine clearance and proteinuria in gout patients.

      (ii) Urate deposition. Renal functional impairment due to urate deposition has been difficult to document and is a late event in severe chronic gout.

      (iii) Lead poisoning can lead to impaired creatinine clearance, hyperuricemia, and gout via an undefined renal defect.

    (b) Clinical features and diagnosis. Proteinuria, impaired ability to concentrate urine, and reduced creatinine clearance have been described in gout patients.

    (c) Therapy for urate nephropathy focuses on controlling factors that can be demonstrated to cause renal functional impairment (i.e., hypertension and, perhaps, chronic pyelonephritis). Correction of hyperuricemia has not been shown to improve or prevent renal dysfunction in gout patients.

  (2) Acute obstructive uropathy

    (a) Incidence. Acute obstructive uropathy may occur in patients with extremely high nucleic acid turnover, which ultimately leads to precipitation of uric acid crystals in the collecting tubules and ureters and, thus, to blockage and renal failure. The typical setting is a patient who develops renal failure after chemotherapeutic treatment of a myeloproliferative or lymphoproliferative malignancy.

    (b) Clinical features and diagnosis. Uric acid-to-creatinine ratios of greater than 1 in random urine samples indicate extremely high urinary uric acid concentrations and, in the setting of acute renal failure, suggest obstructive uropathy due to uric acid crystals.

    (c) Therapy. Prevention is the most important factor. Prophylaxis with allopurinol is important in patients who are scheduled to receive high-dose chemotherapy for myeloproliferative or lymphoproliferative malignancies. Urine alkalinization and maintenance of high urine volumes also may be important preventive measures.

  (3) Nephrolithiasis

    (a) Incidence. As many as 20% of gout patients have a history of either uric acid or calcium oxalate stones. The risk of uric acid stone formation is proportional to both the magnitude and duration of serum uric acid concentration and urinary uric acid excretion.

  (b) **Etiology and pathogenesis**

  (i) **Low urine pH.** A basic defect in patients who form uric acid stones seems to be a persistently low urine pH due to impaired intrarenal production of ammonia.

  (ii) **Hyperuricosuria** (i.e., elevated urinary uric acid concentration) is important for the formation of uric acid stones as well as calcium oxalate stones. Presumably, uric acid crystals can act as a **nidus** for calcium stone formation.

  (iii) **Low urine volume** increases urinary uric acid concentration and the tendency toward stone formation.

  (c) **Therapy for nephrolithiasis** in gout patients is no different than in patients without prior urate deposition. Patients with uric acid stones require a high fluid intake, an alkaline urine, and reduction of uric acid hyperexcretion with allopurinol (not uricosuric agents). Patients with calcium stones also require a dilute urine. Allopurinol has a role in preventing uric acid precipitation, which can act as a nidus for calcium stone formation in patients with hyperuricosuria.

B. Calcium pyrophosphate dihydrate (CPPD) deposition disease

  1. **Definition.** Deposition of CPPD crystals in cartilage and periarticular connective tissues can cause a gamut of articular manifestations, ranging from asymptomatic deposition to acute and chronic inflammatory arthritis. The acute form of CPPD deposition disease is commonly called **pseudogout.**

  2. **Etiologic classification**

  a. **Hereditary CPPD disease.** Many families have been described that have a high prevalence of CPPD disease, with autosomal dominant transmission the typical pattern. Secondary metabolic associations with CPPD disease typically are not present in these families.

  b. **CPPD disease associated with metabolic disorders.** Correction of underlying metabolic disorders, if possible, does not seem to alter the progression of CPPD disease.

  (1) **Probable associations.** CPPD disease occurs at a higher than expected frequency in association with certain diseases and conditions. In many, potential abnormalities of calcium, phosphorus, or cartilage metabolism can explain the associations. These probable associations include:

  (a) Hyperparathyroidism
  (b) Hemochromatosis
  (c) Hypothyroidism
  (d) Osteoarthritis
  (e) Neuropathic joint disorders
  (f) Aging

  (2) **Possible associations.** CPPD disease may or may not occur at a higher than expected frequency in association with:

  (a) Gout
  (b) Diabetes mellitus
  (c) Ochronosis
  (d) Wilson's disease

  3. **Pathogenesis**

  a. **Crystal deposition**

  (1) **Site.** The initial site of CPPD deposition appears to be articular cartilage surrounding lacunae in the midzone. Later, deposition occurs in clefts of degenerated cartilage and in scattered foci in the cartilage matrix and synovial membrane, eventually forming large crystalline masses.

  (2) **Process.** An alteration of cartilage ground substance, the ionic composition of the matrix (i.e., calcium and pyrophosphate), or a combination of these factors is required for crystallization. Possibly, an altered condition of the matrix (e.g., removal of an inhibiting agent or addition of a nucleating agent) allows crystals to form in the microenvironment around the chondrocyte as pyrophosphate is released from the cell. The synovial chondrocyte is the most likely source of the elevated pyrophosphate concentrations found in affected joints.

  b. **Crystal-mediated joint damage.** CPPD deposits stiffen the cartilage, impairing its weight-bearing properties and accelerating osteoarthritic change. The acute arthritic attacks are believed to be induced by the release of crystals from the cartilage into the joint space.

  (1) **Factors mediating crystal release**

  (a) **Matrix loosening.** CPPD crystals in cartilage exist in equilibrium with synovial fluid calcium and pyrophosphate concentrations. Decreases in serum calcium concentration can lead to decreases in synovial fluid pyrophosphate levels and solubilization of joint CPPD crystals as equilibrium is restored. Loss of marginal CPPD deposits may cause loosening of the entire deposit in the matrix and release of large numbers of CPPD crystals into the joint space. Thus, fluctuations of serum calcium concentration in the setting of acute medical illness or during the perioperative period may initiate acute crystal release.

- **(b) Loss of matrix.** Enzymatic erosion of cartilage due to an associated inflammatory arthritis, such as gout or infectious arthritis, also may cause crystal release.
- **(c) Biomechanical forces.** Impaired dissipation of weight-bearing forces on cartilage also may lead to crystal loosening and release into the joint space.

(2) Factors affecting acute attacks

- **(a) Inflammatory response.** Neutrophil and mononuclear phagocytosis of crystals released into the joint space occurs, leading to the release of lysosomal enzymes and neutrophil chemotactic factor (NCF) from the phagocytic cells.
- **(b) Degree of response.** The number of crystals released in the acute attack probably is the most important factor in determining the severity of the attack. To an extent, the degree of inflammatory response is mediated by adsorption of IgG to the CPPD crystal, and CPPD crystals seem to adsorb less IgG than urate crystals and excite a lesser inflammatory response. Finally, CPPD crystals are not membranolytic, as are urate crystals.
- **(c) Amplification of response.** Other inflammatory mediators (e.g., Hageman factor and components of the kinin, plasmin, and complement pathways) may amplify responses to inflammation, but neutrophils are the necessary component for the primary inflammatory response.

4. Clinical syndromes

- **a. Pseudogout** accounts for 25% of cases of CPPD disease. Acute swelling, pain, stiffness, and erythema develop in previously asymptomatic joints. The knee most commonly is involved (i.e., in 50% of cases), but almost any synovial joint can be involved, including the first metatarsophalangeal joint. Spread to adjacent joints can occur, and precipitation of attacks by acute medical or surgical illness is common, occurring in 10%–20% of cases. Systemic findings such as fever and leukocytosis can occur, especially in elderly patients. Joints typically return to normal between attacks, which may last days to weeks.
- **b. Pseudo-rheumatoid arthritis** accounts for 5% of cases of CPPD disease. In some patients, a smoldering chronic arthropathy can occur. Subacute episodes of pain and swelling in one or more joints can be superimposed on a more chronic picture of prolonged morning stiffness, fatigue, synovial thickening, and progressive deformities.
- **c. Pseudo-osteoarthritis** accounts for 50% of cases of CPPD disease. These patients present with a clinical and radiographic picture similar to that of degenerative joint disease, although about half have superimposed acute attacks of pseudogout. Flexion contractures are more common than in typical osteoarthritis, and bilateral knee varus deformities or isolated patellofemoral arthritis may occur more commonly than in osteoarthritis. A small percentage of these patients may have such severe joint destruction (e.g., of the shoulders or knees) that the clinical and radiographic appearance is that of a neuropathic joint disorder, even in the absence of underlying neurologic disease or apparent proprioceptive deficit.
- **d. Asymptomatic CPPD disease** occurs in 20% of cases. These patients do not have joint pain; the disease typically is uncovered by the finding of asymptomatic chondrocalcinosis on radiography. The prevalence of this finding—and of the other, clinically evident, forms of CPPD disease—increases with age and is seen in as many as 7% of elderly people screened.

5. Diagnosis. The finding of typical crystals on synovial fluid analysis is diagnostic of pseudogout. Chondrocalcinosis seen on radiography is evidence for a diagnosis of CPPD deposition. However, chondrocalcinosis may be present in patients who never develop acute pseudogout.

- **a. Synovial fluid findings.** Chunky, rhomboid crystals that exhibit weakly positive birefringence in red-compensated, polarized light are the hallmark of the acute arthritis syndromes associated with CPPD disease. These may be intracellular (in neutrophils) or extracellular, but they usually are much less prevalent than in a typical gout-involved joint. Synovial fluid leukocytosis of 10,000–20,000 cells/mm^3 or greater (mostly neutrophils) is typical.
- **b. Radiographic findings**
  - **(1) Chondrocalcinosis.** Calcification of articular hyaline cartilage, fibrocartilage (most commonly in the knee menisci, intervertebral disk annuli, symphysis pubis, and wrist

triangular disk), synovial membrane, tendons, and bursae can occur, usually in a stippled, linear fashion.

(2) Osteoarthritis. Osteoarthritic changes in atypical joints (e.g., the wrist, elbow, and shoulder and the metacarpophalangeal joints) suggest CPPD disease. Subchondral bone cysts may be more extensive in x-rays of joints affected by CPPD disease, and hook-shaped osteophytes characteristically are present with metacarpophalangeal involvement.

(3) Pseudo-neuropathic joint. Radiographic findings typical of neuropathic joint disorders, including extreme joint disorganization and bone fragments, can be found in severe cases of CPPD disease.

c. Clinical diagnostic distinctions

(1) Clinical or radiographic evidence of osteoarthritis in joints not usually involved by osteoarthritis should suggest CPPD disease as an alternative diagnosis.

(2) Attacks of acute inflammatory arthritis in a setting of apparent osteoarthritis should suggest CPPD disease.

(3) Acute arthritis occurring shortly after a medical illness or surgical procedure should suggest a crystal-mediated arthritis, such as gout or pseudogout.

(4) Radiographic changes more typical of osteoarthritis in a patient thought to have rheumatoid arthritis should suggest CPPD disease as an alternative diagnosis.

(5) Asymmetrical joint inflammation or isolated joints inflamed "out of phase" with other involved joints should suggest CPPD disease.

(6) The presence of diseases commonly associated with CPPD disease (e.g., hyperparathyroidism and hemochromatosis) should suggest CPPD disease as a possible cause of any joint manifestations.

(7) Neuropathic joint presentations should prompt investigation for CPPD disease as well as potentially associated neurologic disorders.

6. Therapy

a. Aspiration of acutely inflamed joints with removal of all obtainable synovial fluid can shorten the duration of acute attacks.

b. Nonsteroidal anti-inflammatory medications, given on tapering schedules as for gout treatment [see section II A 4 b (5) (b)], is a common means of treating the acute inflammatory attack after joint aspiration has been performed. These drugs are used on a more chronic basis for symptoms due to the osteoarthritis-like or rheumatoid arthritis-like presentations.

c. Intravenous colchicine appears to be effective treatment for acute attacks of pseudogout; it is particularly effective in patients who cannot take oral medications or who have contraindications to nonsteroidal anti-inflammatory treatment. The same drug doses and precautions recommended for acute gout apply for treatment of acute pseudogout [see section II A 4 b (5) (a) (ii)].

d. Corticosteroid injections. Intra-articular injection of a long-acting corticosteroid preparation, following aspiration of an inflamed joint, may have an additional anti-inflammatory effect, but this procedure should not be attempted if infection might be present.

e. Screening evaluations for possible associated metabolic diseases should be considered if the clinical situation warrants it.

f. Prophylaxis for recurrent attacks is not known to be effective. However, patients who have chronic symptoms or frequent recurrences usually are treated with chronic nonsteroidal anti-inflammatory therapy.

C. Hydroxyapatite arthritis. Hydroxyapatite crystals, the typical form of calcium in bone, also can cause several rheumatic syndromes.

1. Clinical syndromes

a. Crystal deposition in osteoarthritis. Mineral formation may be a result of abnormal cartilage metabolism in more severe forms of osteoarthritis. Patients with more severe forms of osteoarthritis are more likely to have mineral deposited in articular cartilage, and joint effusions in these patients contain crystals of hydroxyapatite as often as they contain CPPD crystals.

b. Calcific periarthritis. Hydroxyapatite deposition in bursae and tendon sheaths can cause episodes of acute inflammation (i.e., periarthritis and peritendinitis), with acute attacks of pain, swelling, and erythema. Discrete clumped deposits can be found radiographically around the shoulders, greater trochanters, wrists, elbows, and digits and in other periarticular areas. These deposits can be shown to disintegrate gradually on radiographs taken several weeks after the acute periarthritis.

c. Destructive arthritis. Hydroxyapatite crystals can be associated with a chronic destructive arthropathy, which is characterized by erosive radiographic changes, large usually noninflammatory effusions, proliferative synovitis, synovial mineral deposition, and periarticular ligamentous instability. This syndrome occurs most often in the knees and shoulders (the **"Milwaukee shoulder"**) of elderly patients. Synovial fluid analysis shows few cells (500–1000/mm³, with monocytes predominating) and high concentrations of neutral proteases and collagenases.

2. **Diagnosis.** Light microscopic examination of synovial fluid occasionally reveals brownish globules that are large clumps of hydroxyapatite crystals. However, electron-microscopic examination is necessary to reveal isolated crystals. A calcium stain—alizarin red S—can be used as a screening test for the presence of hydroxyapatite or CPPD crystals in effusions. Aspirates from bursae or tendon sheaths may yield milky or pasty material that contains high concentrations of these hydroxyapatite crystals.

3. **Therapy.** Mechanical splinting and nonsteroidal anti-inflammatory agents are used to treat acute episodes of periarthritis. Nonsteroidal anti-inflammatory medications often are used in the chronic hydroxyapatite arthropathy as well. Periodic aspiration of the large synovial effusions that occur in the Milwaukee shoulder may help to preserve ligamentous integrity and remove destructive enzymes. Corticosteroid injections may help to treat acutely symptomatic joints.

III. RHEUMATOID ARTHRITIS

A. **Definition.** Rheumatoid arthritis is a chronic inflammatory disorder of unknown cause, which is typified by polyarticular, symmetrical joint involvement but also is known for its characteristic extra-articular involvement. **Rheumatoid factor** (see section III D 2) frequently is present in the serum of affected individuals.

B. **Epidemiology**

1. **Prevalence and sex distribution.** As many as 1% of adults may have rheumatoid arthritis, depending on the criteria used to make the diagnosis. Clinically meaningful forms of disease are less common—0.5% of women and 0.1% of men have forms of the illness that require ongoing treatment.

2. **Human leukocyte antigen (HLA) associations.** There is an increased prevalence of the B-cell alloantigen HLA-DR4 in patients with seropositive rheumatoid arthritis but not in those with seronegative rheumatoid arthritis.

3. **Seropositivity for rheumatoid factor.** Patients who have rheumatoid factor in their serum appear to have a different illness from patients who are seronegative. The HLA association supports this hypothesis; furthermore, seropositive patients tend to have more severe disease, more erosions, and more extra-articular features.

C. **Etiology.** No single factor or agent is known to cause rheumatoid arthritis. Presumably, an initial insult (possibly infectious) interacting with the host's genetically established immune responses determines whether an initial synovitis is suppressed or perpetuated.

1. **Extra-articular agent.** The earliest inflammatory changes in the rheumatoid joint involve inflammation and occlusion of small subsynovial vessels, suggesting that the agent is carried in the circulation to the joint.

2. **Infectious agent.** An infectious etiology often is suggested because of the presence of virus-like particles in synovial biopsies early in the disease course and because of the occurrence of polyarthritis in several human and animal bacterial or viral illnesses. However, no direct evidence of infection has been discovered.

3. **Genetic factors.** A genetic susceptibility to altered immune responses probably is important in rheumatoid arthritis. There is no known association of HLA-A or HLA-B haplotypes with the disease, but a significant association exists between seropositive rheumatoid arthritis and the presence of **HLA-Dw4** and **HLA-DR4** alloantigens of the major histocompatibility complex. The presence of these and other genetically coded immune response alloantigens may be important in modulating the host's cellular and humoral immune responses to potential etiologic agents.

4. **Effects of Epstein-Barr virus on the immune response.** Rheumatoid arthritis patients have a defect in their ability to regulate B cells infected with Epstein-Barr virus. The virus may act as a polyclonal activator of B-cell autoantibody production in rheumatoid arthritis and, as such, may have a role in perpetuation (not initiation) of the disease.

D. **Pathogenesis.** An unknown etiologic agent (an exogenous one or an "altered" endogenous one) initiates a nonspecific immune response. The joint lesion in rheumatoid arthritis begins as an inflammatory lesion in the synovial membrane that can progress to a proliferative one (the pannus), which can deform by destroying adjacent cartilage and bone. Alternatively, the inflammatory or proliferative lesions can regress, most commonly with disease-altering therapies. Immune response genes may also be important in determining the type, intensity, and chronicity of the immune response.

1. **Synovial cell interactions** are important for maintenance of articular inflammation.
    a. **Macrophage–T cell.** Macrophage and helper T cell interrelationships are central to the amplification of the immune response. Macrophages process antigen and "present" it to the helper T cells, which then become activated by the interaction.
    b. **Helper T cell–B cell.** Activated helper T cells stimulate B-cell proliferation and differentiation into antibody-producing cells. These B cells are "factories" for the production of rheumatoid factor.
    c. **Helper T cell–synovial cell.** Helper T cells produce soluble mediators that can modulate the function of synovial lining cells, both macrophage-like and fibroblast-like. The fibroblast-like lining cell produces collagenase, prostaglandins, and connective tissue, all of which may be important in the destructive effects of the synovial pannus.
    d. **Macrophage–endothelial cell.** The ingrowth of capillaries is important to the propagation of synovitis and the later growth of the pannus. Macrophages may transmit signals to capillary endothelial cells to migrate and replicate, although it is possible that the endothelial cell may operate independently of such signals.

2. **Rheumatoid factor**
    a. **Definition.** B cells and plasma cells in the synovial membrane produce immunoglobulins. One specific type of immunoglobulin produced is rheumatoid factor, an **antibody directed against immunoglobulin G (IgG)**. Conceivably, the IgG has been altered in some way to appear as "nonself," perhaps by binding to another antigen. IgM and IgG rheumatoid factors constitute a large fraction of the immunoglobulin production of the rheumatoid synovial membrane.
    b. **Pathogenicity.** Rheumatoid factor is present in the serum of most (possibly 80%) patients with established rheumatoid arthritis. Patients who have rheumatoid factor generally have more severe disease and a higher frequency of rheumatoid nodules and systemic extra-articular complications such as vasculitis than those without rheumatoid factor. Complexes of IgG rheumatoid factor and complement can be found in synovial tissue and fluid as well as in extra-articular inflammatory lesions. Rheumatoid factor can trigger immune response in two ways.
       (1) **Immune complex activation of complement.** Rheumatoid factor may combine with IgG away from its antibody combining site, leaving the IgG molecule free to combine with other antibodies and form larger "poly-IgG complexes." These aggregates can reach a size large enough to fix complement and activate complement pathways via kinin-mediated chemotaxis.
       (2) **Immune complex ingestion.** Aggregates of IgG rheumatoid factor are phagocytized by macrophages, which release lymphokines, and also by neutrophils, which release digestive enzymes. Both of these effects amplify inflammation. Synovial levels of IgG rheumatoid factor but not IgM rheumatoid factor are relatively reduced compared to the levels in serum, suggesting that phagocytosis of IgG rheumatoid factor may have a specific role in the inflammatory response.

3. **Synovial fluid phase**
    a. **Neutrophil attraction.** Neutrophils are attracted by chemotactic factors (e.g., complement fragments, kallikrein, plasminogen activator, fibrin degradation products, fibronectin, and collagen fragments) that are released in the synovial reaction as well as lymphocyte-derived factors (e.g., interleukin 2) and platelet products. Immune complexes trapped in the collagen matrix also may be important chemoattractants.
    b. **Neutrophil mediator release.** Phagocytosis of immune complexes (e.g., IgG rheumatoid factor) or binding of chemotactic factors on neutrophil membranes initiates release of leukotrienes, prostaglandins, oxygen-free radicals, hydrolytic enzymes, and other chemotactic factors. More inflammatory cells are attracted, and enzymatic destruction of cartilage ensues.
    c. **Inflammatory pathway activation.** Release of the products mentioned above into the joint space incidentally causes activation of the clotting cascade, the fibrinolytic system, and the kinin and complement systems. These reactions further amplify chemotaxis and enzyme release.

4. **Chronic proliferative lesion.** A mass of fibroblastic, vascular, and inflammatory cells called the **pannus** accumulates at the margin of the synovial membrane–cartilage border, driven by

cellular interactions based in the synovial membrane and the soluble mediators generated in the synovial fluid. The mass can cause local erosions of cartilage and bone or produce enzymes that degrade collagen and proteoglycans in the cartilage.

  a. Damage to cartilage
    (1) Proteoglycan depletion. Neutral or acid proteases in inflammatory synovial fluid can leach proteoglycans from cartilage at sites distant from the pannus. The structural integrity of the distant cartilage remains intact because these proteases cannot attack native collagen.
    (2) Collagen destruction. Collagenases from synovial cells and neutrophils in the fluid can cleave the collagen triple helical configuration and allow the proteases to break down the denatured collagen further. Plasmin generated by synovial cell synthesis of tissue plasminogen activator may be involved in cleaving procollagenases into active enzymes. Proteinases inactivate angiogenesis inhibitors and allow the vascular pannus to erode cartilage locally.
  b. Damage to bone
    (1) Solubilization of bone mineral. A component of the pannus may be able to solubilize bone mineral or stimulate osteoclasts to resorb it. Prostaglandins synthesized by synovial cells may be involved since they can stimulate osteoclast activity. Another possible mechanism for bone resorption could be production of osteoclast activating factor (also called interleukin 1) by macrophages in the pannus.
    (2) Direct erosion by the pannus. The vascular pannus can erode bone locally, as it can cartilage.

E. Pathology

  1. Synovial membrane. Synovial lining cells, both type A (macrophage-like) and type B (fibroblast-like), proliferate early. Small blood vessels dilate and proliferate, but focal areas of small vessel inflammatory change or occlusion also can be formed in early lesions. Heterogeneous collections of mononuclear cells (especially T cells and macrophages) occur around blood vessels, with plasma cells arranged around the periphery; neutrophils generally are absent. These collections of inflammatory and vascular tissue enlarge into thickened villi, which protrude into the joint space and erode cartilage and subchondral bone at the joint margins.

  2. Synovial fluid. The volume of the synovial fluid and its protein content increase. Lymphocytes increase in the initial stages, but soon a shift occurs and neutrophils predominate. White blood cell counts of 20,000/mm³ or greater, with neutrophils comprising 70%, are common in active inflammatory stages. Lysosomal enzymes (i.e., acid hydrolases and neutral proteases) are released by neutrophils and accumulate in the fluid. Viscosity and mucin clot integrity are reduced because of alterations in hyaluronic acid caused by the inflammatory products.

  3. Established joint disease. Destructive change is unpredictable, since the inflammatory process can be arrested at any stage. However, unimpeded inflammation and proliferation lead to loss of cartilage and underlying bone, joint capsular thickening, and tendon sheath stretching and infiltration with inflammatory tissue. Cartilage and surrounding tendons and ligaments no longer can dissipate mechanical forces. Mechanical incongruities and pressure from synovial fluid distension are degenerative forces secondary to the inflammatory forces destroying cartilage. The additive effects of inflammatory destruction and altered biomechanical loading eventually can lead to deformities characteristic of rheumatoid arthritis and even to joint ankylosis.

F. Clinical features

  1. Disease onset
    a. Signs and symptoms of disease
      (1) Constitutional symptoms. Weight loss, generalized aching, anorexia, malaise, and fatigue all are complaints that are associated with active inflammatory arthritis and tend to wax and wane with disease activity.
      (2) Articular complaints
        (a) Joint stiffness lasting longer than 30–45 minutes upon arising in the morning (''**morning stiffness**'') is a cardinal symptom of inflammatory arthritis, and duration of the stiffness is a measure of the activity of the arthritis.
        (b) In addition to stiffness, patients also complain of pain in affected joints, which usually is worse with motion. Limitation of joint motion, soft tissue swelling, and mild erythema or warmth also may be features.
        (c) The metacarpophalangeal and proximal interphalangeal joints of the hands, wrists, knees, and the metatarsophalangeal and proximal interphalangeal joints of the feet

are the most common joints involved initially. Typically, patients have polyarticular, bilaterally symmetrical disease. Distal interphalangeal joint involvement is unusual, and significant spinal changes usually are confined to the cervical spine. However, any diarthrodial joint can be involved as the disease progresses.

b. Patterns of onset

(1) **Acute.** Ten to fifteen percent of patients notice that their symptoms begin abruptly, over the course of hours to days. Another 15%–20% notice that their symptoms worsen rapidly, but the period of evolution is days to weeks. Both groups of patients usually have prominent systemic complaints, and the very acutely ill ones may be febrile.

(2) **Insidious.** The symptoms of as many as 60%–70% of patients with rheumatoid arthritis appear gradually, over a period of weeks to months. Sometimes the constitutional complaints precede the joint findings. Brief remissions of symptoms may occur early in the disease course, only to return as sustained inflammatory arthritis later.

(3) **Palindromic rheumatism** is a recurring acute inflammatory arthritis that begins in one or two joints and evolves quickly into intensely inflammatory, gout-like arthritis. The signs and symptoms of inflammation typically last only 2–3 days before the joints become asymptomatic again. Different joints can be involved in a sequential or migratory fashion. This pattern of onset is unusual, but 30%–50% of patients with palindromic rheumatism eventually develop the more chronic disease typical of rheumatoid arthritis.

2. Disease course

a. Early disease. It is difficult to predict the early course of rheumatoid arthritis because as many as 80% of patients who initially fulfill the American Rheumatism Association criteria for probable rheumatoid arthritis either develop another illness or recover completely.

b. Disease present after 1 year. Spontaneous remission of rheumatoid arthritis after 1 year of symptoms is unusual, so this somewhat artificial time standard may be useful in planning treatment decisions.

(1) **Episodic course.** A course of intermittent remissions and exacerbations is more common early in the course of rheumatoid arthritis; however, most patients tend to develop sustained disease over time. Some patients do continue to exhibit episodic attacks of arthritis that return to asymptomatic states throughout their entire illness.

(2) **Sustained course.** The bulk of patients with established rheumatoid arthritis, who comprise the group most in need of disease-modifying treatment, either demonstrate from the beginning or evolve into a pattern of sustained inflammatory activity. A small subset of this group exhibits inexorable progression of disease to severe deformities or death, despite aggressive treatment.

3. Signs and symptoms of established disease

a. Articular manifestations

(1) **Generalized joint involvement.** Pain with motion and joint swelling are common in patients with rheumatoid arthritis as well as other types of inflammatory arthritis, and functional weakness of involved extremities may be present due to the pain. Physical examination may show swelling, tenderness on palpation, slight warmth, and limitation of active and passive motion of the involved joint. Redness is not typically seen, and swelling usually is confined to the periarticular areas (due to joint effusions or thickened synovial membrane). Fairly symmetrical but not bilaterally identical joint involvement is typical.

(2) **Specific joint involvement**

(a) **Cervical spine.** Although zygapophyseal or neurocentral joint inflammation can lead to neck pain, muscle spasm, and limitation of neck motion, the most serious form of cervical spine involvement is **atlantoaxial joint subluxation**. The most common form of this instability is anterior movement of the atlas on the axis, demonstrable by lateral radiographs of cervical spine flexion and extension, which show an increase in the normal 3-mm distance between the anterior arch of the atlas and the odontoid process of the axis when the head is flexed. Up to 20% of patients with rheumatoid arthritis may have disease of spinal level C1–C2, but only rarely is treatment needed in addition to a soft or hard cervical collar. Neurologic symptoms (e.g., progressive spastic tetraparesis, painless sensory loss in the hands, or transient episodes of medullary or pontine dysfunction) may necessitate cervical spinal fusion. Anesthesiologists must take special precautions to avoid neck hyperextension in rheumatoid patients who have subluxation of the C1–C2 spinal level.

(b) **Cricoarytenoid joint.** Synovitis of the joints that allow the vocal cords to rotate can lead to hoarseness in up to 30% of rheumatoid patients. Rarely, these joints can become adducted and immobilized, causing stridor. Fixation in abduction can lead to repeated aspiration pneumonias.

(c) **Shoulder.** Glenohumeral involvement can lead to a large degree of functional impairment in rheumatoid arthritis. **Rotator cuff fraying and rupture** can be just as important as synovitis in eventual morbidity, and abrupt onset of severe pain and profound weakness of the first 90° of shoulder abduction is a typical presentation of a ruptured rotator cuff. Although chronic adhesive capsulitis can be an outcome of severe glenohumeral involvement, marked shoulder instability is the more typical outcome in a patient with severe rotator cuff abnormalities.

(d) **Elbow.** Synovitis of the elbow can occur early and quickly, and it can lead to limitation of extension. Rheumatoid nodules present on the extensor aspect of the forearm can lead to chronic **olecranon bursitis.**

(e) **Hand and wrist**
   (i) Swelling and tenderness of metacarpophalangeal and proximal interphalangeal joints usually are among the earliest findings in rheumatoid arthritis. Distal interphalangeal joints are typically spared.
   (ii) **Swan neck deformities** (flexion of the distal interphalangeal and metacarpophalangeal joints and hyperextension of the proximal interphalangeal joint) due to spasm of the intrinsic muscles and tenosynovitis of hand flexor tendons can develop.
   (iii) Chronic swelling or rupture of the extensor hood at the proximal interphalangeal joint can lead to proximal interphalangeal flexion deformity with distal interphalangeal hyperextension, the so-called "**boutonnière deformity.**"
   (iv) Dorsal wrist swelling is a typical finding in rheumatoid arthritis, sometimes with a ganglion-like presentation.
   (v) **Wrist synovitis** and palmar flexor tenosynovitis (which is very common in rheumatoid arthritis) can lead to medial nerve compression at the wrist, producing the **carpal tunnel syndrome.** Chronic wrist involvement leads to volar and radial hand deviation due to carpal bone rotation. The fingers compensate with an **ulnar drift.** The normal grasp is in a slightly ulnar direction, and chronic metacarpophalangeal joint swelling and intrinsic muscle spasm tend to increase ulnar forces further, with the consequent drift. Advanced synovitis occasionally can lead to extensor tendon rupture, classically at a point where an eroded ulnar styloid can abrade the fourth and fifth extensor tendons.

(f) **Hip. Groin pain** due to hip joint involvement is common in adults with rheumatoid arthritis, but severe involvement with protrusio acetabuli occurs in only about 5% of patients. Physical examination usually shows limitation of hip internal rotation before abduction and adduction are affected.

(g) **Knee** involvement is quite common; quadriceps atrophy and flexion deformities can develop quickly if not prevented by appropriate physical therapeutic measures. Palpable knee swelling often is due to a combination of thickened synovial membrane and effusion. Popliteal cysts (**Baker's cysts**) can form in the popliteal space when fluid accumulates rapidly in the knees. Flexion of the knee in this situation can lead to marked increases in intra-articular pressure and herniation of synovial membrane and fluid posteriorly, most often into a communicating semimembranosus-gastrocnemius tendon sheath. These cysts can dissect, causing calf swelling, or they can rupture, causing an acute thrombophlebitis-like picture.

(h) **Ankle and foot.** Ankle and subtalar joint involvement is common in rheumatoid arthritis. Swelling anterior to the malleoli associated with pain on plantar flexion and dorsiflexion of the ankle suggests ankle involvement. In contrast, pain with inversion or eversion of the foot suggests subtalar joint involvement. Pain in the ball of the foot that occurs with weight bearing suggests metatarsophalangeal joint involvement, which can lead to a **cock-up toe** deformity when it is more advanced.

b. **Extra-articular manifestations.** Rheumatoid arthritis is a systemic disease and, as such, frequently affects tissues other than joints. Generally, extra-articular involvement is present in patients who are seropositive and who have more severe and long-standing arthritis.

(1) **Nodules** probably are the most common manifestation of extra-articular disease, occurring in 20%–25% of patients. They are firm, round masses that can be felt in the subcutaneous tissues, especially in sites of repetitive trauma such as the olecranon bursae and extensor surfaces of the forearms. They also can occur in visceral structures such as the heart and lungs. Histologically, they resemble the proliferative synovial lesions, although the cellular reaction is polarized around a necrotic core. These nodules usually are asymptomatic in subcutaneous locations, and they may appear and disappear rapidly, although a slower evolution is characteristic.

(2) **Eye**
   (a) **Sicca complex.** Ten to fifteen percent of patients with rheumatoid arthritis have the burning, gritty sensation in the eyes that is typical of keratoconjunctivitis sicca. Dry mouth (xerostomia) and salivary gland enlargement are other clinical features. The

pathologic basis of these complaints is lymphocytic infiltration of lacrimal and salivary glands, respectively. Keratoconjunctivitis sicca and xerostomia associated with rheumatoid arthritis and other rheumatic diseases can be differentiated from those occurring in primary Sjögren's syndrome on the basis of specific clinical and HLA associations (see section IX).

(b) **Episcleritis** is a self-limited, sometimes recurrent, and only mildly painful condition that may present as an erythematous or nodular inflammation of the superficial scleral tissues. This condition often is bilateral and does not interfere with vision. If treatment is required, short courses of mild topical corticosteroid preparations can be used.

(c) **Scleritis** is a more serious inflammation of the deeper, relatively avascular tissues of the sclera. It usually is indolent, bilateral, slowly progressive, and painful. Most importantly, it can lead to progressive visual deterioration from secondary uveitis or interstitial keratitis. Unchecked, progressive disease leads to scleral thinning and even **scleromalacia perforans**—a complete loss of scleral tissue in focal areas with uveal tissue bulging through the defect. Close ophthalmologic care is important, and intraocular corticosteroid injections or chronic systemic corticosteroids may be necessary.

(3) **Heart.** Cardiac complications of rheumatoid arthritis often are found postmortem but rarely are clinically significant during life. Acute pericarditis is the most common clinically relevant problem, and recurrent bouts of pericarditis can progress to pericardial tamponade or constriction. Corticosteroid therapy usually controls the acute illness, but surgical intervention may be required for tamponade or constriction. Other potential but unusual cardiac complications are inflammatory granulomas that can resemble rheumatoid nodules; these can occur anywhere in the heart. A focal myocarditis is not uncommon at autopsy, but it is usually indolent and often does not cause congestive heart failure or arrhythmias.

(4) **Lung.** Pulmonary involvement in rheumatoid arthritis resembles cardiac involvement—it is common at autopsy but usually asymptomatic during life.

(a) **Pleural involvement.** Pleural effusions usually accompany the pleuritis that is associated with rheumatoid arthritis, and they often recur or become chronic. Although characterized by an exudative and usually mononuclear cell–predominant fluid, the hallmarks of rheumatoid pleural effusions are low levels of pleural fluid glucose (often less than 10 mg/dl) and low complement levels.

(b) **Interstitial fibrosis** that is indistinguishable from diffuse interstitial pulmonary fibrosis can be seen in patients with rheumatoid arthritis, especially in seropositive men who smoke. Fibrotic involvement is most apparent radiographically at the lung bases, and clinical progression can best be assessed by monitoring pulmonary function tests and measurements of diffusing capacity. Corticosteroids are used to treat disease progression only when an inflammatory component is present and rapid progression can be demonstrated.

(c) **Nodules.** Single or multiple rheumatoid nodules are most common in patients who have nodules elsewhere, and these present as coin lesions on chest x-ray. Rheumatoid patients who have prior exposure to industrial agents (e.g., coal or asbestos) can develop **Caplan's syndrome**—interstitial lung disease and multiple nodules seen on chest x-ray, apparently due to the combined effects of the pneumoconiosis and rheumatoid arthritis.

(5) **Nerve.** Neurologic complications usually are related to vasculitis [see section III F 3 b (7)], although entrapment neuropathies (carpal tunnel syndrome or tarsal tunnel syndrome) can occur when the nerves passing through these rigid tunnels are compressed by swollen tendon sheaths. Amyloid infiltration of nerves can cause a distal sensory neuropathy in chronically active, long-standing disease.

(6) **Blood**

(a) **Red blood cells.** The normochromic normocytic anemia that occurs in chronic diseases is common in rheumatoid arthritis and typically reflects the activity of this illness. Chronic gastrointestinal blood loss from treatment with nonsteroidal anti-inflammatory drugs also can occur, and iron-binding capacity and ferritin levels may be difficult to interpret due to iron deficiency enhanced by the bleeding. Iron levels also are affected by the inflammatory response in rheumatoid arthritis.

(b) **Platelets.** Thrombocytosis in the range of 500,000–700,000/mm³ of blood is quite common in rheumatoid arthritis and may be associated with active disease and extra-articular manifestations. Thrombocytopenia, on the other hand, is unusual unless it is due to a drug side effect or occurs in association with **Felty's syndrome** (a combination of rheumatoid arthritis, thrombocytopenia, leukopenia, and splenomegaly).

(c) **Leukocytes.** Eosinophilia and mild leukocytosis are the only common white cell abnormalities in rheumatoid arthritis and may reflect the presence of active disease or extra-articular manifestations. Leukopenia associated with splenomegaly (Felty's syndrome) is uncommon, but the absolute granulocytopenia associated with Felty's syndrome can be chronic and quite severe. Splenic sequestration, increased granulocyte utilization in joints, and impaired marrow production of granulocytes all can be involved in granulocytopenia. Antibodies adherent to granulocyte membranes can interfere with granulocyte function as well as cause cellular destruction. Splenectomy may be required when treatment for the rheumatoid arthritis does not reverse the low granulocyte count.

(7) Vasculitis of small synovial vessels is a feature of the basic rheumatoid process, but several different extra-articular presentations can occur in chronic, highly expressed rheumatoid arthritis.

(a) Skin. Small vessel vasculitis can result in splinter hemorrhages, palpable purpura, distal digital infarction, or even acro-osteolysis. The course of this vasculopathy can be chronic and in milder cases may not require treatment; when vasculitis is more severe or widespread, corticosteroid or immunosuppressive treatment may be required.

(b) Nerve

(i) Distal sensory neuropathy. In patients with long-standing rheumatoid arthritis, a distal sensory neuropathy may develop that is mildly progressive but usually does not require treatment. Close observation is required to insure that this presentation does not signal generalized vasculitic involvement.

(ii) Sensorimotor neuropathy. Vasculitis of the vasonervorum of the entire peripheral nervous system with consequent sensory and motor dysfunction (**mononeuritis multiplex**) usually occurs acutely and in the context of widespread small and medium-size artery inflammation. Corticosteroid and immunosuppressive treatment usually are instituted promptly.

(c) Visceral lesions. The mononeuritis presentation discussed above often is associated with systemic vasculitis such as coronary and mesenteric arteritis. This grave complication is due to widespread necrotizing lesions in the small and medium-size arteries and requires aggressive treatment.

G. Diagnosis. Two major sets of criteria have been developed for making the diagnosis of rheumatoid arthritis: the American Rheumatism Association and the New York criteria. These criteria are most useful for classifying patients in epidemiologic studies and therapeutic trials; they are less useful for physicians making the diagnosis of rheumatoid arthritis in an individual patient. A period of 1–2 years may pass before characteristic features appear and allow confident diagnosis because the disease often begins atypically. A diagnosis of rheumatoid arthritis is made by considering historical, physical, laboratory, and radiographic information and excluding other disease processes.

1. Historical information. Inquiry into constitutional complaints; the presence and duration of morning stiffness; joint pain, warmth, and swelling; and the duration and chronicity of symptoms is necessary. Many forms of arthritis are self-limited; therefore, a diagnosis of rheumatoid arthritis is more secure when the arthritis has been present for 3 months or more.

2. Physical examination. Generally there is a fairly symmetrical but not identical inflammatory arthritis of extremity joints, specifically sparing distal interphalangeal joints in most cases. The axial skeleton also is spared except for the cervical spine. Rheumatoid nodules are prominent physical findings that suggest rheumatoid arthritis, most commonly present in seropositive patients with established disease.

3. Laboratory findings

a. Hematologic findings. A normochromic normocytic anemia in rheumatoid arthritis is a common indicator of chronic disease. The presence of microcytes and a low mean corpuscular volume should trigger a search for blood loss. Eosinophilia can be seen in patients with rheumatoid arthritis, often in those with more severe disease. Thrombocytosis, a high erythrocyte sedimentation rate, and polyclonal increases in gamma globulin concentration are common findings, reflecting acute and chronic inflammation.

b. Serologic findings. Rheumatoid factor is found in 70%–80% of patients with rheumatoid arthritis, but it is not a specific marker for the disease. It can be found in normal aging individuals and in patients with other chronic diseases. However, its presence in the setting of an inflammatory polyarthritis usually favors the diagnosis of rheumatoid arthritis. Antinuclear antibodies are found in 25% of patients with rheumatoid arthritis, and false-positive results of the Venereal Disease Research Laboratory (VDRL) test are found in 5%–10%.

   c. **Synovial fluid findings.** The typical characteristics of the synovial fluid are those of a moderately inflammatory fluid: The leukocyte count usually is 5000–25,000 cells/mm³ and is mostly neutrophils. Glucose levels can be somewhat low and complement levels depressed, depending on the intensity of the inflammation. Urate and CPPD crystals are not present.

4. Radiographic findings
   a. **Symmetry.** Roughly symmetrical involvement of joints is the rule, although bilateral involvement may not be of equal severity.
   b. **Osteopenia.** Radiographic evidence of bone loss in periarticular areas is one of the earliest findings in rheumatoid arthritis; more generalized osteopenia occurs later in the disease course.
   c. **Soft tissue swelling.** Localized swelling of the soft tissue around particular joints often is an early feature of rheumatoid arthritis. This finding can be especially valuable in pinpointing early involvement of the small joints of the hands.
   d. **Erosions.** Loss of bone at joint margins is caused by pannus formation and is indicative of more advanced disease.
   e. **Joint space narrowing.** Widespread articular cartilage loss caused by persistent inflammation leads to joint space narrowing, a finding of severe or established disease in a particular joint.

5. Differential diagnosis. The diagnosis of rheumatoid arthritis can be made with confidence in a symmetrical, sustained polyarthritis only when other possible causes of similar presentations are excluded.
   a. **Spondylarthropathies** (see section IV). The presence of significant axial spinal involvement, excluding the cervical spine, and prominent **enthesopathic** manifestations should suggest the diagnosis of one of the spondylarthropathies. Sacroiliac joint involvement is particularly suggestive of these disorders. Specific historical evidence or evidence on physical examination (e.g., oral and genital ulcerations, anterior uveitis, recurrent urethritis, bowel disease, and psoriatic plaques) is indicative of spondylarthropathic disease. Finally, reactive new bone formation at involved sites is more typical of spondylarthropathies than rheumatoid arthritis.
   b. **Other connective tissue diseases**
     (1) **Systemic lupus erythematosus (SLE).** A nondeforming polyarthritis often is present in SLE and can mimic rheumatoid arthritis because of its symmetry and involvement of similar joints. Furthermore, ulnar deviation and swan-neck deformities can occur as a result of chronic swelling of the joint capsule (Jaccoud's arthropathy). However, usually there are typical clinical findings of SLE in these patients. Joint fluids in SLE usually are noninflammatory (i.e., a white cell count < 2000/mm³, with lymphocyte predominance), and destructive joint disease (with erosions and joint space narrowing) does not occur.
     (2) **Systemic sclerosis.** Inflammatory joint involvement in this disease rarely is sustained, and the obvious distal skin changes usually allow clear distinction between systemic sclerosis and rheumatic arthritis.
     (3) **Dermatomyositis or polymyositis.** Inflammatory muscle involvement dominates the clinical picture, but an arthropathy can occur similar to that described for SLE.
     (4) **Overlap presentations.** Uncommonly, the presentations of any of these connective tissue diseases can overlap in situations where sustained features of two or more diseases are present (e.g., rheumatoid arthritis and polymyositis).
     (5) **Rheumatic fever** occurs uncommonly in adults, but it should be suspected when a migratory arthritis is associated with a streptococcal pharyngitis. The arthritis in rheumatic fever is self-limited and lasts 1–4 weeks; therefore, diagnostic confusion should be minimal.
     (6) **Polymyalgia rheumatica.** Patients with polymyalgia rheumatica occasionally present with a symmetrical polyarthritis along with the typical hip and shoulder aching and a high erythrocyte sedimentation rate. The arthritis is not sustained or deforming.
     (7) **Vasculitic syndromes.** Vasculitis, especially polyarteritis and Wegener's granulomatosis, can present in the early stages with inflammatory polyarthritis. Evolution of more characteristic organ involvement distinguishes these syndromes from rheumatoid arthritis.
   c. **Infectious diseases**
     (1) **Viral.** Polyarthritis can occur as an initial manifestation of viral illnesses such as rubella, mononucleosis, and hepatitis B. These are typically self-limited.
     (2) **Bacterial.** Bacterial infections (e.g., bacterial endocarditis and disseminated gonorrhea) occasionally can present as symmetrical polyarthritis, but they are diagnosed by

distinctive clinical associations and positive cultures. Cultures from appropriate sites should always be taken in patients with undiagnosed polyarthritis and fever.

(3) Lyme disease. Infection caused by the spirochete *Borrelia burgdorferi* can cause a chronic arthritis that is indistinguishable from rheumatoid arthritis. The history of tick bite; the association of typical skin, cardiac, or central nervous system (CNS) findings; or a rise in antibody titer to the organism helps to distinguish this illness from rheumatoid arthritis.

(4) Whipple's disease. Although sometimes confused with rheumatoid arthritis, the chronic arthropathy of Whipple's disease more closely resembles a spondylarthropathy. The associated chronic diarrhea and weight loss indicate the need for appropriate bowel studies.

d. Crystal-mediated arthritis. In established disease, both gout and CPPD deposition disease can be clinically similar to chronic erosive rheumatoid arthritis. Although the history of early attacks may suggest crystal-mediated disease by the sudden occurrence and rapid disappearance of arthritis, aspirates from involved joints must be examined for crystals to distinguish these diseases from rheumatoid arthritis.

e. Endocrine and metabolic diseases
   (1) Thyroid disorders
      (a) Hypothyroidism has been associated with synovial effusions and widespread aching and stiffness (fibrositis). In addition to typical findings of the primary disorder, noninflammatory joint effusions (often with CPPD crystals) distinguish this presentation from that of rheumatoid arthritis.
      (b) Hyperthyroidism. Patients with this disorder can have the widespread aching and stiffness of fibrositis, or, rarely, they may have **thyroid acropathy**—a syndrome of periostitis and synovitis that is similar to hypertrophic pulmonary osteoarthropathy. The clinical and laboratory features of hyperthyroidism should be sought.
   (2) Hyperlipoproteinemia. Patients with hyperlipoproteinemia types II and IV sometimes can have pauciarticular arthritis as well as subcutaneous and tendon sheath nodules. These patients usually do not manifest the clinical or laboratory findings (including synovial fluid findings) of an inflammatory arthropathy.
   (3) Hemochromatosis. This disease of iron overload commonly presents as an arthropathy, classically an osteoarthritic involvement of the second and third metacarpophalangeal joints and, less commonly, larger joints. CPPD crystals often can be found in superimposed inflammatory effusions, but otherwise the arthritis lacks the typical systemic features or synovial inflammatory features of rheumatoid arthritis. Appropriate iron studies are confirmatory.
   (4) Wilson's disease. Adults with this disease of copper storage can present with an arthropathy similar to that described for hemochromatosis. The associated hepatic and neurologic findings should indicate the need for appropriate tests of copper metabolism.

f. Osteoarthritis. When severe and extensive, osteoarthritis may resemble rheumatoid arthritis with secondary degenerative manifestations. In osteoarthritis, the absence of constitutional complaints and prolonged morning stiffness, the distinctive joint involvement (i.e., most commonly, involvement of the distal interphalangeal joints, knees, and hips), and the typical lack of soft tissue swelling around the joints are distinguishing. Also, laboratory evidence of inflammation is lacking, the synovial fluid is noninflammatory (i.e., a white cell count < 2000/mm³), and radiographic findings are more typical of degenerative joint disease.

g. Fibrositis. Patients with this syndrome of generalized aching and stiffness have tenderness in specific nonarticular areas rather than in the joints. There are no joint or laboratory abnormalities suggesting inflammation.

h. Other conditions
   (1) Oral contraceptive use. Occasionally, patients taking oral contraceptives develop polyarticular aching, often associated with positive antinuclear antibodies or rheumatoid factor. These findings resolve with discontinuation of the drug.
   (2) Multicentric reticulohistiocytosis. The joint manifestations in this disorder are those of a severely destructive polyarthropathy. However, factors distinguishing it from rheumatoid arthritis include characteristic skin lesions, prominent distal interphalangeal joint involvement, a normal erythrocyte sedimentation rate, and the absence of rheumatoid factor.
   (3) Sarcoidosis is associated with periarthritis and an inflammatory polyarthritis similar to rheumatoid arthritis early in the course of the disease. Most patients present with polyarthritis, erythema nodosum, and bilateral hilar adenopathy; the arthritis is self-limited. A chronic asymmetrical articular form of sarcoidosis also exists, but radiographs reveal the cystic changes typical of sarcoid bone lesions.

    (4) Hypertrophic osteoarthropathy. Knee, ankle, and wrist involvement are typical, with prominent distal extremity periostitis evident on x-ray. This entity can be confused with rheumatoid arthritis when clubbing is not present, but the radiographic findings are distinctive. Pulmonary neoplasms are the most common clinical association.

    (5) Amyloidosis and multiple myeloma. Patients with primary amyloidosis or amyloidosis associated with multiple myeloma can manifest an arthropathy from the synovial deposition. The synovial fluid is noninflammatory, and greenish amyloid fibrils can be seen under a polarizing microscope after staining with Congo red.

    (6) Common variable immunodeficiency. Some patients with this syndrome can develop rheumatoid arthritis, but arthralgia with or without noninflammatory effusions is a more common musculoskeletal presentation. These complaints usually resolve during gamma globulin treatment.

    (7) Malignancy. Patients with leukemias, lymphomas, and, occasionally, carcinomas can present with polyarthritis resembling rheumatoid arthritis. Nodules and rheumatoid factor typically are absent in these patients.

H. Therapeutic approach. Effective management of rheumatoid arthritis involves thorough patient education as well as the development of a multidisciplinary treatment plan.

  1. Goals

    a. General. In all patients with rheumatoid arthritis, an attempt is made to control pain and reduce inflammation without causing undesirable side effects. Preservation of joint function and ability to maintain life-style are important long-term goals.

    b. Specific. The goals of a specific patient are important in fashioning treatment for rheumatoid arthritis. More aggressive treatment may be desirable in an individual whose job is threatened, whereas a more traditional approach may be taken for someone who has no such constraints.

  2. Education. Educating the patient about the disease process is particularly important in chronic diseases such as rheumatoid arthritis, in which a patient's compliance with instructions and drug treatment is critical to the outcome.

    a. Description of the illness. The various disease courses of rheumatoid arthritis must be described, emphasizing the fact that most patients do well if they are appropriately treated. The **chronicity** and **intermittency** of symptoms must be discussed so that the patient understands that spontaneous fluctuations in an extended disease course are the norm. The patient must be educated about the **systemic nature** of the disease process, so that both patient and family will understand the fatigue, malaise, and weight loss that often accompany this illness.

    b. Etiology. The physician should explain to the patient that the cause of the disease is unknown and that the disease could not have been caused by any action on the part of the patient. It should be explained that rheumatoid arthritis has poorly defined genetic associations but that the genetic features do not warrant prevention of pregnancy.

    c. Drug treatment. Drug effects, side effects, and dosage schedules should be explained carefully to patients. Patients should understand why a particular medication is being used (i.e., as analgesia, for immediate anti-inflammatory effects, or as disease-modifying therapy) and the trial length of medication use necessary to assess efficacy. The frequency of follow-up visits and laboratory testing needed to monitor potential medication toxicity may be critical in a patient's choice of treatment. The use of ''quack'' remedies (e.g., bee venom or dental extractions) should be discouraged.

    d. Rest and exercise. Patients should be informed about the importance of resting or splinting acutely involved joints to reduce inflammation. Brief periods of bed rest may be useful in patients with severe polyarticular exacerbations, and regular naps may help patients deal with the fatigue of rheumatoid arthritis. Conversely, exercises to strengthen muscles surrounding involved joints should be encouraged when the arthritis is under good control. All joints should be put through a full range of motion once daily to prevent contractures.

  3. Therapy

    a. Drug therapy

      (1) Analgesics. Pure analgesic agents such as acetaminophen, propoxyphene, and codeine sometimes are added to anti-inflammatory agents for additional pain relief in acutely symptomatic periods. However, pure analgesic agents are most useful in rheumatoid arthritis when pain is due to secondary degenerative arthritis rather than to active synovitis. The addiction potential of narcotics in a chronic illness must always be considered.

      (2) Salicylates

        (a) Aspirin is the prototypical anti-inflammatory agent used in the treatment of rheumatoid arthritis, and it is usually the agent tried first. Advantages include the ability to measure serum levels and to use symptoms of ototoxicity as a therapeutic end point. Many physicians feel that, of the nonsteroidal anti-inflammatory drugs, aspirin is the most effective in the treatment of rheumatoid arthritis, and it is certainly the most affordable.

   (i) Administration. Typically, treatment is initiated with a dose of 3 regular (325-mg) aspirin tablets four times a day in adults. The dosage is titrated upward 1–2 pills weekly until adequate response is achieved or symptoms of ototoxicity occur. If patients complain of symptoms of tinnitus or impaired hearing, the drug is stopped until these symptoms resolve; then the drug is restarted at 1 less pill per day. Serum salicylate levels can be drawn if questions about compliance, efficacy, or toxicity arise, and a serum level of 20–30 mg/dl is the therapeutic range.

   (ii) Toxicity. Other than ototoxicity, the most common side effects of aspirin are gastrointestinal, including abdominal pain, mucosal erosions, peptic ulcer disease, and hepatotoxicity. Irreversible abnormalities of platelet function occur as well; these can be quantitated by evaluating prolongation of bleeding times. Reversible drug-related changes in renal function, which are mediated by inhibition of renal prostaglandins, also can occur.

   (b) Nonacetylated salicylates include choline magnesium trisalicylate, salsalate, and others. These drugs cause much less inhibition of prostaglandins than aspirin and as a consequence are less toxic to the gastrointestinal system and platelet function. Unfortunately, in most patients, the anti-inflammatory effects usually are less marked as well.

(3) Other nonsteroidal anti-inflammatory agents. Drugs such as ibuprofen, naproxen, sulindac, and indomethacin often are used in the treatment of rheumatoid arthritis if patients cannot tolerate large amounts of aspirin. These drugs may cause fewer gastrointestinal side effects than aspirin, usually do not cause ototoxicity, and may be as effective as aspirin in a given patient.

   (a) Administration. The levels of these drugs cannot be measured and ototoxicity cannot be relied on, so general dosage guidelines approved by the Food and Drug Administration usually are followed. At least a 2-week trial usually is necessary to assess response.

   (b) Toxicity. Gastrointestinal, hepatic, and renal toxicity occur to varying degrees with these agents.

(4) Corticosteroids have potent anti-inflammatory effects, but they have equally potent and predictable toxicities and do not have disease-modifying effects. These drugs are used most commonly in rheumatoid arthritis to control serious extra-articular manifestations such as vasculitis.

   (a) Systemic administration. In rare situations, such as severe progressive active disease, prednisone doses no higher than 5–10 mg once daily in the morning may be used to allow continued functioning. Continual attempts to taper the dosage of these drugs should be made.

   (b) Local instillation. Injectable corticosteroid preparations can be instilled into one or two joints inflamed "out of phase" with other involved joints. These injections should be performed only occasionally, since osteonecrosis or cartilage loss may result from frequent injections into the same joint.

(5) Disease-modifying agents. Patients with persistent polyarticular synovitis, progressive deformities, erosive radiographic changes, or all three usually require the addition of a disease-modifying agent to their treatment programs. These agents work more slowly (weeks to months) than the anti-inflammatory agents and are employed to alter the basic course of the disease, not just to dampen acute inflammation. Although these drugs function as immunomodulatory agents, their precise mechanisms of action in rheumatoid arthritis remain largely unknown. The decision to employ disease-modifying agents is not always clear-cut. The duration of joint complaints helps in making this decision (arthritis present for less than 3 months often remits spontaneously; arthritis present for more than 1 year rarely does so without treatment). In general, the more disabling and sustained the arthritis, the more likely that a disease-modifying agent will be required. Typically, an ineffective disease-modifying agent is stopped before a new one is started; treatment with a nonsteroidal anti-inflammatory agent usually is continued after the disease-modifying agent is started.

   (a) Antimalarial drugs. Hydroxychloroquine is the most commonly used drug of this type. Antimalarial agents are effective in certain patients with rheumatoid arthritis, and significant side effects are uncommon with these drugs.

   (i) Administration. Hydroxychloroquine is given in doses of 200–400 mg daily. Patients who will respond to this drug usually do so within 12 weeks, so 3 months is an appropriate therapeutic trial.

   (ii) **Toxicity.** The most common side effects are gastrointestinal (nausea, epigastric pain, and diarrhea), but these usually are not severe enough to interfere with treatment. The most serious toxicity is ophthalmologic (macular pigmentary retinopathy, causing visual impairment), which is rare at presently used doses. Patients taking this drug must have baseline eye examination and reexamination every 6 months, because early detection of retinopathy and discontinuation of medication can prevent blindness.

(b) **Gold compounds.** Injectable and oral compounds of gold are effective disease-modifying agents in the treatment of rheumatoid arthritis. The injectable form is more effective but also more toxic than the oral form. A long treatment period (5–6 months) generally is required to assess efficacy.

   (i) **Administration.** A 10-mg test dose of gold preparation typically is injected intramuscularly and is followed by 25 mg 1 week later and 50 mg weekly thereafter until a total dose of 1 g has been given. If the response is unsatisfactory, the drug is stopped. If the response is adequate, the dosage interval gradually is lengthened to every 2, then every 3, then every 4 weeks, if possible. The oral form of the drug is given as a 6-mg dose—either 6 mg once daily or 3 mg twice a day. A 6-month trial should be adequate to assess response.

   (ii) **Toxicity.** The most important toxicities of gold are hematologic, renal, and dermatologic. Thrombocytopenia, leukopenia, and aplastic anemia are serious but uncommon hematologic effects that can occur suddenly at any time during gold treatment. Patients receiving intramuscular gold therapy should have a complete blood count, differential count, and platelet count done before each injection because of this toxicity. A membranous glomerulonephritis can cause profuse proteinuria, so urine should be examined monthly. Pruritic skin rashes and oral ulcers are the most common manifestations of dermatologic toxicity, although exfoliative dermatitis has occurred if gold treatment is continued despite the rash. Oral gold treatment also is a frequent cause of diarrhea.

(c) D-**Penicillamine** is an effective disease-modifying agent in the treatment of rheumatoid arthritis, but its effectiveness is not apparent for weeks to months.

   (i) **Administration.** The drug typically is started at a low oral dose (125–250 mg daily) and is increased at 4-week intervals to an effective dosage, usually no higher than 750–1000 mg. A 6-month therapeutic trial is appropriate.

   (ii) **Toxicity.** Toxicities are quite similar to those that occur in gold therapy; therefore, urinalysis should be done monthly, and the complete blood count, differential count, and platelet count also should be checked monthly.

(6) **Other drug therapies**

   (a) Sulfasalazine may be an effective disease-modifying agent in the treatment of rheumatoid arthritis, although it has not been used as extensively in rheumatoid arthritis as in inflammatory bowel disease.

   (b) Cytotoxic agents (azathioprine and cyclophosphamide) or cytostatic agents (methotrexate) often are used when the drugs mentioned fail.

   (c) Other experimental therapies, such as apheresis and total lymphoid irradiation, sometimes are used in aggressive disease when all other remedies have failed.

b. **Physical medicine**

(1) All patients with rheumatoid arthritis benefit from coordination of their nonpharmacologic treatment by a **physiatrist**.

(2) **Physical therapists** can help patients strengthen weakened muscle groups to protect damaged joints. They can show patients range-of-motion exercises that prevent joint contractures.

(3) **Occupational therapists** can help patients obtain devices to assist them, can construct splints for involved joints, and can aid in rehabilitating patients for activities of daily living and employment.

c. **Surgery.** Surgical intervention may be necessary early as well as late in the course of rheumatoid arthritis. Synovectomies may decrease the inflammatory process in particularly involved joints early in the disease course. Later, arthroplasties or total joint replacements may be appropriate to relieve pain or help restore function in structurally damaged joints.

4. **Assessment of response.** The intensity of the inflammation must be evaluated at each visit to gauge disease activity and therapeutic response so that treatment decisions can be made. The tendency for the activity of rheumatoid arthritis to fluctuate spontaneously must be considered in assessing treatment responses. Definitions of disease remission rely on the absence of or marked improvement in the following indicators of disease activity for a sustained interval.

    a. Morning stiffness longer than 15–30 minutes implies inflammation, and the duration of the stiffness is a useful measure of disease activity.

    b. Systemic complaints. Prominent constitutional complaints in rheumatoid arthritis imply active systemic disease. The time to the onset of fatigue in rheumatoid arthritis is a potential measure of disease activity. Anorexia and weight loss also may reflect new inflammation.

    c. Joint complaints. The number of joints involved as well as the amount of joint pain, limitation of motion, and swelling present are important features of disease activity.

    d. Laboratory findings

        (1) The presence of a normochromic normocytic anemia, an elevated erythrocyte sedimentation rate, and thrombocytosis are laboratory indications of inflammation. To some extent, the degree of these abnormalities varies with the activity of the illness.

        (2) White blood cell counts greater than 2000/mm³ in synovial fluid suggest active disease.

I. Prognosis. The majority of patients with rheumatoid arthritis have a good prognosis, and most of them respond well to appropriate treatment.

    1. Disease course. Attempts to predict disease outcome based on type of disease onset (i.e., sudden versus gradual onset of joint complaints) have not been useful. Spontaneous remission is unusual after the disease has been established for 1 year. Patients with intermittent disease activity tend to have a better outcome than those with chronic, progressive disease.

    2. Sex. Women generally have more severe disease than men.

    3. Rheumatoid factor. Seropositive patients are less likely to have complete remission of symptoms than seronegative patients. Seropositive patients also tend to have more chronic, progressive disease with more extra-articular features than seronegative patients.

    4. Extra-articular features. Patients with nodules and other extra-articular features (i.e., patients with highly-expressed disease) have a more severe and more disabling disease than those without extra-articular features. The mortality rate in this group also is greater than in the average rheumatoid patient population, particularly when patients have cardiopulmonary symptoms, vasculitic complications, or amyloidosis.

    5. Thrombocytosis. In some studies, elevations in platelet count parallel the severity of disease. This value seems to be a marker for chronic inflammation and perhaps for extra-articular features.

IV. SPONDYLARTHROPATHIES

A. Introduction. The spondylarthropathies are **a group of inflammatory arthritides** that are distinct from rheumatoid arthritis. Typical distinguishing features include the following.

    1. Clinical features

        a. Skeletal

        (1) Axial. As a group, the spondylarthropathies prominently involve the **axial skeleton**, particularly the sacroiliac joints. The axial skeleton is not commonly involved in rheumatoid arthritis except for the cervical spine.

        (2) Appendicular. Inflammatory arthritis of the appendicular skeleton also occurs in these disorders, but the involvement tends to be **oligoarticular** and **asymmetrical**. In contrast, rheumatoid arthritis usually is polyarticular and symmetrical.

        (3) Enthesis. In both the axial and appendicular skeletons, inflammation of tendon and ligament sites of attachment to bone is common (e.g., costochondritis, Achilles tendinitis, and plantar fasciitis). Tendon inflammation is less prominent in rheumatoid arthritis.

        b. Extraskeletal

        (1) Nodules. Rheumatoid nodules are not found in the spondylarthropathies.

        (2) Internal organ involvement. The typical eye involvement in the spondylarthropathies (conjunctivitis and anterior uveitis), cardiac involvement (aortitis), and genitourinary involvement (urethritis and prostatitis) are much different from the usual extra-articular features of rheumatoid arthritis.

        c. Laboratory findings. Several cardinal laboratory features of chronic inflammation (i.e., anemia, thrombocytosis, and elevated gamma globulin levels) are not commonly present in the spondylarthropathies as they are in rheumatoid arthritis. Erythrocyte sedimentation rate may be increased but is not a good measure of disease activity. Rheumatoid factor typically is absent.

        d. Radiographic findings. The characteristic changes seen radiographically are those of periosteal new bone formation at the site of the enthesopathic lesions (see section IV A 3), both at axial locations (in the form of syndesmophytes) and appendicular locations. Although erosive changes can occur, they occur most typically in the axial skeleton (in the hips, sacroiliac joints, and shoulders).

    e. Therapeutic response. Disease-modifying agents that are commonly required in treating rheumatoid arthritis (gold, D-penicillamine, or hydroxychloroquine) have no clinical effect on the spondylarthropathies, with the exception of psoriatic peripheral arthropathy. Typically, nonsteroidal anti-inflammatory agents alone are sufficient to treat these illnesses.

2. Genetic factors. The strong association of the histocompatibility antigen **HLA-B27** with clinical expression of the spondylarthropathies provides evidence for genetic transmission of these disorders.

    a. This relationship also is a major reason for grouping these disorders. The independent correlation of HLA-B27 with specific features of spondylarthropathies (e.g., sacroiliitis, aortitis, and anterior uveitis) explains both the clinical overlap among these diseases and their familial clustering.

    b. The role of the antigen in disease causation is not understood. The antigen may be a marker for a disease susceptibility gene, or it may be intimately involved in the interaction of a foreign antigen at the host cell surface and the consequent modulation of the immune response to that foreign antigen.

3. Pathology

    a. The basic pathologic lesion in the spondylarthropathies is an **enthesopathy**—an inflammation occurring at the site where ligaments and tendons attach to bone. This type of inflammation explains the frequency of sacroiliitis, ascending spinal lesions, and peripheral tendon lesions (e.g., Achilles tendinitis) in these diseases.

    b. Although inflammatory synovitis that is indistinguishable from rheumatoid synovitis can be seen in these illnesses, it is not typically as widespread, chronically active, and potentially destructive as it is in rheumatoid arthritis (psoriatic arthritis mutilans is a notable exception).

B. Specific disorders

  1. Ankylosing spondylitis

    a. Definition. Ankylosing spondylitis is the spondylarthropathy that is most closely associated with inflammation of the axial skeleton. Back pain and limited spinal mobility caused by sacroiliitis and variable ascent of the inflammation up the spine dominate the clinical expression of this disease.

    b. Epidemiology

      (1) Prevalence. Ankylosing spondylitis may be as common as 1 in 100 white individuals, since the frequency of disease parallels the prevalence of the HLA-B27 antigen (10%–20% of the 6% of whites with HLA-B27 antigen may have ankylosing spondylitis). The frequency of ankylosing spondylitis is lower in black and Asian populations, paralleling the prevalence of the antigen in these groups.

      (2) Sex distribution. Ankylosing spondylitis may be as prevalent in women as in men if x-ray findings of sacroiliitis are considered to be diagnostic of the disease. However, women tend to have asymptomatic or very mild disease with more peripheral joint manifestations.

    c. Etiology

      (1) The major histocompatibility antigen HLA-B27 occurs in 90%–95% of white patients with ankylosing spondylitis, but the association is less marked in nonwhite populations (40%–50% of blacks with ankylosing spondylitis have HLA-B27).

      (2) Because the gene or genes coding for the expression of HLA-B27 reside on the sixth chromosome, autosomal transmission occurs. Thus, children of a proband who is heterozygous for the gene controlling HLA-B27 production have a 50% probability of eventual expression of the antigen on cell surfaces.

      (3) Only 10%–20% of whites with HLA-B27 develop ankylosing spondylitis, and the incidence is even lower for those without a family history of the disease. Although the presence of HLA-B27 is a marker at least for susceptibility to the disease, it is likely that pathogenic and benign forms of HLA-B27 exist or that other genetic factors are important in determining expression of spondylitic disease. Environmental factors (e.g., viral or bacterial infection and bacterial antigens) may act as foreign antigens to trigger disease expression.

    d. Clinical features

      (1) Disease onset usually occurs in the second or third decade of life.

      (2) Disease course. The disease begins with the gradual onset of chronic low backache, which is associated with prolonged morning stiffness and which improves with exercise. Most patients have prolonged, unremitting low back pain for years as the major feature of their illness. The disease may be mild and cause minimal interference with function, or it may be severe and deforming.

(3) Manifestations of disease

    (a) Axial skeletal involvement

        (i) Sacroiliac joints typically are symmetrically inflamed in ankylosing spondylitis, with this involvement causing the insidious low back pain and limitation of lumbar spinal mobility.

        (ii) Ascending spinal involvement. Zygapophyseal joint inflammation and the enthesopathy occurring in the annulus fibrosus at its attachment to the vertebrae determines the severity of the ascending spinal involvement and the consequent further limitation of thoracic and cervical spinal mobility.

        (iii) Axial ligamentous attachments. Costovertebral, costosternal, and intercostal tendon and ligament inflammation cause chest pain. Fixed limitation of chest expansion suggests prolonged and generalized inflammation of these attachments.

    (b) Peripheral joint involvement. Peripheral joint disease typically is a feature of more severe ankylosing spondylitis. Erosive hip and shoulder involvement is not uncommon and may be severe. More distal synovitis is less common, although 35% of patients with ankylosing spondylitis have some evidence of peripheral joint disease.

    (c) Extraskeletal features. Constitutional complaints, fatigue, and weight loss are not as common in ankylosing spondylitis as in rheumatoid arthritis but may occur. Cardiac involvement, pulmonary abnormalities, and, rarely, amyloid deposition occur in patients with long-standing, more severe disease. On the other hand, the ocular disease does not vary with the severity of the spondylitis but pursues an independent course.

        (i) Eye involvement. Episodic anterior uveitis occurs in approximately one-fourth of patients with ankylosing spondylitis. It also can occur in an association with HLA-B27 that is distinct from ankylosing spondylitis. Conjunctivitis can also occur. Ocular disease usually is self-limited and typically does not lead to visual impairment. Corticosteroids administered locally may be required for severe symptoms.

        (ii) Cardiovascular disease. Inflammation at the root of the aorta can lead to aortic valve insufficiency; the incidence of this complication increases with the duration and severity of the spondylitis. The inflammation can extend into the subaortic area, leading to complete heart block or mitral valve incompetence.

        (iii) Pulmonary disease. Upper lobe pulmonary fibrosis that can mimic tuberculosis can occur in long-standing, severe ankylosing spondylitis, and in rare cases these fibrotic lesions can become extensive. Chest wall enthesopathy can interfere with ventilation and can lead to postoperative pulmonary complications.

        (iv) Genitourinary involvement. Chronic prostatitis occurs commonly in ankylosing spondylitis; however, symptomatic urethritis is not a feature.

e. Diagnosis. The diagnosis of ankylosing spondylitis is made by blending historical, physical, and radiographic evidence as well as by excluding mechanical low back pain, other spondylarthropathies, and other inflammatory arthritides. Laboratory confirmation of HLA-B27 status rarely is needed for the diagnosis.

(1) Historical information

    (a) Inflammatory low back pain can be distinguished from mechanical low back pain. The onset of inflammatory sacroiliitis is gradual, beginning when the patient is in the teens or twenties, and the pain is persistent for more than 3 months. The pain of sacroiliitis is associated with prolonged morning back stiffness, and it is relieved by exercise and worsened by rest. In contrast, the onset of mechanical low back pain usually occurs later in life, with sudden, self-limited episodes. This type of pain is worsened by exercise and improved by bed rest.

    (b) Familial association. Patients with ankylosing spondylitis often have other affected family members.

    (c) Associated complaints. Evidence of prior inflammatory eye symptoms, recurrent oligoarthritis, and inflammatory tendinitis should be sought.

(2) Physical findings

    (a) Various maneuvers should be performed in seeking characteristic spondylitic involvement.

        (i) Sacroiliac joint tenderness. Each sacroiliac joint is evaluated for tenderness as a sign of inflammation.

        (ii) The **Schober test** is a measurement of lumbar spinal mobility. A point is made over the lumbar spine at the intersection of a line between the two posterior il-iac spines. Another point is made along the spine, 10 cm above the first one. The patient attempts to touch toes with knees locked, and the distance be-tween the two points is measured. An increase over the original 10 cm of less than 5 cm indicates limited mobility.

    (iii) Lateral spinal mobility. The spine is flexed from side to side, and limitation of motion is noted. Patients with spondylitis typically have marked limitation of mobility of both lateral flexion and anterior flexion. Patients with mechanical low back pain usually have asymmetrical limitation.

    (iv) Chest expansion. Measurement of chest expansion is a useful means of assess-ing the severity of chest wall enthesopathic lesions. Patients without chest wall involvement should be able to expand the chest more than 5 cm from full ex-piration to full inspiration.

(b) General physical examination. Evidence of associated disorders should be sought, including conjunctivitis, aortic insufficiency murmurs, and peripheral arthritis and tendinitis.

(3) Laboratory findings. The only characteristic laboratory abnormality in ankylosing spondylitis is the variable presence of HLA-B27 in different population groups, and, in general, testing for this antigen is not necessary for the diagnosis.

(4) Radiographic findings.

(a) The anteroposterior x-ray of the pelvis is the most useful radiograph in this disease. Blurred, irregular sacroiliac joint margins are typical of early involvement. Periar-ticular sclerosis of the bone, erosions, and joint space narrowing indicate active sacroiliitis. Bilateral symmetrical sacroiliac joint disease is typical in ankylosing spondylitis; only later in the course of the disease is there ascending spinal involve-ment.

(b) Ascending spinal involvement. Vertebral squaring occurs as inflammation erodes the attachment of the annulus fibrosus at the anterior vertebral corner. **Vertical syndesmophytes** occur later from calcification of these enthesopathic lesions. **Zy-gapophyseal joint fusion** occurs. These changes ascend gradually from the lumbar spine, sometimes resulting in the **bamboo spine**, a vertebral column ensheathed by flowing syndesmophytes from bottom to top.

(c) Periostitis. Periosteal new bone formation may be visible at the sites of chronic en-thesopathies. Attachment sites of the plantar fascia and the Achilles tendon are common places for this bone formation to occur.

(5) Differential diagnosis

(a) Mechanical low back pain, as previously mentioned, must be differentiated from inflammatory low back pain.

(b) Other spondylarthropathies. The presence of the skin lesions of psoriasis or Reiter's syndrome, the recurrent urethritis of Reiter's syndrome, or manifestations of inflammatory bowel disease in a patient with spondylitis is an important indica-tion of an alternative diagnosis to ankylosing spondylitis. Asymmetrical sacroiliitis or atypical, asymmetrical syndesmophytes also should suggest an alternative diagnosis.

(c) Other inflammatory arthritides. Clear-cut sacroiliitis is highly unusual in nonspon-dylitic arthritides. The absence of axial skeletal disease and the presence of a relatively symmetrical polyarthritis should suggest diagnoses other than ankylosing spondylitis.

f. Therapy. Patient education and multidisciplinary treatment are important therapeutic components in ankylosing spondylitis, as they are in rheumatoid arthritis.

(1) Goals. Short-term goals involve control of pain and reduction of inflammation without causing drug toxicity. Prevention of postural deformity and retention of employment are long-term goals.

(2) Education

(a) Cigarette smoking. Individuals with enthesopathic chest wall restriction or fibrotic lung disease should be discouraged from smoking.

(b) Genetic counseling. Patients should be made aware of the familial incidence of the illness so that it can be diagnosed early in children and treatment of spondylitic symptoms begun.

(3) Exercise. Spinal extension exercises and correct posture are important for prevention of deformity. Hard mattresses and small cervical pillows help to prevent excessive spinal flexion during sleep.

(4) Drug treatment. In contrast to rheumatoid arthritis, nonsteroidal anti-inflammatory drugs are the mainstay of treatment. Disease-modifying agents useful in rheumatoid ar-thritis are not effective in ankylosing spondylitis.

      (a) Nonsteroidal anti-inflammatory agents
        (i) Indomethacin, the drug most commonly employed in treatment, is used in the minimal dose found to control symptoms without causing unacceptable toxicity; a total daily dose of 150 mg is typical in an adult.
        (ii) Phenylbutazone is used only when all other nonsteroidal anti-inflammatory agents have been found to be ineffective.
        (iii) Aspirin usually is ineffective in the treatment of ankylosing spondylitis.
      (b) Corticosteroids
        (i) Local joint or peritendinous instillation of a corticosteroid sometimes is beneficial in patients with prominent peripheral disease manifestations that are not controlled by nonsteroidal anti-inflammatory drugs.
        (ii) Systemic glucocorticoids have no place in the treatment of ankylosing spondylitis.
    (5) Surgery. Patients with severe spondylitis who undergo surgical procedures should be screened carefully.
      (a) Cervical spinal complications. Patients with prominent cervical spinal disease lose neck extension and can be extremely difficult to intubate; a nasotracheal approach may be required. The cervical spine can fracture in these patients if excessive force is applied during intubation.
      (b) Pulmonary complications. A higher frequency of postoperative atelectasis and pneumonia can result from the impairment of normal chest wall mechanics.
  g. Complications. Several complications of long-standing spinal disease should be emphasized to preclude mismanagement.
    (1) Fractures. Minimal trauma can cause spinal fractures in patients who have bamboo spines. Increased back pain, local tenderness, and a sudden increased range of motion at the site of possible fracture should suggest the need to obtain a radiograph of the involved area.
    (2) Spondylodiskitis. Intervertebral disk lesions, possibly arising from minimal trauma, can cause local pain and erosive change of the adjoining vertebrae, simulating disk space infection. Bed rest or back bracing is appropriate symptomatic treatment for this condition.
    (3) Spinal stenosis. Symptoms of leg claudication can develop in spondylitic patients without obvious peripheral vascular disease as a result of bone encroachment on the cauda equina. Surgical intervention may be required.
  h. Prognosis. Most patients with ankylosing spondylitis remain employable and continue to function well in society. The progression to severe, deforming disease cannot be predicted on the basis of HLA-B27 status or other criteria. Patients with severe spondylitis tend to have more cardiopulmonary disease and other extraspinal complications, and these patients may have a shortened life span.

2. Reiter's syndrome
  a. Definition. Reiter's syndrome is another spondylarthropathy that is strongly associated with the histocompatibility antigen HLA-B27. Reiter's syndrome is **an eponym for seronegative reactive arthritis**; it is a predominantly lower extremity oligoarthritis triggered by urethritis, cervicitis, or dysenteric infection. The variable features of the typical syndrome include mucocutaneous lesions, inflammatory eye lesions, and sacroiliitis.
  b. Epidemiology
    (1) Incidence. Reiter's syndrome occurs in 1%–3% of patients after nonspecific urethritis and 0.2% of patients after dysentery outbreaks due to *Shigella flexneri*. The HLA-B27 antigen is present in 75%–80% of cases. Patients with the antigen who develop nonspecific urethritis or *S. flexneri* dysentery have a 20%–25% chance of developing Reiter's syndrome.
    (2) Sex distribution. Reiter's syndrome is diagnosed in men much more commonly than in women, in part because cervicitis is less symptomatic than urethritis. However, the arthritis tends to be less severe in women as well.
  c. Etiology. Specific infections trigger the clinical expression of arthritis in susceptible patients. These include both chlamydial and mycoplasmal urethritis as well as dysenteric infections caused by *Shigella*, *Salmonella*, and *Yersinia*. Conceivably, infectious antigens cross-react with self antigens and stimulate an exaggerated immune response that can include a noninfectious arthritis. The presence of the organism does not seem necessary for later exacerbations or chronic activity of the clinical manifestations. The HLA-B27 antigen may be a marker for an involved immune response gene, or the antigen itself may cross-react with a foreign antigen to induce disease.
  d. Clinical features
    (1) Disease onset. Reiter's syndrome begins most often in young adulthood. One to three

weeks after an episode of urethritis or dysentery, any of the typical clinical features of the syndrome can occur. The disease often is misdiagnosed because these features tend to occur serially rather than simultaneously.

(2) Manifestations of disease

(a) Musculoskeletal

(i) Arthritis. A lower extremity oligoarthritis is the most common joint presentation. The arthritis may be acute and self-limited, but it is more commonly relapsing or chronic.

(ii) Enthesopathy. Inflammation of the tendons and ligaments are as much a part of Reiter's syndrome as they are of ankylosing spondylitis. Plantar fasciitis and Achilles tendinitis are most typical. **Dactylitis** (sausage toe), a lesion involving both joint and tendon inflammation in the same digit, also is a common feature of Reiter's syndrome.

(iii) Sacroiliitis. Asymmetrical involvement of sacroiliac joints occurs in about 20% of patients with Reiter's syndrome. Less frequently, asymmetrical ascending spinal disease occurs. The consequent back pain has typical inflammatory characteristics, but only rarely does the ascending spinal disease limit thoracic or cervical spinal mobility.

(b) Genitourinary. Symptomatic or asymptomatic urethritis is extremely common in patients with Reiter's disease. Chronic prostatitis also is common, affecting as many as 80% of patients in some series.

(c) Ocular. Both conjunctivitis and anterior uveitis are common features. The conjunctival inflammation is an acute, usually self-limited manifestation, which may be recurrent. Anterior uveitis occurs in more established forms of disease; it may be chronic and require topical or systemic corticosteroids to prevent visual deterioration.

(d) Mucocutaneous. Fleeting and painless oral ulcers are the typical mucous membrane features of Reiter's syndrome. **Keratoderma blennorrhagica** is the characteristic scaling, plaque-like lesion found anywhere on the body, including the palms and soles. This lesion resembles psoriasis clinically and pathologically. **Circinate balanitis** is a painless, erythematous erosion of the glans penis that may expand to surround the urethral orifice. Each of these skin lesions occurs in about 20%–30% of patients with Reiter's syndrome, although circinate balanitis is the most common.

(e) Cardiovascular. Early cardiovascular changes in Reiter's syndrome include transient pericardial rubs or first-degree heart block. In more severe, long-standing disease, an aortitis identical to that seen in ankylosing spondylitis can cause valvular insufficiency or conduction system lesions.

e. Diagnosis

(1) General considerations. Reiter's syndrome can be difficult to diagnose when the onset of various clinical features is widely separated over time, but it is quite easy if arthritis, urethritis, conjunctivitis, and mucocutaneous lesions appear simultaneously. A tentative diagnosis can be made when a seronegative asymmetrical, oligoarthritis is associated with any of these extra-articular features. Since Reiter's syndrome is strictly speaking, a **reactive arthritis**, the temporal appearance of arthritis after urethritis or a dysenteric illness is especially convincing. Since the mucocutaneous lesions, urethritis, and cervicitis often are asymptomatic, they must be sought specifically while taking the patient history and during the physical examination.

(2) Laboratory findings. Eighty percent of whites with Reiter's syndrome have the HLA-B27 antigen. The synovial fluid typically is mildly to moderately inflammatory, with neutrophil predominance and no particular distinguishing characteristics.

(3) Radiographic findings. Asymmetrical, oligoarticular erosions, joint space narrowing, and periarticular osteopenia can be seen radiographically in established disease. Periosteal new bone formation is a characteristic feature of Reiter's syndrome, especially adjacent to the insertions of the Achilles tendon and plantar fascia. Sacroiliitis, if it occurs, typically is asymmetrical, and the occasional patient with spondylarthropathy has asymmetrical, large syndesmophytes at scattered vertebrae levels.

(4) Differential diagnosis

(a) Diseases most likely to mimic acute Reiter's syndrome are gonococcal arthritis and other infectious arthropathies, even Lyme disease. Thus, appropriate tissues should be cultured and serologies taken. Crystal-mediated arthritis (i.e., gout and pseudogout) and the arthritis of rheumatic fever should be excluded.

(b) Diseases most likely to mimic chronic recurring Reiter's syndrome include other spondylarthropathies, especially psoriatic arthritis, or ankylosing spondylitis. Close attention to the symmetry and severity of sacroiliac and spinal involvement, to extraskeletal features, and to the presence or absence of reactive features may help to differentiate these illnesses. Many cases of so-called "seronegative rheumatoid arthritis" may actually be cases of Reiter's syndrome. Typical clinical features as well as radiographic evidence of sacroiliac joint and periostitic involvement should be sought. The presence or absence of the HLA-B27 antigen may be helpful in diagnosing particularly difficult cases.

f. Therapy
   (1) Goals of treatment are essentially the same as in ankylosing spondylitis [see section IV B 1 f (1)].
   (2) Exercise. Patients should be instructed in exercises that will allow preservation of joint function and prevention of contractures. Extension exercises for preservation of spinal mobility are important in patients with spinal involvement.
   (3) Drug treatment
      (a) Nonsteroidal anti-inflammatory drugs are the mainstay of treatment of Reiter's syndrome. Indomethacin is the drug of choice because aspirin is relatively ineffective in this illness.
      (b) Corticosteroids. Occasional intra-articular instillation may be useful in the management of particular joints that do not respond to treatment with nonsteroidal anti-inflammatory drugs.
      (c) Disease-modifying antirheumatic drugs. Both azathioprine and methotrexate have been used to control particularly severe and chronic disease, although their effects on disease course are not yet known.
      (d) Antibiotics. The disease course of Reiter's syndrome apparently is not altered by the treatment of urethritis or dysentery by antibiotics.

g. Prognosis. Chronic or recurrent disease appears to be common. In 60%–80% of patients with Reiter's syndrome, skeletal or extraskeletal complaints or both recur or become chronic. Neither sex nor the HLA-B27 status appears to affect outcome. Perhaps as many as 25% of patients with Reiter's syndrome are functionally disabled by their illness. Long-term problems with aortic regurgitation and conduction disturbances are unusual but increase with the duration of the disease.

3. Psoriatic arthritis
  a. Definition. Any form of **inflammatory arthritis associated with psoriasis** is called psoriatic arthritis. Rheumatoid factor generally is absent.
  b. Epidemiology
   (1) Psoriatic arthritis occurs much more commonly in patients who have a first-degree relative with the disorder.
   (2) Psoriasis occurs two to three times more commonly in patients with arthritis than in the normal population. Conversely, as many as 10%–20% of patients with psoriasis may have an inflammatory arthritis.
  c. Etiology. Although a hereditary etiology is apparent in psoriatic arthritis, its characteristics are not fully understood. The histocompatibility antigen HLA-B27 is highly associated with sacroiliitis in psoriatics, and HLA-B27, -B13, and -DR7 are independently associated with arthritis and psoriasis at an increased frequency. Unknown environmental factors also may be important in disease expression.
  d. Clinical features
   (1) Disease onset. Most patients with psoriatic arthritis develop the disease in their late thirties to early forties. Most patients develop skin lesions before the arthritis, but as many as 16% develop inflammatory arthritis before the psoriasis.
   (2) Patterns of arthritis. Five patterns of psoriatic arthropathy have been distinguished, although the typical patient often has the skeletal manifestations of several of these patterns. Peripheral joint and tendon involvement may be more severe in the upper than in the lower extremities.
      (a) Distal interphalangeal joint arthritis is the classic form of psoriatic arthritis. It is strongly associated with typical fingernail abnormalities as well as distal interphalangeal joint redness, soft tissue swelling, and erosive changes seen radiographically in a clinical picture resembling primary erosive osteoarthritis.
      (b) Asymmetrical oligoarthritis. Large and small joint oligoarthritis is another clinical form of psoriatic arthritis. Sausage digits are common in this form as a manifestation of joint and enthesis involvement of a single phalanx.
      (c) Symmetrical polyarthropathy. A fairly symmetrical polyarthropathy can occur in conjunction with psoriasis, and it can be difficult to distinguish from rheumatoid arthritis. As many as 25% of these patients may be seropositive for rheumatoid factor.
      (d) Arthritis mutilans is an unusually destructive form of psoriatic arthritis because of the severe periarticular bone resorption that occurs in the small finger joints. "Tele-

scoping digits" characterize the end stage of this uncommon form of arthritis. Widespread joint ankylosis also can occur.

(e) **Sacroiliitis.** As many as 20% of patients with psoriatic arthritis can have clinical or radiographic evidence of sacroiliitis, usually asymmetrical. Ascending spinal syndesmophytes occur in an asymmetrical and patchy fashion.

(3) Extra-articular features

(a) **Skin.** Arthritis is more likely to occur in patients with severe skin involvement than in those with mild psoriasis, although it can occur in the presence of localized cutaneous lesions. In most patients, the disease processes of the skin and joint involvement are independent of one another.

(b) **Nails.** Nail abnormalities most commonly occur in conjunction with distal interphalangeal joint lesions; however, nail changes are noted more frequently in all of the peripheral forms of psoriatic arthritis in comparison to psoriasis uncomplicated by arthritis. Multiple pitting, transverse depressions, and onycholysis are the characteristic abnormalities found.

(c) The only other **extra-articular features** that occur commonly in patients with psoriatic arthritis are conjunctivitis (in 20% of cases) and anterior uveitis (in 10% of cases).

e. Diagnosis

(1) General considerations. An association should be made between the typical skin and nail lesions and the joint and spinal involvement to diagnose psoriatic arthritis. The skin manifestations may be subtle, so particular care must be taken to check the elbows, scalp, groin, navel, and buttock cleft.

(2) Laboratory findings. Laboratory indicators of chronic disease such as anemia and thrombocytosis typically are not present. Patients usually are seronegative for rheumatoid factor, although 25% of the patients with symmetrical polyarthritis are seropositive.

(3) Radiographic findings

(a) **Distal interphalangeal joint erosions** can lead to joint space widening, and proximal phalangeal bone resorption can lead to a "pencil-in-cup" abnormality seen in arthritis mutilans. This severe destruction also can occur in more proximal joints.

(b) **Spinal involvement.** Asymmetrical sacroiliitis and asymmetrical patchy syndesmophytes are seen and are similar to those seen in Reiter's syndrome.

(c) **Enthesopathy.** Calcifications at tendon and ligament insertions occur.

(4) Differential diagnosis

(a) **Reiter's syndrome** is distinguished from psoriatic arthritis by its characteristic extra-articular features and its tendency to involve the lower extremities more than the upper extremities. In psoriatic arthritis, upper extremity peripheral joint involvement may be more common.

(b) **Rheumatoid arthritis.** A presentation of symmetrical polyarthritis, seropositivity for rheumatoid factor, and rheumatoid nodules in a patient with psoriasis may be diagnosed as rheumatoid arthritis. Other overlapping presentations of the two diseases may be difficult to diagnose as being one or the other.

f. Therapy. Drug treatment for psoriatic arthritis differs from that of the other spondylarthropathies in that gold often is administered intramuscularly to treat sustained manifestations of peripheral arthritis. D-Penicillamine and hydroxychloroquine have also been used, but reports of exfoliative dermatitis due to treatment with hydroxychloroquine mandate particular caution with its use. Use of methotrexate has been particularly successful in controlling both the skin disease and refractory arthritis, and other cytotoxic drugs (e.g., azathioprine) also have been used in treatment of severe skin and joint disease.

g. Prognosis. Most patients with psoriatic arthritis are able to avoid significant deformity and remain employed. The 5% or so who develop arthritis mutilans obviously are exceptions.

4. Enteropathic arthropathies

a. Definition. Inflammatory arthritis associated with either Crohn's disease or ulcerative colitis is typified by a seronegative, migratory polyarticular involvement, which waxes and wanes with the activity of the bowel disease. Sacroiliitis and spondylitis can also occur in affected individuals.

b. Clinical syndromes

(1) Peripheral arthritis. In 10%–20% of patients with severe ulcerative colitis or Crohn's disease—usually those with other extra-intestinal manifestations—a predominantly lower extremity arthritis occurs in association with flare-ups of bowel disease. The arthritis often occurs abruptly and usually remits completely within weeks. There is no association with the histocompatibility antigen HLA-B27 in this peripheral arthritis. Treatment is directed at control of the bowel disease, although nonsteroidal anti-inflammatory drugs or local or systemic corticosteroids may help to control the articular complaints.

      (2) **Spondylitis.** The spondylitis of inflammatory bowel disease is associated with the histocompatibility antigen HLA-B27 in about 50% of patients. The radiographic findings are typical of those found in primary ankylosing spondylitis (i.e., symmetrical sacroiliac joint changes and, less commonly, ascending symmetrical spondylitis without skin lesions). Approximately 5% of patients with inflammatory bowel disease develop sacroiliitis or spondylitis, but the activity of these lesions and that of the bowel disease are independent of one another. Nonsteroidal anti-inflammatory drugs usually are effective in controlling symptoms but occasionally can cause increased bowel complaints.

   c. **Differential diagnosis. Whipple's disease** can be confused with enteropathic arthropathies since most patients manifest prominent bowel and joint complaints. In fact, sacroiliitis occurs in about 20% of cases. However, Whipple's disease is quite rare and most commonly presents in middle-aged men with weight loss, skin hyperpigmentation, lymphadenopathy, fever, and symptoms of malabsorption. When suspected, a jejunal biopsy should be performed, and the tissue should be treated with periodic acid-Schiff stain to ascertain the presence of bacteria-like inclusions in macrophages. This disease is treated with long-term antibiotics rather than nonsteroidal anti-inflammatory agents.

V. JUVENILE RHEUMATOID ARTHRITIS

  A. Definition. Juvenile rheumatoid arthritis is a chronic inflammatory arthritis that begins in childhood. Prior to considering a diagnosis of juvenile rheumatoid arthritis, arthritis should be present in one or more joints for more than 6 weeks, and other rheumatic diseases should be excluded.

  B. Epidemiology. The incidence of juvenile rheumatoid arthritis may be as high as 0.01% of children annually. Although the apparent HLA associations would suggest that the altered immune responses are genetically transferable, familial aggregation of cases is uncommon.

  C. Etiology and pathogenesis. The same factors important in the development of adult rheumatoid arthritis also apply to juvenile rheumatoid arthritis. Etiologic factors are unknown but may include **infectious agents. Immune system dysfunction** is apparent in the prolongation and maintenance of synovitis. A subset of patients with juvenile rheumatoid arthritis have immunodeficiency states (e.g., agammaglobulinemia or IgA deficiency), which may be important in disease pathogenesis. **HLA associations** may be important in the pauciarticular forms of arthritis.

  D. Pathology. The synovial lesions cannot be distinguished histologically from those in adult rheumatoid arthritis. The inflammatory lesion can involve the growing epiphysis, however, and can result in involved bones that are longer or shorter than normal. Chronically involved joints exhibit fibrous ankylosis more often than in adult rheumatoid arthritis. Pannus formation can occur, although typically later in the disease course than in adults with rheumatoid arthritis. As a consequence, destructive joint disease also is much less common in juvenile rheumatoid arthritis.

  E. Classification. Three primary subtypes of juvenile rheumatoid arthritis (i.e., **systemic-onset juvenile rheumatoid arthritis**, **pauciarticular arthritis**, and **polyarticular arthritis**) can be distinguished in the first 6 months of illness. Making distinctions between subtypes of illness appears to be important prognostically and therapeutically. Important classification features are the **presence or absence of prominent systemic features** and the **total number of involved joints**. The cervical spine, wrist, and ankle articulations are counted as one joint each for classification purposes; all other joints are counted separately.

  1. Systemic-onset juvenile rheumatoid arthritis, also called **Still's disease**, occurs in approximately 10%–20% of the patients and is characterized by an early pattern of prominent systemic complaints and extra-articular involvement. Boys are affected as commonly as girls, and a peak age of incidence is not evident.

    a. Clinical features

      (1) Typical features of the early disease course are high spiking fevers and marked constitutional complaints. Overt arthritis may not be part of the early course but develops within weeks to months of the onset of illness. A characteristic nonpruritic, fleeting, maculopapular rash occurs in 90% of patients and may be most apparent with fever spikes.

      (2) Common features of active disease include lymphadenopathy, hepatosplenomegaly, and pleuropericarditis.

      (3) The most serious manifestation of systemic-onset juvenile rheumatoid arthritis is myocarditis, sometimes progressing to overt congestive heart failure.

b. **Laboratory findings**
   (1) **Hematologic findings** include a strikingly elevated erythrocyte sedimentation rate, prominent leukocytosis and thrombocytosis, and mild-to-moderate anemia of chronic disease.
   (2) **Serologic findings** only rarely include rheumatoid factor and antinuclear antibodies.
c. **Disease course.** Disease flare-ups are punctuated by relatively symptom-free intervals. Polyarticular arthritis becomes evident at some point in the first 6 months of illness, although some children may have only myalgia and arthralgia at disease onset.
   (1) Approximately 50% of these patients may begin to develop symptoms of disease that resemble the polyarticular arthritis subset, with progressive joint involvement determining disease outcome and systemic features becoming less evident over time.
   (2) The remaining 50% of the patients eventually recover completely.

2. **Polyarticular arthritis** occurs in approximately 30%–40% of patients and involves five or more joints in the first 6 months of illness. Systemic features usually do not dominate the early course of disease. Girls are affected much more often than boys. Polyarticular arthritis can be further separated into **rheumatoid factor–positive** or **–negative** subsets. Patients who are seropositive for rheumatoid factor present most often in late childhood; a peak age of incidence is not evident for patients who are seronegative for rheumatoid factor.
   a. **Clinical features**
      (1) Typically, inflammatory polyarticular arthritis may have an acute or a gradual onset similar to the presentation of adult rheumatoid arthritis. Symmetrical large and small joint involvement also is typical. Prominent features may include cervical spine, sacroiliac joint, and temporomandibular joint disease.
      (2) Occasionally, patients have symptoms and signs of anterior uveitis typical of that seen in spondylarthropathies.
      (3) Patients who are seropositive for rheumatoid factor can have subcutaneous nodules as in adult-onset rheumatoid arthritis.
   b. **Laboratory findings**
      (1) **Hematologic findings** frequently include moderate elevation of erythrocyte sedimentation rate, leukocyte count, and platelet count. Patients usually develop a mild normochromic normocytic anemia of chronic disease.
      (2) **Serologic findings** include rheumatoid factor in 10%–20% and antinuclear antibodies in 20%–40% of patients.
   c. **Disease course.** Polyarticular arthritis can be chronic and persistent or can pursue a more intermittent, relapsing course.
      (1) Patients with polyarticular arthritis who are seropositive for rheumatoid factor are at greatest risk for chronic, erosive, and severe arthritis and significant disability. These patients have disease that is very similar to adult-onset rheumatoid arthritis.
      (2) Patients who are seronegative for rheumatoid factor less often have severe disease or disease that lasts into adulthood.
      (3) A subset of patients with spondylitic presentations may be distinguishable over long-term follow-up.

3. **Pauciarticular arthritis** occurs in about 50% of the patients and involves four or fewer joints in the first 6 months of illness. This patient group is composed of two subsets.
   a. **Oligoarthritis and anterior uveitis** affect girls more often than boys, and peak incidence is in early childhood.
      (1) **Clinical features**
         (a) Typically, the arthritis is asymmetrical, mild, and involves the knee. Other peripheral joints also can be involved, but the axial skeleton usually is spared.
         (b) Systemic symptoms and signs are mild or absent.
         (c) Potentially serious anterior uveitis unrelated to arthritis activity can develop in 20%–40% of patients. This usually chronic eye lesion can be asymptomatic and can lead to blindness if unrecognized or inadequately treated.
      (2) **Laboratory findings**
         (a) **Hematologic findings** usually do not include anemia, thrombocytosis, and leukocytosis. The erythrocyte sedimentation rate is normal or only minimally elevated.
         (b) **Serologic findings** include antinuclear antibody positivity in 60% of these patients, which seems to be a good marker for those at risk for chronic uveitis. Rheumatoid factor typically is not present. Associations with HLA-DR5, -DR6, and -DR8 antigens may be important in this subset.
      (3) **Disease course.** Most patients have pauciarticular involvement that is manageable and not disabling. In approximately one-third of the patients, the disease evolves into a more polyarticular form.
   b. **Axial skeletal oligoarthritis** predominantly affects boys, with disease onset usually beginning in late childhood.

(1) **Clinical features.** The sacroiliac joints are most often involved, but asymmetrical hip or knee arthritis also can occur. Acute anterior uveitis can occur as in adult spondylar-thropathies, but this feature is not the chronic and sight-threatening form seen in the other pauciarticular subset.

(2) **Laboratory findings**

(a) **Hematologic findings** are not distinct in this subset.

(b) **Serologic findings** indicate that 50% of these patients have the HLA-B27 antigen, but few have rheumatoid factor.

(3) **Disease course.** Most of these patients develop features of ankylosing spondylitis, psoriatic arthritis, or Reiter's syndrome in later life.

F. Diagnosis

1. **Difficulties in diagnosis.** Diagnosing arthritis in a child may be difficult. Children may avoid using a painful joint instead of complaining of pain. Irritability, regressive behavior, or emotional withdrawal may be the child's response to the pain of an inflamed joint. Once joint involvement has been discovered, disease should be present for at least 6 weeks before a diagnosis of juvenile rheumatoid arthritis is seriously considered. Within the first 6 months, an attempt should be made to classify the patient into a clinical subset. Synovial fluid and radiographic findings may be useful in classifying patients.

   a. **Synovial fluid findings.** In juvenile rheumatoid arthritis, the synovial fluid usually is mildly inflammatory (i.e., a white blood cell count of 10,000–20,000/mm³); however, the number of white blood cells present may not parallel disease activity. Joint fluid culture and analysis are especially important in pauciarticular forms to exclude infection (bacterial or mycobacterial) or hemorrhage (e.g., due to trauma or hemophilia).

   b. **Radiographic findings.** Radiographic abnormalities are nonspecific.

      (1) **Early findings** may include only soft tissue swelling, periarticular demineralization, or periosteal bone proliferation in early stages.

      (2) **Late findings** include epiphyseal changes (either premature closure or overgrowth, depending on epiphyseal activity at the time of involvement) and articular erosion or joint space narrowing.

      (3) Distinctive long bone periosteal elevation in leukemia may allow differentiation from juvenile rheumatoid arthritis, and localized joint abnormalities (e.g., osteonecrosis or osteochondritis) may have distinct radiographic presentations.

2. **Differential diagnosis**

   a. A variety of genetic or inborn metabolic disorders, as well as nonrheumatic conditions, can superficially resemble juvenile rheumatoid arthritis. It is specifically important to rule out infectious etiologies (e.g., Lyme disease and tuberculosis) and malignancies (e.g., leukemia) as causes of childhood arthritis.

   b. Other rheumatic diseases (e.g., rheumatic fever, SLE , and spondylarthropathies) may require a period of observation for characteristic extra-articular features to evolve.

G. Therapeutic approach

1. **Education** of patients and parents about inflammatory arthritis is important, and the generally favorable course of juvenile rheumatoid arthritis should be emphasized. **Long-term goals** of suppression of disease activity and prevention of deformity should be instituted, and the child's psychological and emotional development should not be neglected.

2. **Therapy.** The use of appropriate therapy is important in relieving pain and maintaining function. Parents should be urged to perform active roles in giving physical therapy and medications, encouraging school attendance, and maintaining the child's ability to be self-sufficient.

   a. **Drug therapy**

      (1) **Salicylates** are the primary drug used in treating juvenile rheumatoid arthritis. **Aspirin** is the most commonly used salicylate, but **nonacetylated versions can be used** in children with bleeding problems or gastrointestinal toxicity. Synovitis can be controlled with anti-inflammatory doses in 75% of patients, although the onset of response can be gradual. Fever, constitutional complaints, and pleuropericardial symptoms in patients with systemic-onset disease usually are treated with salicylates in full anti-inflammatory doses.

         (a) **Administration.** Children weighing less than 25 kg should receive 80–120 mg/kg body weight/day of salicylates in 4–6 divided doses, beginning at the lower end of the dosage range. Children weighing 25 kg or more can take adult doses (i.e., 8–12 adult aspirin/day). Therapeutic serum levels are 20–30 mg/dl.

         (b) **Toxicity.** The major hazard of chronic salicylate treatment in children is overdosage, manifested by respiratory depression or stimulation or CNS depression.

Children usually do not complain of tinnitus or hearing loss, so these warning symptoms are not helpful in avoiding over-dosage.

   (i) **Reye's syndrome** is a potential problem in children on salicylates and must be discussed with parents of children taking these drugs.

   (ii) Nausea or other symptoms of gastrointestinal toxicity and platelet dysfunction are well-known side effects of these agents.

   (iii) Asymptomatic elevation in hepatic enzyme levels can occur but are typically reversible and nonprogressive. Liver function tests should be performed prior to and at regular intervals during therapy with these agents.

(2) **Other nonsteroidal anti-inflammatory agents.** Tolmetin and naproxen are approved for use in children with juvenile rheumatoid arthritis and may be indicated for patients who do not respond to salicylates or who develop toxicity.

(3) **Gold compounds.** Patients with chronically active, progressive disease that is not responsive to salicylate treatment may need a disease-modifying agent such as gold. Many of these patients have a polyarticular syndrome and are seropositive for rheumatoid factor. Details of administration and drug toxicity are the same as in adult rheumatoid arthritis [see section III H 3 a (5) (b)], but dosages are much reduced in children weighing less than 50 kg.

(4) **Corticosteroids.** Systemic corticosteroids are used infrequently in the treatment of juvenile rheumatoid arthritis; however, certain conditions may warrant the use of topical or local corticosteroids.

   (a) In patients with systemic complaints who do not respond to salicylates or who have life-threatening manifestations (e.g., myocarditis), systemic corticosteroids may be required.

   (b) Local corticosteroid injections are used occasionally, especially in oligoarticular disease, but systemic corticosteroids are not used to control synovitis.

   (c) In the treatment of chronic uveitis, systemic corticosteroids may be needed if initial treatment with topical or local corticosteroids and dilating agents is not effective. Patients at high risk for chronic uveitis (oligoarticular subgroup) should be evaluated every 3 months to determine treatment effectiveness.

(5) **Other drugs.** Other disease-modifying agents (e.g., hydroxychloroquine and D-penicillamine) have been used in the treatment of juvenile rheumatoid arthritis, but experience with these agents is limited.

   b. **Surgery.** Patients who most clearly benefit from early orthopedic intervention are those with chronic monoarticular or oligoarticular arthritis, in which a single synovectomy may be very helpful in controlling disease activity. Correction of deformities and total joint replacements may be needed in chronic, severe disease.

   c. **Physical and occupational therapy** are especially important in treating patients with juvenile rheumatoid arthritis. Children must learn and perform exercises that will maintain muscle tone and prevent joint contractures. Temporary splinting may be useful for the control of active synovitis, and serial splinting may improve joint contractures.

H. Prognosis

1. **Disability.** Approximately 75% of patients recover completely by adulthood. About 10% develop severe functional deformities.

2. **Specific complications**

   a. **Joint deformities.** Patients with polyarticular arthritis are most likely to develop joint deformities, especially patients with rheumatoid factor who resemble patients with adult rheumatoid arthritis.

   b. **Chronic uveitis.** As many as 50% of patients with oligoarticular disease who have chronic uveitis develop blindness in the involved eye, even if the problem is carefully treated.

   c. **Growth retardation**

      (1) **General growth retardation** can occur in patients with persistent, widespread inflammatory activity and in those treated with systemic corticosteroids.

      (2) **Local growth abnormalities** from the inflammatory process can lead to micrognathia as well as to leg and finger length discrepancies in some patients.

3. **Death.** In rare cases, patients with particularly severe and protracted disease develop progressive amyloidosis or die of secondary infection. Rarely, overwhelming myocarditis in systemic-onset juvenile rheumatoid arthritis can lead to congestive heart failure and death.

VI. SYSTEMIC LUPUS ERYTHEMATOSUS

A. Definition. Systemic lupus erythematosus (SLE) is a chronic immune disorder characterized by multisystem involvement and clinical exacerbations and remissions. Circulating immune complexes and autoantibodies cause tissue damage and organ dysfunction. Manifestations involving the skin, serosal surfaces, CNS, kidneys, and blood cells are particularly characteristic. Evidence for the autoimmune nature of this disorder lies in the laboratory finding of antibodies to nuclear antigens, the demonstration of immune complexes in tissues, and the utilization of complement.

B. Epidemiology

  1. The prevalence of SLE in **young women** of childbearing age is approximately eight to ten times that in men. Black women are affected approximately three times as often as white women.

  2. The frequency of occurrence of lupus is much higher in the relatives of affected individuals than in the general population, and the disease concordance rate in identical twins approaches 50%.

C. Etiology. No single cause of lupus has been discovered. Complex interrelationships among environmental factors, genetically determined host immune responses, and hormonal influences probably are critical in the initiation as well as the expression of the disease.

  1. Environmental factors. Viruses and drugs or toxins have been pursued as causative agents, but neither has been shown to cause idiopathic SLE. Viral agents might trigger changes in lymphocyte interactions that would allow disease expression (e.g., interference with suppressor T-cell or helper T-cell effects on B-cell regulation).

  2. Genetic factors. Family studies of SLE indicate a genetic component to the disease, evident in the concordance rate in monozygotic twins (50%). The disease occurs commonly in families with hereditary deficiencies of early complement components. Histocompatibility antigens **HLA-DR2** and **HLA-DR3** are present much more commonly in SLE patients than in controls.

  3. Autoimmunity. Loss of tolerance to autoantigens is central to the pathogenesis of SLE, and genetic tendencies toward the development of autoantibodies, B-cell hyperreactivity, and T-cell dysfunction are evident in patients with the disease.

  4. Hormonal influences. Lupus is predominantly a disease of women of childbearing age, but hormonal factors probably are more important in modulation of the expression of disease than in causation.

D. Pathogenesis. All of the clinical features of SLE are manifestations of cellular and humoral immune dysfunction.

  1. Immune complexes. Circulating antigen-antibody (immune) complexes are deposited in blood vessels and the renal glomerulus, initiating a pathologic response that damages these tissues. These complexes are characteristic features of active disease, and their size, solubility, concentration, and complement-fixing properties as well as vessel hydrostatic forces are important in determining tissue deposition.

  2. Reticuloendothelial dysfunction. The chronic circulation of immune complexes seems to be important in their pathogenicity, as occurs in a chronic serum sickness reaction (see Chapter 7, section II C). Conceivably, the ability of the reticuloendothelial system to remove immune complexes from the circulation may be overwhelmed.

  3. Autoantibodies produced to the host's own antigens can cause:
    a. Tissue damage (antibodies to red blood cells or platelets can cause immune cytopenias)
    b. Cellular dysfunction (antibodies to lymphocytes can impair interaction between T cells and B cells)
    c. Immune complex formation (complexes of antibodies and double-stranded DNA are important in mediation of autoimmune renal disease)

  4. Lymphocyte dysfunction. B-cell hyperreactivity, impaired suppressor T-cell function, and augmented helper T-cell activity are present in various combinations in lupus patients, leading to autoantibody production and increased generation of immune complexes.

E. Pathology

  1. Microscopic changes
    a. Hematoxylin bodies. Amorphous masses of nuclear material can be found in connective tissue lesions that become purple-blue when stained with hematoxylin. Neutrophils that ingest these bodies in vitro are called **LE cells.**
    b. Fibrinoid necrosis. In SLE, immune complexes of DNA, antibody to DNA, and comple-

ment may stain with eosin (which can stain immune complexes as well as fibrin) in vessel walls and connective tissue, demonstrating so-called "fibrinoid necrosis."
    c. **Onion skin lesions.** Lesions characteristic of SLE in splenic arteries are called onion skin lesions because of the concentric deposition of collagen around them.

  2. **Tissue changes**
    a. **Skin.** Although some of the milder skin lesions in SLE have only nonspecific lymphocytic infiltration in perivascular locations in the dermis, more typical lupus lesions show dermo-epidermal junction deposits of immunoglobulins and complement as well as necrosis. Classic **discoid lesions** show follicular plugging, hyperkeratosis, and the loss of skin appendages. Frank vasculitic lesions also can occur in small dermal vessels.
    b. **Kidney.** Immune complex deposition in the kidney can lead to various histologic pictures of inflammation. Mesangial disease and **minimal change disease** (lipoid nephrosis) are milder forms of renal involvement, but focal or diffuse proliferative glomerulonephritis and membranous glomerulonephritis are common. Interstitial damage can occur in all of these forms.
    c. **CNS.** Large vessel vasculitic lesions can occur (although they are uncommon) in focal presentations of the disease, but focal areas of bland vascular occlusion or microhemorrhages are more typical and do not correlate well with the clinical features.
    d. **Vasculitis.** Inflammatory lesions of capillaries and small arteries due to immune complex deposition and variable cellular infiltration occur and are responsible for much of the tissue destruction and damage seen in SLE.
    e. **Other tissue lesions.** Nonspecific mild synovitis and lymphocytic infiltration of muscles occur frequently. **Nonbacterial endocarditis** often is present but clinically is asymptomatic.

F. Clinical features
  1. **Manifestations of disease. Fatigue, weight loss,** and **fever** are prominent systemic complaints in this disease.
    a. **Skin.** The butterfly rash (i.e., facial erythema over the cheeks and nose) and the chronic, potentially scarring, discoid lesions (i.e., coin-shaped lesions with hyperemic margins, central atrophy, and depigmentation) are the most classic. Less commonly, bullous and maculopapular eruptions can occur, and nonscarring, psoriasiform lesions (subacute cutaneous lupus) have recently been described. Recurrent mucous membrane ulceration, generalized or focal alopecia, digital vasculitis, and photosensitivity also are potential dermatologic features of SLE.
    b. **Nerve**
      (1) **CNS.** Focal or diffuse neurologic disorders occur in approximately 50% of patients. Generalized manifestations include reactive depressions, psychoses, cognitive disturbances, and seizures. Focal seizures also have been described, and hemipareses, cranial nerve deficits, transverse myelitis, and movement disorders may pinpoint discrete areas of involvement. Diagnostic tests [e.g., lumbar puncture, electroencephalography, and computed tomography (CT)] often are unrevealing. Even severe neurologic findings may improve spontaneously, and although corticosteroids often are used to treat CNS manifestations, their efficacy remains unproven.
      (2) **Peripheral nervous system.** Some patients have sensory or sensorimotor neuropathies, and those with more generalized larger vessel vasculitis may manifest mononeuritis multiplex.
    c. **Heart.** Symptomatic pericarditis occurs in approximately 20% of SLE patients and pericardial effusions on echocardiography in as many as 50%, but tamponade is uncommon. Myocarditis (conduction abnormalities, arrhythmias, and congestive heart failure) is much less common. Although coronary vessel vasculitis can occur in fulminant cases, premature atherosclerosis in steroid-treated patients is a more common cause of myocardial infarction in lupus patients. The nonbacterial endocardial lesions (Libman-Sacks endocarditis) rarely cause clinical features unless they become secondarily infected.
    d. **Lung.** At some time in the disease course, approximately 30% of SLE patients have symptomatic pleuritis and fewer have friction rubs or actual effusions apparent upon ultrasonography. Parenchymal involvement (lupus pneumonitis) can be difficult to distinguish from acute infections, although pulmonary infiltrates may be bilateral, fleeting, and associated with hemoptysis rather than purulent sputum. Diffuse interstitial lung disease is recognized, albeit uncommonly. Pulmonary hypertension due to isolated pulmonary vascular involvement also occurs.
    e. **Gastrointestinal tract.** Although symptoms of nausea, vomiting, and abdominal pain are common, diagnostic testing often is unrevealing. Overt intestinal vasculitis can lead to bowel infarction, perforation, and hemorrhage. Corticosteroid-related pancreatitis and reversible nonsteroidal anti-inflammatory agent–induced hepatitis occur as well.

    f. Kidney. About 50% of lupus patients manifest some form of renal involvement. The most severe form, **diffuse proliferative glomerulonephritis**, often is associated with progressive renal insufficiency, and therapy involves chronic immunosuppressive treatment with corticosteroids and cytotoxic agents. **Membranous glomerulonephritis** can lead to nephrotic syndrome and slowly progressive abnormalities of renal function. Renal biopsy may be useful for treatment decisions and the determination of prognosis.

    g. Muscle and bone. Arthralgia and symmetrical arthritis often are features of acute SLE, but the rare joint deformities that occur are a function of tendon or ligament involvement rather than that of erosive joint disease. Inflammatory muscle involvement usually is subclinical, but clinical inflammatory myopathy can occur.

    h. Other. Photosensitivity can trigger systemic symptoms as well as skin manifestations. Raynaud's phenomenon and secondary Sjögren's syndrome each occur in about 25% of patients.

2. Precipitants of disease activity. Disease exacerbations often can be related to recent viral or bacterial infections, emotional stress, surgery, or exposure to ultraviolet light. Sulfonamides and oral contraceptives may worsen disease in susceptible individuals. Patients with active disease may notice their symptoms worsening during pregnancy and in the postpartum period.

3. Lupus-related syndromes

    a. Mixed connective tissue disease. A syndrome of high titer antibody to ribonucleoprotein (RNP) in patients with clinical features of several connective tissue diseases has been called mixed connective tissue disease. Patients with this disease may have cutaneous features of SLE, dermatomyositis, or systemic sclerosis; inflammatory muscle disease; and a destructive form of arthritis more typical of rheumatoid arthritis. Furthermore, the severe renal and CNS manifestations of SLE usually are not present. When followed for prolonged periods of time, most of these disorders develop into systemic sclerosis or SLE.

    b. Drug-induced lupus. Chronic ingestion of several drugs can precipitate a syndrome of polyserositis and antihistone antinuclear antibodies called drug-induced lupus. Dermal, renal, and CNS diseases are uncommon in this syndrome, which resolves upon discontinuation of the drug. Hepatic acetylation of drugs such as hydralazine, isoniazid, and procainamide is apparently slow in patients who develop this syndrome, although these drugs typically are tolerated well by patients with SLE.

    c. Neonatal lupus syndrome. Infants of mothers who have high-titer IgG antibodies to Ro (SS-A) can develop the neonatal lupus syndrome. In this syndrome, the maternal antibodies apparently cross the placenta, bind to the fetal cardiac tissue, and cause immunologic injury. Clinically, infants present with congenital heart block, typical lupus skin lesions, or both.

    d. Discoid lupus. Patients can have typical skin manifestations of SLE without systemic disease. Fifteen percent of these patients have positive antinuclear antibodies without other clinical features of SLE.

G. Diagnosis. Arriving at a diagnosis of SLE involves careful consideration of historical and physical findings that suggest this multisystem disease. In suspicious settings, the physician seeks laboratory evidence of autoimmunity and attempts to exclude other illnesses. The 1982 American Rheumatism Association revised criteria for classification of SLE (Table 10-1) are useful when the disease is suspected, and the presence over time of any four of the eleven criteria strongly suggests the diagnosis. Although low serum complement levels are not part of the criteria, they may be supportive evidence in individual patients.

1. Criteria for classification (see Table 10-1)

2. Laboratory findings

    a. Hematologic findings. Anemia is common during active disease and more often is the anemia of chronic disease than hemolytic anemia. Antibodies to leukocytes also occur, with autoimmune lymphopenia a common feature of active disease and neutropenia less common. Antibodies to platelets can cause chronic immune thrombocytopenia or more acute falls in the platelet count with active disease. Elevation of the erythrocyte sedimentation rate is common and correlates with disease activity.

    b. Coagulation parameters. Antibodies to the phospholipid components of individual clotting factors can cause interference with coagulation testing (i.e., prolongation of the partial thromboplastin time not correctible by normal plasma). Paradoxically, patients with the partial thromboplastin time prolongation have a higher frequency of thrombosis than bleeding.

    c. Serologic findings. Phospholipid antibodies also can cause false-positive test results for syphilis, more often by interference with reagin testing than with antitreponemal testing.

Table 10-1. Criteria for Classification of Systemic Lupus Erythematosus (SLE)

Criterion	Definition
Malar rash	Fixed erythema, flat or raised, over the malar eminences, tending to spare the nasolabial folds
Discoid rash	Erythematous raised patches with adherent keratotic scaling and follicular plugging; atrophic scarring may occur in older lesions
Photosensitivity	Skin rash as a result of unusual reaction to sunlight—documented by patient history or observed by a physician
Oral ulcers	Oral or nasopharyngeal ulceration, usually painless—observed by a physician
Arthritis	Nonerosive arthritis involving two or more peripheral joints, characterized by tenderness, swelling, or effusion
Serositis	Pleuritis—convincing history of pleuritic pain or friction rub heard by a physician or evidence of pleural effusion **or** Pericarditis—documented by ECG or friction rub or evidence of pericardial effusion
Renal disorder	Persistent proteinuria exceeding 0.5 g/day or greater than 3+ if quantitation not performed **or** Cellular casts—may be red cell, hemoglobin, granular, tubular, or mixed
Neurologic disorder	Seizures—in the absence of offending drugs or known metabolic derangements (e.g., uremia, ketoacidosis, or electrolyte imbalance) **or** Psychosis—in the absence of offending drugs or known metabolic derangements (e.g., uremia, ketoacidosis, or electrolyte imbalance)
Hematologic disorder	Hemolytic anemia—with reticulocytosis **or** Leukopenia—less than 4000/mm³ total on two or more occasions **or** Lymphopenia—less than 1500/mm³ on two or more occasions **or** Thrombocytopenia—less than 100,000/mm³ in the absence of offending drugs
Immunologic disorder	Positive LE cell preparation **or** Antibody to native DNA in abnormal titer **or** Antibody to Sm nuclear antigen **or** False-positive serologic test for syphilis known to be positive for at least 6 months and confirmed by *Treponema pallidum* immobilization or fluorescent treponemal antibody absorption test
Antinuclear antibody	An abnormal titer of antinuclear antibody by immunofluorescence or an equivalent assay at any point in time and in the absence of drugs known to be associated with drug-induced lupus syndrome

Note.—The classification is based on eleven criteria. For the purpose of identifying patients in clinical studies, an individual is said to have SLE if any four or more of the eleven criteria are present, serially or simultaneously, during any interval of observation. (Adapted from Tan EM, Cohen AS, Fries JF, et al: The 1982 revised criteria for the classification of systemic lupus erythematosus (SLE). *Arthritis Rheum* 25:1271–1277, 1982.)

    d. Immune reactions
        (1) General considerations. Depression of levels of complement components (C3 and C4) by immune complex activation is common, and in some patients, falls in complement levels parallel disease flare-ups. Hypergammaglobulinemia reflects B-cell hyperreactivity.
        (2) Autoantibodies
            (a) Antinuclear antibodies. Approximately 95% of patients with SLE have antinuclear antibodies. These antibodies are detectable by an immunofluorescence technique that involves rat kidney or liver tissue. When the test serum is applied to rat tissue

that has been frozen and cut to expose nuclear components, the patient's anti-nuclear antibodies interact with the rat's nuclear material, and this interaction can be detected by fluorescence microscopy.

- **(i) Antibodies to double-stranded DNA** are found in over 50% of SLE patients, and their presence and titer may vary with the disease activity. When present, they are fairly specific for diagnosis. Some of these antibodies give a "rim" pattern of nuclear fluorescence on rat tissue sections.
- **(ii) Antibodies to histones.** Patients with SLE, especially the drug-induced lupus syndrome, can have antibodies to the structural proteins of DNA. These antibodies often yield homogeneous or diffuse staining on rat tissue.
- **(iii) Antibodies to single-stranded DNA** are found in a variety of connective tissue diseases, SLE, and even in normal populations. They are not detectable by routine immunofluorescence techniques.
- **(iv) Antibodies to small ribonucleoproteins.** Antibodies to the **Sm antigen** and the related **RNP antigen** usually give speckled patterns of immunofluorescence. Antibody to Sm is relatively specific for SLE, but antibody to RNP is commonly present in mixed connective tissue disease, which is a specific overlap syndrome with SLE (see section VI F 3 a). **Antibody to Ro (SS-A)** typically is associated with forms of SLE that have prominent dermatologic and photosensitive components and also is a marker for Sjögren's syndrome. Antibody to Ro (SS-A) is not detectable by routine immunofluorescence and is present in most of the cases of antinuclear antibody-negative SLE. The presence of antibodies to both Ro (SS-A) and La (SS-B) can occur in SLE but is more closely associated with Sjögren's syndrome.
- **(v) Antibodies to nucleolar components.** These antinuclear antibodies give "nucleolar" fluorescence on routine antinuclear antibody testing and are found in some patients with SLE as well as systemic sclerosis.

- **(b) Antibodies to membrane and cytoplasmic components.** Antibodies to **transfer RNA (tRNA)** and ribosomal nucleoproteins can be found in SLE. Other cytoplasmic autoantibodies possibly are made to cell membrane constituents (e.g., phospholipids) and are responsible for the **tissue specificity** of some autoantibodies (e.g., antibodies to gastric parietal cells, thyroid epithelial cells, and blood cellular elements).

3. **Differential diagnosis.** The physician must be careful to exclude other chronic rheumatic diseases, especially rheumatoid arthritis, overlap syndromes, and vasculitic syndromes, in arriving at the diagnosis of SLE. Drug exposure causing drug-induced lupus should be excluded. Chronic discoid lupus with positive antinuclear antibodies should be considered to be SLE only when other appropriate clinical features are present (see Table 10-1).

H. Therapy. Treatment of SLE must be individualized to the features that a particular patient exhibits, and it need not always include corticosteroids. Patients must understand that the prognosis in this chronic disease generally is better than they fear and that their compliance with medication regimens and avoidance of disease precipitants (e.g., ultraviolet light and emotional stress) often can favorably affect the disease course.

1. **Sunscreens.** Topical sunscreens containing para-aminobenzoic acid or benzophenones are effective in protecting the one-third of lupus patients who are photosensitive.

2. **Nonsteroidal anti-inflammatory drugs.** Aspirin and other nonsteroidal anti-inflammatory drugs are used in full anti-inflammatory doses for fever, joint complaints, and serositis. Mild elevation in transaminase levels often develops in SLE patients on nonsteroidal anti-inflammatory drugs, and aseptic meningitis has been reported in lupus patients on ibuprofen and sulindac.

3. **Antimalarial drugs.** Hydroxychloroquine, chloroquine, and other antimalarial drugs often are used to treat skin disease (especially discoid lupus erythematosus) and arthritis in patients with SLE. These drugs often work slowly (8–12 weeks may be required to establish efficacy), and they may cause macular pigmentary retinopathy, leading to blindness, if not monitored properly. Hydroxychloroquine is the most commonly used drug, usually taken in doses of 200–400 mg daily, with lower doses used when the disease is controlled.

4. **Corticosteroids**
   a. **Topical preparations.** Some of the skin manifestations are improved by treatment with topical glucocorticoids two to three times daily, although discoid lesions usually require additional treatment with antimalarial agents.
   b. **Systemic corticosteroids**
      (1) **Glucocorticoids in varying doses** often are required to control severe manifestations of SLE and less severe symptoms when they are persistent and disabling. These drugs

should be used cautiously, because long-term treatment usually is needed and typical side effects ensue. Chronic arthritis and serositis may require glucocorticoids if nonsteroidal anti-inflammatory agents are not sufficient. Severe hemolysis, life-threatening thrombocytopenia, pneumonitis, central or peripheral nervous system disease, clinically evident cardiac or skeletal muscle disease, renal disease, and vasculitis are typical indications for systemic glucocorticoids. Usually the drug dosage selected is proportionate to the severity of the illness; the dosage is tapered as manifestations subside. Alternate-day therapy is difficult to achieve in lupus patients because of worsening of systemic complaints on off-days.

(2) "Pulse" corticosteroids. Large doses of corticosteroids sometimes are administered intravenously for particularly severe cases of SLE. Serious renal and CNS manifestations have been the typical indications for pulse treatment, but dangerous cardiopulmonary and hematologic involvement also might warrant this aggressive treatment. Daily doses of 250–1000 mg of methylprednisolone are infused in 1–3 day courses; however, evidence for greater efficacy or lesser side effects of this approach remains to be proven.

5. Cytotoxic agents such as azathioprine and cyclophosphamide sometimes are employed to treat severe, refractory features of lupus, particularly renal disease.

6. Ancillary drugs are important in managing particular features of the disease. Dilantin and phenobarbital may be useful in the control of seizure disorders, and antipsychotic agents may prove more useful than corticosteroids in treating acute or chronic psychoses.

I. Prognosis. The prognosis clearly is better today than in the presteroid era; milder forms of disease are recognized and, presumably, appropriate drug treatment improves morbidity and mortality rates. Renal disease and infectious complications are still major causes of death, and prominent CNS disease can lead to severe disability. Steroid-related complications can be crippling (e.g., avascular necrosis of the femoral head and osteoporotic vertebral fractures) or fatal (e.g., premature coronary atherosclerosis).

VII. SYSTEMIC SCLEROSIS

A. Definition. Systemic sclerosis (**scleroderma**) is a connective tissue disease characterized by widespread small vessel obliterative disease and fibrosis of the skin and multiple internal organs, including the heart, lungs, kidneys, and gastrointestinal tract.

B. Epidemiology. Systemic sclerosis is a relatively rare disease, with familial clustering being uncommon. The disease is three to four times more common in women than in men. Coal miners have a high frequency of the disease, presumably as a result of exposure to silica dust.

C. Etiology. The etiology of systemic sclerosis is unknown, although similar pathologic lesions can be found in **autoimmune syndromes** (e.g., graft-versus-host disease of bone marrow transplantation), **overlap connective tissue diseases**, and **toxin exposures** (e.g., toxic oil syndrome, vinyl chloride exposures, and silicosis).

D. Pathogenesis. Vascular endothelial cell injury, mediated through several possible mechanisms (e.g., serum cytotoxic factors, cellular or humoral autoimmunity, or toxins), appears to be the basic process in systemic sclerosis.

1. Intimal damage in capillaries and small arteries leads to increased vascular permeability and consequent tissue edema. Eventually, fibrin deposition and microthrombosis lead to vessel occlusion and ischemic damage.

2. Fibroblast proliferation occurs, perhaps due to the same cytotoxic factors that injure the endothelial cell. Increased collagen production by these cells leads to connective tissue fibrotic lesions.

3. Vascular hyperreactivity. The injured vessels are hyperreactive to stimuli causing vessel constriction; consequent spasm can lead to **Raynaud's phenomenon** and, potentially, further increases in ischemic damage.

4. Renin-angiotensin axis. In patients with renal involvement, reduced renal blood flow and volume contraction can lead to increased production of renin and angiotensin, leading to further vasoconstriction.

E. Clinicopathologic features

1. Organ involvement
a. Skin. Ninety-five percent of patients with systemic sclerosis have skin involvement. An ear-

ly edematous phase of small vessel endothelial injury and increased permeability may progress through an indurative phase as increasing amounts of collagen are produced in the subcutaneous tissue. Epidermal and skin appendage atrophy may occur in late forms of the disease as the skin becomes progressively bound to underlying tissue.

(1) **Distribution.** Changes most often begin in the fingers and hands and may spread to involve more proximal tissues including the trunk and face. The lower extremities often are less severely involved.

(2) **Associated features**

(a) **Raynaud's phenomenon** occurs in 95% of patients with systemic sclerosis. Episodic vasospasm of the damaged small vessels in the digits results in a triphasic color change of the involved area as blood flow ceases (white), returns sluggishly (blue), and exhibits reactive hyperemia (red).

(b) **Telangiectasia** can occur in involved areas as well as on mucous membranes.

(c) **Subcutaneous calcifications** can occur, especially in finger tips.

(d) **Salt-and-pepper changes.** The skin can become taut, shiny, and immobile, and hyperpigmented areas can alternate with depigmented areas.

(e) **Microcapillary abnormalities.** The distal nail bed proliferates and the capillary bed becomes visibly abnormal, with dilatation, tortuosity, and loss of vessels.

(f) **Skin ulcers.** Distal digital ulcers and finger tapering occur due to distal infarctions and consequent loss of digital pulp, sometimes resulting in infection.

b. **Gastrointestinal tract**

(1) In the upper one-third of the esophagus, striated muscles are relatively unaffected. Esophageal motility dysfunction and reflux are common features of systemic sclerosis as collagen replaces smooth muscle in the lower two-thirds of the esophagus, and esophageal strictures can result from the constant reflux. Ulceration can occur at the gastroesophageal junction. More prominent than the amount of fibrotic replacement of muscle is the atrophy of the esophageal muscularis tissue.

(2) Similar small bowel involvement leads to intestinal hypomotility and intermittent cramping, diarrhea, and bacterial overgrowth **malabsorption syndrome**. Wide-mouth diverticuli can be seen in the transverse and descending colon in areas of patchy muscularis involvement.

c. **Lung.** Pleural inflammatory change is quite uncommon compared to other rheumatic diseases such as rheumatoid arthritis and SLE. Widespread small pulmonary arterial narrowing and fibrotic change eventually can lead to pulmonary hypertension. More commonly, a fibrotic proliferation in the peribronchial and perialveolar tissues leads to progressive interstitial lung disease. Patients may only have symptoms of progressive shortness of breath on exertion, with moderately severe pulmonary function abnormalities.

d. **Heart.** Cardiac involvement by an interstitial myocardial fibrotic process can take several forms. Clinically, acute and chronic pericarditis are unusual, but effusions often can be seen on ultrasonography and are associated with myocardial involvement. If interstitial disease is extensive, frank cardiomyopathy can result with the occurrence of symptoms of congestive heart failure, arrhythmias, and conduction disturbances. Small coronary artery involvement can lead to angina and arrhythmias with normal large coronary vessels being found on angiography.

e. **Kidney.** Renal failure is the leading cause of death in patients with systemic sclerosis. Clinically silent, interlobular arterial intimal proliferation and periarterial fibrosis can proceed slowly. However, collapse of renal blood flow due to small artery spasm with consequent renal cortical ischemia, massive renin-angiotensin release, and malignant hypertension with microangiopathic hemolytic anemia can occur suddenly and result in acute renal failure. Some patients develop hypertension, proteinuria, or creatinine clearance impairment before this malignant phase, and some episodes of acute renal failure are precipitated by volume contraction states (e.g., diuresis, blood loss, or surgery). In many episodes, however, no precipitant or clue can be identified, and chronic renal failure or even death occurs.

f. **Muscle.** In many patients, a mild indolent myopathy manifested by minor enzyme elevations and perhaps mild weakness occurs but does not require treatment. In others, a clinically evident inflammatory myopathy with interstitial cellular infiltrates indentical to polymyositis occurs and requires similar treatment.

g. **Joint and tendon** involvement causes swelling, stiffness, and pain in finger, wrist, and knee joints in more than 50% of patients with systemic sclerosis. Mild, self-limited inflammatory arthritis can occur early in the disease, but typical joint involvement is limited to synovial fibrosis and impaired range of motion due to the generalized restriction of the fibrotic process. Tendon sheath involvement is not unusual, and complaints due to tendon sheath fibrosis often are accompanied by audible rubs. **Carpal tunnel syndrome** can result from extensive tendon sheath fibrosis in the wrist.

h. Nerve. Neurologic involvement typically is limited to fibrotic entrapment neuropathies of the median and trigeminal nerves.

2. Clinical syndromes

a. Diffuse systemic sclerosis. The central features of the diffuse form of systemic sclerosis are **widespread and proximal skin involvement** (skin proximal to the metacarpophalangeal joints or forearms in various definitions) as well as **early visceral organ involvement**. Diffuse pulmonary fibrosis, cardiac involvement, and renal disease are more common in this group, and the progression of disease can vary from a very acute to a slowly progressive form.

b. CREST syndrome. The CREST syndrome (involving the coexistence of subcutaneous **C**alcinosis, **R**aynaud's phenomenon, **E**sophageal motility dysfunction, **S**clerodactyly, and **T**elangiectasia) has been described as a syndrome distinct from diffuse systemic sclerosis. Skin disease in this form typically is limited to distal areas (often just the fingers and the face), visceral involvement is very slowly progressive, and severe kidney and myocardial involvement are uncommon. Pulmonary fibrosis is common but indolent; many cases of pulmonary involvement resemble the diffuse form by the third or fourth decade of disease.

c. Local forms of disease. Two forms of purely local disease—**morphea** and **linear scleroderma**—have very similar clinical and pathologic appearances to sclerodermatous skin. These forms present as localized fibrotic plaques (morphea) or longitudinal bands (linear scleroderma). Infiltration of the fibrotic lesions with chronic inflammatory cells can occur but is inconsistently present. Linear scleroderma and morphea may resolve spontaneously and have neither the characteristic distal hand involvement of systemic sclerosis nor the visceral organ changes.

F. Diagnosis

1. Clinical approach. A diagnosis of systemic sclerosis should be entertained in the presence of symptoms of Raynaud's phenomenon, distal skin thickening, and visceral organ involvement. In addition to physical evidence of internal organ change, the physician should evaluate distal nail beds for suggestive capillary abnormality and attempt to document the location and extent of the skin thickening to differentiate local from generalized forms. Characteristic antinuclear antibody test results may also be useful in classifying patients.

2. Laboratory findings

a. Nonspecific. Anemia of chronic disease is common in patients with visceral organ changes. The erythrocyte sedimentation rate often is elevated but is not useful in following disease activity. Creatine kinase (CK) or aldolase elevations occur in patients with muscle involvement. Urinalysis abnormalities (e.g., proteinuria, red blood cells, and casts) reflect renal involvement. Hypergammaglobulinemia (primarily elevated IgG levels) and positive tests for rheumatoid factor occur in 30%–40% of patients.

b. Specific. Antinuclear antibodies are found frequently in patients with systemic sclerosis when human tumor cell lines are used as substrate. Positivity for either **antibody to Scl-86** or **antibody to Scl-70** is very common in diffuse systemic sclerosis, and antibodies to the nucleolus can be found in diffuse systemic sclerosis and the CREST syndrome but occur infrequently in other rheumatic diseases. **Antibody to centromere** is highly associated with the CREST syndrome.

3. Differential diagnosis. Exclusion of **pseudoscleroderma** and **mixed connective tissue disease** is an important consideration in the diagnosis of systemic sclerosis.

a. Pseudoscleroderma

(1) Skin biopsy results are different in some **scleroderma-like conditions** from the characteristic disease features (e.g., prominent dermal collagen, fibrosis, and loss of skin appendages) that support a diagnosis of scleroderma.

(a) **Diffuse fasciitis with eosinophilia** is a pseudoscleroderma syndrome that typically occurs in an extremity after vigorous exercise. Tenderness and skin induration resembling scleroderma develop, but without Raynaud's phenomenon or sclerodactyly. A full-thickness skin biopsy (including underlying fascia and muscle) reveals deep fascial eosinophil and chronic inflammatory cell infiltrate.

(b) **Scleredema (Buschke's scleredema adultorum)** is a chronic disorder occurring in both children and adults that is characterized by edematous induration of the face, scalp, neck, trunk, and proximal extremities (i.e., not the hands and feet). Skin biopsy results demonstrate mucopolysaccharide deposits in the dermis and skeletal muscle when appropriate staining techniques are used.

(c) **Scleromyxedema (lichen myxedematosus)** is a rare disorder that involves the face and hands and is characterized by yellowish nodules and thickening of the skin. An appropriately stained skin biopsy specimen reveals dermal mucopolysaccharide deposits.

    (d) Primary amyloidosis diffusely infiltrates the dermis of the face and extremities and can be differentiated by biopsy using appropriate stains.

  (2) Toxic environmental, occupational, and drug exposures can have important prognostic and therapeutic implications.

    (a) Environmental and occupational exposures include factors such as vinyl chloride, silica dust, toxic oil, and vibration-associated disease ("jackhammer disease"). These exposures may cause scleroderma-like skin lesions, Raynaud's phenomenon, or nail-fold capillary abnormalities.

    (b) Exposure to drugs such as intramuscular pentazocine, L-tryptophan, carbidopa, or bleomycin may cause scleroderma-like skin characteristics.

  (3) Metabolic disturbances. Collections of 5-hydroxytryptophan or urinary porphyrins can be obtained in appropriate clinical settings to investigate possible metabolic defects causing skin thickening (i.e., carcinoid syndrome or porphyria cutanea tarda).

b. Mixed connective tissue disease is a rheumatic syndrome characterized by clinically overlapping features of systemic sclerosis, SLE, and polymyositis (see section VI F 3 a).

  (1) Features of systemic sclerosis include a typical scleroderma-like skin on the hands, telangiectatic lesions, Raynaud's phenomenon, esophageal motility dysfunction, and pulmonary abnormalities.

  (2) Features of SLE include the typical erythematous rash, immunoglobulin deposits at the dermoepidermal junction, and high titers of antibody to nuclear ribonucleoprotein.

  (3) Features of polymyositis include muscle weakness, elevated muscle enzyme levels, myalgia, and the erythematous patches typical of dermatomyositis.

G. Therapy

1. Education. Patient education should focus on information about specific organ involvement and the tendency for spontaneous fluctuation in disease activity to occur. Distinctions between diffuse and CREST subsets should be made for prognostic and perhaps therapeutic purposes.

2. Monitoring organ involvement. Specific ancillary investigations may be useful in certain patients in attempting to document or follow visceral involvement.

  a. Barium swallow and esophageal manometry may be helpful in documenting esophageal involvement, and lower gastrointestinal contrast radiographic studies or malabsorption testing may demonstrate small bowel or colonic involvement.

  b. Pulmonary function testing with diffusion capacity measurements is useful in documenting pulmonary involvement not visible on chest x-ray.

  c. Noninvasive cardiac testing (e.g., ultrasonography, nuclear medicine procedures, and Holter monitoring) may show pericardial effusions, myocardial function abnormalities, arrhythmias, or conduction disturbances not found on routine testing.

  d. Routine urinalyses and 24-hour urine collections of creatinine and protein may help to quantitate renal involvement.

3. Drug therapy

  a. General disease. Patients with diffuse systemic sclerosis have been treated with D-penicillamine orally in daily dosages of 500–1500 mg, and some studies have suggested an improvement in skin disease and stabilization or improvement of visceral organ involvement. D-Penicillamine has not yet been proven effective in randomized trials or approved by the FDA for this use; therefore, it should be administered only by physicians experienced in its use and toxicity. It may function by preventing collagen cross-linking or by immunomodulatory effects. **Colchicine** also has been used to block procollagen–collagen transformation, but evidence for efficacy is lacking.

  b. Specific disease features

    (1) Raynaud's phenomenon is managed by controlling vasospasm. Patients should understand the need to cover their head, hands, and trunk when exposed to the cold. Avoidance of smoking may help to relieve vasospasm. Calcium channel blockers (e.g., nifedipine) have been added to the armamentarium of ganglionic blocking agents, α-blockers, and vasodilators and may be more effective than these agents if vascular obstruction has not occurred.

    (2) Pulmonary involvement has been managed by the use of corticosteroids and D-penicillamine, but the results have been uncertain. Tobacco smoking may be synergistic in pulmonary injury, and should be discouraged.

    (3) Esophageal involvement should be managed by the usual antireflux measures. Mucosal protective agents (e.g., sucralfate) and histamine$_2$ (H$_2$)-receptor blockers such as cimetidine may be added to antacids for symptomatic reflux esophagitis.

(4) **Lower gastrointestinal involvement.** Bacterial overgrowth malabsorption may be improved by treatment with broad-spectrum antibiotics such as tetracycline.

(5) **Muscle involvement.** When inflammatory myositis occurs in overlap syndromes, corticosteroids are used, as in polymyositis. Nonsteroidal anti-inflammatory agents such as aspirin should be used in treating articular symptoms and indolent muscle disease forms.

(6) **Renal involvement** is best managed by aggressive control of hypertension. The angiotensin-converting enzyme (ACE) inhibitors captopril and enalapril are major advances in controlling blood pressure in patients with systemic sclerosis. The avoidance of hypovolemia and the use of hemodialysis for acute or chronic renal failure also are important management considerations.

(7) **Cardiac involvement.** Medications useful for control of angina, congestive heart failure, and arrhythmias are employed when these complications occur.

H. Prognosis. Prognosis is difficult to estimate because of the variable natural history of the disease, with spontaneous relapses and remissions in activity being common. In general, patients with diffuse disease have a poorer prognosis than those with the CREST syndrome. Cardiac, renal, and pulmonary involvement are poor prognostic indicators, particularly when present early in the disease, and are the most common causes of death in patients with systemic sclerosis.

VIII. POLYMYOSITIS AND DERMATOMYOSITIS

A. Definition. **Polymyositis** is an idiopathic inflammatory muscle disease associated with prominent proximal muscle weakness, muscle enzyme elevations, characteristic myopathic electromyographic patterns, and inflammatory infiltrates on muscle biopsy. When this complex is accompanied by a characteristic rash it is called **dermatomyositis.** Dermatomyositis is much more common than polymyositis in children.

B. Classification. Inflammatory muscle diseases are grouped into the following categories so that potential differences in disease subsets can be studied.*

1. Adult polymyositis

2. Adult dermatomyositis

3. Polymyositis or dermatomyositis associated with malignancy

4. Juvenile dermatomyositis (or polymyositis)

5. Polymyositis or dermatomyositis associated with other rheumatic diseases (overlap syndromes)

C. Epidemiology. Polymyositis is a rare disease, occurring in about 1 in 200,000 individuals, with a peak incidence in childhood and in late adulthood. It is twice as common in females as in males and may be associated with malignancy in the adult-onset form.

D. Etiology and pathogenesis. The basic cause of polymyositis is unknown. However, it is believed that chronic viral infection and altered immune responses are potentially important in causation and pathogenesis. Lymphocyte-mediated muscle cell damage is thought to be the central pathogenetic factor in this disease.

1. Viral infections can cause acute myositis.
   a. Elevated titers of antibodies to coxsackie B virus have been found in some juvenile dermatomyositis patients, and high titers of antibodies to *Toxoplasma gondii* have been found in some adult polymyositis patients.
   b. Isolation of these organisms from muscle of patients with polymyositis or dermatomyositis has not been accomplished, and antibiotic treatment for toxoplasmosis has not improved myositis in patients with high titers of antibody to *T. gondii.*

2. Autoimmunity
   a. Humoral. Most patients with polymyositis demonstrate autoantibodies when human tumor cell lines are used as testing substrate. The role of autoantibodies in the pathogenesis of polymyositis is unclear, however. Vascular deposits of immune complexes and complement are associated with endothelial cell injury and small vessel obstruction in some cases of juvenile dermatomyositis.

*Adapted from Bohan A and Peter JB: Polymyositis and dermatomyositis. *N Engl J Med* 292:344, 1975.

b. Cellular. Peripheral blood lymphocytes from polymyositis patients produce a lymphotoxin that is cytotoxic to muscle cells. In addition, lymphocytes are the predominant cell type found in the inflammatory infiltrate in muscle.

E. Pathology. The major sites of inflammation are skeletal muscle and, less commonly, cardiac muscle. Skin involvement is a minor pathologic feature.

1. **Inflammatory infiltrate.** Lymphocytes and plasma cells are the predominant inflammatory cells, although macrophages, eosinophils, and neutrophils also can be seen in muscle tissue. Lymphocytes infiltrate muscle fibers and cluster around small blood vessels within the muscle.

2. **Muscle fiber damage.** Spotty muscle fiber necrosis and degeneration occur, with loss of cross-striations and variation in the size of surviving fibers. Increased numbers of muscle nuclei and enhanced basophilic staining of fibers indicate regeneration in the midst of cell death. Interstitial fibrotic infiltrates occur in chronic cases.

F. Clinical features

1. **Organ involvement**
   a. **Skin.** The rash of dermatomyositis consists of erythematous patches, which sometimes are scaling or atrophic and are distributed over the face, neck, upper chest, and extensor surfaces. Characteristic skin findings include **heliotrope lids** (a violet discoloration and swelling of the eyelids) and **Gottron's sign** (heaped-up erythematous papules over the metacarpophalangeal or proximal interphalangeal joints). Only scattered inflammatory infiltrates in the dermis are evident on biopsy.
   b. **Lung.** Chronic interstitial lung disease can occur, particularly in the presence of antibody to Jo-1. Aspiration pneumonitis and ventilatory insufficiency also can occur.
   c. **Joint.** A mild, symmetrical inflammatory arthritis occurs uncommonly and rarely is destructive.
   d. **Muscle.** Most patients have gradual but steady progression of muscle weakness; however, some patients have such fulminant courses that acute respiratory failure or myoglobinuric renal failure can ensue.
      (1) **Skeletal muscle weakness** is the primary manifestation of polymyositis.
         (a) Symmetrical, proximal, upper and lower extremity weakness occurs, causing difficulty with rising from a chair, sitting up in bed, or combing one's hair.
         (b) **Pharyngeal muscle involvement** can lead to swallowing difficulties and aspiration, and **respiratory muscle dysfunction** can lead to respiratory failure.
      (2) **Cardiac muscle involvement** is not as common, but when it occurs it presents as cardiomyopathy with congestive heart failure, arrhythmias, and conduction disturbances.

2. **Clinical syndromes**
   a. **Adult polymyositis or dermatomyositis.** Both forms of disease are characterized by all of the clinical features noted above with the exception of skin manifestations, which occur only in dermatomyositis. No differences in clinical presentation, therapeutic response, or prognosis have been convincingly shown to exist between polymyositis and dermatomyositis in the adult.
   b. **Polymyositis or dermatomyositis associated with malignancy.** Visceral malignancies occur more frequently than expected in elderly individuals with late-onset polymyositis (or dermatomyositis). The association appears equally strong for both forms of muscle disease and not just dermatomyositis, as was originally believed. The malignancies that are most common in polymyositis or dermatomyositis are those that are most common in elderly individuals (i.e., cancers of the lung, gastrointestinal tract, breast, and ovaries). Removal of the malignancy occasionally results in remission of the muscle disease.
   c. **Juvenile dermatomyositis.** Most children have dermatomyositis rather than polymyositis. Young patients may develop muscle **contractures** (from large **calcific deposits** in the chronically damaged muscle) and a widespread small artery and capillary **vasculitis**, which can lead to serious skin, muscle, and bowel ischemic lesions.
   d. **Overlap syndromes.** Muscle disease that is identical to polymyositis can occur in SLE, rheumatoid arthritis, systemic sclerosis , and Sjögren's syndrome.

G. Diagnosis

1. **Clinical approach**
   a. The diagnosis of polymyositis is based on finding symmetrical proximal muscle weakness, elevated muscle enzymes, a myopathic electromyogram, and a typical muscle biopsy specimen. The characteristic rash also is supportive if found and sometimes precedes

clinical evidence of muscle involvement. Muscle biopsy should be performed in a symptomatic deltoid or quadriceps muscle that is not already atrophic.

b. A search for a malignancy is warranted in middle-aged or elderly polymyositis or dermatomyositis patients. Thorough physical examination and chest x-ray as well as routine hematologic and biochemical testing and urinalysis and stool testing for occult blood should be performed in these patients and abnormalities pursued through additional testing.

2. Laboratory findings

a. Muscle enzymes. An increased concentration of enzymes typically present in skeletal muscle is prominent in polymyositis. **CK** and **aldolase** are the enzymes that are routinely measured, and CK fractionation may suggest myocardial involvement if the **MB fraction** (i.e., the CK isoenzyme found mainly in the myocardium) is increased. Enzyme elevations usually correlate with the activity of the muscle disease and its response to treatment.

b. Autoantibodies. Routine antinuclear antibody testing usually is negative in polymyositis. However, newly discovered autoantibodies to **intermediate filament cytoskeletal proteins** and **tRNA synthetases** have been associated with polymyositis.

(1) One of the tRNA synthetase antibodies—**antibody to Jo-1**—is associated with interstitial lung disease in polymyositis; it rarely is found in dermatomyositis.

(2) Another autoantibody—PM_1 **(PM-Scl)**—is directed against a nucleolar protein and is associated with an overlap syndrome with characteristics of both polymyositis and systemic sclerosis.

3. Differential diagnosis. The diagnosis of polymyositis is likely if three of the four muscle criteria are present. However, the following diseases or factors also must be considered, especially if the presentations are not classic.

a. Endocrine disorders

(1) Hyperthyroidism or hypothyroidism

(2) Cushing's syndrome

b. Polymyalgia rheumatica

c. Myasthenia gravis

d. Muscular dystrophies

e. Metabolic disorders of muscle (e.g., periodic paralysis and glycogen storage diseases)

f. Drug effects

(1) Alcohol

(2) Clofibrate

(3) Hydroxychloroquine

(4) D-Penicillamine

g. Trichinosis

h. Sarcoidosis

i. Amyotrophic lateral sclerosis

H. Therapy

1. Corticosteroids. Large doses of corticosteroids appear to be effective in controlling the muscle disease in most patients. Prednisone usually is begun at a dose of 60 mg/day and is reduced gradually over several months as muscle strength improves and CK level falls. Alternate-day regimens can be used to prevent steroid toxicity but only after the normalization of CK level and return of muscle strength.

2. Cytotoxic agents. Patients who do not respond to the above-mentioned corticosteroid schedules within 3 months are considered to be nonresponders to treatment. Frequently, the addition of methotrexate or azathioprine allows control of the muscle disease and gradual tapering of the steroids. These and other cytotoxic agents should be used only by practitioners who are experienced in their actions and toxicity.

I. Prognosis. Most patients respond to treatment, although lasting remission is unusual. The presence of cardiac involvement or malignancy indicates an unfavorable outcome. Patients who are on potent immunosuppressive regimens are at an increased risk of death due to opportunistic infections.

IX. SJÖGREN'S SYNDROME

A. Definition. Dry mouth (**xerostomia**), dry eyes (**keratoconjunctivitis sicca**), and variable **salivary gland enlargement** result from lymphocytic infiltration of lacrimal and salivary glands in this idiopathic, autoimmune disorder. Sjögren's syndrome, which also is called **sicca syndrome**, may occur in a primary form (associated with characteristic organ and exocrine glandular features) and a secondary form (associated with another rheumatic disease, such as rheumatoid arthritis, SLE, or systemic sclerosis).

B. Distinctions between primary and secondary Sjögren's syndrome. The two forms of Sjögren's syndrome can be distinguished on the basis of clinical features and HLA associations.

  1. Clinical features
  a. Primary Sjögren's syndrome can present as a wide variety of clinical manifestations that are uncommon in the secondary form, mainly due to a wider attack on exocrine glands. Specific organ involvement is as follows:
    (1) Skin: Dry skin and vagina, Raynaud's phenomenon, and purpura (vasculitis)
    (2) Lung: Recurrent infections and interstitial fibrosis
    (3) Gastrointestinal tract: Recurrent parotitis, dysphagia, atrophic gastritis, chronic active hepatitis, biliary cirrhosis, and pancreatitis
    (4) Kidney: Renal tubular acidosis and interstitial nephritis
    (5) Muscle: Indolent myositis
    (6) Nerve: CNS vasculitis (with a spectrum of clinical manifestations similar to CNS lupus) and peripheral neuropathy
    (7) Hematologic system: Splenomegaly with neutropenia, lymphomas, and pseudolymphomas
    (8) Endocrine system: Chronic thyroiditis
  b. Secondary Sjögren's syndrome. Patients with the secondary form of the disorder usually have symptoms that are limited to lacrimal and salivary gland abnormalities.

  2. HLA associations. Primary Sjögren's syndrome has a significantly increased association with HLA-DR3 rather than the higher frequency of HLA-DR4 that is seen in the secondary form.

C. Diagnosis

  1. Clinical approach
  a. Chronic complaints of gritty eyes and dry mouth can be investigated by:
    (1) Ophthalmologic slit-lamp examination or rose bengal staining to examine for keratoconjunctivitis sicca
    (2) Biopsy of the minor salivary glands of the lip to search for characteristic lymphocytic infiltration of salivary glands.
    (3) Autoantibody testing [for **antibody to Ro (SS-A)** or **antibody to La (SS-B)**]
  b. Schirmer's test, which measures the degree of tear wetting on filter paper, gives unacceptably high false-positive and false-negative results.

  2. Laboratory findings
  a. Nonspecific findings. Anemia of chronic disease, elevated erythrocyte sedimentation rate, hypergammaglobulinemia, rheumatoid factor, and antinuclear antibodies often are found in Sjögren's syndrome, whether primary or secondary.
  b. Autoantibody findings. Antibodies to the small RNA proteins Ro (SS-A) and La (SS-B) frequently are seen in patients with either form of Sjögren's syndrome. Salivary duct antibodies are common only in the secondary form.

  3. Differential diagnosis
  a. Salivary gland enlargement also may be caused by lymphoid or parotid gland neoplasm, granulomatous infiltration (sarcoidosis), cirrhosis, diabetes, or infection.
  b. Xerostomia may be caused by the use of certain drugs, including tricyclic antidepressants, phenothiazines, and antihistamines.

D. Therapy

  1. General considerations
  a. Scrupulous oral hygiene is important to prevent rampant dental caries.
  b. Patients with primary Sjögren's syndrome who demonstrate salivary gland or lymphoid tissue enlargement must be considered at risk for lymphoma, since non-Hodgkin's lymphomas occur at 40 times the normal rate in these patients.

  2. Symptomatic treatment
  a. Xerostomia. Avoidance of drugs that dry out the mouth and frequent drinks of water or other liquids to keep the mouth wet are the usual symptomatic measures for this condition.
  b. Keratoconjunctivitis sicca. Artifical tears (methyl cellulose) are used as often as needed to keep the eyes lubricated.

E. Prognosis for patients with primary Sjögren's syndrome is dependent on the severity of involvement of organs other than the salivary glands. Also, the risk of lymphoma is higher in more severe cases. Features of the primary rheumatic disease determine the prognosis for patients with secondary Sjögren's syndrome.

Table 10-2. Vasculitic Syndromes: Clinicopathologic Distinctions

Syndrome	Clinical Features	Pathology — Vessel Size	Pathology — Cellular Infiltrate	Diagnosis	Therapy
Hypersensitivity vasculitis (serum sickness; drug reactions; Henoch-Schönlein purpura)	Skin involvement predominant Visceral involvement minimal and self-limited	Small (capillaries; venules)	Leukocytoclastic vasculitis with all lesions at the same developmental stage	Skin biopsy	Supportive
Polyarteritis nodosa	Multisystem illness Major arterial ischemic lesions that spare lungs and spleen Nodose skin lesions uncommon	Small and medium-size arteries	Necrotizing arteritis at vessel branch points Simultaneous lesions at various stages	Biopsy of involved organ Visceral angiography	Corticosteroids; cytotoxic agents added if no response
Allergic angiitis (Churg-Strauss disease)	Prominent allergic, asthmatic history Lung involvement Blood eosinophilia common	Varying (capillaries; venules; small arteries)	Granulomatous infiltrates with eosinophils	Lung biopsy	Corticosteroids; cytotoxic agents added if no response
Wegener's granulomatosis	Respiratory tract involvement Prominent renal abnormalities	Small (arteries; veins)	Necrotizing granulomas in upper and lower airways Focal necrotizing arteritis in lungs Necrotizing glomerulonephritis in kidneys	Lung biopsy (sinus biopsy usually non-diagnostic)	Cyclophosphamide; corticosteroids added if disease is fulminant
Giant cell arteritis (temporal arteritis)	Polymyalgia rheumatica common Occurs in the elderly Signs and symptoms of cranial artery involvement High erythrocyte sedimentation rate	Large (especially temporal artery)	Giant cell and chronic mononuclear infiltrates	Temporal artery biopsy	Corticosteroids
Takayasu's arteritis	Large vessel claudication Occurs in young (often oriental) women	Large (aortic arch)	Giant cell and chronic mononuclear infiltrates	Aortography	Corticosteroids Large vessel reconstructive surgery
Vasculitis associated with rheumatic diseases	Overlap syndromes with severe manifestations of rheumatoid arthritis, SLE, and others	Vessel involvement typical of hypersensitivity vasculitis or polyarteritis		Biopsy of involved organ	Control of basic disease; possibly corticosteroids and cytotoxic agents added

X. VASCULITIS

A. Definition. Clinically disparate disorders characterized by necrosis and inflammation of blood vessel walls are called **vasculitic syndromes**. Vasculitis can exist as the primary feature of an idiopathic condition or as a secondary manifestation of an infectious or rheumatic disease.

B. Etiology. Most of the vasculitic syndromes are idiopathic, although **hepatitis B surface antigen** (HB_sAg) has been found in the immune complexes of several different syndromes, including polyarteritis nodosa and essential mixed cryoglobulinemia. Methamphetamine abuse also has been implicated in the causation of vessel lesions in some cases of polyarteritis.

C. Pathogenesis. Although aberrant cellular immune responses also may be involved, disordered humoral immune responses appear to play a central role in these syndromes. Soluble immune complexes deposit in vessel walls, fix complement, and attract inflammatory cells; this sequence leads to vessel damage. Multiple factors are important in determining the size of the vessel involved and the type of immune response mounted. These include physical and biochemical properties of the immune complexes, variations in blood pressure, changes in blood vessel permeability, the ability of the reticuloendothelial system to remove immune complexes, the persistence of the antigen in the circulation, and the genetically determined variations in the host's immune response.

D. Classification. The currently used systems for classifying vasculitic syndromes use clinical features, size of the involved vessel, and type of cellular infiltrate to separate the syndromes (Table 10-2). Nonspecific hematologic and immunologic abnormalities (e.g., anemia, leukocytosis, elevated erythrocyte sedimentation rate, and hypocomplementemia) often exist in many of these syndromes, but these are not noted in Table 10-2 unless they are specifically important for the diagnosis of a particular syndrome.

STUDY QUESTIONS

Directions: Each question below contains five suggested answers. Choose the **one best** response to each question.

1. Which of the following findings is definitive evidence of calcium pyrophosphate dihydrate (CPPD) deposition disease (pseudogout) as the cause of an acute inflammatory arthritis?

(A) Negatively birefringent, needle-shaped crystals on microscopic examination of the synovial fluid
(B) Chondrocalcinosis on radiographic examination of the involved joint
(C) Extensive osteophytes on radiographic examination of the involved joint
(D) Positively birefringent, rectangular crystals on microscopic examination of the synovial fluid
(E) Large numbers of neutrophils in the synovial fluid

2. What is the most serious manifestation of the pauciarticular form of juvenile rheumatoid arthritis?

(A) Inflammatory muscle disease
(B) Joint deformity or contracture
(C) Cardiomyopathy
(D) Central nervous system disease
(E) Chronic anterior uveitis

3. Which human leukocyte antigen is most closely associated with rheumatoid arthritis?

(A) HLA-DR3
(B) HLA-DR4
(C) HLA-DR7
(D) HLA-B27
(E) HLA-B13

4. The most important factor in the etiology and pathogenesis of adult polymyositis is believed to be

(A) autoantibody attack on muscle fibers
(B) lymphocyte-mediated destruction of muscle cells
(C) vasculitis of the small arteries of the muscles
(D) chronic viral infection of muscle
(E) chronic toxoplasmosis of muscle

5. Which of the following factors is believed to be central to the pathogenesis of systemic sclerosis?

(A) Vascular endothelial cell injury
(B) Vascular hyperreactivity
(C) Chronically increased production of renin and angiotensin
(D) Microangiopathic hemolytic anemia
(E) Inflammatory vasculitis

6. Which of the following manifestations is more likely to be found in the diffuse form of systemic sclerosis than in the CREST form?

(A) Esophageal motility dysfunction
(B) Pulmonary involvement
(C) Distal skin thickening and Raynaud's phenomenon
(D) Renal disease
(E) Telangiectasias

Directions: Each question below contains four suggested answers of which **one or more** is correct. Choose the answer

A if **1, 2, and 3** are correct
B if **1 and 3** are correct
C if **2 and 4** are correct
D if **4** is correct
E if **1, 2, 3, and 4** are correct

7. Systemic glucocorticoids may be necessary in systemic lupus erythematosus for the treatment of

(1) mucous membrane ulcerations
(2) central nervous system manifestations
(3) photosensitivity
(4) renal disease

8. Patients with rheumatoid arthritis may exhibit which of the following extra-articular manifestations of disease?

(1) Nodules
(2) Aortitis
(3) Interstitial lung disease
(4) Anterior uveitis

9. Patients with rheumatoid arthritis may require treatment with a disease-modifying agent such as gold. Good reasons for beginning treatment with one of these drugs include

(1) persistent polyarticular synovitis
(2) progressive deformities
(3) radiographic evidence of erosive joint disease
(4) chronic joint pain

10. Antimalarial drugs are useful for treating certain rheumatic diseases. These include

(1) rheumatoid arthritis
(2) systemic sclerosis
(3) systemic lupus erythematosus
(4) Sjögren's syndrome

11. Factors thought to be important in causing or perpetuating rheumatoid arthritis and systemic lupus erythematosus include

(1) disordered cellular immune responses
(2) familial, genetic, or HLA associations
(3) environmental agents (e.g., viruses and drugs)
(4) disordered humoral immune responses

Directions: The groups of questions below consist of lettered choices followed by several numbered items. For each numbered item select the **one** lettered choice with which it is **most** closely associated. Each lettered choice may be used once, more than once, or not at all.

Questions 12–16

Patients with inflammatory arthritis may have extra-articular findings on history or physical examination that give clues to the eventual diagnosis. Match the extra-articular feature with the disease it is most likely to be associated with.

(A) Rheumatoid arthritis
(B) Ankylosing spondylitis
(C) Systemic lupus erythematosus
(D) Enteropathic arthritis
(E) Reiter's syndrome

12. Malar erythema in a butterfly pattern

13. Painless erosive erythema of the glans penis

14. Severe limitation of lumbar spinal range of motion in all planes

15. Painless subcutaneous nodules on the extensor aspects of the forearms

16. Gastrointestinal bleeding, chronic diarrhea, and weight loss

Questions 17–21

Autoantibodies are important markers for several rheumatic diseases. Match the autoantibody with the disease it is most closely associated with.

(A) Mixed connective tissue disease
(B) Sjögren's syndrome
(C) Polymyositis and dermatomyositis
(D) Systemic lupus erythematosus
(E) CREST form of systemic sclerosis

17. Antibody to Jo-1

18. Antibody to centromere

19. Antibody to ribonuclear protein (RNP)

20. Antibodies to Ro (SS-A) and La (SS-B)

21. Antibody to double-stranded DNA

ANSWERS AND EXPLANATIONS

1. The answer is D. [*II B 5 a, b (1)*] The best evidence that pseudogout is the cause of an acute arthritis is the finding of chunky, rhomboid or rectangular crystals that exhibit positive birefringence in red-compensated, polarized light on microscopic examination of synovial fluid. Chondrocalcinosis on x-ray of the involved joint certainly is suggestive evidence of calcium pyrophosphate dihydrate (CPPD) deposition; however, this finding is so common in some elderly populations that it may be misleading. The finding of large numbers of neutrophils in the synovial fluid suggests only an inflammatory arthritis, not a specific cause.

2. The answer is E. [*V E 3 a (1)*] Chronic anterior uveitis occurs in 20%–40% of patients with the pauciarticular form of juvenile rheumatoid arthritis. This eye disease can be entirely asymptomatic and can progress to blindness. The form of anterior uveitis often seen in the spondylarthropathies can be distinguished from that seen in the pauciarticular arthritis because it is acute, relapsing, and remitting rather than chronic and because it responds to treatment rather than leading to severe visual impairment. Further, the serologic association is with HLA-B27 in the spondylarthropathies and with antinuclear antibodies in the pauciarticular form of juvenile rheumatoid arthritis.

3. The answer is B. (*III B 2, C 3*) Rheumatoid arthritis patients who are seropositive for rheumatoid factor have an increased frequency of the B-cell alloantigen HLA-DR4, but those who are seronegative do not. HLA-DR3 is more closely associated with systemic lupus erythematosus, HLA-B27 with the spondylarthropathies, and HLA-B13 and HLA-DR7 with psoriatic arthritis. These HLA associations suggest genetic susceptibility to certain rheumatic diseases.

4. The answer is B. (*VIII D*) The central pathogenetic mechanism in polymyositis seems to be a leukocyte-mediated attack against muscle cells. Although tissue autoantibodies are demonstrated by most patients with polymyositis, these may be only markers for disease and have not been shown to participate in the muscle damage. Vasculitis can be a feature of the childhood form of the disease but rarely is found in the adult form. Ongoing viral or toxoplasmal infections have not been shown to be the cause of polymyositis.

5. The answer is A. (*VII D*) Vascular endothelial cell injury by unknown mechanisms (possibly toxins or autoimmune attack) is believed to be the pathologic basis of systemic sclerosis. Vascular hyperreactivity apparently occurs as a response of the endothelial cell to injury, although severe skin or visceral Raynaud's phenomenon could result in additional injury. Increased production of renin and angiotensin occurs in some patients as a response to renal ischemia, and microangiopathic hemolysis can occur in severe cases, usually in association with malignant hypertension and renal failure. Inflammatory vasculitis rarely is present in systemic sclerosis.

6. The answer is D. (*VII E 2 a–b*) Of the clinical manifestations listed, only renal disease is more likely to be found in diffuse systemic sclerosis than in the CREST syndrome. Both forms are characterized by esophageal motility dysfunction, distal skin thickening, and Raynaud's phenomenon. Telangiectasias also can occur in both forms of systemic sclerosis, although they are more common and widespread in the CREST syndrome. Pulmonary involvement may be less severe early in the CREST syndrome, beginning as pulmonary hypertension, but it becomes more prominent as the disease progresses. Diffuse pulmonary fibrosis occurs commonly in the diffuse form and has a variable progression.

7. The answer is C (2, 4). (*VI H 4 b*) Systemic glucocorticoids often are necessary for the treatment of central nervous system and renal manifestations of systemic lupus erythematosus (SLE). Photosensitivity and mucous membrane ulcerations are features of SLE that do not require corticosteroids for treatment. In general, less toxic drugs are used to control milder lupus symptoms. Corticosteroids in adequate doses are used for more severe manifestations, and the dosage is tapered when the disease is controlled.

8. The answer is B (1, 3). [*III F 3 b (1), (4) (b)*] Extra-articular manifestations are features of highly-expressed rheumatoid arthritis, and subcutaneous nodules and interstitial lung disease are two of the more common of these expressions. Aortitis and anterior uveitis, on the other hand, are extra-articular features of spondylarthropathies. Finding such features in an inflammatory arthritis may be important for diagnosis, therapy, and prognosis.

9. The answer is A (1, 2, 3). [*III H 3 a (5)*] Inflammatory synovitis in rheumatoid arthritis that does not respond to nonsteroidal anti-inflammatory agents and conservative measures in the first few months of illness usually requires disease-modifying treatment. Certainly, active inflammatory joint disease that is present for longer than 1 year is unlikely to remit spontaneously and typically requires long-term treatment with a drug such as gold. Progressive deformities and radiographic evidence of erosive disease suggest more advanced, destructive disease and are even more compelling reasons to begin treatment with a disease-modifying drug. Chronic joint pain in rheumatoid arthritis can be caused by factors other than inflammatory synovitis (e.g., degenerative joint disease secondary to previous inflammation) and, therefore, does not require treatment with disease-modifying agents in all cases.

10. The answer is B (1, 3). [*III H 3 a (5) (a); VI H 3*] Antimalarial drugs, especially hydroxychloroquine, have proven to be effective for treating the joint complaints of rheumatoid arthritis and systemic lupus erythematosus (SLE) as well as the skin disease of SLE. These drugs are slow acting; a period of 3 months may be needed to evaluate their effectiveness. Ophthalmologic examination at 6-month intervals is required to monitor for macular pigmentary retinopathy—the most serious toxic effect of antimalarial drugs.

11. The answer is E (all). (*III C; VI C*) Of all the inflammatory rheumatic diseases, the pathogenesis of rheumatoid arthritis and systemic lupus erythematosus (SLE) is best understood. Although no single cause can be identified for these diseases, several factors are believed to interact to cause or perpetuate rheumatoid arthritis and SLE, including altered immune responses (humoral and cellular) and genetic and environmental factors. It is likely that a combination of some or all of these factors also is important in causing or perpetuating other, less-understood rheumatic diseases, such as vasculitic syndromes, polymyositis, systemic sclerosis, and Sjogren's syndrome.

12–16. The answers are: 12-C, 13-E, 14-B, 15-A, 16-D. [*III F 3 b (1); IV B 1 d (3) (a), 2 d (2) (d), 4 b (1); VI F 1 a*] Malar erythema in systemic lupus erythematosus (SLE) can be either flat or raised, but it is fixed—not evanescent as in a blush. Patients with seborrheic dermatitis can have malar erythema, but the nasolabial folds are prominently involved by a scaling erythema; these folds typically are not involved in SLE.

Circinate balanitis is a typical feature of Reiter's syndrome that often is asymptomatic and must be searched for on physical examination. The lesion may appear as a superficial erosion or a scaling, hyperkeratotic plaque of the glans penis.

The lumbar spine and sacroiliac joints characteristically are severely involved in the axial skeletal inflammation of ankylosing spondylitis. Although other spondylarthropathies (e.g., Reiter's syndrome) can have sacroiliac or lumbar spine inflammation, severe limitation of lumbar spinal mobility is unusual in these disorders.

Painless, subcutaneous nodules characteristically are found on extensor surfaces of the forearms in both rheumatoid arthritis and gout. Needle aspiration of a nodule and microscopic inspection of its contents for uric acid crystals should distinguish these disorders.

The peripheral arthritis that occasionally occurs in inflammatory bowel disease usually varies with the activity of the bowel disease. Episodes of gastrointestinal bleeding, chronic diarrhea, and weight loss in an arthritis patient's history should suggest this possible unifying diagnosis.

17–21. The answers are: 17-C, 18-E, 19-A, 20-B, 21-D. [*VI G 2 d (2) (a) (i) (iv); VII F 2 b; VIII G 2 b (1); IX C 2 b*] Precipitating antibody to the acidic nucleoprotein Jo-1 is found in the serum of approximately 30% of polymyositis patients and 10% of dermatomyositis patients; it may be a marker for interstitial lung disease. Antibody to Jo-1 is not detectable by routine antinuclear antibody testing and is not found in patients with systemic lupus erythematosus (SLE), systemic sclerosis, or rheumatoid arthritis.

Antibodies to centromere components are found in 90% of patients with the CREST form and 50% of patients with the diffuse form of systemic sclerosis, when antinuclear antibody determinations are performed against human tissue culture lines (e.g., Hep 2). This antibody may help to identify those patients with Raynaud's phenomenon who are at risk for developing a form of systemic sclerosis.

Antibodies to two closely related RNA-protein complexes—Sm and RNP—can be demonstrated in patients who have high titers of speckled antinuclear antibodies. Isotonic buffer extraction of antibodies after passive hemagglutination discloses the presence of one of these two extractable nuclear antigens (ENA). The Sm form of ENA is characterized by resistance to destruction by RNAse and trypsin and typically is found in patients with SLE. On the other hand, the RNP form of ENA, is destroyed by incubation with RNAse or trypsin and classically is found in mixed connective tissue disease.

Antibodies to the soluble nucleoproteins Ro (SS-A) and La (SS-B) most often are found together in Sjögren's syndrome. Antibody to Ro also is a marker for SLE and for the neonatal lupus syndrome, but when it is found in these diseases antibody to La usually is not present.

Antibody to native (double-stranded) DNA is commonly present in patients with SLE and may be a relatively specific finding in this disorder. In some patients, the presence and titer of the antibody varies with disease activity. Antibody to double-stranded DNA is thought to be important in the immune complexes that cause renal damage in SLE.

Post-test

QUESTIONS

Directions: Each question below contains five suggested answers. Choose the **one best** response to each question.

1. Which of the following statements best characterizes the physical signs noted in aortic regurgitation?
(A) A large increase in stroke volume occurs acutely, producing many of the physical signs present in this disease
(B) Concentric left ventricular hypertrophy is the major compensatory mechanism
(C) A low-pitched, diastolic blowing murmur is heard best when the patient is lying down
(D) The presence of an Austin Flint murmur indicates moderate-to-severe insufficiency
(E) Quincke's pulse is elicited best in the femoral artery

2. Cellular immunodeficiencies are diagnosed by

(A) inability to demonstrate T-cell functional activity in vivo, in vitro, or both
(B) demonstration of diminished antibody-forming ability
(C) inability of T cells to change the dye nitroblue tetrazolium from yellow to blue
(D) failure of neutrophils and macrophages to migrate in response to chemotactic stimuli
(E) failure to produce hemolysis when the patient's serum is added to a system of red cells and anti-red cell antibody

3. Osteomalacia caused by excessive urinary loss of phosphate is characteristic of

(A) vitamin D deficiency
(B) hereditary vitamin D dependency
(C) familial vitamin D resistance
(D) anticonvulsant drugs
(E) severe liver disease

4. A 27-year-old man is referred for evaluation of hematuria. The patient has noted painless gross hematuria two to three times per year for the last 6 years, which has always remitted spontaneously within 1–2 days. On this occasion, bright red blood has appeared in his urine for the past 8 days. He denies any trauma to his kidneys or any other recent illnesses. Although he has a younger brother with sickle cell anemia, the patient has been free from any symptoms of this abnormality, and there is no other known family history or evidence of any other renal disease, including kidney stones and infection. Urinalysis reveals red-to-pink urine, with numerous red blood cells per high-power field, and no proteinuria on ortho-toluidine dipstick test. At this point, the most likely diagnosis is

(A) nephrolithiasis
(B) carcinoma of the kidney
(C) renal vein thrombosis
(D) prostatitis
(E) sickle cell trait

5. All of the following statements concerning therapy for congestive heart failure are true EXCEPT

(A) diuretics act primarily to reduce cardiac filling pressure
(B) catecholamines are administered intravenously to treat acute reversible heart failure
(C) digoxin is the drug of choice for the chronic treatment of heart failure
(D) captopril acts to reduce ventricular end-diastolic volume
(E) amrinone is a potent inotropic agent useful in the acute treatment of heart failure

6. Patients in which of the following subsets of juvenile rheumatoid arthritis are at greatest risk for developing chronic, erosive, disabling arthritis?

(A) Oligoarthritis and anterior uveitis
(B) Axial skeletal oligoarthritis
(C) Systemic-onset juvenile rheumatoid arthritis
(D) Polyarticular arthritis, seropositive for rheumatoid factor
(E) Juvenile-onset ankylosing spondylitis

7. A 50-year-old woman complains of redness, swelling, and stiffness in the distal interphalangeal joints of the hands without other joint complaints. The most likely diagnosis is

(A) erosive osteoarthritis
(B) rheumatoid arthritis
(C) systemic lupus erythematosus
(D) ankylosing spondylitis
(E) systemic sclerosis

8. A renal biopsy to determine the nature of glomerular disease in a patient with heavy proteinuria is absolutely contraindicated if the patient

(A) has a diastolic blood pressure of 120 mm Hg
(B) has a serum creatinine level of 2.5 mg/dl (normal = 0.8–1.4 mg/dl)
(C) is 65 years of age or older
(D) has nephrotic syndrome with no evidence of renal tubular casts
(E) has undergone a previous renal biopsy

9. When specimens are collected for the microbiology laboratory, all of these rules should be followed EXCEPT

(A) specimens should be delivered as quickly as possible
(B) specimens should be refrigerated if immediate transport is not possible
(C) large specimens should be submitted when possible
(D) specimens should be marked when *Francisella* is considered a likely pathogen
(E) prereduced transport vessels should be used when anaerobes are considered likely pathogens

10. A 23-year-old man is evaluated because of a diagnosis of hypogonadism. Which of the following findings would suggest primary testicular disease rather than hypothalamic or pituitary disease?

(A) Anosmia
(B) Increased levels of follicle-stimulating hormone (FSH) and luteinizing hormone (LH)
(C) Eunuchoidal habitus
(D) Loss of libido and potency
(E) Decreased sperm number and motility

11. A patient receiving high-dose corticosteroid therapy is more susceptible to infection than a similar patient not receiving steroids by all of the following microorganisms EXCEPT

(A) *Cryptococcus* species
(B) *Mycobacterium* species
(C) *Nocardia* species
(D) *Neisseria* species
(E) *Listeria* species

12. A 55-year-old man who has smoked 30 cigarettes daily since he was 25 is seen because of hemoptysis. He denies symptoms except for cough, which produces 5–10 ml of sputum each morning. Results found on physical examination and x-ray are normal. The most likely cause of this man's hemoptysis is

(A) bronchogenic carcinoma
(B) pulmonary tuberculosis
(C) bronchiectasis
(D) α_1-antitrypsin deficiency
(E) chronic bronchitis

13. In a patient with primary lung carcinoma, all of the following factors would preclude surgical cure EXCEPT

(A) growth in a bronchus within 2 cm of the carina
(B) invasion of the chest wall
(C) metastases to the ipsilateral hilar lymph nodes
(D) associated vocal cord paralysis
(E) metastases to the mediastinal lymph nodes

14. All of the following statements concerning gastric carcinoma are true EXCEPT

(A) the incidence in the United States has continued to increase over the past 60 years
(B) the 5-year survival rate is only 12%
(C) atrophic gastritis and gastric polyps are considered premalignant lesions
(D) family members of patients with gastric carcinoma have an increased risk
(E) gross gastrointestinal bleeding is rare

15. A 30-year-old pregnant woman complains of urinary frequency and urgency as well as painful urination, but she has no fever or flank pain. Urinalysis reveals pyuria, and *Klebsiella pneumoniae* is identified on urine culture (bacterial count = 10^5/ml). Blood culture, however, is negative. Which of the following infections is this woman most likely suffering from?

(A) Cystitis
(B) Vaginitis
(C) Urethritis
(D) Pyelonephritis
(E) None of the above

16. The syndrome of painless thyroiditis can best be distinguished from Graves' disease by the finding of

(A) thyroid enlargement
(B) low blood thyroid-stimulating hormone (TSH) levels
(C) elevated blood thyroxine levels
(D) low radioactive iodine uptake
(E) tenderness and pain involving the thyroid gland

17. Which of the following statements best describes amebic liver abscess?

(A) It must be drained surgically
(B) It can be caused by any of the six *Entamoeba* species
(C) In the United States, it is most common in homosexual men and institutionalized patients
(D) It usually is suggested by a history of intestinal amebiasis
(E) It usually is seen in patients with normal serum alkaline phosphatase but elevated serum transaminases

18. All of the following are mediators of immediate hypersensitivity EXCEPT

(A) serotonin
(B) bradykinin
(C) eosinophil chemotactic factors of anaphylaxis
(D) basophil chemotactic factor
(E) neutrophil chemotactic factor

19. What feature do hepatitis A, hepatitis B, and non-A, non-B hepatitis have in common?

(A) Transmission by contaminated food or water
(B) Association with blood transfusions
(C) Increase of serum transaminase levels
(D) They may lead to a chronic carrier state
(E) They may be accompanied by delta virus infection

20. A 28-year-old architect is referred for evaluation of a cause of nephrolithiasis. The patient has had six kidney stones over the last 5 years, with the most recent one requiring surgical removal. He denies any history of urinary tract infections, but his father and paternal grandfather both had kidney stones. On physical examination, he is found to be normotensive; all other findings are normal. Laboratory studies reveal normal serum chemistries, including calcium, phosphorus, and magnesium determinations. Urinary determinations of calcium phosphate, uric acid, and protein also are normal. Urinalysis reveals a urine pH of 5 and occasional hexagonal crystals. What is the most likely etiology of this patient's nephrolithiasis?

(A) Calcium oxalate stones
(B) Uric acid stones
(C) Cystine stones
(D) Calcium phosphate stones
(E) Magnesium-ammonium-calcium phosphate (struvite) stones

21. All of the following clinical findings are seen in patients with pulmonary embolism EXCEPT

(A) hypoxia
(B) right-sided heart failure
(C) cyanosis
(D) deep venous thrombosis
(E) bradycardia

22. A patient with chronic renal failure due to long-standing, severe hypertension is seen because of chest pain. The patient has received hemodialysis twice weekly for the last 2 years. The major problem on dialysis has been recent episodes of hypotension at the beginning of treatment. The chest pain is located over the trapezius muscle and is moderately reduced by assuming the upright position but exacerbated by deep breathing. The most likely cause of this patient's chest pain is

(A) pericarditis
(B) coronary artery disease
(C) diffuse esophageal spasm
(D) pulmonary embolism
(E) costochondritis

Directions: Each question below contains four suggested answers of which **one or more** is correct. Choose the answer

A   if **1, 2, and 3** are correct
B   if **1 and 3** are correct
C   if **2 and 4** are correct
D   if **4** is correct
E   if **1, 2, 3, and 4** are correct

23. A young woman has episodes of sweating and palpitations and is suspected of having an insulinoma. Findings that support this diagnosis include

(1) low serum glucose level and undetectable serum insulin level during a typical attack
(2) occurrence of attacks several hours after meals
(3) low serum level of proinsulin
(4) high serum level of C-peptide following insulin infusion

24. Urate deposition in tissues of gout patients can be reversed with administration of

(1) colchicine
(2) allopurinol
(3) indomethacin
(4) probenecid

25. Physical signs of pulmonary embolism include

(1) wheezing
(2) loud aortic component (A_2) of the second heart sound (S_2)
(3) neck vein distension
(4) bradycardia

26. Signs of severe aortic stenosis noted on physical examination include

(1) a harsh, late-peaking systolic ejection murmur
(2) a loud aortic component (A_2) of the second heart sound (S_2)
(3) a delayed carotid upstroke
(4) a diastolic rumble

27. Disseminated intravascular coagulation is an acquired coagulopathy that is associated with which of the following conditions?

(1) Amniotic fluid embolism
(2) Lowered platelet levels
(3) Infections with gram-negative organisms
(4) Elevated levels of fibrin degradation products

28. Independent prognostic factors in breast carcinoma include

(1) estrogen receptor status
(2) size of primary tumor
(3) pathology of primary tumor
(4) presence of lymph node metastasis in axillae

29. Urticarial lesions usually demonstrate which of the following characteristics?

(1) They blanch with pressure
(2) They last longer than 48 hours
(3) They are circumscribed
(4) They do not coalesce

30. When used to treat hypertension, β-adrenergic blocking agents act to

(1) block the conversion of angiotensin I to angiotensin II
(2) decrease cardiac output
(3) decrease intravascular volume
(4) decrease renin release from the kidney

31. Drugs that are believed to be disease-modifying agents in rheumatoid arthritis include

(1) D-penicillamine
(2) glucocorticoids
(3) gold compounds
(4) nonsteroidal anti-inflammatory drugs

32. The two major forms of acute meningitis—bacterial and aseptic—both are characterized by

(1) headache and stiff neck
(2) leukocyte pleocytosis
(3) increased cerebrospinal fluid (CSF) protein
(4) decreased CSF glucose (i.e., to less than half of the serum level)

33. Gastroenteritis may produce which of the following simple acid-base disturbances?

(1) Respiratory alkalosis
(2) Metabolic alkalosis
(3) Respiratory acidosis
(4) Metabolic acidosis

34. Factors that have been associated with an increased incidence of head and neck carcinomas include

(1) alcohol
(2) tobacco
(3) Epstein-Barr virus
(4) hepatitis B virus

35. A patient with a recent change in mental status is found to have a serum sodium level of 119 mmol/L. The serum osmolality is 265 mOsm/kg, and the urine osmolality is 350 mOsm/kg. Urine sodium excretion is 85 mmol/24 hr. Possible causes for this syndrome include

(1) pulmonary tuberculosis
(2) demeclocycline
(3) chlorpropamide
(4) sodium depletion

36. A 25-year-old woman comes to the emergency room with an acutely tender, swollen, and red left knee. Aspiration yields 30 ml of cloudy joint fluid, and Gram staining reveals only an abundance of white cells. The diagnostic workup of this patient should include

(1) examination for tenosynovitis
(2) cervical and pharyngeal cultures for *Neisseria gonorrhoeae*
(3) bacterial cultures of joint fluid
(4) careful cutaneous examination for skin lesions

37. Causes of thrombocytopathia (i.e., reduced platelet function) include

(1) uremia
(2) hemophilia A
(3) aspirin ingestion
(4) idiopathic thrombocytopenic purpura

38. True statements regarding nephrotic syndrome in patients under the age of 15 include

(1) the prognosis is poor, with most children developing chronic renal failure
(2) children who receive glucocorticoids for minimal change disease have a 10% remission rate for nephrotic syndrome
(3) the light microscopic findings from renal biopsies unequivocally reveal the nature of the underlying disease
(4) the most common etiology is minimal change disease

39. Colonic diverticula may be asymptomatic, but when symptoms do occur they are likely to

(1) result from bacterial overgrowth within the diverticula
(2) include crampy lower abdominal pain with alternating diarrhea and constipation
(3) respond to metoclopramide
(4) mimic symptoms of acute appendicitis when in the presence of infection

40. Features of chest pain that suggest it is due to coronary artery disease include

(1) radiation to the forehead
(2) sudden onset
(3) exacerbation with nitroglycerin
(4) onset with exertion and relief with rest

41. Findings in patients with Turner's syndrome are likely to include

(1) a chromatin-positive buccal smear
(2) lack of breast development
(3) normal ovaries
(4) amenorrhea

42. The complexity of the immune system is evident through its capability of

(1) specific and nonspecific immunity
(2) a stronger response to an antigen when it is encountered a second time
(3) response to an unlimited number of antigens
(4) response both with production of a specific antibody and with committed small lymphocytes

Directions: The groups of questions below consist of lettered choices followed by several numbered items. For each numbered item select the **one** lettered choice with which it is **most** closely associated. Each lettered choice may be used once, more than once, or not at all.

Questions 43–47

The table below shows arterial blood gas data for 5 patients who are denoted by the letters A–E. For each of the following clinical conditions, select the patient with the appropriate group of data.

	PO_2 (mm Hg)	O_2 Saturation (%)	PCO_2 (mm Hg)	$[HCO_3^-]$ (mmol/L)	pH
(A)	120	99	20	19	7.60
(B)	104	99	24	12	7.25
(C)	81	95	51	45	7.58
(D)	62	92	34	23	7.46
(E)	38	65	65	26.2	7.22

43. Fulminant status asthmaticus

44. Long-standing pyloric obstruction

45. Hysterical hyperventilation

46. Diabetic ketoacidosis

47. Emphysematous chronic obstructive pulmonary disease

Questions 48–52

For each clinical situation, select the disease state with which it is most closely associated.

(A) Chronic lymphocytic leukemia (CLL)
(B) Chronic myeloid leukemia (CML)
(C) Both CLL and CML
(D) Neither CLL nor CML

48. Elevated leukocyte alkaline phosphatase level

49. Elevated lymphocyte count

50. Slow, steady disease progression

51. Termination in acute leukemia

52. Splenomegaly

Questions 53–56

Match the variant of Hodgkin's disease to its appropriate histologic classification.

(A) Lymphocyte predominance
(B) Lymphocyte depletion
(C) Nodular sclerosis
(D) Mixed cellularity

53. Hodgkin's disease that involves the mediastinum, is characterized by an early age of onset, and is more common in women than in men

54. Hodgkin's disease that occurs most commonly in men over age 50 and has a poor prognosis

55. Hodgkin's disease that is localized and has an excellent prognosis

56. Hodgkin's disease that is characterized by a variable age of onset and a fair prognosis

Questions 57–60

For each description of a patient with allergic rhinitis, select the most appropriate therapeutic intervention.

(A) Antigen avoidance
(B) Immunotherapy against known offending antigens
(C) Antihistamine-decongestant preparation
(D) Nasal cromolyn sodium
(E) Topical sympathomimetic agent

57. A 34-year-old woman with significant perennial allergic rhinitis loses 10–15 days of work each year as a result of secondary sinusitis. Immediate skin tests show significant positive reactions to house dust, *Cladosporium*, and grass and ragweed pollens. A variety of pharmacologic preparations are only partially successful in controlling symptoms.

58. A 20-year-old man has mild but persistent year-round symptoms of nasal congestion, rhinorrhea, and watery eyes. Immediate skin tests show positive reactions to house dust, *Alternaria*, and grass and ragweed pollens.

59. A 10-year-old girl develops rhinorrhea and nasal pruritus whenever she visits the home of a friend whose family has just acquired a kitten.

60. An 8-year-old boy regularly experiences moderate sneezing spells and watery eyes in May and June, September and October, and occasionally during January through March. Immediate skin tests show positive reactions to *Alternaria*, *Cladosporium*, house dust, and grass and ragweed pollens.

ANSWERS AND EXPLANATIONS

1. The answer is D. [*Chapter 1 III C 3 b (2)–(4)*] An Austin Flint murmur (diastolic rumble) probably occurs when a large amount of regurgitation from the aortic valve strikes the mitral valve, generating the murmur. In acute aortic regurgitation, there is little time for ventricular dilatation and, thus, little increase in stroke volume; therefore, many of the signs of aortic regurgitation often are absent acutely. Eccentric rather than concentric hypertrophy is the rule in aortic regurgitation. Eccentric hypertrophy allows for increased chamber size and reestablishment of forward stroke volume. A diastolic blowing murmur is characteristic of aortic insufficiency, but it is high-pitched and best heard when the patient is sitting up and leaning forward. Quincke's pulse is seen in the nail beds.

2. The answer is A. (*Chapter 7 I C 1 b*) The cellular immunodeficiencies are characterized by dysfunction of the T cells, and this defect is demonstrated by methods that examine T-cell functioning. Diagnostic procedures include both in vivo methods of skin testing to ubiquitous antigens and observation of the time needed to reject a skin homograft and in vitro tests quantifying lymphocyte responses to mitogens, antigens, and allogeneic cells. Since the prognosis is serious, the cellular immunodeficiencies usually are tested by multiple methods. Diminished antibody-forming ability is an indication of an antibody deficiency syndrome—not a cellular immunodeficiency. The nitroblue tetrazolium dye (NBT) test is used to identify microbicidal disorders of phagocytes (neutrophils and microphages); failure of these cells to migrate toward a chemotactic stimulus indicates a chemotactic disorder such as lazy leukocyte syndrome. One way to diagnose complement component deficiencies is through functional assays that measure hemolysis.

3. The answer is C. [*Chapter 9 VIII A 2 a, b, c (2)*] Familial vitamin D-resistant rickets is characterized by excessive excretion of phosphate in the urine; the cause of this is not understood. Vitamin D deficiency prevents normal gastrointestinal absorption of calcium and phosphorus. Liver disease and anticonvulsant drugs may impair the hepatic conversion of vitamin D to 25-hydroxyvitamin D_3. In hereditary vitamin D-dependent rickets, there is impaired conversion of 25-hydroxyvitamin D_3 to 1,25-dihydroxyvitamin D_3.

4. The answer is E. [*Chapter 6 Part I: VI B; VIII C 2; X C 1; XV B 1, F 2 (b); XVI A 2 a (2)*] Sickle cell trait, nephrolithiasis, carcinoma of the kidney, renal vein thrombosis, and prostatitis all may be associated with hematuria. The finding of gross hematuria in a young man with a family history of sickle cell anemia, however, strongly suggests that, in the absence of other stigmata of sickle cell disease, he suffers from sickle cell trait. This abnormality commonly is associated with hematuria and is due to sickling of red blood cells in the vessels on the surface of the renal pelvis and papilla, leading to small areas of infarction and bleeding. Renal tumor can produce bleeding, but it is rarely so persistent in the absence of other symptoms. Renal vein thrombosis can produce hematuria but usually in the setting of severe pain and proteinuria. Nephrolithiasis also may produce relatively silent hematuria if the stone has been present for a long period of time, but pain typically is associated. Urinary tract infection also can be associated with hematuria, but symptoms of infection (e.g., dysuria and fever) should be present.

5. The answer is C. [*Chapter 1 I F 2 a (1)–(3), c (1)*] The use of digoxin in the chronic treatment of congestive heart failure is controversial, and digoxin is not necessarily the drug of choice (e.g., in Great Britain). By reducing intravascular volume, diuretics also reduce cardiac filling pressure. Captopril, which reduces both preload and afterload, allows for reduced cardiac filling and increased cardiac emptying, with a resultant decrease in both end-diastolic and end-systolic cardiac volumes. The use of β-adrenergic agonists (e.g., catecholamines) is limited to intravenous treatment of acute reversible heart failure.

6. The answer is D. [*Chapter 10 V E 2 c (1)*] The subset of juvenile rheumatoid arthritis patients most likely to develop chronic, erosive, and severe arthritis is the polyarticular group that is seropositive for rheumatoid factor. This form of the disease also is the one that is most similar to adult rheumatoid arthritis and most likely to require disease-modifying treatment such as gold.

7. The answer is A. (*Chapter 10 I E 1 b*) Erosive osteoarthritis typically involves the distal interphalangeal joints in middle-aged women. It is unlikely that such prominent distal joint symptoms would occur in a patient with rheumatoid arthritis or systemic lupus erythematosus without more generalized joint complaints. No evidence is presented to suggest ankylosing spondylitis or systemic sclerosis.

8. The answer is A. (*Chapter 6 Part I: I D 2*) Hypertension is an absolute contraindication to performing a renal biopsy since there is a high (75%) incidence of subclinical bleeding at the site of a renal biopsy. In a hypertensive patient, this bleeding may lead to a major, life-threatening hemorrhage. Mild renal insufficiency (as evidenced by a small decrease in creatinine clearance), nephrotic syndrome without urinary casts, and moderately advanced age are not contraindications to performing a renal biopsy.

9. The answer is B. (*Chapter 8 III A 1–3*) All efforts should be directed toward preserving the viability of potential pathogens after specimen collection. Large specimens prevent drying and provide more organisms to start with. Fresh specimens allow the laboratory to make an identification more quickly, and time spent in transport should be under favorable conditions of atmosphere, humidity, and temperature. Refrigeration is permissible for some specimens (e.g., urine) but is forbidden for others (e.g., cervical cultures for *Neisseria gonorrhoeae*). When there is doubt, a technologist should be consulted for information about appropriate transport. It is important to provide information about potential hazards such as tularemia (caused by *Francisella tularensis*) so as not to jeopardize the health of laboratory workers.

10. The answer is B. (*Chapter 9 VII A 1, 2*) Increased gonadotropin production indicates primary testicular failure with negative-feedback stimulation of the hypothalamic-pituitary axis. Hypogonadism, whether caused by hypothalamic-pituitary disease or by testicular disease, is associated with loss of libido and potency and abnormalities of sperm production. A eunuchoidal habitus results from continued growth of long bones due to delay in testosterone-induced epiphyseal closure. Anosmia is sometimes associated with hypothalamic failure to secrete GnRH.

11. The answer is D. (*Chapter 8 IV I*) Corticosteroid administration results in increased susceptibility to a variety of microorganisms. The list resembles the list of agents to which patients with Hodgkin's disease or acquired immune deficiency syndrome (AIDS) are vulnerable. Cryptococcal infection, most commonly meningitis, is a rare infection overall, but at least half of all patients have some type of immune depression. Because steroids can unmask latent infection caused by *Mycobacterium tuberculosis*, prophylactic isoniazid is recommended for those steroid recipients who have had prior exposure to the tubercle bacillus and who are skin test (PPD) positive. Nocardial infections, usually involving the lungs or brain, occur in patients receiving long-term corticosteroids for a variety of indications including immune diseases (e.g., systemic lupus erythematosus) and organ transplantation. *Listeria monocytogenes* causes serious infection in infants who are otherwise healthy and in adults who are immunosuppressed by steroids or lymphoreticular malignancy. Neisserial infections occur most commonly in previously healthy individuals without immune dysfunction. A rare condition, the deficiency of one of the terminal complement components (i.e., C5–C9) may predispose to such infections, but steroids seldom are implicated.

12. The answer is E. [*Chapter 2 I A 1 a, B 3, E 2 a (1), (2), F; III A 3, 4; IX E 1 b*] By definition (i.e., cough and sputum production), this patient has chronic bronchitis. Normal results on chest x-ray do not absolutely rule out carcinoma but make it unlikely. The same is true for tuberculosis and bronchiectasis. A smoker in this age-group would require bronchoscopy for evaluation if the hemoptysis did not subside soon or if the clinical situation changed. Alpha$_1$-antitrypsin deficiency is a genetic factor that is known to predispose to emphysema. Unlike chronic bronchitis, emphysema is associated with little or no cough and expectoration.

13. The answer is C. [*Chapter 4 IX F a (1)*] Surgery is the primary therapy for non-oat cell lung cancers. Patients with such tumors are evaluated to determine whether they are candidates for surgery. Accepted criteria for nonresectability include invasion of the mediastinum (e.g., recurrent laryngeal nerve with vocal cord paralysis and metastases to the mediastinal and contralateral hilar lymph nodes), invasion of the chest wall or pleural effusions, and local growth that precludes an adequate surgical margin (e.g., growth within 2 cm of the carina). Metastases to the ipsilateral hilar lymph nodes do not preclude surgery.

14. The answer is A. (*Chapter 5 II B 1*) The incidence of gastric carcinoma in the United States has decreased over the past 60 years, although it remains high in eastern Europe and Japan. The etiology is unknown, but several premalignant conditions have been identified, and a genetic factor is implied by the increased incidence in family members. Anemia from chronic low-grade blood loss is common, but gross gastrointestinal blood loss occurs in only 10% of patients. The prognosis is poor, with only 12% of patients surviving for 5 years.

15. The answer is A. (*Chapter 8 V H 1 c; I 3–5*) Infections associated with the genitourinary systems are distinguished clinically and on the basis of a few laboratory tests. Lower urinary tract infections, which present with irritative voiding symptoms but no fever or flank pain, are arbitrarily divided into cystitis (when the urine bacterial count exceeds 10^5/ml) or the urethral syndrome (when the urine bacterial count is less than 10^5/ml). Pyelonephritis may be difficult to distinguish from cystitis but often causes flank pain and fever; in addition, positive blood cultures occur only in upper tract infections. Patients with the urethral syndrome may have illnesses that mimic urinary tract infections, such as vaginitis or urethritis. However, both of these infections may cause a discharge, which does not occur in urinary tract infections. A urine bacterial count exceeding 10^5/ml may be noted in a patient without irritative voiding symptoms. This entity—termed asymptomatic bacteriuria—should be treated in certain clinical settings (e.g., pregnancy).

16. The answer is D. [*Chapter 9 II D 3 b (3)*] Inflammation and injury to thyroid cells as well as lack of thyroid-stimulating hormone (TSH), inhibit radioactive iodine uptake in painless thyroiditis, while the uninjured and immunoglobulin-stimulated thyroid cells in Graves' disease concentrate radioactive iodine at an increased rate. Enlargement of the thyroid gland and increased blood levels of thyroid hormone, with suppression of TSH, may occur in both Graves' disease and painless thyroiditis. The gland is not tender or painful in either condition.

17. The answer is C. (*Chapter 5 IX B 3 a*) Amebic liver abscess is common in areas of the world where intestinal amebiasis is endemic. In the United States, it usually is seen in institutionalized patients and homosexual men, among whom there is a high incidence of intestinal amebiasis. Despite this, only 50% of patients with amebic liver disease have a clear history of intestinal disease. As with most other mass lesions of the liver, the serum alkaline phosphatase is elevated more often (in 80% of patients) than are the transaminases (in 50% of patients). Medical therapy usually is adequate.

18. The answer is D. (*Chapter 7 II A 2 d*) There is no mediator designated as basophil chemotactic factor, but factors chemotactic for basophils, neutrophils, monocytes, and eosinophils have been described. A factor augmenting the chemotactic response of basophils may play an important role in certain delayed hypersensitivity reactions. Mediators of immediate hypersensitivity include histamine, eosinophil chemotactic factors of anaphylaxis, neutrophil chemotactic factor, serotonin, slow-reacting substance of anaphylaxis, platelet activating factor, bradykinin, kallikrein (which cleaves kininogen to form bradykinin), and prostaglandins.

19. The answer is C. (*Chapter 8 V F 1 a, c*) Acute viral hepatitis is a disease that is characterized by jaundice and elevation of serum transaminase and bilirubin levels; serum levels of alkaline phosphatase and other inducible enzymes of the biliary system are normal or mildly increased. The route of transmission distinguishes these infections. Hepatitis A virus is excreted in the feces and can be transmitted by direct fecal-oral contact or by food or water that has been contaminated by infective feces. Hepatitis B and non-A, non-B hepatitis are transmitted by contact with human blood. These forms of hepatitis can give rise to a chronic carrier state. Hepatitis B virus uniquely is associated with the delta agent—a defective RNA virus that requires hepatitis B proteins to form its coat.

20. The answer is C. (*Chapter 6 Part I: VIII B 1–5*) The patient's clinical presentation is typical of any patient with kidney stone disease. In more than 90% of patients, nephrolithiasis is due to calcium oxalate stone formation. In 50% of those individuals, hypercalciuria is present. In the absence of hypercalciuria and with the finding of hexagonal crystals in the urine, the physician must be highly suspicious that this patient has cystinuria. A urinalysis revealing cystine crystals is seen in approximately 40%–50% of patients; however, negative urinalysis should not deter the physician from measuring a 24-hour urinary cystine excretion. An initial presentation of cystinuria at age 25 or 30 is not unusual; in fact, patients in their 70s and 80s who passed their first cystine-containing stone have been described. The condition is an autosomal dominant trait, but a variety of phenotypic forms may be seen.

Treatment of cystine stones includes maintaining high urine flow rates (i.e., up to 4–5 L/day) and urine alkalinization if a urine pH value over 7.5 can be achieved by sodium bicarbonate administration. Cystine solubility is approximately 100 mg/L; therefore, if an individual excretes between 300 and 400 mg/24 hr, high fluid intake may prevent further stone formation. If, however, excretion is greater than 700 or 800 mg/24 hr, patients often may require D-penicillamine, a compound that forms mixed disulfides with cystine and renders cystine much more soluble in the urine.

If the patient in question had not had cystine demonstrated in his urine, the next critical test would have been an analysis of the kidney stone.

21. The answer is E. [*Chapter 2 VII E 1 a (1)–(2), F 1 b, 4 a*] Patients with pulmonary embolism can demonstrate all of the clinical findings listed with the exception of bradycardia. Some degree of hypoxia is noted in most patients, and evidence of deep venous thrombosis is seen in about 50% of patients with pulmonary embolism. Right-sided heart failure and cyanosis are apparent only in cases of massive pulmonary embolism, when more than 50% of the pulmonary circulation is compromised. Tachycardia, not bradycardia, is one of the most frequent electrocardiographic findings in patients with pulmonary embolism.

22. The answer is A. (*Chapter 6 Part I: III E 2*) The chest pain experienced by this patient is typical of pericarditis and inflammation of the pericardium, which are common complications in chronic renal failure patients on hemodialysis. These patients also may have inflammation in various serosal linings, including the peritoneum, the pleura, and various joint spaces; the mechanism of this complication is unknown. Although coronary artery disease is common in dialysis patients, the characteristics of the pain in this individual suggest that this is not the diagnosis. Esophageal disease also is common in dialysis patients and should be specifically excluded as a possible cause. In addition, musculoskeletal pain due to various causes is typically seen in dialysis patients and may be due to the abnormalities of calcium and phosphorous metabolism, which lead to calcific deposits in various components of the musculoskeletal system.

23. The answer is D (4). (*Chapter 9 IV B 1 b*) When hypoglycemia is caused by an insulinoma, the serum insulin level remains high despite the low glucose level. Attacks typically occur in the fasting state. Proinsulin is produced by insulinomas to a greater extent than it is produced by normal beta cells, and serum levels of proinsulin are usually increased in patients with an insulinoma. Persistence of C peptide in the circulation despite insulin-induced hypoglycemia indicates autonomous endogenous insulin production, and supports the diagnosis of an insulinoma.

24. The answer is C (2, 4). [*Chapter 10 II A 4 d (4)*] Both allopurinol and probenecid decrease the serum level of uric acid—allopurinol by decreasing uric acid production and probenecid by increasing renal excretion of uric acid. In patients with gout, tissue deposition of urate can be reversed by employing such drugs, if a serum uric acid level below 7 mg/dl can be maintained. At such levels, the serum no longer is saturated with uric acid and tissue deposits can be mobilized. Colchicine and indomethacin affect only the inflammatory response excited by the uric acid crystals and have no effect on serum uric acid level or tissue deposition of urate.

25. The answer is B (1, 3). [*Chapter 1 VII C 3 b (4), (5)*] Wheezing and neck vein distension both are signs of pulmonary embolism. Wheezing occurs due to bronchial constriction, probably as a result of histamine and other humoral agents released at the time of the embolization. Neck vein distension occurs due to right heart strain imposed by obstruction of the pulmonary arteries. Pulmonary embolism may lead to pulmonary hypertension and the finding of a loud pulmonary component (P_2) of the second heart sound (S_2) on physical examination. Tachycardia, not bradycardia, commonly is produced by pulmonary embolism.

26. The answer is B (1, 3). (*Chapter 1 III A 3 b*) A delayed carotid upstroke is the most reliable sign of severe aortic stenosis. The ejection murmur in severe aortic stenosis usually is harsh and peaks late in systole, when outflow from the left ventricle is at a maximum. However, the murmur may be quite soft, as decreased outflow in the later stages of the disease reduces the intensity of the murmur. The aortic component (A_2) of the second heart sound (S_2) usually is soft or absent due to limited motion of the valve.

27. The answer is E (all). [*Chapter 3 V D 2 b (1)–(4)*] Disseminated intravascular coagulation (DIC) is initiated by activation of factor VII by abnormal entry of tissue thromboplastins into the circulation (e.g., in obstetric complications and carcinomatosis). DIC also is initiated by abnormal activation of factor XII due to endothelial damage (e.g., with gram-negative sepsis and viremia). The excess thrombin in the circulation consumes coagulation moieties (e.g., platelets, factor VIII, and fibrinogen), which causes plasma levels to drop. Also, secondary activation of fibrinolysis results in elevated levels of fibrin degradation products.

28. The answer is E (all). (*Chapter 4 VIII C 1*) Different pathologic subtypes of breast carcinoma carry different prognoses. For example, patients with medullary carcinomas do well whereas those with inflammatory carcinomas do poorly. The tumor size, the presence or absence of lymph node metastasis in the axillae, and the estrogen receptor status of the tumor all are independent prognostic variables in the cure rate and the 5- to 10-year survival rate of patients with breast carcinoma.

29. The answer is B (1, 3). (*Chapter 7 IV A 1 a*) Urticarial lesions are well-circumscribed, blanch with pressure, occasionally coalesce, and seldom last longer than 48 hours. Acute urticaria is self-limited. Chronic urticaria often persists for years and may occur at variable intervals of time up to 10 years or more.

30. The answer is C (2, 4). [*Chapter 1 VII B 2 b (3), (4), (6), (8)*] After diuretics, β-adrenergic blocking agents are the most-used drugs in the treatment of hypertension. These agents reduce both cardiac output and renin release, which may partly explain their antihypertensive effect. They do not, however, prevent the conversion of angiotensin I to angiotensin II, which is the mechanism of captopril therapy. Intravascular volume may be reduced by the action of diuretic agents.

31. The answer is B (1, 3). [*Chapter 10 III H 3 a (5) (b)–(c)*] Gold and D-penicillamine are two agents that are believed to be disease-modifying in rheumatoid arthritis. These agents have slow-acting, immunomodulatory effects on the joint disease of rheumatoid arthritis without being generally immuno-suppressive. In contrast, glucocorticoids and nonsteroidal anti-inflammatory agents are short-acting agents that suppress pain and acute inflammation but do not suppress the chronic inflammatory lesion of rheumatoid arthritis.

32. The answer is A (1, 2, 3). [*Chapter 8 V B 1 a (1)*] Acute meningitis is an inflammatory process in-volving the arachnoid layer of the meninges and the cerebrospinal fluid (CSF). Two major forms of acute meningitis are recognized—bacterial and aseptic. Because the two forms have a similar clinical presentation of fever, headache, and stiff neck, the interpretation of CSF findings is important in the management of acute meningitis. Aside from a diagnostic Gram stain, lowered CSF glucose (i.e., to less than half of the simultaneous serum level) and the presence of a neutrophil pleocytosis are the most characteristic findings in bacterial meningitis. An increased CSF protein level also is a consistent finding in bacterial meningitis; however, CSF protein may be mildly elevated in the aseptic form as well. The pleocytosis in aseptic meningitis is modest (usually < 100 cells/mm³) and is characterized by a preponderance of lymphocytes.

33. The answer is C (2, 4). [*Chapter 6 Part II: IV D 2 b (2) (a) E 2 a*] Gastroenteritis that is characterized by excessive diarrhea results in bicarbonate loss with the generation of a hyperchloremic metabolic acidosis. Gastroenteritis that is characterized by protracted vomiting with loss of gastric hydrochloric acid leads to a metabolic alkalosis, which is usually maintained by the extracellular fluid volume that results.

34. The answer is A (1, 2, 3). (*Chapter 4 I B 1–3*) The incidence of squamous cell cancers of the head and neck is related strongly to the use of tobacco and to alcohol consumption, and these factors may have a synergistic effect. Epstein-Barr virus is associated with the uncommon nasopharyngeal carcino-ma that occurs in oriental populations.

35. The answer is B (1, 3). [*Chapter 9 I B 1 c, d (2), 2 d*] Pulmonary disorders such as tuberculosis cause the syndrome of inappropriate secretion of antidiuretic hormone (SIADH) through unknown mecha-nisms. Chlorpropamide potentiates the secretion and the renal effects of ADH; it may produce SIADH and may be useful for the treatment of diabetes insipidus. Demeclocycline, on the other hand, blocks the action of ADH and may be used in the treatment of the SIADH. When hyponatremia results from sodium depletion, rather than ADH excess, renal homeostatic mechanisms retain sodium, and urinary sodium excretion is low, usually less than 20 mmol/24 hr.

36. The answer is E (all). (*Chapter 8 V K 1 a–d*) This patient's clinical presentation should suggest bacterial arthritis. Of the most common causes of septic arthritis, *Neisseria gonorrhoeae* is seen most frequently in young, sexually active adults. Although culture of the joint fluid seldom yields this organism, it often is found at other body sites. Even when the Gram stain is negative, bacterial cultures are warranted to help identify the cause of the bacterial arthritis. Disseminated gonococcal infection is characterized by peripheral vesicopustular skin lesions, which may be few in number and must be searched for carefully. Tenosynovitis also is quite common in this syndrome and if present would strongly suggest the diagnosis.

37. The answer is B (1, 3). (*Chapter 3 V C 2 a, b*) Although the exact mechanism is unclear, uremia is believed to cause platelet dysfunction by toxins that alter the factor VIII antigen polymers required for normal platelet function. Aspirin causes thrombocytopathia by inhibiting synthesis of thromboxane A_2, a strong inducer of platelet aggregation. Hemophilia A and hemophilia B are diseases involving coagu-lation factors VIII and IX, respectively; platelet function is not affected in these diseases. Idiopathic thrombocytopenic purpura (ITP) lowers platelet numbers by excessive destruction; individual platelet function, however, is normal or possibly enhanced in ITP.

38. The answer is D (4). (*Chapter 6 Part I: XI B*) In childhood nephrotic syndrome, the most common etiology is minimal change disease, in which no specific histologic findings are seen with light microscopy. Electron microscopy may reveal fusion of the epithelial cell foot processes but no other findings. The prognosis for this condition is quite good with the majority of children going into remis-sion following initial treatment with glucocorticoids. In a small number of patients (10%), progressive renal disease occurs, particularly if nephrotic syndrome recurs throughout childhood and early adulthood. Renal biopsy is not unequivocal in establishing this diagnosis since light microscopic changes in membranous nephropathy or focal glomerulosclerosis may not be evident early in the course of disease.

39. The answer is C (2, 4). (*Chapter 5 V B*) Colonic diverticula are outpouchings of the mucosa of the colon. Although the etiology of colonic diverticula is not fully established, their presence predominant-ly in the descending colon and sigmoid may reflect LaPlace's law since the sigmoid is the narrowest segment of the colon. When uncomplicated by inflammation, colonic diverticula are referred to as diverticulosis, a condition that is associated with only vague symptoms. Inflammation of diverticula, or diverticulitis, causes a clinical picture similar to that seen in acute appendicitis; however, it is the left lower abdomen—not the right—that is involved in diverticulitis. Unlike jejunal diverticula, colonic diverticula are not a site for bacterial overgrowth as the normal colon already is heavily colonized. Metoclopramide causes increased bowel motility and is not used in the treatment of colonic diverticula.

40. The answer is D (4). [*Chapter 1 II A 5 a (1), (3) (a)*] The classic characteristic of angina (chest pain) is its onset with exertion—which increases myocardial oxygen consumption demands beyond coronary arterial capabilities—and its relief with rest. Angina may radiate anywhere from the bridge of the nose to the umbilicus; thus, radiation to the forehead would be distinctly unusual. Typically, angina builds gradually over several minutes and rarely is sudden in onset. Nitroglycerin usually relieves angina due to a fall in wall stress, which diminishes oxygen demands.

41. The answer is C (2, 4). (*Chapter 9 VI A 1 a, b*) The 45,X karyotype of patients with gonadal dysgenesis, or Turner's syndrome, results in a buccal smear that is chromatin-negative, since there is only one X chromosome. In patients with this syndrome, ovaries fail to develop normally. This results in amenorrhea and lack of estrogen-dependent secondary sexual characteristics, such as breast development.

42. The answer is E (all). (*Chapter 7 I A 1; Chapter 8 I B*) Although most discussions of the immune system attempt to present it in a simplified form, it is in reality a very complex system. There are nonspecific barriers such as skin and mucous membranes that can resist infectious agents, and there are highly specific immune defenses that react with the production of specific antibody or with small lymphocytes that attack the potential pathogen. These specific host defenses can respond to any antigen, and they demonstrate immunologic memory in the sense that response to a previously encountered antigen is more rapid and more efficient than the response to the initial encounter.

43–47. The answers are: 43-E, 44-C, 45-A, 46-B, 47-D. [*Chapter 2 I E 2 a (1) (a); II E 2, F 5; Chapter 6 Part II: IV C 1, 2 a, D 2 a (1), 4 b, E 1, 2 a; Chapter 9 IV A 6 a*] The patient denoted by (E) has status asthmaticus with respiratory failure. The patient has retained carbon dioxide from severe airway obstruction (as indicated by an arterial PCO$_2$ above the normal level of 40 mm Hg). The combination of abnormally high PCO$_2$ and abnormally low PO$_2$ (i.e., below the normal level of 80–100 mm Hg) in this patient indicates the presence of respiratory failure.

The blood gas data for the patient denoted by (C) exemplify hydrochloric acid loss from pyloric-outlet obstruction. The high arterial pH (i.e., above the normal value of 7.40), increased arterial PCO$_2$, and increased bicarbonate level (i.e., above the normal level of 24 mmol/L) indicate the presence of metabolic alkalosis with a compensatory respiratory acidosis.

A patient with hysterical hyperventilation has no obvious pulmonary disease and, therefore, should have no alveolar-arterial PO$_2$ gradient. This is the case in the patient denoted by (A). The excessive elimination of carbon dioxide by this patient results in pure respiratory alkalosis, which is characterized by below normal arterial PCO$_2$ and bicarbonate levels and increased arterial pH.

The patient denoted by (B) represents an individual without lung disease but with a primary metabolic acidosis with a compensatory respiratory alkalosis. This condition is defined by a decrease in both arterial pH and arterial bicarbonate concentration and a lower than predicted arterial PCO$_2$ value (as determined using Winter's formula). This condition is seen in patients with diabetic ketoacidosis.

The patient denoted by (D) shows signs of the emphysematous type of chronic obstructive pulmonary disease (COPD). (The other classic type of COPD—bronchitic COPD—is dominated by signs and symptoms of chronic bronchitis.) Pulmonary function testing in patients with emphysematous COPD reveals only mild hypoxia and hypocapnea, which are demonstrated in this patient by slight decreases in oxygen saturation and arterial PCO$_2$. In contrast, patients with bronchitic COPD demonstrate severe hypoxia and hypocapnea on pulmonary function testing.

48–52. The answers are: 48-D, 49-A, 50-A, 51-B, 52-C. [*Chapter 3 III A 2, B 3 a (3)*] Chronic lymphocytic leukemia (CLL) is a steadily progressive disease characterized by an accumulation of mature lymphocytes in the tissues and peripheral blood. Clinical manifestations of CLL vary with the extent of disease progression, which is broken down into stages (0 through 4). Examples include splenomegaly (a stage 2 CLL presentation) and anemia (a stage 3 CLL presentation). In time, CLL causes marrow failure and death.

Chronic myeloid leukemia (CML) is characterized by excessive granulocytes and granulocyte precursors in the blood and tissues. These cells lack the normal leukocyte alkaline phosphatase level. Splenomegaly is a common finding with CML. This disease, which often terminates in acute leukemia, is characterized by an accelerated progression.

53–56. The answers are: 53-C, 54-B, 55-A, 56-D. (*Chapter 4 XI C; Table 10-1*) Four histologically distinct forms of Hodgkin's disease exist, all of which have the common characteristic of the presence of Reed-Sternberg cells.

The nodular sclerosis variety of Hodgkin's disease classically presents as mediastinal involvement in young women. Usually, patients respond very well to therapy but have a higher risk of relapse than patients with the lymphocyte-predominant form of Hodgkin's disease.

The lymphocyte-depleted variety of Hodgkin's disease most often occurs in men over age 50. This disease is quite refractory to therapy, with a long-term survival rate of less than 40%. In contrast, lymphocyte-predominant Hodgkin's disease classically presents as localized disease (either stage IA or stage IIA) and has a cure rate in excess of 90%.

The mixed-cell variety of Hodgkin's disease is characterized by the presence of Reed-Sternberg cells with eosinophils and lymphocytes. Patients with this disease have a long-term survival rate that is higher than that for patients with lymphocyte depletion and lower than that for patients with lymphocyte predominance.

57–60. The answers are: 57-B, 58-C, 59-A, 60-C. (*Chapter 7 III F 1–3*) Immunotherapy significantly ameliorates symptoms and is used when allergic rhinitis is severe, when medical complications or intolerance to medication occurs, and when various types of medications have been only partially successful.

Antihistamine-decongestant preparations remain the most often initially used medications. These drug preparations usually control moderate symptoms; however, some patients have intolerable side effects such as drowsiness.

Antigen avoidance usually is most successful when only one antigen is responsible for symptoms. Complete avoidance of animal dander often is possible but thorough avoidance of multiple outdoor antigens is impossible. Any sensible environmental precautions, however, will help to limit exacerbations.

Topical sympathomimetic preparations have no role in the regular management of allergic rhinitis and should be used for no longer than 2–3 days to treat acute nasal congestion leading to sinusitis or, perhaps, before air travel in individuals who are susceptible to barotitis media.

Nasal cromolyn sodium now is available for management of seasonal allergic rhinitis; it appears to be most effective when used four times daily prior to expected antigen exposure. Although cromolyn sodium may be as effective as oral antihistamine-decongestant preparations, the need to carry a nasal pump and to administer this medication intranasally four times a day is an unpleasant burden for the patient. For patients who are intolerant to oral medications, however, cromolyn sodium may be an attractive alternative. It is also effective for perennial allergic rhinitis but probably less so than for acute seasonal symptoms.

Index

Note: Page numbers in *italics* denote illustrations; those followed by (t) denote tables; those followed by Q denote questions; and those followed by E denote explanations.